I0057319

Orthopedic Surgery in Clinical Practice

Orthopedic Surgery in Clinical Practice

Edited by Kristian Gilmore

hayle medical

New York

Hayle Medical,
750 Third Avenue, 9th Floor,
New York, NY 10017, USA

Visit us on the World Wide Web at:
www.haylemedical.com

© Hayle Medical, 2019

This book contains information obtained from authentic and highly regarded sources. Copyright for all individual chapters remain with the respective authors as indicated. All chapters are published with permission under the Creative Commons Attribution License or equivalent. A wide variety of references are listed. Permission and sources are indicated; for detailed attributions, please refer to the permissions page and list of contributors. Reasonable efforts have been made to publish reliable data and information, but the authors, editors and publisher cannot assume any responsibility for the validity of all materials or the consequences of their use.

ISBN: 978-1-63241-715-2

Trademark Notice: Registered trademark of products or corporate names are used only for explanation and identification without intent to infringe.

Cataloging-in-Publication Data

Orthopedic surgery in clinical practice / edited by Kristian Gilmore.
    p. cm.
Includes bibliographical references and index.
ISBN 978-1-63241-715-2
1. Orthopedic surgery. 2. Orthopedics. 3. Surgery, Operative. I. Gilmore, Kristian.
RD731 .O78 2019
617.47--dc23

Table of Contents

Preface

The field of surgery that deals with the disorders associated with the musculoskeletal system is called orthopedic surgery. Some of the common procedures associated with orthopedic surgery include astragalectomy, bone grafting and corpectomy. Astragalectomy refers to the surgical procedure used for removing the talus bone for the stabilization of the ankle. The surgical procedure which is used to replace a missing bone for repairing complex bone fractures is called bone grafting. Corpectomy is a type of surgical operation which is concerned with the removal of all or part of the vertebral body. This book brings forth some of the most innovative concepts and elucidates the unexplored aspects of orthopedic surgery. The objective of this book is to give a general view of the different areas of orthopedic surgery and its applications. A number of latest researches have been included to keep the readers up-to-date with the global concepts in this area of study.

The information contained in this book is the result of intensive hard work done by researchers in this field. All due efforts have been made to make this book serve as a complete guiding source for students and researchers. The topics in this book have been comprehensively explained to help readers understand the growing trends in the field.

I would like to thank the entire group of writers who made sincere efforts in this book and my family who supported me in my efforts of working on this book. I take this opportunity to thank all those who have been a guiding force throughout my life.

Editor

Relationship between the social support and self-efficacy for function ability in patients undergoing primary hip replacement

Kuan-Ting Wu[1†], Pei-Shan Lee[2†], Wen-Yi Chou[1*], Shu-Hua Chen[2] and Yee-Tzu Huang[3]

Abstract

Background: The World Health Organization (WHO) reported that nearly 25% of people will suffer from physical disability owing to the bone and joint problems until 2050. The condition of patients with this type of difficulty could be improved by increasing positive self-efficacy and instigating suitable medical treatment to implement self-efficacy for functional ability (SEFA) and physical functional ability self-care. In this study, we aim to evaluate the influence of social support on SEFA in patients after total hip arthroplasty.

Methods: This cross-sectional study used structural questionnaires, telephone appointments, and data collection to obtain patient characteristics, such as gender, age, educational level, and marital status. Questionnaires about social support and self-efficacy for functional ability (SEFA) were sent to 200 patients at 3 months following a primary total hip replacement from September 2011 to December 2014. Factor analysis was used to categorize the dimensions of social support; the t test, analysis of variance (ANOVA), and correlation analysis were applied to screen factors influencing SEFA. Multiple regression analysis was employed to ascertain the relationships between patient characteristics, social support, and SEFA.

Results: In total, 134 patients responded to the questionnaires. Lower SEFA scores were observed in patients of an older age, unmarried patients, and those with a low level of education. Correlation analysis showed that emotional information and appraisal support, instrumental support, and SEFA were positively correlated. Multiple regression analysis was applied to ascertain the relationships between patient characteristics, social support, and SEFA. We identified significant coefficient values of − 0.187 for age, 5.344 for emotional information and appraisal support, and 1.653 for instrumental support.

Conclusion: The results of this study demonstrated that in patients undergoing primary hip replacement, positive impacts on SEFA were observed in relation to emotional information, appraisal support and instrumental support. The results indicated that enhancing emotional information and appraisal support could improve a patient's self-efficacy for functional ability.

Keywords: Self-efficacy for functional ability, Social support, Primary hip replacement, Arthroplasty

* Correspondence: murraychou@yahoo.com.tw
†Kuan-Ting Wu and Pei-Shan Lee contributed equally to this work.
[1]Department of Orthopaedic Surgery, Kaohsiung Chang Gung Memorial Hospital, No.123, Dapi Rd., Niaosong Dist., Kaohsiung city 833, Taiwan, Republic of China
Full list of author information is available at the end of the article

Background

Degenerative hip disease is the most common form of hip discomfort. According to the World Health Organization (WHO), bone and joint diseases may result in physical disability in nearly 25% of the population until 2050. Degenerative osteoarthritis can be diagnosed via physical examination in almost 80% of patients older than 55–65 years, and 20% of these patients already have a disability [1]. Based on research conducted by the Centers for Disease Control and Prevention (CDC) in the USA, the number of patients with osteoarthritis will double in the population over 65 years of age by 2030 [2].

Degenerative osteoarthritis often results in pain and limitation of daily activity, which are the leading causes requiring medical assistance [3]. Initially, these discomforts can be alleviated by appropriate medical management and self-care modification. In addition, caregivers play a key role in psychological support by providing patients with company [4]. In patients who are refractory to conservative treatment, a total hip replacement (THR) is usually indicated. According to the literature, THR yields excellent pain relief, with a survival rate from 90 to 99.8% during a 10–15-year follow-up period [5–7]. However, functional outcome varies according to preoperative characteristics, such as age, comorbidities, and activity level [8]. In addition to surgical technique, postoperative rehabilitation, activity adjustment, and posture limitation are also important for better functional recovery. Psychosocial factors are also associated with recovery after THR [9, 10].

Pain from degenerative osteoarthritis has a negative effect on patients in terms of psychosocial issues in the long term, such as effects on mood and sleep, which interact with activity level [11]. Langford and Bowsher [12] pointed out that adequate social support has positive effects on health status and behavior. In patients with a hip fracture, social support is also correlated with the function of the lower limbs [13]. Self-efficacy represents a patient's personal confidence in completing specific tasks and also brings about a sense of accomplishment. After lower limb arthroplasty, Moon and Backer identified significant correlations between self-efficacy, walking distance, and lower limb activity frequency [14]. In the elderly population, health status and physical function are key factors affecting the execution of regular exercise; therefore, the condition of patients with this type of difficulty may be improved by increasing positive self-efficacy and social support following THR [15].

In this study, we aimed to examine the relationships between social support, self-efficacy level, and functional ability in patients undergoing primary THR after discharge from the hospital.

Methods

Study design and sample

This cross-sectional study used structural questionnaires, telephone appointments, and data collection to obtain patient characteristics, such as gender, age, educational level, and marital status. The Institutional Review Board at our hospital approved this analysis. Patients who had undergone THR due to osteoarthritis of the hip were enrolled from September 2011 to December 2014. Patients with the following conditions were excluded: dementia, psychological disorders, or postoperative complications such as cardiovascular accident, fat embolism, vascular or nerve injury, intraoperative acetabulum, or femur fracture. We used modified versions of the self-efficacy for functional ability (SEFA) scale and the social support scale for patient evaluation.

Questionnaires

We collected patient characteristics such as gender, age, educational level, and marital status. Self-efficacy for functional ability (SEFA) and social support questionnaires were completed by the patients 3 months following primary THR. As the average age of the patients was greater than 65 years, we used modified versions of the questionnaires for simplification.

Social support scale

The modified social support scale [16] was revised from the Inventory of Socially Supportive Behaviors (ISSB) developed by Barrera et al. [17] for the measurement of assistance provided in the areas of emotional information, appraisal support, and instrumental support by a spouse, family, friends, and relatives. The patients were asked to respond to 15 items using a Likert scale from 0 to 3 points, representing no assistance, little assistance, much assistance, and very much assistance, respectively. Hence, the global score ranged from 0 to 90, with higher scores indicating better social support. In addition, we categorized social support into two dimensions. Dimension 1 represented emotional information and appraisal support, with a Cronbach's alpha of 0.973, while dimension 2 represented instrumental support, with a Cronbach's alpha of 0.767.

Self-efficacy for functional ability scale

The SEFA scale is usually employed to assess patient confidence in performing daily activities. In this study, we used a modified SEFA proposed by Resnick [18]. Nine items were included in the modified SEFA questionnaire, which assessed functional ability in terms of dressing, getting out of and into bed, using the toilet, bathing, walking, and climbing stairs. Items were scored from 1 to 4, representing patient levels of confidence of less than 20%, 20–50%, 50–80%, and greater than 80%, respectively, in performing the activities by themselves. The total score ranged from 9 to 36, with higher scores representing greater confidence in performing daily activities. The Cronbach's alpha for this scale was 0.969.

Statistical analysis

Factor analysis was used to categorize dimensions of social support. The Kaiser-Meyer-Olkin value was 0.898, and the Barlett test showed a p value < 0.001. Furthermore, the t test, analysis of variance (ANOVA), and correlation analysis were applied to screen the factors influencing SEFA. Multiple regression analysis was employed to ascertain the relationships between patient characteristics, social support, and SEFA. The reliability of the questionnaires was assessed using Cronbach's alpha; the higher the Cronbach's alpha value, the greater the internal consistency.

Results

From September 2011 to December 2014, 200 patients underwent THR for advanced osteoarthritis. Following the exclusion of 66 patients who met the exclusion criteria, 134 patients were enrolled in this study, 51.5% of whom were male; 21.6% of the patients were under 55 years of age, 23.1% were aged between 51 and 64, 35.1% between 65 and 75, and 20.1% were over 75 years of age. 38.1% of the patients had an educational level ranging from elementary school to junior high school, and 26.9% were uneducated. 86.6% of the patients were married (Table 1).

In terms of social support, the average score for the dimension of emotional information and appraisal support was 1.81 ± 0.7, while that for the dimension of

Table 1 Characteristics of primary THR patients ($n = 134$)

	Number	Percentage (%)
Sex		
Male	69	51.5
Female	65	48.5
Age (years)		
< 51	29	21.6
51–64	31	23.1
65–75	47	35.1
> 75	27	20.1
Educational level		
Uneducated	36	26.9
Primary/secondary school	51	38.1
> Senior high school	47	35.1
Marital status		
Single	18	13.4
Married	116	86.6

instrumental support was 1.56 ± 0.77. The highest score (2.08 ± 0.65) of the items in the dimension of emotional information and appraisal support was obtained for "expressed interest and concern in your well-being," followed by "reminded you of follow-up hospital appointments" (2.02 ± 0.77). Furthermore, the lowest score was obtained for the item "assisted you in appropriate exercise" (1.37 ± 0.85). In the dimension of instrumental support, the lowest score (1.50 ± 0.75) was obtained for the item "listened to you talk about your private feelings" (Table 2).

The average SEFA score of the patients after THR was 3.33 ± 0.84. The lowest-scored items in terms of self-efficacy were "wash your lower body (3.24 ± 0.95)," "dress your lower body (3.19 ± 1.00)," and "climb up and down four stairs (2.78 ± 1.21)." The highest score (3.53 ± 0.28) was obtained for "get in and out of bed and chairs" (Table 3). Male patients scored 19.97 ± 8.21 and female patients 21.95 ± 6.84 on average, with a p value < 0.01.

A positive correlation between emotional information and appraisal support with instrumental support was observed, with a Pearson correlation coefficient of 0.6. In addition, a positive relationship between emotional information and appraisal support with SEFA was seen, with a Pearson correlation coefficient of 0.635 (Table 4).

Scores on the scales of self-efficacy (17.58 ± 8.98) and emotional information and appraisal support (1.46 ± 0.80) were lower in the uneducated patients ($p < 0.01$), as was the instrumental support score ($p < 0.05$). In addition, the elderly patients had lower SEFA scores ($p < 0.01$) (Table 5).

We included predictors selected from t tests and ANOVA, such as sex, age, educational level, marital status, emotional information, appraisal support, and instrumental support in stepwise multivariable regression analysis. After the elimination procedure, age, educational level, emotional information and appraisal support, and instrumental support were selected as significant predictors. These significant predictors were analyzed using an all-possible regression procedure. It was found that an older age was related to a lower self-efficacy ($b = - 0.187$, $p < 0.001$). Emotional information and appraisal support had a positive influence on self-efficacy ($b = 5.344$, $p < 0.001$), as did instrumental support ($b = 1.653$, $p < 0.05$). The model explained approximately 52.6% of the variance in SEFA 3 months after THR, and the final regression model explained 50.7% of the variance (Table 6).

Discussion

Social support is a key factor related to the daily activity of geriatric patients. Friedland and McColl [19] pointed out that interventions to increase social support in critical patients can improve chronic stress and physical

Table 2 Descriptive analysis of social support after THR

	No assistance (0) Number (%)	Little assistance (1)	Much assistance (2)	Very much assistance (3)	Mean ± SD
Emotional information and appraisal support					1.81 ± 0.70
Expressed interest and concern in your well-being	0 (0%)	23 (17%)	78 (57.8%)	34 (25.2%)	2.08 ± 0.65
Was right there with you in a stressful situation	5 (3.7%)	32 (23.7%)	76 (56.3%)	22 (16.3%)	1.85 ± 0.73
Joked and kidded to try to cheer you up	4 (3%)	23 (17%)	82 (60.7%)	26 (19.3%)	1.96 ± 0.69
Agreed that what you want to do was right	8 (6%)	35 (13.4%)	73 (26.1%)	18 (54.5%)	1.75 ± 0.76
Let you know you did something well	8 (6%)	25 (18.7%)	34 (25.4%)	67 (50%)	1.81 ± 0.80
Expressed esteem or respect for a competency or personal quality of yours	6 (4.5%)	29 (21.6%)	32 (23.9%)	67 (50%)	1.93 ± 0.79
Provided some advice on medical treatment	8 (6%)	30 (22.4%)	31 (23.1%)	65 (48.5%)	1.87 ± 0.82
Provided some advice on daily living	6 (4.5%)	25 (18.7%)	36 (26.9%)	67 (50%)	1.83 ± 0.78
Reminded you of follow-up hospital appointments	6 (4.5%)	20 (14.9%)	35 (26.1%)	73 (54.4%)	2.02 ± 0.77
Assisted you in setting a goal for yourself	13 (9.7%)	26 (19.4%)	47 (35.1%)	48 (35.8%)	1.65 ± 0.90
Did some activity together to help you get your minds off things	24 (17.9%)	26 (19.4%)	27 (20.1%)	57 (42.5%)	1.59 ± 0.99
Helped you in adjustment of daily activities	8 (6%)	32 (23.9%)	42 (31.3%)	52 (38.8%)	1.81 ± 0.87
Assisted you in appropriate exercise	12 (9%)	21 (15.7%)	46 (34.3%)	55 (41%)	1.37 ± 0.58
Instrumental support					1.56 ± 0.77
Listened to you talk about your private feelings	9 (6.7%)	62 (45.9%)	52 (38.5%)	12 (8.9%)	1.50 ± 0.75
Loaned or gave you something that you needed	14 (10.4%)	32 (23.9%)	34 (25.4%)	54 (40.3%)	1.63 ± 0.96

disability. Social support also has positive effects on health status and behavior [12] and can enhance execution of healthy behaviors, such as taking medicines on time, engaging in regular exercise, and diet control [20]. In studies of patients with hip fractures, a significant relationship was also identified between social support and lower limb functional activity [13], especially when supported by their spouse and family [21]. Social support is usually provided by the patient's family members who live with them. Kiefer identified a higher level of social support in patients living with a spouse, adult child,

or friends while the singles had a lower level of social support [22]. In this study, we found that the item with the highest score (2.08 ± 0.65) was "expressed interest and concern in your well-being." Because it is easier for a caregiver or family to focus on the patient's disease-related health status, as they can directly observe their gait, muscle power, and agility following THR. Sveikata et al. [23] demonstrated better postoperative functional results 12 months after total knee arthroplasty in patients who had better social support. McHugh et al. [24] also identified key psychosocial factors and

Table 3 Descriptive analysis of SEFA after THR

Confidence (score) Item	< 20% (1) Number (%)	20–50% (2)	50–80% (3)	> 80% (4)	Mean ± SD
Wash your upper body	8 (6%)	10 (7.5%)	28 (20.9%)	88 (65.7%)	3.46 ± 0.87
Wash your lower body	9 (6.7%)	21 (15.7%)	33 (24.6%)	71 (53%)	3.24 ± 0.95
Dress your upper body	4 (3%)	12 (9%)	26 (19.4%)	92 (68.7%)	3.48 ± 0.92
Dress your lower body	9 (6.7%)	24 (17.9%)	29 (21.6%)	72 (53.7%)	3.19 ± 1.00
Get on and off the toilet and manage your clothes	8 (6%)	13 (9.7%)	20 (14.9%)	93 (69.4%)	3.48 ± 0.90
Get in and out of bed and a chair	4 (3%)	8 (6%)	31 (23.1%)	91 (67.9%)	3.53 ± 0.82
Walk 50 ft	4 (3%)	12 (9%)	32 (23.9%)	86 (64.2%)	3.43 ± 0.92
Walk 120 ft	6 (4.5%)	12 (9%)	37 (27.6%)	79 (59%)	3.37 ± 0.93
Climb up and down four stairs	22 (16.4%)	26 (19.4%)	31 (23.1%)	55 (41%)	2.78 ± 1.21
Total score					29.96 ± 7.6
Total average score					3.33 ± 0.84

Table 4 Pearson's correlations with SEFA scale

Variable	Correlation coefficient, r	p value
Emotional information and appraisal support	0.635	< 0.001
Instrumental support	0.489	< 0.001

biomedical predictors of pain, anxiety, and depression related to recovery following THR in 206 patients. Social support can affect self-efficacy in terms of verbal encouragement. In a randomized control study, improved general self-efficacy and physical function were observed in the group who received telephone follow-up appointments conducted by a nurse, which was structured along the lines of the VIPS model (the Swedish acronym for the concepts of Well-being, Integrity, Prevention and Safety) [25]. We also identified a significant positive correlation between social support and self-efficacy in our study, with a coefficient of 5.344 for emotional information and appraisal support and 1.653 for instrumental support.

Physical activity is crucial in the elderly and can prevent chronic disease, promote physical health, and help to maintain the quality of life [26]. Elderly persons who engage in regular exercise will perform better in functions of daily activity and will have an improved health status and reduce few chronic diseases such as stroke, cardiovascular disease, osteoporosis, hypertension, and diabetes [27, 28]. If patients are restricted in terms of the execution of physical activity, they will be unwilling to perform daily activities [29]. Similar with social support, increase self-efficacy is associated with higher physical activity levels [30, 31]. Poor self-efficacy usually leads to greater distress in patients during their recovery; they often worry about their condition getting worse after executing a specific task because they are not confident in their course of rehabilitation. In research into self-efficacy, self-efficacy was taken as an evaluation of capability in terms of achievement in specific tasks, a significant correlation between self-efficacy and personal success was identified [32, 33]. Dominick et al. demonstrated a significant correlation between low self-efficacy for exercise and less improvement in functional recovery over time after total knee arthroplasty [34]. Waldrop et al. [35] also addressed self-efficacy predicted significant variance in rehabilitation outcomes in orthopedic surgery. They concluded that augmenting self-efficacy beliefs by psychologists could improve functional recovery. The higher the level of induced self-efficacy, the greater the performance accomplishments.

Patients who undergo THR are usually discharged home directly. Therefore, it is easy to assess the correlation of functional outcome with the quality of home care. Self-efficacy was identified as a significant predictor of recovery after joint arthroplasty by Moon and Backer et al. [14]. They also found that walking distance and the

Table 5 Group comparison of emotional information and appraisal support, instrumental support and SEFA

Variable	Emotional information and appraisal support		Instrumental support		Self-efficacy of functional ability	
	M ± SD	t, F value	M ± SD	t, F value	M ± SD	t, F value
Sex (T)		4.454		0.563**		3.487**
Male	1.66 ± 0.75		1.35 ± 0.73		19.91 ± 8.21	
Female	1.97 ± 0.61		1.80 ± 0.75		21.95 ± 6.84	
Age (years)(A)		0.954		0.197		8.123**
(1) < 50	1.88 ± 0.74		1.64 ± 0.91		23.83 ± 4.65	
(2) 51–64	1.74 ± 0.56		1.48 ± 0.46		21.27 ± 9.18	
(3) 65–75	1.90 ± 0.68		1.55 ± 0.79		22.10 ± 4.63	
(4) > 75	1.64 ± 0.83		1.58 ± 0.91		15.04 ± 9.74	
Post hoc Scheff					(4) < (1), (2), (3)	
Educational level (A)		8.978**		4.430*		7.476*
(1) Uneducated	1.46 ± 0.80		1.39 ± 0.73		17.58 ± 9.00	
(2) Primary to secondary school	2.07 ± 0.50		1.81 ± 0.73		23.65 ± 4.97	
(3) > Senior high school	1.79 ± 0.72		1.43 ± 0.80		20.12 ± 8.16	
Post hoc Scheff	(1) < (2)		(1) < (2)		(1) < (2)	
Marital status (T)		3.502		0.284		8.182*
Single	1.88 ± 0.46		1.64 ± 0.68		20.51 ± 7.90	
Married	1.80 ± 0.73		1.55 ± 0.79		23.83 ± 4.40	

A represents ANOVA and T represents independent t test
p < 0.05, **p < 0.01

Table 6 Multivariable regression analysis of SEFA

SEFA			
Variable	B	S(B)	VIF
Patient characteristics			
Age	− 0.187***	− 0.333	1.355
Educational level			
Uneducated (reference)			
Primary/secondary school	− 0.039	− 0.003	2.038
> Senior high school	− 2.644	− 0.161	1.875
Social support			
Emotional information and appraisal support	5.344***	0.491	1.714
Instrumental support	1.653*	0.166	1.609

$R^2 = 0.526$, adjust $R^2 = 0.507$, $n = 134$
*$p < 0.05$, **$p < 0.01$, *** $p < 0.0001$

frequency of lower limb activity increased as self-efficacy improved. In our study, the SEFA item with the highest score was "get in and out of bed and chairs," while the lowest-scored item was "climb up and down four stairs". As climbing stairs requires high levels of coordination and strength, it is difficult for patients to complete this task with ease. Self-efficacy might be affected in several ways. According to the literature, there exist two factors that influence the daily activity and self-efficacy of patients who have undergone THR: patient characteristics and disease characteristics. In terms of patient characteristics, confidence in self-efficacy decreases with aging [36, 37]. Janiszewska et al. demonstrated that older age deteriorated general health and decreased general self-efficacy level in women who undergone osteoporosis treatment [38]. With regard to the level of education, Lien and Wei studied 350 patients separated into diabetic and non-diabetic groups, and a better self-efficacy was associated with a higher educational level [39]. Marital status also affects self-efficacy in correlation with social support. Fitzgerald et al. [40] evaluated 222 patients 12 months after joint replacement surgery, and better social support and self-efficacy were noted in patients who were married or living with someone. Regarding disease characteristics, patients have difficulties in performing daily activities owing to specific posture limitations during the first 6 to 12 weeks following THR [41, 42]. In our study, we evaluated patients 3 months following THR in order to minimize bias and observed better SEFA in married patients and those with a higher level of education.

Some studies have identified different contributions of preoperative and postoperative self-efficacy to patient outcome following THR [43–45]. A higher preoperative self-efficacy means that the patient has more confidence in their recovery and is willing to undergo THR; furthermore, preoperative self-efficacy has also been identified as a predictor of better recovery. However, in a systemic review regarding the influence of self-efficacy on functional recovery, the effect of preoperative self-efficacy was inconclusive, while in contrast, the effect of postoperative self-efficacy was consistent and was found to be associated with functional recovery in terms of distance ambulation, exercise repetition, and frequency [45, 46]. Some studies have indicated that self-efficacy is associated with emotional outcomes [47]. In our study, we attempted to identify factors correlated with postoperative SEFA; therefore, we evaluated the relationships of emotional information and instrumental support with postoperative SEFA and identified significant correlations, with Pearson coefficients of 0.635 and 0.483, respectively.

Limitations
First, we used modified questionnaires in order to make it easier for the elderly participants to respond to items. The validity of the SEFA and social support questionnaires was examined, and both had a high internal consistency, with Cronbach's alpha values greater than 0.7; however, these values were still lower than those of the primary versions of the questionnaires. Second, all patients were enrolled from a single hospital, and differences in culture in other cities might result in differences in social support and self-efficacy.

Conclusion
This study concluded that in patients undergoing primary hip replacement, emotional information, appraisal support, and instrumental support had positive impacts on self-efficacy for functional ability. The results indicated that enhancing emotional information and appraisal support could improve self-efficacy for functional ability and lead to a better recovery following THR.

Abbreviations
CDC: Centers for Disease Control and Prevention; SEFA: Self-efficacy for functional ability; THR: Total hip replacement; WHO: World Health Organization

Acknowledgements
We would like to acknowledge Y. H Chuang for formatting the draft and Chang Gung Statistical Analysis Center for the counsel.

Authors' contributions
PSL contributed to the planning of the study, recruitment of the patients, data interpretation, writing of the draft, and literature review and revised and analyzed the data and statistics. KTW contributed to the data interpretation, writing of the draft, literature review, and critical revision of the paper and revised and analyzed the data and statistics. YTH contributed to the data

interpretation and writing of the draft and revised and analyzed the data and statistics. SHC organized the study and contributed to the clinical analysis of the data and critical commenting and improvement of the manuscript. WYC contributed to the critical revision of the paper and submitted revisions. All authors read and approved the final manuscript. PSL and KTW contributed equally to the article and listed as the co-first author.

Competing interests
The authors declared that they have no competing interests.

Author details
[1]Department of Orthopaedic Surgery, Kaohsiung Chang Gung Memorial Hospital, No.123, Dapi Rd., Niaosong Dist., Kaohsiung city 833, Taiwan, Republic of China. [2]Department of Orthopedics Operation Room, Kaohsiung Chang Gung Memorial Hospital, No.123, Dapi Rd., Niaosong Dist., Kaohsiung city 833, Taiwan, Republic of China. [3]Department of Hospital and Health Care Administration, Chia Nan University of Pharmacy and Science, No.60, Sec. 1, Erren Rd., Rende Dist, Tainan city 717, Taiwan, Republic of China.

References
1. Baird CL, Schmeiser D, Yehle KT. Self-caring of women with osteoarthritis living at different levels of independence. Health Care Women Int. 2003;24: 617–34.
2. Public health and aging. projected prevalence of self-reported arthritis or chronic joint symptoms among persons aged >65 years—United States, 2005–2030. MMWR Morb Mortal Wkly Rep. 2003;52:489–91.
3. Murphy L, Helmick CG. The impact of osteoarthritis in the United States: a population-health perspective: a population-based review of the fourth most common cause of hospitalization in US adults. Orthop Nurs. 2012;31: 85–91.
4. Chen Y-C, Yuan S-C. The effectiveness of an intervention program among total hip replacement patients. Chung Shan Medical Journal. 2003;14:109–18.
5. Williams HD, Browne G, Gie GA, Ling RS, Timperley AJ, Wendover NA. The Exeter universal cemented femoral component at 8 to 12 years. A study of the first 325 hips. J Bone Joint Surg Br. 2002;84:324–34.
6. Clohisy JC, Harris WH. The Harris-Galante porous-coated acetabular component with screw fixation. An average ten-year follow-up study. J Bone Joint Surg Am. 1999;81:66–73.
7. Lee YK, Ha YC, Yoo JJ, Koo KH, Yoon KS, Kim HJ. Alumina-on-alumina total hip arthroplasty: a concise follow-up, at a minimum of ten years, of a previous report. J Bone Joint Surg Am. 2010;92:1715–9.
8. Fortin PR, Penrod JR, Clarke AE, St-Pierre Y, Joseph L, Belisle P, et al. Timing of total joint replacement affects clinical outcomes among patients with osteoarthritis of the hip or knee. Arthritis Rheum. 2002;46:3327–30.
9. Keefe FJ, Smith SJ, Buffington AL, Gibson J, Studts JL, Caldwell DS. Recent advances and future directions in the biopsychosocial assessment and treatment of arthritis. J Consult Clin Psychol. 2002;70:640–55.
10. Brembo EA, Kapstad H, Van Dulmen S, Eide H. Role of self-efficacy and social support in short-term recovery after total hip replacement: a prospective cohort study. Health Qual Life Outcomes. 2017;15:68.
11. Neogi T. The epidemiology and impact of pain in osteoarthritis. Osteoarthr Cartil. 2013;21:1145–53.
12. Langford CP, Bowsher J, Maloney JP, Lillis PP. Social support: a conceptual analysis. J Adv Nurs. 1997;25:95–100.
13. Mock C, MacKenzie E, Jurkovich G, Burgess A, Cushing B, deLateur B, et al. Determinants of disability after lower extremity fracture. J Trauma. 2000;49: 1002–11.
14. Moon LB, Backer J. Relationships among self-efficacy, outcome expectancy, and postoperative behaviors in total joint replacement patients. Orthop Nurs. 2000;19:77–85.
15. Struck BD, Ross KM. Health promotion in older adults. Prescribing exercise for the frail and home bound. Geriatrics. 2006;61:22–7.
16. Wang YH. Study on life quality and its associated factors of rheumatoid arthritis patients. Journal of Chang Gung Institute of Nursing. 2000;2:71–95.
17. Barrera M, Sandler IN, Ramsay TB. Preliminary development of a scale of social support: studies on college students. Am J Community Psychol. 1981;9:435–47.
18. Resnick B. Efficacy beliefs in geriatric rehabilitation. J Gerontol Nurs. 1998;24: 34–44.
19. Friedland JF, McColl M. Social support intervention after stroke: results of a randomized trial. Arch Phys Med Rehabil. 1992;73:573–81.
20. Chiang W-Y, Chung H-H. Hemodialysis patients' fatigue relating to depression, social support and blood biochemical data. The Journal of Nursing Research. 1997;5:115–26.
21. Saltz CC, Zimmerman S, Tompkins C, Harrington D, Magaziner J. Stress among caregivers of hip fracture patients. J Gerontol Soc Work. 1999;30:167–81.
22. Kiefer RA. The effect of social support on functional recovery and wellbeing in older adults following joint arthroplasty. Rehabil Nurs. 2011;36:120–6.
23. Sveikata T, Porvaneckas N, Kanopa P, Molyte A, Klimas D, Uvarovas V, et al. Age, sex, body mass index, education, and social support influence functional results after total knee arthroplasty. Geriatr Orthop Surg Rehabil. 2017;8:71–7.
24. McHugh GA, Campbell M, Luker KA. Predictors of outcomes of recovery following total hip replacement surgery: a prospective study. Bone Joint Res. 2013;2:248–54.
25. Szots K, Konradsen H, Solgaard S, Ostergaard B. Telephone follow-up by nurse after Total knee arthroplasty: results of a randomized clinical trial. Orthop Nurs. 2016;35:411–20.
26. Lee YS, Laffrey SC. Predictors of physical activity in older adults with borderline hypertension. Nurs Res. 2006;55:110–20.
27. Nelson ME, Rejeski WJ, Blair SN, Duncan PW, Judge JO, King AC, et al. Physical activity and public health in older adults: recommendation from the American College of Sports Medicine and the American Heart Association. Circulation. 2007;116:1094–105.
28. Haskell WL, Lee IM, Pate RR, Powell KE, Blair SN, Franklin BA, et al. Physical activity and public health: updated recommendation for adults from the American College of Sports Medicine and the American Heart Association. Circulation. 2007;116:1081–93.
29. Resnick B, Spellbring AM. Understanding what motivates older adults to exercise. J Gerontol Nurs. 2000;26:34–42.
30. Lewis BA, Marcus BH, Pate RR, Dunn AL. Psychosocial mediators of physical activity behavior among adults and children. Am J Prev Med. 2002;23:26–35.
31. Trost SG, Owen N, Bauman AE, Sallis JF, Brown W. Correlates of adults' participation in physical activity: review and update. Med Sci Sports Exerc. 2002;34:1996–2001.
32. Peeters GM, Brown WJ, Burton NW. Psychosocial factors associated with increased physical activity in insufficiently active adults with arthritis. J Sci Med Sport. 2015;18:558–64.
33. Stubbs B, Hurley M, Smith T. What are the factors that influence physical activity participation in adults with knee and hip osteoarthritis? A systematic review of physical activity correlates. Clin Rehabil. 2015;29:80–94.
34. Dominick GM, Zeni JA, White DK. Association of psychosocial factors with physical activity and function after total knee replacement: an exploratory study. Arch Phys Med Rehabil. 2016;97:S218–25.
35. Waldrop D, Lightsey OR Jr, Ethington CA, Woemmel CA, Coke AL. Self-efficacy, optimism, health competence, and recovery from orthopedic surgery. J Couns Psychol. 2001;48:233–8.
36. Scult M, Haime V, Jacquart J, Takahashi J, Moscowitz B, Webster A, et al. A healthy aging program for older adults: effects on self-efficacy and morale. Adv Mind Body Med. 2015;29:26–33.
37. Liu N, Liu S, Yu N, Peng Y, Wen Y, Tang J et al. Correlations among Psychological Resilience, self-efficacy, and Negative Emotion in Acute Myocardial Infarction Patients after Percutaneous Coronary Intervention. Front Psychiatry. 2018;9:1.
38. Janiszewska M, Kulik T, Zolnierczuk-Kieliszek D, Drop B, Firlej E, Gajewska I. General self-efficacy level and health behaviours in women over the age of 45 years who have undergone osteoporosis treatment. Prz Menopauzalny. 2017;16:86–95.
39. Lien R-Y, Wei J, Li J-Y, Tung H-H, Chen C-Y. Difference in predictors of self efficacy and compliance between diabetic and non diabetic patients who underwent coronary artery bypass surgery. The Journal of Nursing. 2012;59: 40–50.

40. Fitzgerald JD, Orav EJ, Lee TH, Marcantonio ER, Poss R, Goldman L, et al. Patient quality of life during the 12 months following joint replacement surgery. Arthritis Rheum. 2004;51:100–9.

41. Peak EL, Parvizi J, Ciminiello M, Purtill JJ, Sharkey PF, Hozack WJ, et al. The role of patient restrictions in reducing the prevalence of early dislocation following total hip arthroplasty: a randomized, prospective study. J Bone Joint Surg Am. 2005;87:247–53.

42. Peters A, Tijink M, Veldhuijzen A, Huis in 't Veld R. Reduced patient restrictions following total hip arthroplasty: study protocol for a randomized controlled trial. Trials. 2015;16:360.

43. van den Akker-Scheek I, Stevens M, Groothoff JW, Bulstra SK, Zijlstra W. Preoperative or postoperative self-efficacy: which is a better predictor of outcome after total hip or knee arthroplasty? Patient Educ Couns. 2007;66: 92–9.

44. Wylde V, Dixon S, Blom AW. The role of preoperative self-efficacy in predicting outcome after total knee replacement. Musculoskeletal Care. 2012;10:110–8.

45. Magklara E, Burton CR, Morrison V. Does self-efficacy influence recovery and well-being in osteoarthritis patients undergoing joint replacement? A systematic review. Clin Rehabil. 2014;28:835–46.

46. de Vries H, Kremers SP, Smeets T, Brug J, Eijmael K. The effectiveness of tailored feedback and action plans in an intervention addressing multiple health behaviors. Am J Health Promot. 2008;22:417–25.

47. Ayers DC, Franklin PD, Ring DC. The role of emotional health in functional outcomes after orthopaedic surgery: extending the biopsychosocial model to orthopaedics. AOA critical issues. J Bone Joint Surg Am. 2013;95:e165.

2

Clinical experience of debridement combined with resorbable bone graft substitute mixed with antibiotic in the treatment for infants with osteomyelitis

Zhiqiang Zhang[†], Hao Li[†], Hai Li, Qing Fan, Xuan Yang, Pinquan Shen, Ting Chen, Qixun Cai, Jing Zhang and Ziming Zhang[*]

Abstract

Background: Osteomyelitis (OM) is an uncommon disease that originates from many different mechanisms in children. Treatment often involves a combination of surgical debridement combined and antibiotic therapy. The purpose of this article is to evaluate the effect of debridement combined with a new resorbable bone graft substitute (RBGS) mixed with antibiotics in the treatment of infants with OM.

Methods: Twenty-two patients diagnosed with OM at our institution underwent debridement combined with implantation of RBGS mixed with vancomycin within 48 h after admission. Clinical and epidemiological factors, preoperative and postoperative radiographs, and laboratory parameters, including white blood cell (WBC), C-reactive protein (CRP), erythrocyte sedimentation rate (ESR), and neutrophil percentage (NEU%), were documented. The function of the involved extremity was evaluated at the final follow-up.

Results: The mean age was 6.3 ± 4.8 months (range, 0.5 to 12 months). The mean duration of the symptoms was 14.5 ± 8.4 days (range, 2 to 30 days). The average length of hospitalization was 13.7 ± 6.2 days (range, 6 to 28 days). 13.64% (3/22) had positive results of purulent material obtained at the time of open biopsy and 18.18% (4/22) had positive blood cultures. The most common sites were located in the proximal femur (12), the distal femur (3), and the proximal humerus (3). Ten patients presented with concurrent pyogenic arthritis, while another 12 infants suffered from simple isolated hematogenous OM. The mean follow-up time was 3.0 ± 1.6 years (range, 1.0 to 6.0 years). Seven of 22 patients (31.82%) had complications such as limb length deformity (LLD), avascular necrosis (AVN), and pathologic subluxation of the hip. Fifteen out of 22 (68.18%) patients achieved good results. Additionally, patients who had concomitant pyogenic arthritis were more likely to develop complications than those with isolated OM ($p = 0.02$).

Conclusions: Early debridement combined with implantation of RBGS mixed with vancomycin in the treatment of infants with OM achieved acceptable results in this series. Compared to those with simple isolated OM, patients with secondary pyogenic arthritis had a more virulent course.

Keywords: Infants, Osteomyelitis, Pyogenic arthritis, Debridement, Resorbable bone graft substitute, Antibiotics

* Correspondence: zhangziming@xinhuamed.com.cn
[†]Zhiqiang Zhang and Hao Li contributed equally to this work.
Department of Pediatric Orthopedics, Xinhua Hospital, School of Medicine, Shanghai Jiao Tong University, 1665 Kongjiang Road, Yangpu District, Shanghai 20092, China

Background

Osteomyelitis (OM) is postulated to occur as a result of bacteremia and local trauma and occurs in children because of the rich blood supply to the growing bones. The clinical features and severity may differ somewhat based on the causative organism, children's age, immune level, and other factors [1]. The long bone metaphysis is the most vulnerable part. If the infection has not been effectively controlled or treated, the whole bone will become involved and may lead to bone defects [2]. Concomitant pyogenic arthritis in infants occurs in the hip, knee, and other large joints, mostly as the result of OM extended to the adjacent joints. Due to the presence of the transphyseal vessels, as well as immature immune system, an epiphyseal OM secondary to septic arthritis could occur in an infant, especially without a timely and effective treatment [3].

Despite intervention with antibiotic therapy, the treatment of OM is still challenging on account of delays in treatment, drug-resistant bacteria, and inadequate treatment. Administration of antibiotics by local delivery with "filling agents" can result in an increased local concentration of antibiotics at the infection site. This technique has been described as an option to treat some conditions. For example, calcium sulfate pellets impregnated with antibiotics were applied successfully in the treatment of chronic OM and non-union in adults [4, 5].

To our knowledge, there are no previous reports focusing on infants with OM treated with debridement combined with resorbable calcium sulfate mixed with antibiotics. Therefore, the objective of this study was to evaluate the outcome of early debridement combined with implantation of resorbable bone graft substitute (RBGS) mixed with antibiotics for the treatment of OM in infants.

Methods

After the institution's Ethics Committee approval, a retrospective review was performed and all patients with the diagnosis of OM between January 1, 2012, and December 31, 2016, at our institution were enrolled. The inclusion criteria were (1) infants younger than 1 year old; (2) diagnosed with OM, (3) patients who underwent debridement combined with RBGS mixed with antibiotics, and (4) surgery within 48 h after admission.

OM was defined as having symptoms for several days with clinical and radiological features. Contrary to common belief, the main clinical symptom in infants may be as subtle as local irritability (e.g., a child crying on changing of diapers or touching the affected extremity) [6]. Laboratory findings such as increased WBC, ESR, and CRP plus radiological investigations supplement the clinical symptoms. A diagnosis of concurrent septic arthritis was made in patients who were found to have purulent material in the joint capsule at the time of surgical treatment of the OM.

Clinical and laboratory data were documented during and after admission. Physical examination data points including increased body temperature, local swelling, and limited range of motion. Meanwhile, radiological and laboratory tests were performed preoperatively. Namely, plain radiographs, CT scan, or MRI were taken to determine the site and area of the lesion. WBC, ESR, and CRP were tested immediately after hospitalization. Blood samples and cultures of purulent material obtained on aspiration or at the time of open exploration, debridement, or arthrotomy were collected for bacteria culture and sensitivities of the causative organism.

Antibiotic treatment by intravenous or oral therapy was started after admission, and the options of antibiotics were guided by local microbiology advice wherever possible to facilitate a more focused therapeutic regimen.

Surgical intervention was warranted if the child had persistent pain and fever after 48 h or bone lesion identified by MRI or plain radiograph or if there was evidence of a collection of purulent material by physical exam or advanced imaging. Patients who were observed to have bone lesions were given the treatment of RBGS combined antibiotics. Other interventions such as multiple surgical debridements and the usage of vacuum sealing drainage (VSD) were more often used for severe septic arthritis in our institution. Cultures from bone or joint fluid samples were processed during the surgeries. Open biopsy was done in cases where other diagnostic entities were considered (i.e., sarcoma). Antibiotic susceptibility test was taken simultaneously to guide for adjustment of the antibiotic regime. The necrotic and infectious bone lesion was excised completely and flushed with hydrogen peroxide, chlorhexidine, or saline repeatedly. After irrigation and debridement, the bone defect was filled with RBGS (OSTEOSET resorbable bead kit, Wright Medical Group, NV.), which was mixed with 0.5 g vancomycin. To prepare the RBGS, all the diluent was added to both calcium sulfate and antibiotic powders in a mixing bowl and mixed to a "dough"-- like consistency (mixed thoroughly for 30–45 s). After molded and dried on the template, the molded RGBS beads were filled into the bone defect as many as possible. The affected limb was immobilized by a cast or brace to prevent possible pathologic fracture.

Postoperatively, multidisciplinary management included pediatric surgery intensive care unit, orthopedics, microbiology/infectious disease consultants, radiology, and nursing. Based on the results of bacteria culture, the antibiotic therapy was adjusted. If the results were negative, the previous regime was continued. WBC, CRP, ESR, and NEU% were noted every 48 h postoperatively.

Complications were documented at the final follow-up. Good outcomes were defined as no complications and without recurrence until the latest follow-up. Fisher exact test was used to compare the rates of complication between both groups (OM concurrent with pyogenic arthritis group and isolated OM group). Outcomes are expressed with p value. A 5% level of significance was used in analyses (SPSS19.0, IBM, USA).

Results

Thirty-four patients were treated for OM in our hospital between January 2012 to December 2016. Seven patients who had repeated surgeries, using Vacuum Sealing Drainage (VSD) rather than RBGS, were excluded in this series. There were five patients lost to follow-up. Finally, 22 infants were included in the present study (16 boys and 6 girls). The mean follow-up time was 3.0 ± 1.6 years (range, 1.0 to 6.0 years). The mean age was 6.3 ± 4.8 months (range, 0.5 to 12 months). The mean duration of the symptoms was 14.5 ± 8.4 days (range, 2 to 30 days). 13.6% (3/22) had positive surgical cultures, and 18.2% (4/22) had positive blood cultures. The average

length of hospitalization was 13.7 ± 6.2 days (range, 6 to 28 days). The most common sites affected by infection were the proximal femur (12), the distal femur (3), and the proximal humerus (3). The right proximal fibula and the right proximal radius were involved in one case, respectively. Ten patients had OM concurrent with pyogenic arthritis, while 12 infants suffered from isolated OM (Table 1).

All patients had a clinical examination and laboratory tests upon admission. The mean temperature on admission was 37.0 ± 0.4 °C. One patient (4.5%) had a temperature over 37.8 °C. All patients had decreased activity and cried on the passive movement of the extremity. Limb tenderness was present in 40.9% (9/22). The mean WBC was $14.1 \pm 6.7 \times 10^9$/L (5.5–33.8×10^9/L), ESR was 33.5 ± 23.2 (2–85) mm/h, CRP was 15.5 ± 13.6 (7–55) mg/L (CRP was recorded as 7 when the result was less than 8.), and NEU% was 45.5 ± 19.5% (7.5.0–87.5%). In our study, children who undergo a surgical debridement are then serially monitored every 48 h with repeated inflammatory indices (WBC, ESR, and CRP) [7]. The tendency of WBC and CRP had risen on the first day after

Table 1 Demographic data of enrolled patients

Number	Sex	Age(months)	Location	Septic arthritics	Pathogen	The last time follow-up	Follow-up time(years)
1	M	2	RDF	N	N	Good	2.0
2	M	12	LDF	N	N	LLD	5.7
3	F	1.5	LDF	N	Staphylococcus aureus	Good	6.0
4	F	2.5	RPF	N	Staphylococcus aureus	Good	5.7
5	M	1	LPH	N	N	Good	3.2
6	F	10	LPT	N	N	Good	4.9
7	M	12	RF	N	N	Good	2.0
8	M	0.4	RPH	N	N	Good	3.3
9	M	9	RPT	N	N	Good	1.1
10	M	7	RPF	N	Gram-positive cocci	Good	3.5
11	M	10	RPH	N	N	Good	3.5
12	M	8	RPF	N	N	Good	1.1
13	M	1	LPF	Y	Acinetobacter baumannii	PHD LLD	1.0
14	M	1	LPF	Y	Staphylococcus aureus	AVN	1.1
15	M	0.67	RPF,	Y	N	Good	4.3
16	F	1	LPF	Y	Staphylococcus aureus	LLD	2.7
17	M	11	LPF	Y	N	LLD,	1.5
18	M	11	LPF	Y	N	Good	4.5
19	F	12	RPR	Y	N	Good	1.8
20	F	11	LPF	Y	N	Good	3.3
21	M	2	LPF	Y	Staphylococcus warneri	AVN	1.9
22	M	12	RPF	Y	N	AVN	2.4

F female, *M* male, *Y* yes, *N* no, *RDF* right distal femur, *LDF* left distal femur, *RPF* right proximal femur, *LPF* left proximal femur, *LPH* left proximal humerus, *LPT* left proximal tibia, *RF* right fibula, *RPH* right proximal humerus, *RPT* right proximal tibia, *RPR* right proximal radius, *LLD* limb length discrepancy, *PHD* pathological hip dislocation, *AVN* avascular necrosis

surgery, maybe due to the stress response. In the postoperative course, the trend of lab biomarkers was generally decreased. ESR and CRP had a similar tendency, which recovered within 6 days. WBC trend was slower, with a mean time of 2 weeks to return to normal range, whereas that of NEU% showed no trend (Fig. 1).

The most common complication was LLD, which was occurred in four patients by review of available imaging. Other complications included AVN of the femoral head in three patients and pathologic subluxation of the hip in one patient. At the final follow-up, 15 patients (68.2%) had no complications and were graded as good outcomes, while seven patients (31.8%) had complications.

There were no differences in complications occurrence between sexes ($P = 0.62$), temperatures (($P = 0.09$), duration of symptoms ($P = 0.93$), WBC ($P = 0.58$), CRP ($P = 0.97$), NEU% ($P = 0.71$), ESR ($P = 0.47$), or the length of hospitalization ($P = 0.29$). However, patients who had concomitant pyogenic arthritis were more likely to develop complications than those with isolated osteomyelitis ($P = 0.02$). (Table 2).

Discussion

The occurrence of OM is uncommon but missed or delayed diagnosis can lead to catastrophic consequences due to the unique vascular structure in infants. Because the transphyseal vessels persist until 15 to 18 months of age, infection in the metaphysis can spread into the epiphysis and produce concurrent septic arthritis [8–10]. Furthermore, joint effusion or empyema may be associated with joint dislocation and AVN [11]. Therefore, prompt diagnosis and early treatment are essential for good outcomes [12].

The diagnosis of OM might be difficult in infants because the clinical manifestations are not as evident as in older children and adults. In our study, one child (5.00%) had a temperature over 37.8 °C. All patients had decreased activity and cried on the passive movement of the extremity. Limb swelling and erythema were noted on the affected limb in 40.9% (9/22) of subjects. In comparison with patients from 1968 to 1972, Goergens [13] found that most patients suffering from OM and septic arthritis presented with only mild symptoms instead of the traditional symptoms of infection, such as fever, swelling, and clear decreased range of motion. In that study, the most common symptom was (> 90% of patients) refusal to move the affected limb, whereas only 50% of children showed local swelling and 32% children had no fever. Therefore, even if with normal body temperature and laboratory parameters, the diagnosis of OM should

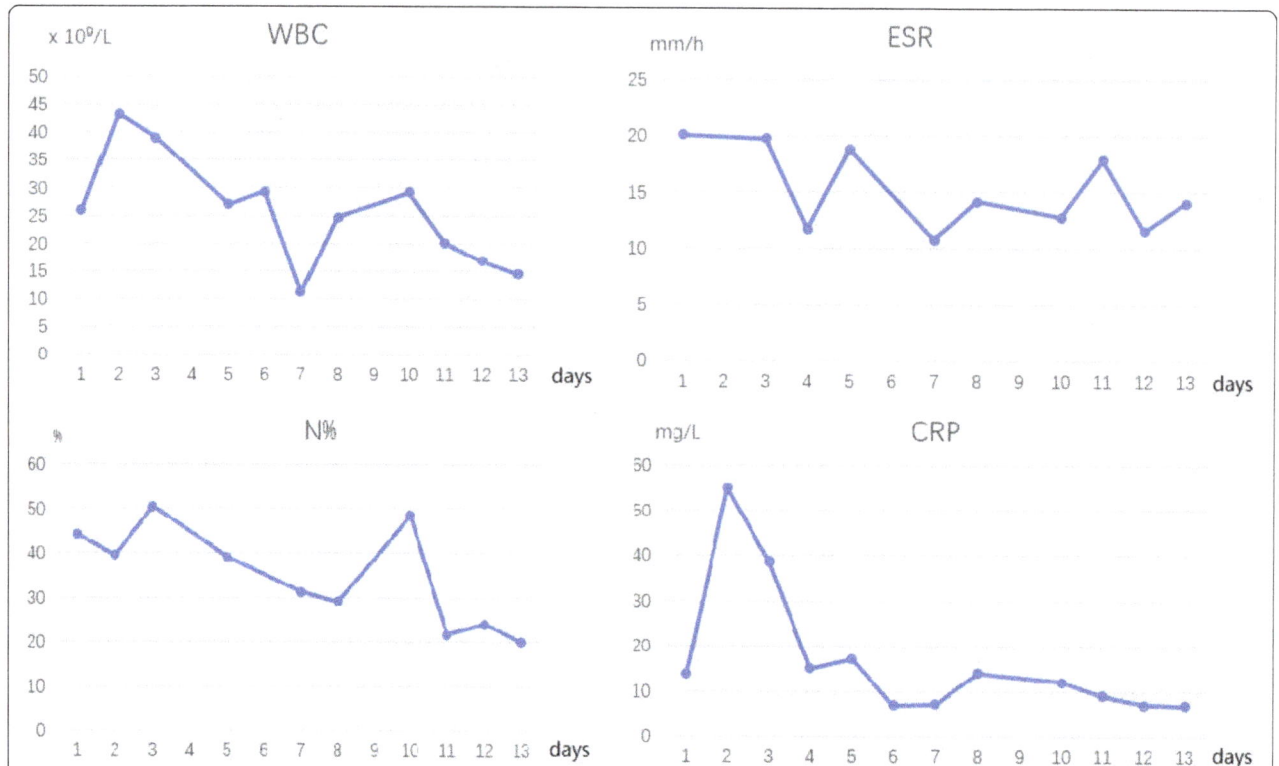

Fig. 1 Changes of patients' laboratory markers. The mean value of each laboratory marker consisted of those plots. WBC, white blood cell; ESR, erythrocyte sedimentation rate; NEU%, neutrophil%; CRP, C-reactive protein

Table 2 Comparison between cases with complications and those without complications

	Good outcomes	Complications	P
Cases, no.	15	7	
Sex, no.			0.62
F	5	1	
M	10	6	
Ages, average (range), months	6.5 ± 4.6 (0.5–12)	5.7 ± 5.6 (1–12)	0.73
Temperature, average (range), °C	36.9 ± 0.3 (36.5–37.5)	37.3 ± 0.5 (36.8–38.2)	0.09
WBC, average (range), × 10^9/L	13.4 ± 5.8 (5.5–28.2)	15.5 ± 8.7 (9.3–33.8)	0.58
CRP, average (range), mg/L	15.5 ± 14.1 (7–55)	15.3 ± 13.3 (7–38)	0.97
ESR, average (range), mm/h	30.7 ± 20.3 (2–70)	39.7 ± 29.2 (10–85)	0.47
NEU%, average (range), %	45.2 ± 23.9 (7.5–87.5)	43.7 ± 11.2 (28.1–62.1)	0.71
Duration of symptoms, average (range), days	14.4 ± 8.7 (2–30)	14.7 ± 8.3 (7–30)	0.93
Hospitalization, average (range), days	12.7 ± 5.0 (6–23)	15.7 ± 8.3 (7–28)	0.29
Septic arthritis, no.			0.02
Y	11	1	
N	4	6	

F female, *M* male, *WBC* white blood cell, *CRP* C-reactive protein, *ESR* erythrocyte sedimentation rate, *Y* yes, *N* no

not be ruled out. MRI and bone scan were recommended to search for evidence of infection.

We quantified the biochemical markers in the recovery of postoperative course. CRP was found to be a better match for recovery, which was compatible with other reports [14]. Evidence has suggested that the CRP has a half-life of 19 h, rising and normalizing faster, and is easily tested, which makes it an ideal parameter for monitoring the improvement of pediatric infections [15]. Unkila-Kallio et al. [16] elaborated that the level of CRP usually decreased rapidly if the children have isolated OM. If it does not decrease, associated septic arthritis should be suspected. In our study, the trend of NEU% showed no trend, which was less meaningful for the assessment of change of infection. Both WBC and CRP increased on the first day after surgery probably due to stress response. CRP and ESR decreased and reached normal range in about 1 week postoperatively. However, an irregular phenomenon was noticed on day 7, when all the parameters showed an increase after they gradually decreased. The reasons might be that the plots were the average value of each laboratory marker, which reported the central tendency. Thus, it is greatly influenced by outliers (values that are very much larger or smaller than most of the values).

OM occurring in the metaphysis in infants younger than 18 months old has a potential risk of physeal plate injury and growth disturbance [8, 10, 17]. Kao [18] reported three cases of physeal plate injury in his 12 years of clinical experience, which all required debridement for further treatment. Longjohn et al. [17] also reported poor outcome when OM concurred with septic arthritis.

In the present study, patients were diagnosed with septic arthritis if a purulent material was found in the joint capsule during the operation. Other patients in whom pus was not found during the operation were diagnosed as isolated OM. Moreover, patients who had concurrent pyogenic arthritis were more likely to have complications than those with OM alone ($P = 0.02$). Therefore, once the diagnosis of OM is made, appropriate antibiotics should be started as soon as possible, because of the tendency for OM of metaphysis to develop secondary septic arthritis due to the unique structure of vessels in infants [19].

The treatment of OM often begins with an antibiotic intravenously. A more specific antibiotic should be chosen according to bacteria culture and drug sensitivity results as soon as possible [20]. Initial antibiotic choice should cover *Staphylococcus aureus* which is the most common pathogen [21, 22]. Subsequent administration of antibiotics should be adjusted according to the results of drug sensitivity test, clinical manifestations, and laboratory tests. Usually, 4-to 6-week course of antibiotics is required [18]. Nikolas A et al. [23] reported that only 50% of patients had positive blood culture in their 70-person study. In the current study, the overall positive rate of blood and pus culture was 31.82% (7/22). This might be associated with previous use of antibiotics prior to admission. Systemic administration of antibiotics may cause systemic side effects, such as diarrhea and liver function damage, as well as low concentration at the infection site, especially in infants. For these reasons, combining antibiotic therapy with surgical intervention is warranted.

OM without bone lesions has traditionally been treated with 4–6 weeks of antibiotics. In the current study, debridement surgery combined with RBGS was performed when a bone lesion was observed by radiological investigations in our institution. The choice of initial antibiotics was guided by local microbiology. Broad spectrum coverage was generally utilized in this population as infants may be infected with a wider variety of organisms. [24]

The use of a local delivery of antibiotics has advantages over traditional debridement because it increases the local concentration at the infection sites [25]. In previous animal studies, Penn-Barwell and Wencke [26] showed that local delivery of antibiotics into an infected bone defect was superior to systemic antibiotics alone at 14 days after surgery. Branstetter et al. [27] confirmed that calcium sulfate mixed with antibiotics eradicated bacteria better after debridement when compared with calcium sulfate alone. The use of RBGS mixed with vancomycin has been shown to be a successful outcome in the management of chronic osteomyelitis and non-union in adults [28, 29]. McNally MA et al. described effective results in the treatment of deep bone infection using a new antibiotic-loaded biocomposite in

the eradication of infection from bone defects [30]. Also, a systematic review of 15 studies to access the utility of anti-infective bone graft substitutes in osteomyelitis treatment suggested that such treatment could be a good option [25]. Based on these reports, we were interested to determine if this treatment regimen would be effective in treating OM in infants.

In the current study, RBGS mixed with antibiotics were implanted in the local defect after debridement. There are multiple benefits to this technique. The local delivery allows for a slow-release effect and can maintain a relatively higher antibiotic concentration locally. Local use of antibiotics has previously been shown to improve local concentrations. The use of tobramycin had local concentrations of about 1000 times above the minimal inhibitory concentration (MIC) for most strains of *Staphylococcus* [31]. Gentamicin-PMMA beads also showed high local concentrations, around 100 times above the MIC, and remained bactericidal several days later [32]. Local sustained availability of drugs is more effective in achieving prophylactic and therapeutic outcomes. It could also help to avoid high systemic levels of parenteral antibiotics which can lead to additional adverse effects, such as toxic liver injury and fungal

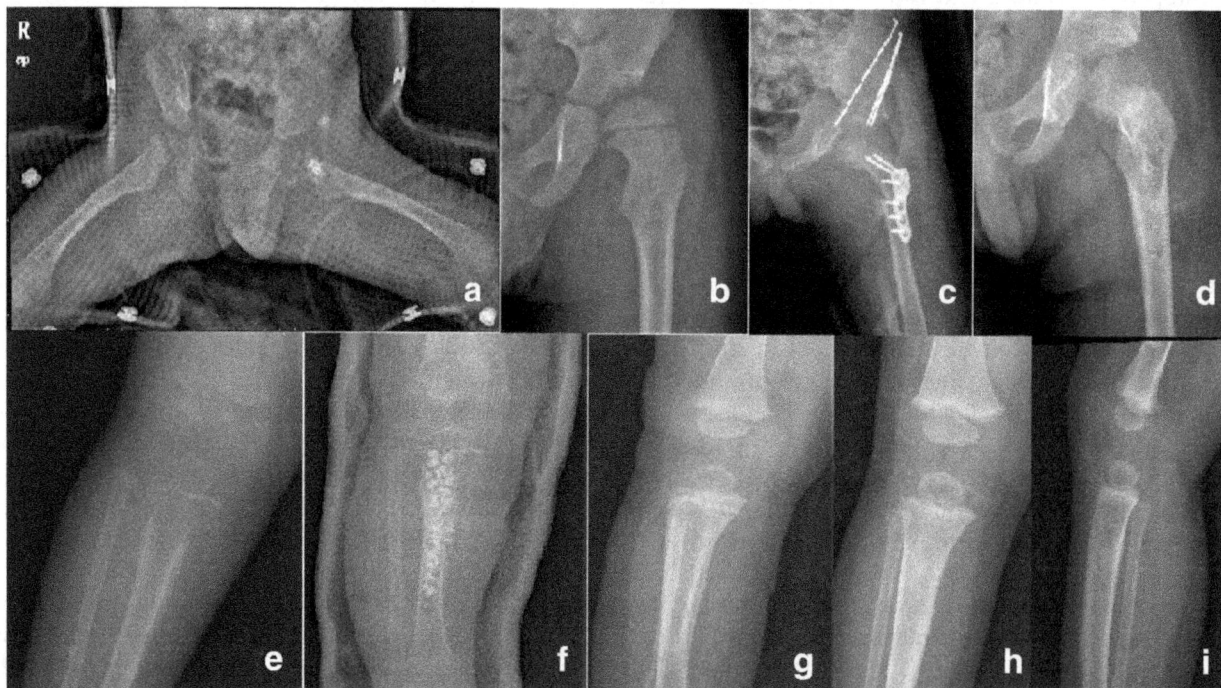

Fig. 2 AHO with or without a secondary septic arthritis. **a** An 11-month-old boy, who suffered from osteomyelitis concurred with septic arthritis on the left proximal femur, had received debridement combined with RBGS mixed with antibiotics. The hip was immobilized with a brace postoperatively. **b** Pathological subluxation was observed after 3 years postoperatively. **c** An innominate osteotomy and varus derotational osteotomy of the proximal femur were performed to correct residual deformities **d** A limb shortening of 1 cm was noted at the final follow-up. **e** A 9-month-old boy who suffered from osteomyelitis on the right proximal tibia. **f** After being debrided, bone defect was filled with RBGS, which was mixed with 0.5 g vancomycin. The affected limb was immobilized by a cast postoperatively. **g** The bone lesion healed after 2 months postoperatively. **h,i** The outcome of the involved limb was good at the final follow-up

infection [33]. Additionally, after debridement, a large defect usually occurred, which weakens the strength of the bone (Fig. 2). Filling the cavity with RBGS mixed with antibiotics can provide mechanical support as well as stimulate bone regrowth [34]. Furthermore, we stressed the importance of immobilization postoperatively to prevent pathological fractures.

Adult OM is commonly seen with contiguous infection caused by open fractures or joint replacement surgeries and vascular or neurologic insufficiency [35]. Antibiotic therapy is the first-choice treatment for acute OM, while debridement is indicated in chronic OM [36]. In infants, however, OM tends to occur in the site of the metaphysis, which has a potential risk of physeal plate injury. Based on that, aggressive surgical intervention is warranted to prevent the devastating complications such as LLD and AVN.

Recently, a new technology named supercritical emulsion extraction (SEE) had been confirmed to be a green, flexible way to make a multiloaded poly-lactic-co-glycolic acid (PLGA) microdevice for gentamicin (Gen) sustained release in an in vitro study. Gen molecules were not chemically changed by such technology and maintained their biological activity [37]. In the future, other new technologies may provide alternative treatment options by delivering in situ in a dose- and time-controlled manner pharmacologically active molecules to tackle bone infection.

There were some limitations in this study. Firstly, a small sample size decreased the power of our statistical analysis. However, this is the first study focused on infants with OM treated with RBGS mixed with antibiotics. Secondly, this retrospective study contained patients with different lesion sites which introduced bias into the results. Thirdly, lack of a control group of other treatment options and loss of follow-up also affected the statistical efficiency. At the final follow-up, we only observed seven patients with complications. Longer-term close follow-ups until skeletal maturity of those patients with good outcomes are necessary in our subsequent works. Finally, a multi-center and prospective study should be performed in the future to obtain more powerful evidence about this issue.

Conclusions

We reported a single-stage protocol for treatment of infantile OM including early operative debridement and the use of RBGS mixed with vancomycin as a space filler. This protocol showed a low recurrence rate and few complications over one- to six-year follow-up period. These results suggest that this option in the treatment of OM might achieve acceptable results and merits further investigations.

Abbreviations
AVN: Avascular necrosis; CRP: C-reactive protein; ESR: Erythrocyte sedimentation rate; Gen: Gentamicin; LLD: Limb length deformity; MIC: Minimal inhibitory concentration; NEU%: Neutrophil percentage; OM: Osteomyelitis; PLGA: Poly-lactic-co-glycolic acid; RBGS: Resorbable bone graft substitute; SEE: Supercritical emulsion extraction; WBC: White blood cell

Funding
The project is sponsored by the Natural Science Foundation of Shanghai No. 17411965800 and Shanghai Jiao Tong University, School of Medicine, Improvement Project of Clinical Research Capability for Clinical Medicine Graduate in Scarcity Major No. JQ201707.

Authors' contributions
ZQZ and HOL made substantial contributions to the conception, reviewed the case, collected the data, carried out the initial analyses, and drafted the initial manuscript. HIL and QF collected the data and performed the surgeries. XY, PQS, TC, QXC, and JZ performed the surgeries. ZMZ coordinated and supervised data collection and critically reviewed the revised the manuscript. All authors read and approved the final manuscript.

Competing interests
The authors declare that they have no competing interests.

References
1. Green NE, Edwards K. Bone and joint infections in children. Orthop Clin North Am. 1987;18(4):555–76.
2. El-Rosasy MA. Ilizarov treatment for pseudarthrosis of the tibia due to haematogenous osteomyelitis. J Pediatr Orthop B. 2013;22(3):200–6.
3. Matic A, et al. Acute osteomyelitis and septic arthritis of the shoulder in premature neonates--report of two cases. Med Pregl. 2012;65(1–2):59–64.
4. Humm G, et al. Adjuvant treatment of chronic osteomyelitis of the tibia following exogenous trauma using OSTEOSET®-T: a review of 21 patients in a regional trauma Centre. Strategies Trauma Limb Reconstr. 2014;9(3):157–61.
5. Fleiter N, et al. Clinical use and safety of a novel gentamicin-releasing resorbable bone graft substitute in the treatment of osteomyelitis/osteitis. Bone Joint Res. 2014;3(7):223–9.
6. Agarwal A, Aggarwal AN. Bone and joint infections in children: acute hematogenous osteomyelitis. Indian J Pediatr. 2016;83(8):817–24.
7. Tuason DA, et al. Clinical and laboratory parameters associated with multiple surgeries in children with acute hematogenous osteomyelitis. J Pediatr Orthop. 2014;34(5):565–70.
8. Rosenbaum DM, Blumhagen JD. Acute epiphyseal osteomyelitis in children. Radiology. 1985;156(1):89–92.
9. Kramer SJ, Post J, Sussman M. Acute hematogenous osteomyelitis of the epiphysis. J Pediatr Orthop. 1986;6(4):493–5.
10. Green NE, Beauchamp RD, Griffin PP. Primary subacute epiphyseal osteomyelitis. J Bone Joint Surg Am. 1981;63(1):107–14.
11. Montgomery CO, et al. Concurrent septic arthritis and osteomyelitis in children. J Pediatr Orthop. 2013;33(4):464–7.
12. Porat S, et al. Complications of suppurative arthritis and osteomyelitis in children. Int Orthop. 1991;15(3):205–8.
13. Goergens ED, et al. Acute osteomyelitis and septic arthritis in children. J Paediatr Child Health. 2005;41(1–2):59–62.
14. Arnold JC, et al. Acute bacterial osteoarticular infections: eight-year analysis of C-reactive protein for oral step-down therapy. Pediatrics. 2012;130(4):e821–8.
15. Chou AC, Mahadev A. The use of C-reactive protein as a guide for transitioning to oral antibiotics in pediatric osteoarticular infections. J Pediatr Orthop. 2016;36(2):173–7.
16. Unkila-Kallio L, Kallio MJ, Peltola H. The usefulness of C-reactive protein levels in the identification of concurrent septic arthritis in children who have acute hematogenous osteomyelitis. A comparison with the usefulness of the erythrocyte sedimentation rate and the white blood-cell count. J Bone Joint Surg Am. 1994;76(6):848–53.

17. Longjohn DB, Zionts LE, Stott NS. Acute hematogenous osteomyelitis of the epiphysis. Clin Orthop Relat Res. 1995;316:227–34.

18. Kao FC, et al. Acute primary hematogenous osteomyelitis of the epiphysis: report of two cases. Chang Gung Med J. 2003;26(11):851–6.

19. Bar-On E, et al. Chronic osteomyelitis in children: treatment by intramedullary reaming and antibiotic-impregnated cement rods. J Pediatr Orthop. 2010;30(5):508–13.

20. Paakkonen M, et al. C-reactive protein versus erythrocyte sedimentation rate, white blood cell count and alkaline phosphatase in diagnosing bacteraemia in bone and joint infections. J Paediatr Child Health. 2013;49(3):E189–92.

21. Stone B, et al. Pediatric tibial osteomyelitis. J Pediatr Orthop. 2016;36(5):534–40.

22. Belthur MV, et al. Prospective evaluation of a shortened regimen of treatment for acute osteomyelitis and septic arthritis in children. J Pediatr Orthop. 2010;30(8):942.

23. Jagodzinski NA, et al. Prospective evaluation of a shortened regimen of treatment for acute osteomyelitis and septic arthritis in children. J Pediatr Orthop. 2009;29(5):518–25.

24. Yeo A, Ramachandran M. Acute haematogenous osteomyelitis in children. Bmj. 2014;348(jan20 3):g66.

25. van Vugt TA, Geurts J, Arts JJ. Clinical application of antimicrobial bone graft substitute in osteomyelitis treatment: a systematic review of different bone graft substitutes available in clinical treatment of osteomyelitis. Biomed Res Int. 2016;2016:6984656.

26. Rand BC, Penn-Barwell JG, Wenke JC. Combined local and systemic antibiotic delivery improves eradication of wound contamination: an animal experimental model of contaminated fracture. Bone Joint J. 2015;97-B(10):1423–7.

27. Branstetter JG, et al. Locally-administered antibiotics in wounds in a limb. J Bone Joint Surg Br. 2009;91(8):1106–9.

28. Vazquez M. Osteomyelitis in children. Curr Opin Pediatr. 2002;14(1):112–5.

29. Humm G, et al. Adjuvant treatment of chronic osteomyelitis of the tibia following exogenous trauma using OSTEOSET((R))-T: a review of 21 patients in a regional trauma Centre. Strategies Trauma Limb Reconstr. 2014;9(3):157–61.

30. McNally MA, et al. Single-stage treatment of chronic osteomyelitis with a new absorbable, gentamicin-loaded, calcium sulphate/hydroxyapatite biocomposite: a prospective series of 100 cases. Bone Joint J. 2016;98-B(9):1289–96.

31. Wahl P, et al. Systemic exposure to tobramycin after local antibiotic treatment with calcium sulphate as carrier material. Arch Orthop Trauma Surg. 2011;131(5):657–62.

32. Walenkamp GH, Vree TB, van Rens TJ. Gentamicin-PMMA beads. Pharmacokinetic and nephrotoxicological study. Clin Orthop Relat Res. 1986;205:171–83.

33. Zalavras CG, Patzakis MJ, Holtom P. Local antibiotic therapy in the treatment of open fractures and osteomyelitis. Clin Orthop Relat Res. 2004;427:86–93.

34. Canavese F, et al. Successful treatment of chronic osteomyelitis in children with debridement, antibiotic-laden cement spacer and bone graft substitute. Eur J Orthop Surg Traumatol. 2017;27(2):221–8.

35. Waldvogel FA, Medoff G, Swartz MN. Osteomyelitis: a review of clinical features, therapeutic considerations and unusual aspects. N Engl J Med. 1970;282(4):198–206.

36. Maffulli N, et al. The management of osteomyelitis in the adult. Surgeon. 2016;14(6):345–60.

37. Della Porta G, et al. Injectable PLGA/hydroxyapatite/chitosan microcapsules produced by supercritical emulsion extraction technology: an in vitro study on teriparatide/gentamicin controlled release. J Pharm Sci. 2016;105(7):2164–72.

3

Factors affecting intraosseous pressure measurement

Michael Beverly*[ID] and David Murray

Abstract

Background: Although a raised intraosseous pressure (IOP) has been found in osteoarthritis and osteonecrosis, the normal physiology of subchondral circulation is poorly understood. We developed an animal model and explored the physiology of normal subchondral perfusion and IOP.

Methods: In 21 anaesthetised rabbits, 44 intraosseous needles were placed in the subchondral bone of the femoral head ($n = 6$), femoral condyle ($n = 7$) or proximal tibia ($n = 31$). Needles were connected to pressure transducers and a chart recorder. In 14 subjects, the proximal femoral artery and vein were clamped alternately. In five subjects, arterial pressure was measured simultaneously in the opposite femoral artery.

Results: The average IOP at all 44 sites was 24.5 mmHg with variability within SD 6.8 and between subjects SD 11.5. IOP was not significantly influenced by gender, weight, site or size of a needle. Needle clearance by flushing caused a prolonged drop in IOP whereas after clearance by aspiration, recovery was rapid. IOP recordings exhibited wave patterns synchronous with the arterial pulse, with respiration and with drug circulation time. There was a correlation between IOP and blood pressure (13 sites in 5 subjects, Pearson correlation 0.829, $p < 0.0005$). There was a correlation between IOP and the associated pulse pressure (PP) in 44 sites among 21 subjects (Pearson correlation 0.788, $p < 0.001$). In 14 subjects (31 sites), arterial occlusion caused a significant reduction in IOP and loss of PP ($p < 0.0001$). Venous occlusion significantly raised IOP with preservation of the PP ($p < 0.012$).

Conclusion: Our study shows that subchondral cancellous bone behaves as a perfused tissue and that IOP is mainly a reflection of arterial supply. A single measure of IOP is variable and reflects only perfusion at the needle tip rather than being a measure of venous back pressure. Alternate proximal vessel clamping offers a new means of exploring the physiology of subchondral perfusion. We describe a model that will allow further study of IOP such as during loading.

Keywords: Intraosseous pressure, Physiology, Subchondral, Bone blood flow, Vascular occlusion, Osteoarthritis, Osteonecrosis

Background

Intraosseous pressure (IOP) and bone blood flow have been studied by authors interested in bone circulation and physiology for more than 50 years. Varying techniques using different needles, flushing and recording methods have produced differing results, and there has been limited progress in understanding IOP physiology since Azuma reported IOP fluctuation in a rabbit model in 1964 [1–7]. Measurement of IOP in man has also proved variable [8]. IOP has generally been found to be raised in bone diseases such as osteonecrosis and after steroid use [9–13]. A raised

IOP has been associated with pain in osteoarthritic joints, chondromalacia patellae and with cartilage degeneration. IOP may also be important in driving fluid through canaliculi, hence governing osteocyte activity and bone turnover [14, 15]. It has usually been thought that IOP had a static or fixed value which was due to venous back pressure, intramedullary pressure or interstitial pressure [2]. IOP has been measured experimentally in animals and in man. Steroid-induced models of avascular necrosis have been developed in order to study IOP and its treatment [16, 17]. Ficat and others developed a technique for the 'functional exploration' of bone in patients with early osteonecrosis [10]. However, the factors that control IOP at rest and

* Correspondence: michael.beverly@btinternet.com
Botnar Research Centre, Nuffield Department of Orthopaedics, Rheumatology & Musculoskeletal Sciences, University of Oxford, Nuffield Orthopaedic Centre, Headington, Oxford OX3 7LD, UK

during activity and the physiology of subchondral bone circulation remain largely unknown [18].

In a preliminary unpublished clinical work, we measured IOP prior to forage, osteotomy or decompression. The findings were variable. The rationale for our study was to explore the physiology of IOP in healthy subchondral cancellous bone at rest in an animal model.

Methods
Experimental measurements

IOP was measured experimentally using intraosseous needles in the subchondral cancellous bone of the femoral head, femoral condyle and proximal tibia of 21 adult New Zealand White rabbits (Royal Postgraduate Medical School, Home Office licence ELA 24/4994). The rabbits were anaesthetized through an ear vein with intravenous Sublimaze (fentanyl, Janssen-Cilag Pty Ltd., NSW 2113, Australia) and Valium (diazepam, Genentech Inc., San Francisco, CA 94080, USA). Induction of anaesthesia was by IV Sublimaze (fentanyl) 2 ml of 0.05 mg/ml solution depending on the size of the animal with top up IV infusion of Valium (diazepam) 0.5 ml of 5 mg/ml solution alternating with Sublimaze (fentanyl) 0.5–1.0 ml given slowly on approximately a ½ hourly basis. The initial recordings were mainly from the right femoral head with later recordings mainly from the femoral condyles and proximal tibia as in Fig. 1 as these were more reliable. There were 44 different IOP recordings, six at the femoral head, seven from the femoral condyles and 31 from the proximal tibiae. The femoral head was approached by dissection anteriorly through the femoral triangle. A saline-filled 21G ($n = 13$) or 23G ($n = 31$) venesection needle was pushed by hand into the femoral head subchondral bone by rocking the needle through a 5° to 10° arc along the line of the bevel of the needle. The needles were placed under direct vision in the approximate centre of the subchondral region within a few millimetres of the subchondral surface. For the femoral condyle, insertion was a few millimetres proximal to the visible and palpable surface. The same was applied to the proximal tibia. In 14 subjects, the right femoral artery and vein were selectively clamped at the inguinal ligament. The needles were connected by saline-filled lines to pressure transducers (Druck PDCR75, Druck Ltd., Leicester LE6 0FH, UK) and to a four-channel chart recorder (Lectromed MX4P-31, Lectromed Ltd., Jersey, Channel Islands, UK). The transducers were calibrated on a 0–100 mmHg scale. In five animals, the arterial blood pressure was measured by cannulating the left femoral artery and recording pressure using the same transducer system.

The experimental set up was as illustrated in Fig. 1.

Statistical analysis

Experimental time varied from about 15 min to over 2 h. Intraosseous pressure and the associated pulse pressure

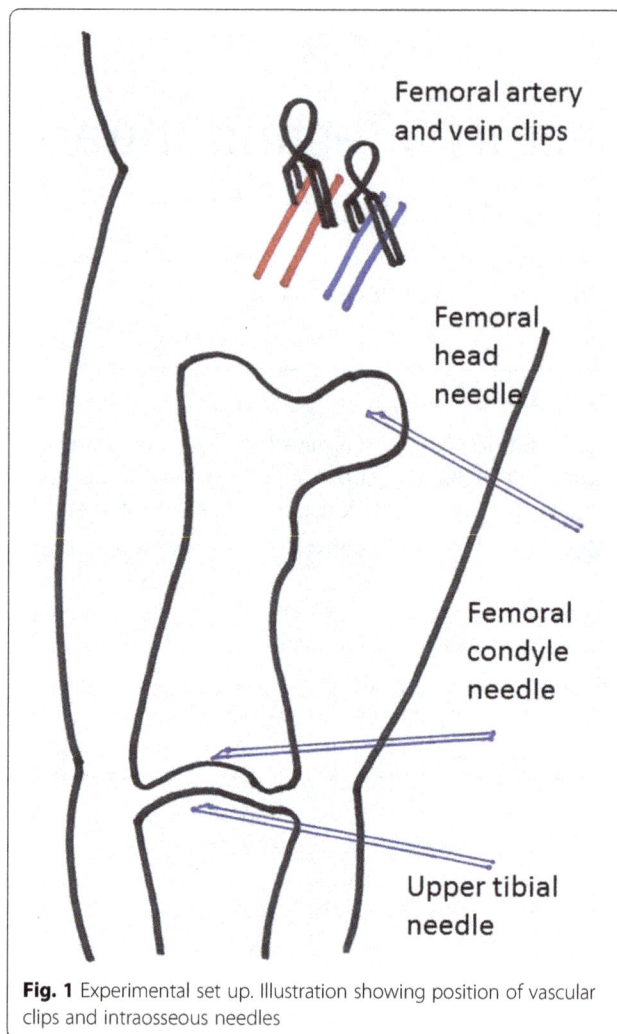

Fig. 1 Experimental set up. Illustration showing position of vascular clips and intraosseous needles

(PP) were measured at all 44 sites on three occasions, early, middle and late during each experiment and were averaged. Results were expressed as means, standard deviations and ranges. Student's t test was used to determine if there were significant differences. When each subject was used as its own control, paired tests were used. Otherwise, unpaired tests were used. The Pearson test was used to assess correlations. $P < 0.05$ was considered to be statistically significant.

Experimental plan

A series of experiments was undertaken to investigate the following:

1. Normal baseline IOP: The normal IOP was measured at all 44 sites and the influence of factors relating to animal, including gender, weight, site and size of needle were explored.
2. Method of measuring: The Ficat method in which a 0.5 ml clearance bolus of saline was

injected was compared with a method using needle clearance by aspiration [10].

3. IOP wave forms: IOP wave forms were explored at different chart speeds, 12.5 mm/sec and 12.5 mm/min. The traces were compared with the directly visible pulse and respiratory waves. The chart speed was 12.5 mm/minute in subsequent experiments.

4. Drug administration: The effect of a bolus drug administration of Valium (diazepam 2.5 mg) or Sublimaze (fentanyl 0.05 mg) on IOP was recorded.

5. Relationship between systemic blood pressure, IOP and the pulse pressure (PP)
The relationship between systemic blood pressure and IOP in 13 sites among 5 subjects was explored.

6. The relationship between IOP and pulse pressure: The relationship between IOP and the associated pulse pressure was explored at 44 sites among all 21 subjects. The pulse pressure was taken as the difference between the top and bottom of the wave on the IOP tracing at that point.

7. Vascular occlusion: The effect on IOP of clamping the femoral artery or femoral vein was recorded in 31 sites among 14 subjects. The clamps were small 'bulldog' sheathed vascular clips. They were applied to the proximal femoral artery or vein under direct vision.

Results
Normal IOP
Basal intraosseous pressure was measured at 44 sites among 21 subjects as in Fig. 2. At each site, the early, middle and late IOP and the corresponding PP were averaged. The averaged IOP at different sites varied considerably (mean 23.4 mmHg, SD 13.7, range 3–55). Gender (female $n = 14$, male $n = 7$) had no effect on IOP (t test $p = 0.537$). Weight (2920–5560 g) had no effect on IOP (Pearson correlation $p = 0.368$). Needle size 21G ($n = 13$) and 23G ($n = 31$), t test 0.14, had no effect on IOP.

Several subjects had two or more sites measured. There was variation between subjects (SD 11.5 mmHg) and variation between sites within subjects (SD 6.8 mmHg). Where paired measurements were available ($n = 7$), there was no difference (t test $p = 0.52$) between the femoral condyle (mean 9.8, SD 3.6, range 5–16) and proximal tibia (mean 12, SD 7.4, range 5.7–16.7). There were insufficient paired data for femoral head comparisons.

Method of measurement of IOP
Previous investigators have used a saline bolus or 'clearance' injection [10] before recording IOP. We found that in healthy bone this caused a marked fall in IOP which was followed by a gradual recovery taking up to 10 min. Aspiration was followed by faster recovery which took less than 1 min as in Fig. 3.

IOP wave forms
The majority of recordings showed a pulsatile wave form. At a fast chart speed of 12.5 mm/sec, the wave was seen to be synchronous with the cardiac arterial pulse by direct observation. At a speed 60 times slower or 12.5 mm/min, the arterial pulse was obliterated but an underlying slower wave form was observed. This wave was seen to be synchronous with respiration by direct observation as in Fig. 4.

Drug administration
Systemic administration of anaesthetic agents affected the IOP. For example, in the representative trace shown, the administration of an intravenous bolus of Valium (diazepam 2.5 mg) lowered the IOP and PP waves for about 90 s. Sublimaze (fentanyl 0.05 mg) caused a variable effect. In this representative trace, there was an excitatory effect. The IOP and PP rose for about 90 s with another lesser peak following. This double-wave pattern corresponds to the expected circulation time of the drug bolus as in Fig. 5.

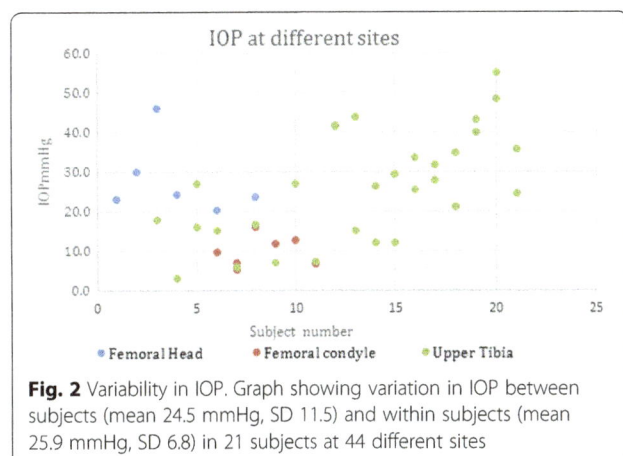

Fig. 2 Variability in IOP. Graph showing variation in IOP between subjects (mean 24.5 mmHg, SD 11.5) and within subjects (mean 25.9 mmHg, SD 6.8) in 21 subjects at 44 different sites

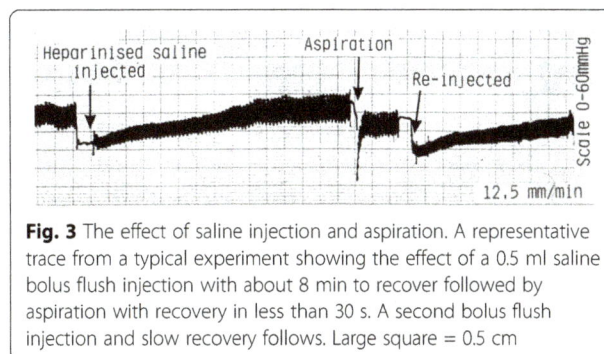

Fig. 3 The effect of saline injection and aspiration. A representative trace from a typical experiment showing the effect of a 0.5 ml saline bolus flush injection with about 8 min to recover followed by aspiration with recovery in less than 30 s. A second bolus flush injection and slow recovery follows. Large square = 0.5 cm

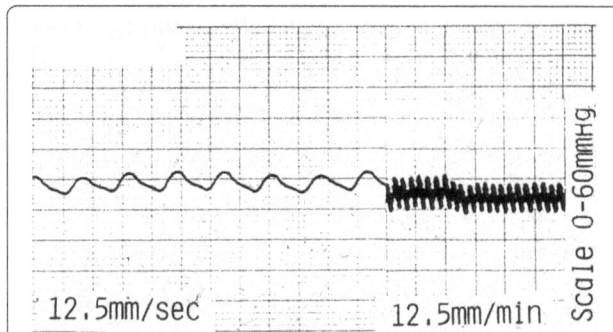

Fig. 4 Cardiac and respiratory waves. A representative IOP recording at different speeds. On the left (12.5 mm/sec, eight pulses in 6 s, pulse rate 80/min), a wave which was seen to be synchronous with the arterial pulse is observed. On the right (at a speed 60 times slower (12.5 mm/min), for 3 min, eight respirations per minute), an underlying wave which was seen to be synchronous with respiration was observed. Large squares are 0.5 cm

Relationship between IOP and blood pressure and IOP and PP

Arterial blood pressure (BP) was measured in the left femoral artery in five animals using a pressure transducer. The mean BP was 62.8 mmHg, SD 8.2, range 55–73. Intraosseous pressure was measured at the same time at 13 different sites among the five subjects. The mean IOP was 11.7 mmHg, SD 7.2, range 5–27. There was a significant relationship ($p < 0.0005$) between blood pressure and IOP, Pearson correlation 0.829 as in Fig. 6.

Relationship between IOP and pulse pressure

IOP was compared with the associated pulse pressure (PP) at all sites ($n = 44$) among the 21 subjects. The pulse pressure was taken as the difference between the top and bottom of the IOP trace wave. There was a significant correlation ($p < 0.0001$) between IOP and the associated PP, Pearson correlation 0.788 as in Fig. 7.

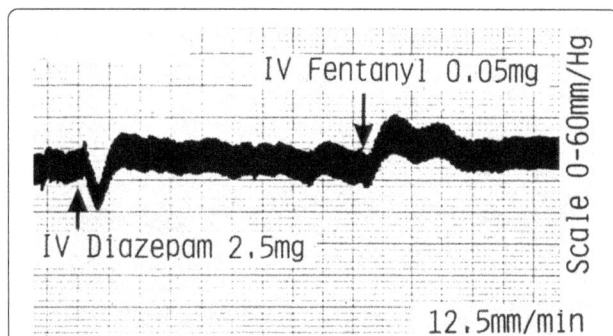

Fig. 5 Effect of systemic drug administration. Systemic administration of anaesthetic agents such as diazepam and fentanyl affected the IOP as in this representative trace. Large square = 0.5 cm

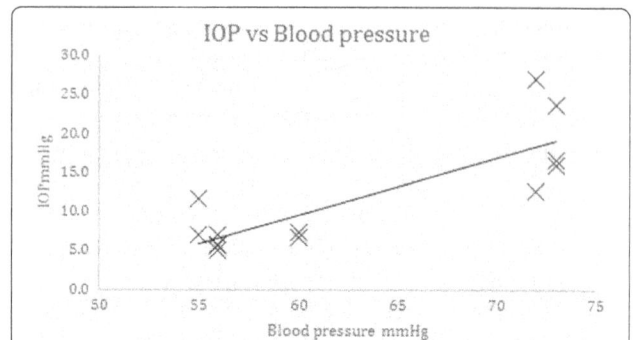

Fig. 6 Correlation of IOP with blood pressure. Effect of blood pressure on IOP. Intraosseous pressure was measured at 13 sites among 5 subjects

Effect of clamping supplying artery or draining vein

In 14 subjects (31 sites), when the proximal femoral artery was clamped at the inguinal ligament, there was a fall in IOP with loss of the pulse pressure immediately. IOP stabilised within about 1 min as in Fig. 8. Recovery in IOP and restoration of the pulse pressure wave following release of the arterial clip was seen after less than 1 min. When the proximal femoral vein was clamped, the IOP rose and the pulse pressure was preserved as in Fig. 8. With clamping the proximal femoral vein, there was a pressure rise taking up to 30 s to stabilise and a similar time after venous release before the IOP returned to normal. During proximal venous clamping, the pulse pressure or respiratory wave was preserved. The period during which the clamp was applied was typically 3–5 min as shown in the representative traces in Fig. 8.

For 31 sites among the 14 subjects, the mean basal IOP (IOPb) was 20.4 mmHg (SD 13.5 mmHg). The mean arterial occlusion IOP (IOPa) was 7.5 mmHg (SD 4.6 mmHg), and the mean venous occluded IOP (IOPv) was 28.8 mmHg (SD 12.0 mmHg). We compared IOPb vs IOPa and IOPv using paired t tests. Each subject was its own control. There were significant differences between them, IOPb vs IOPa $p < 0.00001$, IOPb vs IOPv $p < 0.012$, and IOPa vs IOPv $p < 0.00001$ as shown in Fig. 9.

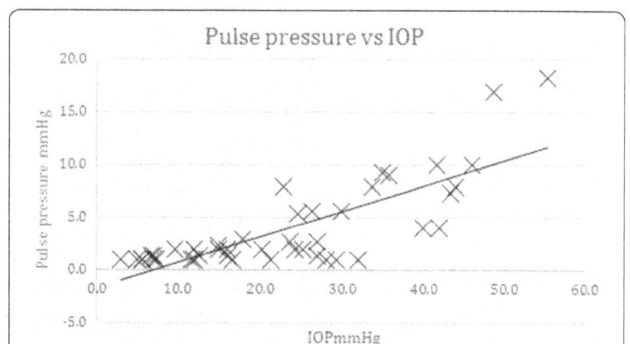

Fig. 7 Correlation of pulse pressure with IOP. Pulse pressure (mmHg) with IOP (mmHg) for 44 separate sites among 21 subjects

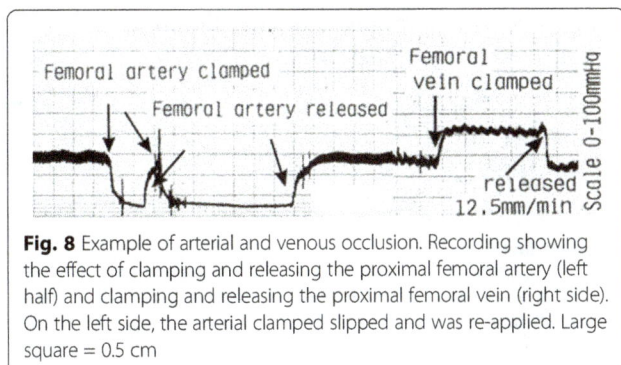

Fig. 8 Example of arterial and venous occlusion. Recording showing the effect of clamping and releasing the proximal femoral artery (left half) and clamping and releasing the proximal femoral vein (right side). On the left side, the arterial clamped slipped and was re-applied. Large square = 0.5 cm

Discussion

This study of the physiology of resting intraosseous pressure measurement in a healthy animal model gives insights which contradict some current views. IOP has usually been thought to have a fixed or static value which reflects an interstitial pressure, tissue turgor or venous back pressure [2, 10]. We found variation in IOP between and within normal subjects even when using a standardised approach. Although IOP was not related to gender, weight, size or site of needle, it was proportional to blood pressure. In addition, pulse pressure was proportional to IOP. The demonstration of variability in IOP and proportionality between IOP and PP shown by our 44 different sites in otherwise normal bone strongly suggests that the needle tip strikes different vessels within the cancellous bone by chance and that the IOP and PP reflect conditions in the blood pool at the needle tip rather than IOP being of a fixed value for any whole bone or subject. In the blood pool at the needle tip, we assume that IOP from the highest pressure vessel will be recorded. Larger arterioles will give a higher IOP and PP as they are nearer the arterial side of the vascular tree. Smaller vessels or capillaries give a lower IOP and lower PP. Venules, fat and trabeculae may return virtually no pressure.

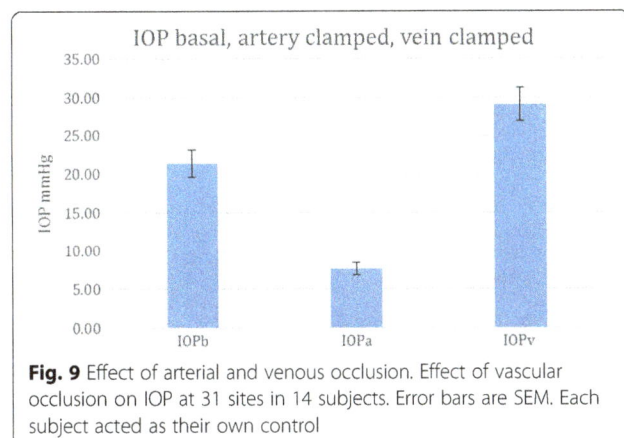

Fig. 9 Effect of arterial and venous occlusion. Effect of vascular occlusion on IOP at 31 sites in 14 subjects. Error bars are SEM. Each subject acted as their own control

IOP not only correlated with pulse pressure, but IOP also correlated with blood pressure, and was seen to correspond to respiratory waves and systemic or drug circulatory effects further suggesting that IOP is governed mainly by the arterial circulation. Moreover, there was a greater fall in IOP with arterial occlusion than a rise with venous occlusion. This would also indicate that the majority of the recorded IOP is due to the arterial supply side. The disappearance from the trace of the pulse pressure with arterial occlusion also demonstrates that the IOP and both the associated pulse and respiratory waves are mediated through the arterial supply. Both are preserved when the proximal femoral vein is clamped. Once again this suggests that IOP is therefore a 'supply' side phenomenon rather than a venous back pressure or measure of drainage. We found no previous references to this analysis of the physiology of IOP [8].

We have shown that IOP is not a constant but varies between and within subjects and also depends on the method and timing of measurement. Within that variability, there are recognisable wave forms with arterial, respiratory and drug or circulatory time patterns.

Whilst trying to optimise the method of measuring IOP, we compared the usual standard method, which involves injecting a small clearance bolus of saline (Ficat technique), with a novel method in which the needle was aspirated prior to IOP measurement. In healthy bone, both techniques resulted in an initial decrease in IOP which recovered but not necessarily to exactly the same starting point (Fig. 2). The recovery after aspiration was quicker and was usually stable within 1 min. After saline injection up to 10 min was required for recovery. Saline bolus injection appears to be harmful to the local microcirculation [19]. The delay in return to normal IOP may reflect a washout or recovery period. The subsequent slightly higher IOP may reflect renewed contact with larger arterial supply vessels following local destruction. The use of forced saline injection should probably be avoided. The aspiration method appears preferable. Previous workers assessing IOP after using the bolus injection method may in fact have been measuring an IOP which was temporarily lowered as a result of their saline injection [2, 7, 9, 10]. It is equally possible that in osteonecrotic bone the IOP recorded would be high because of the pressure of the injection itself into poorly drained or ischaemic bone. A third possibility is that the flushing of heparinised saline, blood, fat and bone fragments backwards into the delicate subchondral vascular tree is physically damaging or toxic [19]. The slower recovery after injection may represent a prolonged washout or recovery phase which is not required after less damaging aspiration.

The residual pressure after arterial clamping, for example in Fig. 8, probably does represent a real residual venous or tissue back pressure at the needle tip. Similarly with proximal venous occlusion, the IOP recorded may represent the best obtainable arterial supply pressure at that needle tip. For the first time, this simple approach gives a means of assessing the perfusion pressure range obtainable at the needle tip deep in the cancellous bone.

There are several potential limitations in this study. X-rays were not available for needle placement, but under direct vision hand placement of the needle tip was to within a few millimetres of the subchondral surface as illustrated in Fig. 1. The animals used were similar healthy adults but were not identical. Different sites were used, initially mainly the femoral head and later mainly at the femoral condyle and proximal tibia which were technically easier. We could not always obtain tracings from all sites in all subjects. The subject's blood pressures inevitably varied during the experiments. Needle insertion could never be identical at all sites. The experiments varied in duration from about 15 min to over 2 h. Because IOP inevitably fluctuated during that time, an average of the early, middle and late values was used for each of the 44 sites. There was a learning curve but generally anaesthetic control and experimental duration increased with experience [7, 20, 21]. Although the known experimental differences resulted in some variability in results, our experimental conditions were generally representative of the clinical situation. The analysis was based on data from different sites. It could be argued that these are not completely independent as in some subjects there were two or three sites. However, the IOP was not significantly different at different anatomical sites. If the analysis was based on subjects alone, the numbers would be smaller. The work was primarily qualitative and designed to develop a standardised model. Nevertheless, some useful insights on perfusion physiology have been derived from our study. This may in turn allow better use of IOP measurement in the study of circulation in diseased bone states such as osteoarthritis and avascular necrosis. Future work will measure IOP under load and with vascular occlusion to give a better understanding of subchondral perfusion physiology.

Conclusion

In conclusion, we have developed a model for IOP study. Flushing of saline and other material into the bone is probably harmful and causes a prolonged drop in IOP [19]. Aspiration clearance is likely to be better. Our work shows that IOP at rest in vivo mainly reflects physiological arterial pressure at the needle tip in a perfused organ. Whilst a single isolated measure of IOP is therefore of little value even in a standardised model, by alternate proximal arterial and venous clamping, a more useful idea of circulation at the needle tip deep in cancellous bone may be achieved.

Abbreviations
IOP: Intraosseous pressure; PP: Pulse pressure

Acknowledgements
The authors would like to thank Dr. Joseph Pflug for his advice and support with early work at the Hammersmith Hospital and Dr. Jill Urban for her advice and support. We thank Mrs. Barbara Marks for her support and assistance with submission.

Funding
This work was funded by the Wellcome Trust Grant 12425/1.5/SC/wj.

Authors' contributions
MB designed the project, carried out the work and wrote the paper. DM advised and assisted in the presentation and reviewed the paper. Both authors read and approved the final manuscript.

Competing interests
The authors declare that they have no competing interests.

References
1. Azuma H. Intraosseous pressure as a measure of hemodynamic changes in bone marrow. Angiology. 1964;15:396–406.
2. Arnoldi CC, Linderholm H, Mussbichler H. Venous engorgement and intraosseous hypertension in osteoarthritis of the hip. J Bone Joint Surg. 1972;54(3):409–21.
3. Bourne GH. The Biochemistry and Physiology of Bone, Vol. 2. Structure. 2nd Edition. Xvi+376p. Illus. New York; London: Academic Press; 1972.
4. Wilkes CH, Visscher MB. Some physiological aspects of bone-marrow pressure. J Bone Joint Surg Br. 1975;A57(1):49–57.
5. Hungerford DS, Lennox DW. The importance of increased intraosseous pressure in the development of osteonecrosis of the femoral head: implications for treatment. Orthop Clin North Am. 1985;16(4):635–54.
6. Beverly M, Pflug J, Mathie R. Bone—a flexible perfused sponge. J Bone Joint Surg Br. 1987;69:494.
7. Frascone RJ, Salzman JG, Adams AB, Bliss P, Wewerka SS, Dries DJ. Evaluation of intraosseous pressure in a hypovolemic animal model. J Surg Res. 2015;193(1):383–90. https://doi.org/10.1016/j.jss.2014.07.007.
8. Salzman JG, Loken NM, Wewerka SS, Burnett AM, Zagar AE, Griffith KR, Bliss PL, Peterson BK, Ward CJ, Frascone RJ. Intraosseous pressure monitoring in healthy volunteers. Prehosp Emerg Care. 2017;21(5):567–74. https://doi.org/10.1080/10903127.2017.1302529.
9. Green NE, Griffin PP. Intra-osseous venous pressure in Legg-Perthes disease. J Bone Joint Surg Am. 1982;64(5):666–71.
10. Ficat RP. Idiopathic bone necrosis of the femoral head. Early diagnosis and treatment. J Bone Joint Surg Br. 1985;67(1):3–9.
11. Pedersen NW, Kiaer T, Kristensen KD, Starklint H. Intraosseous pressure, oxygenation, and histology in arthrosis and osteonecrosis of the hip. Acta Orthop Scand. 1989;60(4):415–7.
12. Uchio Y, Ochi M, Adachi N, Nishikori T, Kawasaki K. Intraosseous hypertension and venous congestion in osteonecrosis of the knee. Clin Orthop Relat Res. 2001;384:217–23.
13. Ho KY, Hu HH, Colletti PM, Powers CM. Running-induced patellofemoral pain fluctuates with changes in patella water content. Eur J Sport Sci. 2014;14(6):628–34. https://doi.org/10.1080/17461391.2013.862872.
14. Verbruggen SW, Vaughan TJ, McNamara LM. Fluid flow in the osteocyte mechanical environment: a fluid-structure interaction

approach. Biomech Model Mechanobiol. 2014;13(1):85–97. https://doi.org/10.1007/s10237-013-0487-y.

15. Cardoso L, Fritton SP, Gailani G, Benalla M, Cowin SC. Advances in assessment of bone porosity, permeability and interstitial fluid flow. J Biomech. 2013;46(2):253–65. https://doi.org/10.1016/j.jbiomech.2012.10.025.

16. Drescher W, Li H, Jensen SD, Ingerslev J, Hansen ES, Hauge EM, Bunger C. The effect of long-term methylprednisolone treatment on the femoral head in growing pigs. J Orthop Res. 2002;20(4):662–8. https://doi.org/10.1016/S0736-0266(01)00183-8.

17. Miyanishi K, Yamamoto T, Irisa T, Yamashita A, Jingushi S, Noguchi Y, Iwamoto Y. Bone marrow fat cell enlargement and a rise in intraosseous pressure in steroid-treated rabbits with osteonecrosis. Bone. 2002;30(1):185–90.

18. Simkin PA. Marrow fat may distribute the energy of impact loading throughout subchondral bone. Rheumatology (Oxford). 2017; https://doi.org/10.1093/rheumatology/kex274.

19. Taylor CC, Clarke NM. Amputation and intraosseous access in infants. Bmj. 2011;342:d2778. https://doi.org/10.1136/bmj.d2778.

20. Frascone RJ, Salzman JG, Bliss P, Adams A, Wewerka SS, Dries DJ. Intraosseous pressure tracings mimics arterial pressure tracings in timing and contour. Ann Emerg Med. 2013;62(4):S13–4.

21. De Lorenzo RA, Ward JA, Jordan BS, Hanson CE. Relationships of intraosseous and systemic pressure waveforms in a swine model. Acad Emerg Med. 2014;21(8):899–904. https://doi.org/10.1111/acem.12432.

4

The effects of graft shrinkage and extrusion on early clinical outcomes after meniscal allograft transplantation

Jae-Hwa Kim[1], Soohyun Lee[1], Doo Hoe Ha[2], Sang Min Lee[2], Kyunghun Jung[1] and Wonchul Choi[1]* ⓘ

Abstract

Background: Graft shrinkage or radial extrusion is a reported complication after meniscus allograft transplantation (MAT). Whether shrinkage or extrusion progress after surgery and whether they are associated with the clinical outcome of MAT remain debatable. In this study, graft shrinkage and extrusion were measured in the coronal and sagittal planes using serial postoperative magnetic resonance imaging (MRI). The purpose of this study was to evaluate if graft shrinkage or extrusion is correlated to the clinical outcome of MAT.

Methods: MRIs acquired at 3 and 12 months postoperatively in 30 patients (21 men and 9 women) who underwent MAT (6 medial and 24 lateral menisci) from 2010 to 2016 were analyzed. Two orthopedic surgeons and two musculoskeletal specialized radiologists each performed the MRI measurements. Allograft shrinkage was measured by the width and thickness of the graft at the coronal and sagittal planes. To determine the graft extrusion, distances between the proximal tibia cartilage margin and the extruded graft margin were measured in both coronal (either lateral or medial) and sagittal (both anterior and posterior) plane and relative percentage of extrusion (RPE) were calculated. Subjective International Knee Documentation Committee (IKDC) scores at 12 months were evaluated as a clinical outcome measurement, and correlations between shrinkage or extrusion of allograft and IKDC score were analyzed.

Results: In the coronal plane, radial RPE averaged 43.6% at postoperative 3 months, but there was no significant progression of extrusion at 12 months (average 42.0%) ($P = 0.728$). In the sagittal plane, there were no significant progressions of anterior and posterior RPE ($P = 0.487$ and 0.166, respectively) between postoperative 3 and 12 months. Shrinkage was calculated by multiplying the width and height of the three sections and summing these values. There was no significant progression of shrinkage between postoperative 3 and 12 months ($P = 0.150$). RPE in the radial ($R = 0.147$, $P = 0.525$), anterior ($R = 0.249$, $P = 0.264$), and posterior ($R = 0.230$, $P = 0.315$) directions and shrinkage ($R = 0.176$, $P = 0.435$) were not correlated to IKDC score at postoperative 12 months.

Conclusions: In the coronal and sagittal planes, extrusion and shrinkage did not progress from 3 months to 1 year. Extrusion and shrinkage had no correlation with early clinical outcomes. This finding suggests that graft extrusion or shrinkage may be not a great concern especially in early postoperative period of MAT, and multiple, serial MRI may be not necessary.

Keywords: Meniscus allograft transplantation, Extrusion, Shrinkage

* Correspondence: wcosdoc@gmail.com
[1]Department of Orthopaedic Surgery, CHA Bundang Medical Center, CHA University, 351 Yatap-dong, Bundang-gu, Seongnam-si, Gyeonggi-do, Republic of Korea
Full list of author information is available at the end of the article

Background

The meniscectomized knee is associated with early onset of knee osteoarthritis due to a decrease in tibiofemoral contact area and an increase in joint contact pressures, especially among people who are physically active [1–4]. When treating meniscus injury patients, efforts are made to preserve the meniscus by meniscal repair or leave the meniscus as much as possible to prevent degenerative arthritis. However, not all meniscal tears can be repaired or saved, and total meniscectomy is often unavoidable. To address the problems of meniscectomized patients, there are ongoing efforts to develop techniques for meniscus regeneration or meniscus scaffold using tissue engineering strategies [5–7]. However, most of them are preclinical studies and evidences are limited to be a standard treatment option. On the other hand, meniscal allograft transplantation (MAT) has become an alternative treatment option in relatively young and active, but symptomatic, meniscectomized patients. Although evidence of cartilage protection after MAT and long-term studies are still insufficient, studies on MAT have shown pain reduction and functional improvement [8–10].

One of the known problems of MAT is extrusion or shrinkage of allograft. Several studies have reported that extrusion and shrinkage occur at various degrees after MAT by arthroscopic findings or analyses of serial magnetic resonance imaging (MRI) data after surgery [9, 11, 12]. In addition, extrusion and shrinkage of the allograft after MAT may be a biomechanical disadvantage of the knee joint due to ineffective positioning of the allograft [13]. Therefore, adequate anatomic restoration and accurate sizing of the allograft are important for the transplant to function appropriately [14–17]. Whether extrusion or shrinkage progresses with time after surgery and whether they are associated with clinical outcome of MAT remain unclear. Moreover, graft extrusion has been evaluated mainly from the coronal plane, but rarely in the sagittal plane.

The purpose of this article is to evaluate whether extrusion or shrinkage of meniscal allograft progresses during short-term follow-up and to find out if the change of graft position or volume affects the clinical outcome. It was hypothesized that extrusion and shrinkage of the graft do not progress or affect the clinical outcome during short-term follow-up period.

Methods

Clinical and radiographic data of consecutive 50 patients who underwent MAT between 2010 and 2016 were prospectively collected. This study protocol was approved by our institutional review board, and informed consent was acquired from each patient. The indications for MAT were age $18 \leq$ years ≤ 50, history of prior subtotal or total meniscectomy, persistent localized pain that did not resolve even after conservative treatment, well-aligned mechanical axis of lower extremity, correctable ligamentous stability, relatively healthy cartilage status (Outerbridge grade II or less), and preserved joint space (> 2 mm) on a 45° of flexion weight-bearing posteroanterior radiograph. Contraindications for MAT were complete disappearance of the joint space or more than 5° of mechanical axis deviation or uncorrected joint instability.

MRI scans acquired using a SIGNA™ HDxt 3T apparatus (GE Healthcare, Waukesha, WI, USA) were performed at 3 and 12 months postoperatively. The acceptable time limit for MRI at each time point was within 1 month. Patients were excluded if the time was exceeded. Among the 50 patients, 16 patients were excluded because they did not receive MRI according to the schedule. Also, one patient who underwent anterior cruciate ligament reconstruction at the same time as the MAT and three patients who underwent anterior cruciate ligament reconstruction before the MAT operation were excluded. Finally, 30 patients were included in the study.

The 30 patients consisted of 21 males and 9 females with an average age of 35 years (range, 18 to 50). The mean time interval between meniscectomy and MAT was 22 months (range, 6 to 74). Among them, 6 received medial and 24 received lateral meniscal transplantation (Table 1).

Preoperative planning

Plain radiographs were used to measure meniscal dimensions before surgery using the Pollard method [18]. In order to minimize the magnification error, a 100-mm radiopaque rod was attached to the lateral epicondyle of the femur for anterior-posterior radiograph and perpendicularly to the center of the patella for lateral images. Fresh-frozen allograft of size within 10% of the measured value was prepared.

Surgical technique

All MAT procedures were performed by a single surgeon. Before the operation, the allografts were thawed in normal saline solution at room temperature. Medial menisci were transplanted using the double bone plug

Table 1 Demographics of patients

	Patients ($n = 30$)
Age (years)	35 (18–54)
Gender (male:female)	21:9
Body mass index (kg/m^2)	25.5 ± 1.7
Height (cm)	167.7 ± 5.8
Weight (kg)	71.8 ± 7.1
Lateral:medial MAT	24: 6
Time from meniscectomy (months)	15.8 ± 19.3

technique, and lateral menisci were transplanted using the keyhole technique [19, 20]. Diagnostic arthroscopy was first performed to check the states of meniscus, ligaments, and cartilage. The remaining meniscus was removed to within 1–2 mm of the peripheral rim, and a bleeding bed was made using a shaver. For medial meniscus, tibial tunnels were reamed over the guidewires positioned in the anatomic anterior and posterior horn attachments. Each bone plug was anchored with a non-absorbable suture in advance. Three vertical mattress sutures were placed in the posterior horn, and two vertical mattress sutures were placed in the anterior horn at 5 mm intervals using inside-out repair technique. For the lateral meniscus, a keyhole slot parallel to the posterior tibial slope was made just under the lateral tibial spine. After the graft was introduced into the joint through the anterior mini-arthrotomy site, inside-out meniscal suture fixation was performed at 5 mm intervals.

Postoperative care

Immediately after surgery, patients were encouraged to perform quadriceps set and calf pumping as much as possible and straight leg raising exercise was begun 1 day after surgery. Two days after the operation, patients started passive knee range-of-motion exercise using continuous passive motion machine with hinged knee brace on. The goals were to achieve full extension within 1 week, 90° of flexion within 3 weeks, and 120° of flexion at 6 to 8 weeks. Toe-touch weight bearing with crutch was allowed up to 3 weeks and gradually increased to 50% of body weight until 6 weeks. Patients were then allowed full weight-bearing without crutches and hinged knee braces when one leg squatting was possible. Engaging in heavy exercise and competitive sports was prohibited until postoperative 1 year.

Evaluation criteria

All the radiographic measurements were done by two orthopedic surgeons and two musculoskeletal radiology specialists. One of the observers (SL) measured twice at 1-month interval to evaluate intra-observer reliability. Picture Archiving Communication System (Marosis, Infinity, Seoul, Republic of Korea) was used for the measurements. Anterior and posterior extrusions were measured in the mid-sagittal section, and the radial extrusion was measured in the mid-coronal section. The mid-coronal and mid-sagittal sections were pre-determined under the agreement of observers and each observer measured from the same section. The extrusion was defined as the distance between the outer edge of the articular cartilage of the tibial plateau and the outer edge of the meniscus. The relative percentage of extrusion (RPE) of anterior (RPEa), posterior (RPEp), and radial (RPEr) directions were calculated to evaluate the degree of extrusion (Fig. 1). The

intruded meniscus was described as negative value. Shrinkage was evaluated by measuring the height and width of the meniscus in each sections and multiplying them to estimate the volume. Subjective International Knee Documentation Committee (IKDC) scores at preoperative and postoperative 1-year periods were recorded as clinical outcome measurements.

Data analyses

Statistical analyses were performed using SPSS 16.0 for Windows (SPSS, IBM, Chicago, Illinois, USA), with $P < 0.05$ considered statistically significant. The inter- and intra-observer reliabilities of measurements were analyzed by intra-class correlation coefficient (ICC). Change of anterior, posterior, radial RPE and shrinkage between 3 and 12 months after MAT were analyzed by paired t test. Also, the difference between preoperative and postoperative 1 year subjective IKDC scores was compared using paired t test. The differences of RPE and shrinkage between the medial and lateral menisci were analyzed by Mann-Whitney U test. Correlations between demographics or radiographic measurements and IKDC score were analyzed using Pearson's correlation analysis.

Results

Inter- and intra-observer reliabilities of extrusion and shrinkage were excellent (Table 2). There were no significant progressions of anterior ($P = 0.487$) and posterior RPE ($P = 0.166$) between postoperative 3 and 12 months. Also, in the coronal plane, there was no significant progression of radial RPE between postoperative 3 and 12 months ($P = 0.728$). Shrinkage was calculated by multiplying the width and height of the three sections and adding them together, and there was no significant progression of shrinkage between postoperative 3 and 12 months ($P = 0.150$) (Table 3).

Preoperative subjective IKDC score (average 37.7 ± 12.4 points, range 18 to 50 points) significantly improved after 1 year (average 69.0 ± 11.9 points, range 50 to 92 points) ($P < 0.001$).

The difference in RPE changes and shrinkage between 6 medial and 24 lateral MATs were compared. There was no statistical difference in progression of anterior ($P = 0.823$), posterior ($P = 0.218$), and radial ($P = 0.576$) extrusion between the medial and lateral directions. Shrinkage was also statistically insignificant ($P = 0.145$) (Fig. 2).

RPE in radial ($R = 0.147$, $P = 0.525$), anterior ($R = 0.249$, $P = 0.264$), and posterior ($R = 0.230$, $P = 0.315$) directions and shrinkage ($R = 0.176$, $P = 0.435$) were not correlated to IKDC scores at postoperative 12 months. Possible confounding factors that can influence the clinical outcome including age, sex, body mass index, laterality of

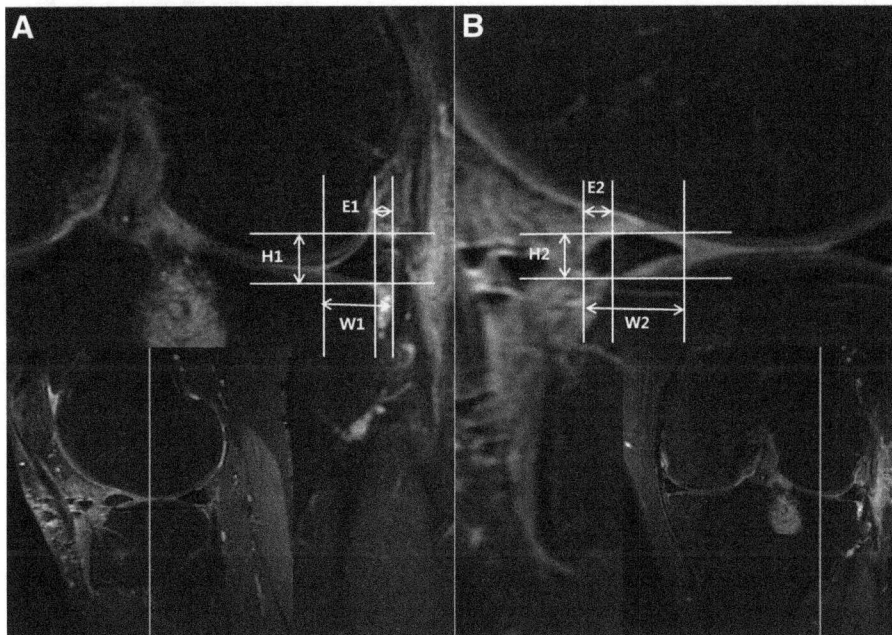

Fig. 1 Measurements of graft extrusion or intrusion in the mid-sagittal plane and mid-coronal plane. From the mid-coronal knee MRI section (**a**), the radial extrusion (E1) was measured as the distance between the outer edge of the articular cartilage of the tibial plateau and the outer edge of the allograft. Also, the height (H1) and the width (W1) of the graft were measured. The radial relative percentage of extrusion (RPEr) was defined as the percentage of the width of extrusion relative to the width of the entire allograft (E1/W1 × 100). Similarly, the anterior relative percentage of extrusion (RPEa) was calculated after measuring the anterior extrusion (E2) and graft width (W2) from the mid-sagittal section (**b**). Graft height in sagittal section (H2) was also measured. Extrusion was expressed as a positive value and intrusion as a negative value

MAT (medial or lateral), or time from previous meniscectomy did not show any significant correlation.

Discussion

In this study, the graft extrusion and shrinkage did not progress between 3 months and 1 year period after MAT in both coronal and sagittal planes. In addition, shrinkage and extrusion of the graft were not related to early clinical outcomes of MAT.

Table 2 Intra-class correlation coefficients (ICC) for measurement of relative percentage of extrusion (RPE) and shrinkage

	Months	Inter-observer ICC	Intra-observer ICC
RPEa[a]	3	0.897 (0.806–0.946)	0.928 (0.897–0.952)
	12	0.871 (0.758–0.936)	0.947 (0.934–0.959)
RPEp[b]	3	0.900 (0.812–0.950)	0.917 (0.895–0.924)
	12	0.863 (0.740–0.933)	0.888 (0.796–0.902)
RPEr[c]	3	0.954 (0.914–0.977)	0.966 (0.953–0.978)
	12	0.921 (0.851–0.962)	0.918 (0.897–0.926)
Shrinkage	3	0.935 (0.878–0.968)	0.976 (0.966–0.990)
	12	0.914 (0.839–0.957)	0.944 (0.929–0.955)

Values are expressed as ICC and 95% CI in parentheses
[a]*RPEa* relative percentage of extrusion at anterior meniscus
[b]*RPEp* relative percentage of extrusion at posterior meniscus
[c]*RPEr* relative percentage of extrusion at radial meniscus

Graft shrinkage is a potential complication of MAT and understood as a change in the graft property during the remodeling process, and several studies have shown that meniscal allografts lose normal collagen architecture during early remodeling periods, and a loss of microarchitecture may cause morphologic alterations [13, 21, 22]. Although it has been regarded as a less frequent problem with the advent of the current (deep-frozen) preservation technique, few studies reported the shrinkage still occurs with deep-frozen grafts [21]. Moreover, studies on the effect of graft shrinkage on the clinical outcome after MAT are surprisingly rare, and it is still unclear whether the graft shrinkage is a progressive phenomenon. A laboratory study by Dienst et al. [14] showed that undersized graft causes increased forces across the articular cartilage and allograft itself. A serial

Table 3 Progression of relative percentage of extrusion (RPE) and shrinkage

	3 months	12 months	P
RPEa	40.3 ± 4.6	41.7 ± 5.4	0.487
RPEp	− 27.7 ± 6.1	− 21.2 ± 5.6	0.166
RPEr	43.6 ± 3.1	42.0 ± 3.7	0.728
Shrinkage	172.0 ± 8.2	180.6 ± 11.5	0.150

Values are expressed as mean ± SD unless otherwise indicated

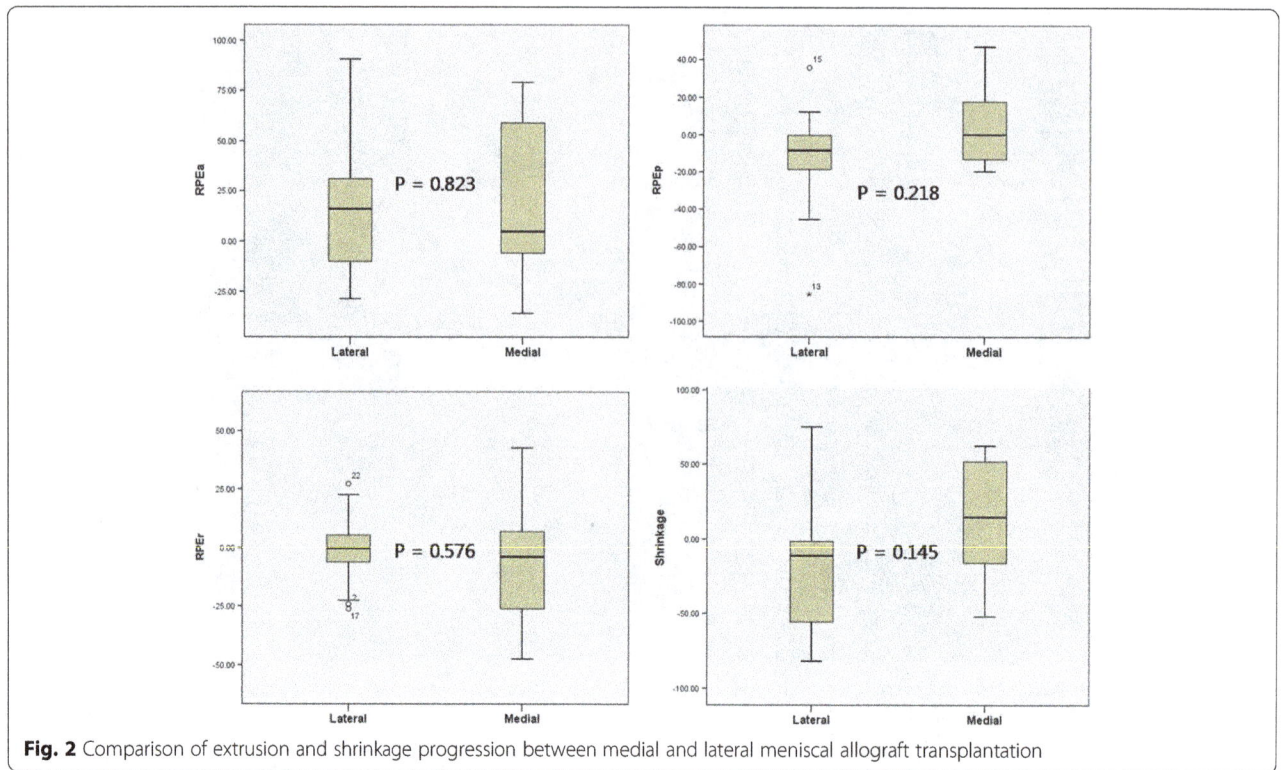

Fig. 2 Comparison of extrusion and shrinkage progression between medial and lateral meniscal allograft transplantation

MRI study by Lee et al. [23] reported that although 65% of cases showed graft shrinkage, it occurred during the first 3 months but stabilized thereafter. Another serial MRI study by Carter and Economopoulos [24] reported that graft shrinkage was observed until 6 months after MAT. In our study, there was no significant progression of shrinkage after 3 months and shrinkage showed no effect on the clinical outcome after 1 year of surgery. This finding suggests that shrinkage may be an initial or early phenomenon after surgery caused by micro-architectural remodeling, but does not progress after the remodeling ends.

The extrusion of the graft is regarded as another complication after MAT, and relatively more studies have investigated this issue compared to the shrinkage. Several studies have investigated the change of graft extrusion after MAT using serial MRI. Lee et al. [25] found that the graft extrusion occurred in early (< 6 weeks) after MAT, while it did not progress until postoperative 1 year. Recently, a mid-term follow-up study reported that early (< 6 weeks) graft extrusion did not progress until 3- to 5-year MRI follow-up [26]. In addition, Ha et al. [27] reported no significant difference in graft extrusion between 1 and 4 years after MAT. It is noteworthy that the graft extrusion was evaluated from both coronal and sagittal MRI images. Most of the studies focused on the graft extrusion in radial direction observed on coronal plane, while only few studies from the same study group [26, 28] evaluated the graft extrusion in anterior or posterior direction. In our study, the graft extrusion in both

coronal and sagittal directions did not progress between 3 months and 1 year post-MAT. Based on this finding, it is supposed that the graft "extrusion" may be not a progressive problem, but rather may be a problem that already existed immediately after surgery due to assumed reasons including graft size mismatch or inadequate graft position. There were studies on efforts to prevent graft extrusion by reducing the graft size [29] or using different approach for graft placement [30–32]. In this respect, the authors recently modified medial MAT technique as tensioning the anterior horn of the graft using suture anchor after bone fixation (unpublished data).

Association between the extrusion of native meniscus and progression of symptomatic knee osteoarthritis has been reported [33–35]. However, many studies on the extrusion after MAT reported that the extent of extrusion did not correlate with the clinical outcomes, although they have confirmed the occurrence of extrusion [26, 28, 36, 37]. Our study result is in accordance with previous MAT studies that even though the graft extrusion was observed, there was no significant correlation between the extrusion and the clinical outcome.

The difference in progression of extrusion and shrinkage between the medial and lateral MAT cases was also compared, and no significant difference was found out. Although there were reports showing more graft extrusion after medial MAT compared to lateral MAT [28, 38], it has not been studied if there are any differences in the progression of extrusion or shrinkage between lateral and medial MATs. However, this issue was not one of our study purposes and our finding cannot be generalized since it may be underpowered with considerably different number of lateral and medial MAT cases.

This study has some limitations. First, the follow-up period was relatively short to evaluate the long-term clinical outcomes of the procedure. Second, the possible early change of the graft within weeks after MAT could not be evaluated, since MRI was first taken 3 months after the surgery. It would be beneficial as reference if immediate postoperative MRI was available. However, it was concerned that early postoperative changes including increased joint effusion, soft tissue swelling may obscure accurate MRI evaluation. In addition, it may be difficult for patient to maintain an adequate position to take MRI at immediate postoperative period. Third, the accuracy of determining the meniscal margin on sagittal images is known to be lower than the measurement from coronal images [39]. Four observers measured all parameters in same, predetermined sections to compensate this possible error, and inter- and intra-observer reliabilities were excellent in our study.

Conclusion

In the coronal and sagittal planes, extrusion and shrinkage did not progress from 3 months to 1 year after meniscal allograft transplantation. This finding suggests that graft extrusion or shrinkage is not progressive, but rather is a static phenomenon. Not the characteristics of the graft itself, but the techniques for graft sizing, fixation, and positioning may be determinants of the early graft change after MAT. In addition, shrinkage and extrusion of the graft did not correlate with early clinical outcomes of MAT. Therefore, multiple, serial MRI may be not necessary in early period after MAT, even though the graft extrusion or shrinkage occurs. However, future studies will be required to determine the effects of the graft extrusion or shrinkage on long-term clinical outcome of MAT.

Abbreviations

ICC: Intra-class correlation coefficient; IKDC: International Knee Documentation Committee; MAT: Meniscus allograft transplantation; MRI: Magnetic resonance imaging; RPE: Relative percentage of extrusion; RPEa: Relative percentage of extrusion of anterior direction; RPEp: Relative percentage of extrusion of posterior direction; RPEr: Relative percentage of extrusion of radial direction

Authors' contributions

J-HK and WC contributed to the study design, data analysis, and manuscript preparation. SL contributed to the data collection and manuscript preparation. DHH and SML contributed to the data collection and data analysis. KJ contributed to the data collection. All authors read and approved the final manuscript.

Competing interests

This manuscript has not been published elsewhere in part or in entirety and is not under consideration by another journal. The authors declare that they have no competing of interests.

Author details

[1]Department of Orthopaedic Surgery, CHA Bundang Medical Center, CHA University, 351 Yatap-dong, Bundang-gu, Seongnam-si, Gyeonggi-do, Republic of Korea. [2]Department of Radiology, CHA Bundang Medical Center, CHA University, 351 Yatap-dong, Bundang-gu, Seongnam-si, Gyeonggi-do, Republic of Korea.

References

1. Longo UG, Ciuffreda M, Candela V, Rizzello G, D'Andrea V, Mannering N, Berton A, Salvatore G, Denaro V. Knee osteoarthritis after arthroscopic partial meniscectomy: prevalence and progression of radiographic changes after 5 to 12 years compared with contralateral knee. J Knee Surg. 2018; [Epub ahead of print]
2. Stein T, Mehling AP, Welsch F, von Eisenhart-Rothe R, Jager A. Long-term outcome after arthroscopic meniscal repair versus arthroscopic partial meniscectomy for traumatic meniscal tears. Am J Sports Med. 2010;38: 1542–8.
3. Verdonk R, Madry H, Shabshin N, Dirisamer F, Peretti GM, Pujol N, Spalding T, Verdonk P, Seil R, Condello V, et al. The role of meniscal tissue in joint protection in early osteoarthritis. Knee Surg Sports Traumatol Arthrosc. 2016; 24:1763–74.
4. Xu C, Zhao J. A meta-analysis comparing meniscal repair with meniscectomy in the treatment of meniscal tears: the more meniscus, the better outcome? Knee Surg Sports Traumatol Arthrosc. 2015;23:164–70.
5. Pillai MM, Gopinathan J, Selvakumar R, Bhattacharyya A. Human knee meniscus regeneration strategies: a review on recent advances. Curr Osteoporos Rep. 2018;16:224–35.
6. Bilgen B, Jayasuriya CT, Owens BD. Current concepts in meniscus tissue engineering and repair. Adv Healthc Mater. 2018;7:e1701407.
7. Dangelmajer S, Familiari F, Simonetta R, Kaymakoglu M, Huri G. Meniscal transplants and scaffolds: a systematic review of the literature. Knee Surg Relat Res. 2017;29:3–10.
8. Rosso F, Bisicchia S, Bonasia DE, Amendola A. Meniscal allograft transplantation: a systematic review. Am J Sports Med. 2015;43:998–1007.
9. Samitier G, Alentorn-Geli E, Taylor DC, Rill B, Lock T, Moutzouros V, Kolowich P. Meniscal allograft transplantation. Part 2: systematic review of transplant timing, outcomes, return to competition, associated procedures, and prevention of osteoarthritis. Knee Surg Sports Traumatol Arthrosc. 2015;23: 323–33.
10. Rongen JJ, Hannink G, van Tienen TG, van Luijk J, Hooijmans CR. The protective effect of meniscus allograft transplantation on articular cartilage: a systematic review of animal studies. Osteoarthr Cartil. 2015;23:1242–53.
11. Verdonk PC, Verstraete KL, Almqvist KF, De Cuyper K, Veys EM, Verbruggen G, Verdonk R. Meniscal allograft transplantation: long-term clinical results with radiological and magnetic resonance imaging correlations. Knee Surg Sports Traumatol Arthrosc. 2006;14:694–706.
12. Ahn JH, Kang HW, Yang TY, Lee JY. Multivariate analysis of risk factors of graft extrusion after lateral meniscus allograft transplantation. Arthroscopy. 2016;32:1337–45.
13. Samitier G, Alentorn-Geli E, Taylor DC, Rill B, Lock T, Moutzouros V, Kolowich P. Meniscal allograft transplantation. Part 1: systematic review of graft biology, graft shrinkage, graft extrusion, graft sizing, and graft fixation. Knee Surg Sports Traumatol Arthrosc. 2015;23:310–22.
14. Dienst M, Greis PE, Ellis BJ, Bachus KN, Burks RT. Effect of lateral meniscal allograft sizing on contact mechanics of the lateral tibial plateau: an experimental study in human cadaveric knee joints. Am J Sports Med. 2007;35:34–42.
15. Lee DH, Kim JM, Lee BS, Kim KA, Bin SI. Greater axial trough obliquity increases the risk of graft extrusion in lateral meniscus allograft transplantation. Am J Sports Med. 2012;40:1597–605.
16. Sekaran SV, Hull ML, Howell SM. Nonanatomic location of the posterior horn of a medial meniscal autograft implanted in a cadaveric knee adversely affects the pressure distribution on the tibial plateau. Am J Sports Med. 2002;30:74–82.

17. von Lewinski G, Kohn D, Wirth CJ, Lazovic D. The influence of nonanatomical insertion and incongruence of meniscal transplants on the articular cartilage in an ovine model. Am J Sports Med. 2008;36:841–50.

18. Pollard ME, Kang Q, Berg EE. Radiographic sizing for meniscal transplantation. Arthroscopy. 1995;11:684–7.

19. Lee DW, Park JH, Chung KS, Ha JK, Kim JG. Arthroscopic lateral meniscal allograft transplantation with the key-hole technique. Arthrosc Tech. 2017;6:e1815–20.

20. Lee DW, Park JH, Chung KS, Ha JK, Kim JG. Arthroscopic medial meniscal allograft transplantation with modified bone plug technique. Arthrosc Tech. 2017;6:e1437–42.

21. Mickiewicz P, Binkowski M, Bursig H, Wrobel Z. Preservation and sterilization methods of the meniscal allografts: literature review. Cell Tissue Bank. 2014;15:307–17.

22. Hommen JP, Applegate GR, Del Pizzo W. Meniscus allograft transplantation: ten-year results of cryopreserved allografts. Arthroscopy. 2007;23:388–93.

23. Lee BS, Chung JW, Kim JM, Cho WJ, Kim KA, Bin SI. Morphologic changes in fresh-frozen meniscus allografts over 1 year: a prospective magnetic resonance imaging study on the width and thickness of transplants. Am J Sports Med. 2012;40:1384–91.

24. Carter T, Economopoulos KJ. Meniscal allograft shrinkage-MRI evaluation. J Knee Surg. 2013;26:167–71.

25. Lee SH, Kim TH, Lee SH, Kim CW, Kim JM, Bin SI. Evaluation of meniscus allograft transplantation with serial magnetic resonance imaging during the first postoperative year: focus on graft extrusion. Arthroscopy. 2008;24:1115–21.

26. Kim NK, Bin SI, Kim JM, Lee CR, Kim JH. Meniscal extrusion does not progress during the midterm follow-up period after lateral meniscal transplantation. Am J Sports Med. 2017;45:900–8.

27. Ha JK, Jang HW, Jung JE, Cho SI, Kim JG. Clinical and radiologic outcomes after meniscus allograft transplantation at 1-year and 4-year follow-up. Arthroscopy. 2014;30:1424–9.

28. Lee DH, Lee CR, Jeon JH, Kim KA, Bin SI. Graft extrusion in both the coronal and sagittal planes is greater after medial compared with lateral meniscus allograft transplantation but is unrelated to early clinical outcomes. Am J Sports Med. 2015;43:213–9.

29. Jang SH, Kim JG, Ha JG, Shim JC. Reducing the size of the meniscal allograft decreases the percentage of extrusion after meniscal allograft transplantation. Arthroscopy. 2011;27:914–22.

30. Kim YS, Kang KT, Son J, Kwon OR, Choi YJ, Jo SB, Choi YW, Koh YG. Graft extrusion related to the position of allograft in lateral meniscal allograft transplantation: biomechanical comparison between parapatellar and transpatellar approaches using finite element analysis. Arthroscopy. 2015;31:2380–2391.e2382.

31. Yoon JR, Kim TS, Lee YM, Jang HW, Kim YC, Yang JH. Transpatellar approach in lateral meniscal allograft transplantation using the keyhole method: can we prevent graft extrusion? Knee Surg Sports Traumatol Arthrosc. 2011;19:214–7.

32. Ren S, Zhang X, You T, Jiang X, Jin D, Zhang W. Clinical and radiologic outcomes after a modified bone plug technique with anatomical meniscal root reinsertion for meniscal allograft transplantation and a minimum 18-month follow-up. J Orthop Surg Res. 2018;13:97.

33. Berthiaume MJ, Raynauld JP, Martel-Pelletier J, Labonte F, Beaudoin G, Bloch DA, Choquette D, Haraoui B, Altman RD, Hochberg M, et al. Meniscal tear and extrusion are strongly associated with progression of symptomatic knee osteoarthritis as assessed by quantitative magnetic resonance imaging. Ann Rheum Dis. 2005;64:556–63.

34. Furumatsu T, Kodama Y, Kamatsuki Y, Hino T, Okazaki Y, Ozaki T. Meniscal extrusion progresses shortly after the medial meniscus posterior root tear. Knee Surg Relat Res. 2017;29:295–301.

35. Kaplan DJ, Alaia EF, Dold AP, Meislin RJ, Strauss EJ, Jazrawi LM, Alaia MJ. Increased extrusion and ICRS grades at 2-year follow-up following transtibial medial meniscal root repair evaluated by MRI. Knee Surg Sports Traumatol Arthrosc. 2017;

36. Ha JK, Shim JC, Kim DW, Lee YS, Ra HJ, Kim JG. Relationship between meniscal extrusion and various clinical findings after meniscus allograft transplantation. Am J Sports Med. 2010;38:2448–55.

37. Lee BS, Chung JW, Kim JM, Kim KA, Bin SI. Width is a more important predictor in graft extrusion than length using plain radiographic sizing in lateral meniscal transplantation. Knee Surg Sports Traumatol Arthrosc. 2012;20:179–86.

38. Yoon KH, Lee SH, Park SY, Kim HJ, Chung KY. Meniscus allograft transplantation: a comparison of medial and lateral procedures. Am J Sports Med. 2014;42:200–7.

39. Hunter DJ, Zhang YQ, Niu JB, Tu X, Amin S, Clancy M, Guermazi A, Grigorian M, Gale D, Felson DT. The association of meniscal pathologic changes with cartilage loss in symptomatic knee osteoarthritis. Arthritis Rheum. 2006;54:795–801.

5

Clinical experiences with a PEEK-based dynamic instrumentation device in lumbar spinal surgery: 2 years and no more

Stavros Oikonomidis[1,2]* , Ghazi Ashqar[1], Thomas Kaulhausen[1], Christian Herren[3], Jan Siewe[2] and Rolf Sobottke[1,2]

Abstract

Background: Dynamic spine implants were developed to prevent adjacent segment degeneration (ASD) and adjacent segment disease (ASDi). Purpose of this study was to investigate the clinical and radiological outcomes of "topping off" devices following lumbar spinal fusion procedure using a PEEK-based dynamic rod system. Moreover, this study focused on the hypothesis that "topping off" devices can prevent ASD.

Methods: This prospective nonrandomized study included patients with indication for single-level lumbar fusion and radiological signs of ASD without instability. The exclusion criteria were previous lumbar spine surgery and no sign of disc degeneration in the adjacent segment according to magnetic resonance imaging. All patients were treated with single-level lumbar interbody fusion and dynamic stabilization of the cranial adjacent segment. Patients underwent a clinical examination and radiographs preoperatively and at 1 and 2 years after surgery. Analyses were performed on clinical data collected with the German Spine Registry using the core outcome measure index (COMI) and visual analogue scale (VAS) scores for back and leg pain.

Results: A total of 22 patients (6 male and 16 female) with an average age of 57.6 years were included in the study; 20 patients completed the follow-up (FU). The average COMI score was 9.0 preoperatively, 4.2 at the 1-year FU, and 4.7 at the 2-year FU. The average preoperative VAS scores for back and leg pain were 7.7 and 7.1, respectively. At the 1-year FU, the scores were 4.25 for back pain and 2.2 for leg pain, and at the 2-year FU, the scores were 4.7 for back pain and 2.3 for leg pain. At FU, failure of the dynamic topping off implant material was verified in four cases, and ASD of the segment cranial to the topping off was confirmed in three cases.

Conclusions: These results demonstrate significant improvements in clinical outcomes and pain reduction after lumbar spinal fusion with topping off at 2 years after surgery. However, the implant failed due to the high rate of implant failure and the development of ASD in the segment cranial to the dynamic stabilized segment.

Keywords: Topping off, Hybrid posterior fixation, Adjacent segment disease, Material failure, Hybrid lumbar instrumentation

Background

Lumbar and lumbosacral spinal fusion is a state of the art in lumbar spinal surgery for treating several degenerative disorders caused by changes in the lumbar spine (i.e., spinal disc herniation, lumbar spinal stenosis, and spondylolisthesis) [1, 2]. The well-known posterior rigid pedicle screw fixation system offers initial stability, a high fusion rate, and good recovery of normal sagittal parameters in the lumbar spine. Stability is restored with surgical posterior fusion using pedicle screw and rod-based systems combined with an intervertebral cage following decompression (e.g., TLIF/PLIF technique). Furthermore, this procedure has been well documented in terms of its good and excellent long-term outcomes [3].

More recent research revealed that the stiffness caused by the posterior fusion operation often results in a redistribution of stress at the neighboring level, which leads

* Correspondence: stavros.oikonomidis@uk-koeln.de
[1]Department of Orthopaedics and Trauma Surgery, Rhein-Maas Klinikum GmbH, Mauerfeldchen 25, 52146 Wuerselen, Germany
[2]Department of Orthopaedics and Trauma Surgery, University Hospital Cologne, Joseph-Stelzmann-Str. 24, 50931 Cologne, Germany
Full list of author information is available at the end of the article

to extended mobility and increased intradiscal pressure in the adjacent segments. These biomechanical changes can lead to new complications, such as adjacent segment degeneration (ASD) accompanied by facet hypertrophy, facet arthritis, and a higher risk of adjacent segment disease (ASDi) [4–7].

The general incidence of ASD varies from 5.2 to 18.5% at 2–5 years after lumbar fusion; however, Moreau et al. reported a rate > 20% for degenerative spondylolisthesis at 2 years after lumbar fusion [8, 9]. Risk factors for the manifestation of ASD are being > 60 years old, having an increased body mass index, preexisting disc and facet joint degeneration, the length of the fusion, and decreased postoperative lumbar lordosis in the sagittal alignment [10]. In the literature, the impact of ASD on clinical outcome is unclear [10]; however, ASDi may result in new clinical symptoms that are detectable adjacent to the previously fused segment.

Dynamic spine implants were developed to prevent ASD. These devices provide dynamic stabilization of the instrumented segment and, in focus to the adjacent segment, reduce load sharing and prevent hypermobility of the adjacent segment. Biomechanical studies reported a reduced range of motion (ROM) and load sharing of the adjacent segment when dynamic stabilization devices were used [11]. Khoueir et al. classified posterior dynamic stabilization devices into three groups: (1) interspinous spacer devices, (2) pedicle screw/rod-based devices, and (3) total facet replacement systems [12]. Many dynamic spine implants have been introduced in recent years, including purely dynamic or hybrid (semi-rigid) implants; however, it is uncertain whether patients benefit from these implants. Topping off systems provide dynamic stabilization for the segment cranially adjacent to the fusion.

The aim of this study was to assess the patient-dependent clinical and radiological outcomes within a 2-year follow-up (FU) period following lumbar interbody fusion using a dynamic instrumentation device to stabilize the segment superior to the rigid instrumented segment (topping off). Furthermore, this study also focused on the development of ASD in the segment superior to the dynamic instrumented level.

Methods
Study design
An observational prospective nonrandomized cohort study of patients with monosegmental degenerative alteration or spondylolisthesis of the lumbar spine and an indication for lumbar fusion was conducted (Table 1). Further inclusion criteria were radiological signs of degeneration without instability in the cranially adjacent segment (Pfirrmann grade 2–4) [13]. Detailed inclusion and exclusion criteria are listed in Table 1 [14]. Diagnosis was based on

Table 1 Inclusion and exclusion criteria

Inclusion criteria	Exclusion criteria
• Indication for monosegmental lumbar spinal fusion with osteochondrosis (Modic grades I–III) or spondylolisthesis (Meyerding grades I–III) with instability • Radiological signs of degeneration without instability in the level cranially adjacent to the intended fusion • Definition of adjacent segment degeneration using MRI (Pfirrmann grades II–IV)	• No degeneration in the segment cranial to the segment intended for fusion • Previous lumbar surgery • Motor deficits • Scoliosis with a Cobb angle > 25° • Spondylolisthesis (Meyerding grade > III) • No prior history of metabolic bone disease • No previous osteoporotic fracture of the lumbar vertebrae

clinical and radiological examinations as well as magnetic resonance imaging (MRI). All patients underwent single-level lumbar interbody fusion using the transforaminal lumbar interbody fusion (TLIF) or posterior lumbar interbody fusion (PLIF) technique and additional dynamic instrumentation (topping off) of the segment superior to the rigid instrumented level according to segment pathology (Table 2). Three senior and "Master-certified" (German Spine Society) spinal surgeons performed the operations. Indications for lumbar spinal fusion were performed based on the radiological and clinical findings, and the Modic classification was used to characterize the grade of osteochondrosis [15].

The implant
The CD Horizon BalanC™ (Medtronic Co., Minneapolis, USA) is a dynamic posterior pedicle screw/rod-based stabilization device, with the dynamic part of the rod constructed of polyether ether ketone (PEEK) and silicone (Ø 6.0; lordotic bend). The fusion portion is entirely made of PEEK (Fig 1). The silicon and PEEK hinge is designed to reduce stress on the adjacent level by restricting extreme ROM. The pedicle screws are made of standard titanium and are comparable to the screws used in the rigidly stabilized level.

Data collection and outcomes
Patients underwent clinical examinations and radiographs preoperatively and at 1 and 2 years after surgery. Evaluation of the clinical data was based on the German Spine Registry using the Core Outcome Measure Index (COMI) score, the Operation 2011 form, and a visual analogue scale (VAS) for back and leg pain. Data regarding length of hospital stay, operation time, perioperative and postoperative complications, blood loss, and ASA classification were collected by the German Spine Registry. Patients filled out the questionnaires (COMI and VAS) preoperatively and at the 1- and 2-year FU examinations.

The radiological examination contained X-rays of the lumbar spine in anterior–posterior and lateral views taken

Table 2 Pathology of the index (fusion) and adjacent segment

Cases	Pathology of the index segment	Pathology of the adjacent segment (Pfirrmann classification)
1	Degenerative spondylolisthesis II° L4–5 and absolute LSS	L3–4: grade III
2	Erosive osteochondrosis L5–S1 Modic III° and foraminal stenosis L5 right	L4–5: grade II
3	Degenerative spondylolisthesis II° L4–5 and absolute LSS	L3–4: grade II
4	Isthmic spondylolisthesis I° L5–S1	L4–5: grade III
5	Erosive osteochondrosis L5–S1 Modic III° and absolute LSS L5–S1	L4–5: grade III
6	Degenerative spondylolisthesis II° L4–5 and erosive osteochondrosis L4–5 Modic III°	L3–4: grade III
7	Isthmic spondylolisthesis II° L5–S1	L4–5: grade III
8	Erosive osteochondrosis L5–S1 Modic III°	L4–5: grade III
9	Degenerative spondylolisthesis II° L4–5 with disc herniation	L3–4: grade II, LSS
10	Degenerative spondylolisthesis II° L4–5	L3–4: grade IV, LSS
11	Erosive osteochondrosis L4–5 Modic III° and absolute LSS	L3–4: grade III, LSS
12	Erosive osteochondrosis L4–5 Modic III° and absolute LSS	L3–4: grade IV
13	Degenerative spondylolisthesis II° L4–5 and absolute LSS	L3–4: grade III
14	Degenerative spondylolisthesis II° L4–5	L3–4: grade II, foraminal stenosis bilateral
15	Erosive osteochondrosis L4–5 Modic II° and absolute LSS	L3–4: grade II
16	Erosive osteochondrosis L5–S1 Modic III°	L4–5: grade II
17	Degenerative spondylolisthesis I° L5–S1 and absolute LSS	L4–5: grade III
18	Degenerative spondylolisthesis I° L5–S1	L4–5: grade IV, disc herniation
19	Degenerative spondylolisthesis II° L4–5 and absolute LSS	L3–4: grade III
20	Erosive osteochondrosis L5–S1 Modic III° and absolute LSS	L4–5: grade III
21	Erosive osteochondrosis L5–S1 Modic III° and absolute LSS	L4–5: grade II
22	Degenerative spondylolisthesis I° L4–5 and absolute LSS	L3–4: grade III, relative LSS

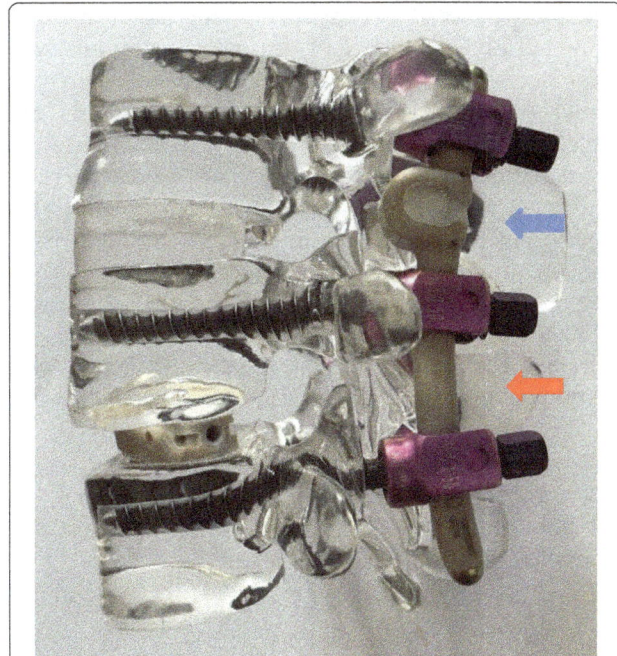

Fig. 1 CD Horizon BalanC™. The dynamic section is composed of PEEK and silicon (blue marker), while the fusion section is composed of PEEK (red marker)

preoperatively and at 1 and 2 years after surgery. All X-rays were performed in a standing position. Radiological signs of degeneration in the segment adjacent to the fusion (topping off segment) and the segment cranial to the topping off were recorded. Degeneration was categorized according to Weiner's classification [16], and a segment was classified as degenerated if it achieved a score of two or more.

Weiner's classification:

Radiographic scoring system for osteoarthritis of the lumbosacral spine:

Intervertebral disc:

0 = no disease. Defined by normal disc height, no spur formation, no eburnation, and no gas present.

1 = mild disease. Defined by < 25% disc-space narrowing, small spur formation, minimal eburnation, and no gas present.

2 = moderate disease. Defined by 25–75% disc-space narrowing, moderate spur formation, moderate eburnation, and no gas present.

3 = advanced disease. Defined by > 75% disc-space narrowing, large spur formation, marked eburnation, and gas present [16].

In addition, the pre- and postoperative sagittal parameters (e.g., the segmental endplate angle of the instrumentation and the topping off segment, lumbar lordosis, pelvic incidence, sacral slope, and pelvic tilt) were also compared.

Statistical analysis

SPSS (version 25, 76 Chicago, IL, USA) was used to evaluate the data. Descriptive and frequency analyses were used to describe the demographic data, clinical data, and outcomes. The COMI score and the radiological sagittal parameter were analyzed using

Student's t test for dependent samples, while the VAS scores for back and leg pain were analyzed using the Wilcoxon test. Line diagrams were used to depict the COMI and VAS scores as well as the radiological parameters, with whiskers indicating standard deviation. All reported P values have a two-tailed significance level of alpha = 0.05. No adjustment for multiple testing was performed.

Results

A total of 22 patients (16 female and 6 male) with symptomatic degenerative disease or spondylolisthesis of the lumbar spine met the inclusion criteria; 20 patients attended the FU examinations at 1 and 2 years after the procedure. The average age of the patients was 57.6 ± 11.5 (range 41–78) years at the time of surgery.

Clinical data
The average hospitalization time was 11.8 ± 6.5 (range 5–34) days. PLIF was performed in 18 cases, and TLIF was performed in four cases. Decompression by laminotomy and flavectomy was performed in the topping off (dynamic) segment in four cases. Clinical data are presented in Table 3.

Clinical outcomes
The average COMI and VAS scores preoperatively and at the 1- and 2-year FU are presented in Table 4. There was a significant reduction in the COMI score at the 1-year ($P < 0.001$) and 2-year ($P < 0.001$) FU compared to preoperatively. VAS scores for both back and leg pain significantly reduced at the 1- and 2-year FU (back pain: $P = 0.002$ at 1 year and $P = 0.003$ at 2 years vs. preoperatively; leg pain: $P = 0.001$ at 1 and 2 years vs. preoperatively). Figs. 2, 3,

Table 3 Clinical data

Case	Operation	Age	Sex	BMI (kg/m²)	ASA	Operation time (h)	Intraoperative blood loss (mL)
1	PLIF L4–5 with topping off L3–4	56	F	26–30	2	2–3	100–500
2	TLIF L5–S1 right with topping off L4–5 and foraminotomy L5 right	50	F	26–30	2	2–3	100–500
3	PLIF L4–5 with topping off L3–4	65	F	26–30	2	2–3	500–1000
4	PLIF L5–S1 with topping off L4–5	66	M	20–25	2	2–3	500–1000
5	TLIF L5–S1 left with topping off L4–5	48	F	31–35	2	2–3	500–1000
6	PLIF L4–5 with topping off L3–4	56	F	26–30	2	3–4	500–1000
7	PLIF L5–S1 with topping off L4–5	50	F	> 35	2	2–3	100–500
8	PLIF L5–S1 with topping off L4–5	50	M	20–25	2	2–3	100–500
9	PLIF L4–5 with topping off L3–4, flavectomy and laminotomy L3–4 bilateral	72	F	26–30	2	3–4	500–1000
10	TLIF L4–5 left with topping off L3–4, flavectomy and laminotomy L3–4 left	71	F	31–35	2	2–3	1000–2000
11	PLIF L4–5 with topping off L3–4	78	M	< 20	3	1–2	500–1000
12	PLIF L4–5 with topping off L3–4	43	F	> 35	2	2–3	100–500
13	PLIF L4–5 with topping off L3–4	58	M	26–30	2	3–4	500–1000
14	PLIF L4–5 with topping off L3–4, laminotomy and foraminotomy L3–4 bilateral	61	F	20–25	2	2–3	500–1000
15	PLIF L4–5 with topping off L3–4	43	M	< 20	1	2–3	100–500
16	PLIF L5/S1 with topping off L4–5	41	M	31–35	2	2–3	500–1000
17	PLIF L5–S1 with topping off L4–5, laminotomy and flavectomy L3–4 left	64	F	31–35	3	3–4	1000–2000
18	PLIF L5–S1 with topping off L4–5 and sequestrectomy L4–5 left	58	F	< 20	1	2–3	100–500
19	PLIF L4–5 with topping off L3–4	71	F	26–30	3	3–4	1000–2000
20	TLIF L5–S1 right with topping off L4–5	45	F	20–25	2	1–2	100–500
21	PLIF L5–S1 with topping off L4–5	45	F	20–25	2	2–3	1000–2000
22	PLIF L4–5 with topping off L3–4	76	F	> 35	3	3–4	500–1000

Table 4 Clinical outcomes: mean COMI score, mean VAS score for back pain, and mean VAS score for leg pain preoperatively and at the 1-year and 2-year FU

	Preoperatively	1-year FU	2-year FU
COMI score	9.0 ± 0.9 (range 6.7–10.0)	4.2 ± 2.5 (range 0–7.5)	4.7 ± 2.7 (range 0.2–8.3)
VAS back pain	7.7 ± 2.4 (range 0–10)	4.25 ± 2.4 (range 0–8)	4.7 ± 2.3 (range 0–9)
VAS leg pain	7.1 ± 2.9 (range 0–10)	2.2 ± 3.2 (range 0–8)	2.3 ± 2.35 (range 0–8)

and 4 illustrate the development of clinical outcomes during the FU.

Radiological outcome

The detailed radiological results of lumbar lordosis, the sagittal segmental endplate angle of the instrumentation, the sagittal segmental endplate angle of the dynamic segment, pelvic incidence, pelvic tilt, and sacral slope are presented in Table 5. Figs. 5 and 6 illustrate the development of the radiological parameters preoperatively, directly after the operation and during the FU.

Interestingly, a 2.2° reduction in the mean sagittal segmental endplate angle of the dynamic segment was observed directly after surgery. The segmental kyphosis remained during the FU examinations. A reduction in the segmental lordosis of the dynamic segment could have a negative effect on the sagittal balance of the lumbar spine; however, no influence was observed in the development of lumbar lordosis. This reduction tended to be significant ($P = 0.063$). At the 2-year FU, there was a significant reduction ($P = 0.044$) of the sagittal segmental angle.

Complications

An incidental durotomy was documented as a perioperative complication in one case. Surgical postoperative complications were reported in three patients. One patient developed a lumbar radiculopathy without a neurological deficit. One patient needed revision surgery because of a misplaced pedicle screw. The pedicle screw misplacement was diagnosed after a computed tomography scan of the lumbar spine was performed due to a persistent radiculopathy without a neurological deficit. One case reported a superficial wound infection. A general complication of pulmonary disease (pneumonia) was reported in one case.

Obvious signs of material failure in the dynamic part of the implant were identified in four cases (18%) (Figs. 7 and 8). In one of these cases, revision surgery was necessary due to persisting back pain during the FU visits (Fig. 9). The other three patients with material failure within the dynamic portion of the implant did not require any revision surgery due to a reduction in back pain and a sufficient clinical outcome.

In addition, radiological signs of ASD within the segment cranially adjacent to the dynamic instrumented segment were evident in three cases (15%). These cases had a Weiner's grade of three (Fig. 10). The COMI scores in these three cases at the 2-year FU were 6.2, 1.15, and 1.6. The VAS scores for back pain were 2, 3, and 6, and the VAS scores for leg pain were 0, 0, and 1. No cases of ASD were documented in the topping off segment.

Discussion

The development of ASDi has prompted the introduction of new operating methods, such as dynamic and semi-rigid implants, for the treatment of degenerative diseases and spondylolisthesis of the lumbar spine. These implants differ in terms of the materials used and the design and biomechanical properties of the dynamic section [12]. Dynamic spine implants allow mobility of the instrumented segment; however, some biomechanical studies have reported small differences in the mechanical performance of posterior dynamic and rigid implants [17].

Many studies reported adequate long-term clinical outcomes after posterior dynamic stabilization of the lumbar spine. In one retrospective study of 299 patients

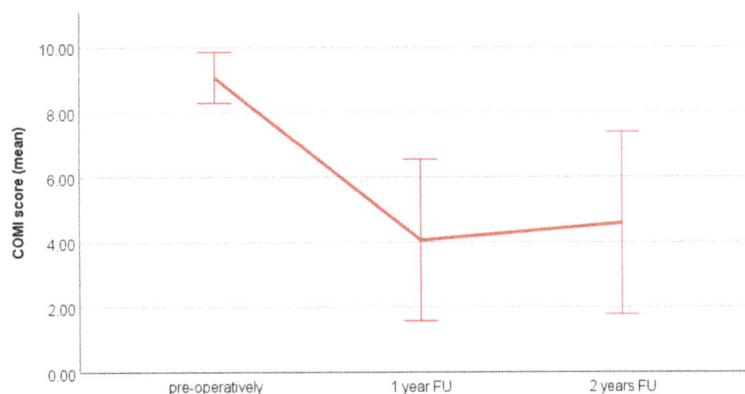

Fig. 2 The COMI score preoperatively and at the 1- and 2-year FU. The whiskers indicate the standard deviation. The COMI score is significantly improved at 1 and 2 years after surgery

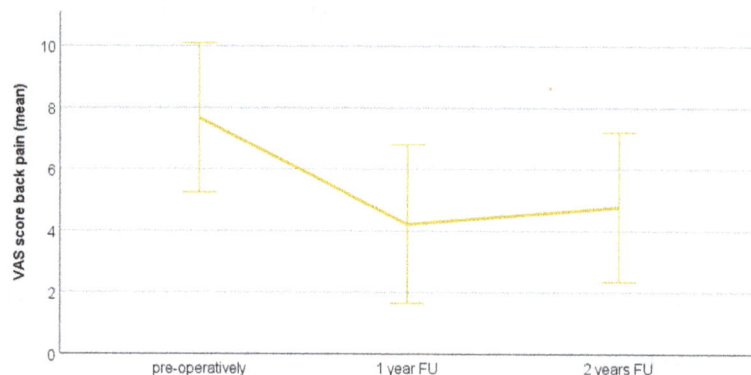

Fig. 3 The VAS score for back pain preoperatively and at the 1- and 2-year FU. The whiskers indicate the standard deviation. The VAS score for back pain is significantly improved at 1 and 2 years after surgery

with a mean FU of 9 months, Greiner-Perth et al. achieved good and stable clinical results using the DSS device (Paradigm Spine, LCC, New York, NY, USA) [18]. In a 2-year FU study of 20 patients treated with the Accuflex (Globus Medical, Inc.) posterior dynamic stabilization device, Reyes-Sanchez et al. reported improvements in pain and quality of life [19]. Overall, dynamic posterior stabilization devices appear to provide convincing clinical results [20, 21]. Nonetheless, it remains uncertain whether dynamic posterior stabilization provides better results than traditional lumbar spinal fusion.

In addition, there is no convincing data regarding the hybrid posterior stabilization systems (topping off) during long-term FU [22]. The findings in this study indicate a significant reduction in back and leg pain as well as a significant improvement in clinical outcomes (according to COMI measurement) at 2 years after hybrid lumbar spine stabilization. These clinical results correlate with the outcomes of lumbar fusion and decompression that are summarized in the literature [1, 2].

However, the aim of this study was to examine whether the use of a hybrid lumbar spinal stabilization system and the resulting supplementary instrumentation

of a segment offered any benefit to the patient. Hybrid posterior stabilization systems were developed to protect the adjacent segment from hypermobility after lumbar spinal fusion, as hypermobility of the adjacent segment can lead to ASDi [23, 24]. Biomechanical studies examining hybrid dynamic lumbar stabilization reported reduced mobility of the adjacent segment after hybrid dynamic stabilization [11]. However, this precautionary fixation is not far from a two-level fusion [25]. This can lead to hypermobility of the segment adjacent to the dynamic stabilization [11, 26]. Thus, ASD can occur in the next cranial segment, as was reported in this study. In this sense, hybrid posterior stabilization can lead to bisegmental fusion and patients underwent supplementary iatrogen operation morbidity.

One possible advantage of hybrid fusion versus single-level fusion is the option to perform extended decompression of the neural structures in the cranial segment and protect the segment from instability [27]. A long-term clinical study comparing single-level lumbar spinal fusion with hybrid lumbar spinal instrumentation identified no clinical benefits of hybrid fusion. In a prospective study comparing single-level fusion and hybrid

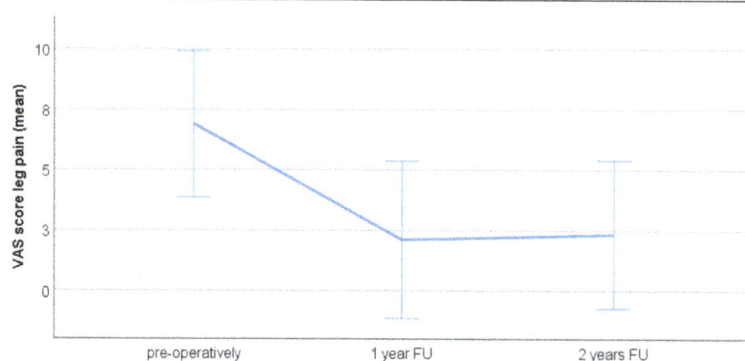

Fig. 4 The VAS score for leg pain preoperatively at the 1- and 2-year FU. The whiskers indicate the standard deviation. The VAS score for leg pain is significantly improved at 1 and 2 years after surgery

Table 5 Radiological outcomes: directly after surgery, at 1-year and 2-year FU (* = significant)

	Preoperatively	Directly after surgery	1-year FU	2-year FU
Lumbar lordosis (°)	− 48.4 ± − 13.0 (range − 25.0 to − 77.0)	− 48.0 ± − 9.9 (range − 27.0 to − 73.0) $P = 0.886$	− 50.6 ± − 11.2 (range − 27.0 to − 73.0) $P = 0.562$	− 49.6 ± − 10.4 (range − 30.0 to − 65.0) $P = 0.835$
Pelvic incidence (°)	63.8 ± 11.8 (range 38.0–85.0)	61.5 ± 9.9 (range 38.0–85.0) $P = 0.141$	63.4 ± 7.5 (range 51.0–72.0) $P = 0.332$	63.3 ± 9.5 (range 40.0–76.0) $P = 0.681$
Pelvic tilt (°)	26.8 ± 8.7 (range 10.0–40.0)	26.8 ± 8.7 (range 10.0–40.0) $P = 0.561$	24.8 ± 6.6 (range 9.0–34.0) $P = 0.018*$	23.2 ± 5.9 (range 10.0–35.0) $P = 0.027*$
Sacral slope (°)	37.3 ± 9.6 (range 20.0–56.0)	37.3 ± 9.6 (range 20.0–56.0) $P = 0.329$	38.8 ± 6.3 (range 30.0–52.0) $P = 0.244$	40.4 ± 9.7 (range 23.0–58.0) $P = 0.060$
Sagittal segmental endplate angle of the instrumentation (°)	− 30.3 ± − 10.3 (range − 7.0 to − 50.0)	− 31.3 ± − 5.2 (range − 20.0 to − 40.0) $P = 0.949$	− 31.1 ± − 7.6 (range − 15.0 to − 46.0) $P = 0.609$	− 31.1 ± − 7.0 (range − 12.0 to − 43.0) $P = 0.622$
Sagittal segmental endplate angle of the dynamic segment (°)	− 18.6 ± − 6.8 (range −6.0 to − 35.0)	− 16.4 ± − 5.0 (range − 9.0 to − 30.0) $P = 0.063$	16.5 ± − 6.0 (range − 7.0 to − 30.0) $P = 0.170$	− 16.1 ± − 5.5 (range − 10.0 to − 28.0) $P = 0.044*$

instrumentation in the lumbar spine, Putzier et al. followed patients for 6 years and reported comparable functional outcomes. These authors used the Allospine Dynesys Transition device (Zimmer, Winterthur, Switzerland) [22]; however, biomechanical studies using Dynesys reported increased stiffness applied to the adjacent segment. Thus, Dynesys performs comparably to rigid implants [28, 29]. In a retrospective study, Baioni et al. assessed clinical and radiological outcomes after hybrid lumbar spinal fusion using the Dynesys implant. They reported satisfying clinical outcomes at the 5-year FU. In addition, the prevalence of radiographic ASD was 10% (3/30 patients) [30]. In contrast, the results reported in our study show a radiographically detectable ASD rate of 15% within the segment superior to the dynamic instrumented level and, interestingly, no radiological or clinical signs of ASD or ASDi within the dynamic instrumented level. The prevalence of ASD in the segment cranially adjacent to the dynamic instrumented level (15%) correlates with the incidence of ASD after lumbar spine fusion reported in the literature [8, 9]. In this respect, the

results show that hybrid lumbar spinal fusion using the CD Horizon BalanC™ rod system is not able to prevent the development of ASD. One possible reason for the development of ASD in the segment cranial to the dynamic instrumentation could be the reduction of lordosis of the dynamic instrumented segment affecting the sagittal balance of the lumbar spine. In our study, we reported a mean reduction of the sagittal endplate angle of the dynamic instrumentation of 2.2.

In a retrospective study of 24 patients (mean FU of 8 months), Maserati et al. assessed clinical and radiological outcomes after hybrid lumbar instrumentation with the DTO. They found improvements in pain and symptomatic degeneration at the dynamically stabilized segment in one case and above the dynamically stabilized segment in two cases [31].

A biomechanical study examining the performance of the dynamic part of the CD Horizon BalanC™ rod reported stiffness in the ROM (except for axial rotation) that was similar to that seen with rigid implants [25].

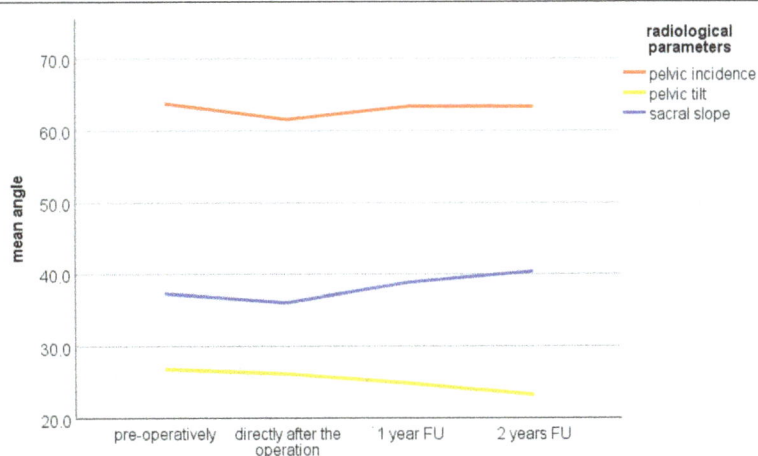

Fig. 5 The positive-valued radiological parameters preoperatively, directly after the operation at the 1- and 2-year FU. Pelvic incidence (PI; orange line), pelvic tilt (PT; yellow line), and sacral slope (SS; blue line). The figure shows a slight reduction in the PI after the operation (2.3°); however, this was comparable to the preoperative value at the 1- and 2-year FU

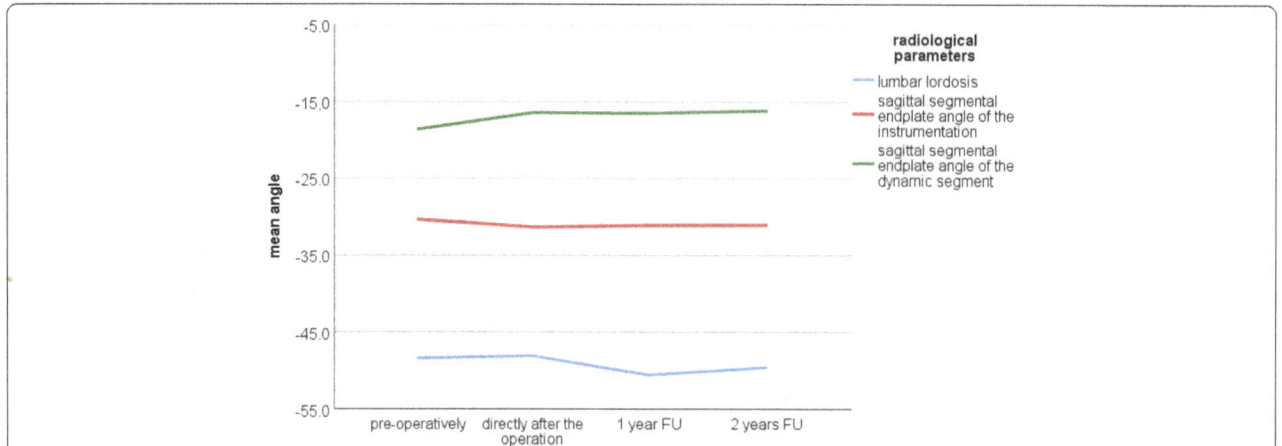

Fig. 6 The negative-valued radiological parameters preoperatively, directly after the operation and at the 1- and 2-year FU. Lumbar lordosis (LL; light blue), sagittal segmental endplate angle of the instrumentation (SSEI; purple line), and sagittal segmental endplate angle of the dynamic segment (SSED; green line). The mean SSED was reduced after the operation. The reduction in segmental lordosis remained during the follow-up. Mean SSEI increased slightly after the operation and remained during the follow-up

According to the radiological findings reported in this study, this biomechanical study supports the hypothesis that load sharing is transferred to one level above the instrumented segments. To the author's knowledge, there has been no published data regarding clinical outcomes after hybrid lumbar instrumentation with the CD Horizon BalanC™ rod system. The dynamic part of the CD Horizon BalanC™ rod is constructed of PEEK and silicone, making it different from the DTO. The results reported here show that there were significant improvements with regard to back and leg pain 2 years after surgery.

The prevalence of material failure in the dynamic implant section was 18% in this study. In these cases, the adjacent segment was no longer protected by the topping off part of the implant. In the author's opinion, this high prevalence indicates a weak area of the implant. Material failure in other dynamic implants has also been reported [19, 32]; for example, Hoff et al. performed a prospective study over a 24-month period to compare single-level dynamic and hybrid instrumentation with the CD Horizon Agile spinal system (Medtronic, Memphis, TN, USA) and reported not only satisfactory functional outcomes but also a high failure

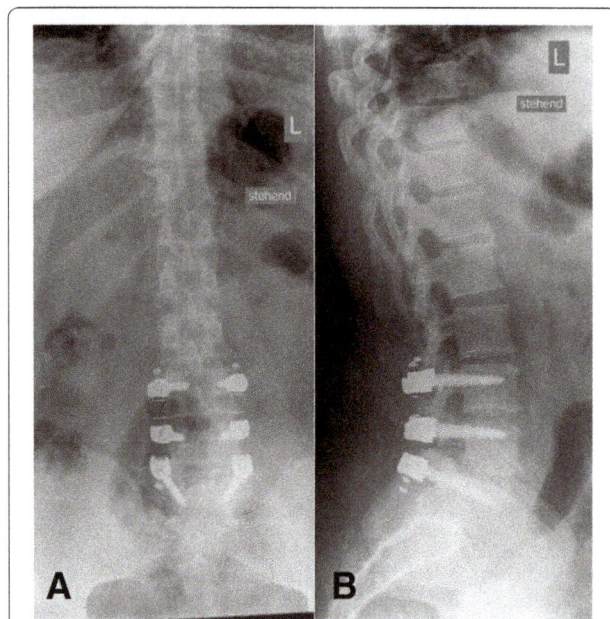

Fig. 7 Lumbar spine anterior–posterior (**a**) and lateral (**b**) radiographs immediately after surgery

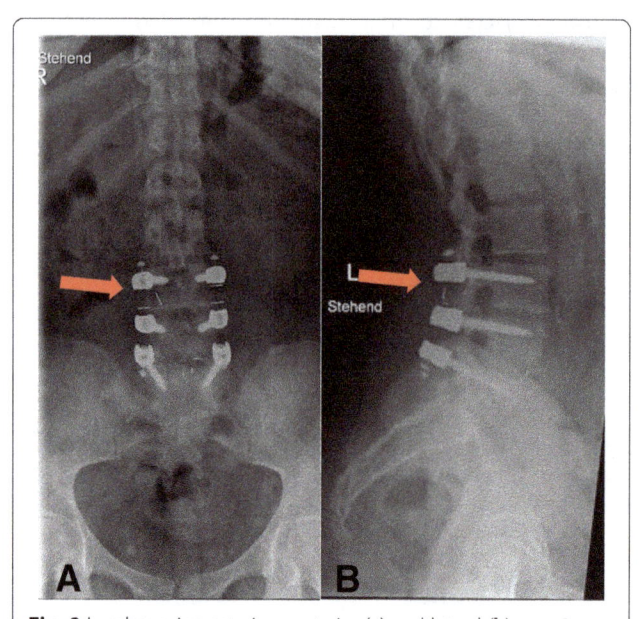

Fig. 8 Lumbar spine anterior–posterior (**a**) and lateral (**b**) radiographs at the 2-year FU. The red marker shows breakage of the PEEK and silicone C-shaped dynamic part at segment L3–4

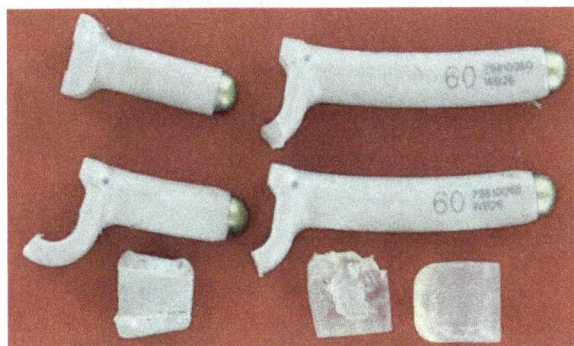

Fig. 9 A BalanC rod implant removed from a patient who required surgical revision due to back pain. Broken dynamic (PEEK and silicone) C-shaped part of both rods

rate of the dynamic portion of the implants [32]. Reports of material failure in dynamic spine implants raise concerns about the use of these devices. In addition, the reliability of before-market implant tests is questionable.

Limitations

First, there was no control group, and due to the fact that the data were obtained from patients who underwent surgery in a single center, there may also have been selection bias. Therefore, a further randomized controlled study should be conducted in multiple hospitals. Second, pathoanatomic risk factors (e.g., facet tropism and sagittalization and horizontalization of the lamina) were not observed.

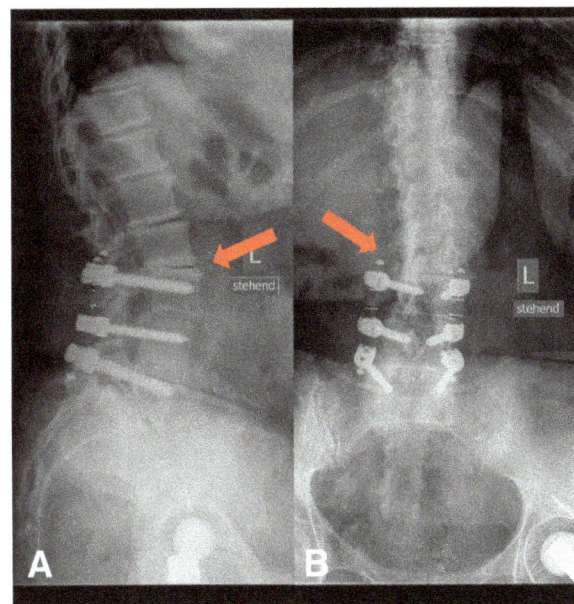

Fig. 10 Lumbar spine lateral (**a**) and anterior–posterior (**b**) radiographs at 2 years after surgery. Radiological signs of degeneration (red marker) in the segment cranially adjacent to the topping off segment

Conclusion

The high rate of material failure (18%) and the onset of adjacent segment alteration superior to the dynamic instrumented level (15%) suggests that the use of a "topping off" device is not able to reduce the incidence of ASD, whereas the reported pain decrease in the study correlates with the outcomes of lumbar fusion and decompression summarized in the literature [1, 2]. Furthermore, the implant is obsolete due to the high failure rate. In this aspect, we conclude that supplementary dynamic instrumentation of the segment cranial to the rigid instrumentation does not offer any benefits to the patient.

Abbreviations
ASA: American Society of Anesthesiologists; ASD: Adjacent segment degeneration; ASDi: Adjacent segment disease; COMI: Core outcome measure index; FU: Follow-up; LSS: Lumbar spinal stenosis; MRI: Magnetic resonance imaging; PEEK: Polyether ether ketone; PLIF: Posterior lumbar interbody fusion; ROM: Range of motion; TLIF: Transforaminal lumbar interbody fusion; VAS: Visual analogue scale

Authors' contributions
SO contributed to the writing of the paper, searched for references, and collected and analyzed the data. GA and TK performed the surgeries. CH contributed to the writing of the paper and designed the study. JS contributed to the study design and data analysis. RS contributed to the study design, performed the surgeries, and performed data analysis. All authors reviewed and approved the final submitted version of the paper.

Competing interests
The authors declare that they have no competing interests.

Author details
[1]Department of Orthopaedics and Trauma Surgery, Rhein-Maas Klinikum GmbH, Mauerfeldchen 25, 52146 Wuerselen, Germany. [2]Department of Orthopaedics and Trauma Surgery, University Hospital Cologne, Joseph-Stelzmann-Str. 24, 50931 Cologne, Germany. [3]Department of Trauma and Reconstructive Surgery, University Hospital RWTH Aachen, Pauwelsstraße 30, 52074 Aachen, Germany.

References
1. Fritzell P, Hägg O, Wessberg P, Nordwall A; Swedish Lumbar Spine Study Group. 2001 Volvo Award Winner in Clinical Studies: Lumbar fusion versus nonsurgical treatment for chronic low back pain: a multicenter randomized controlled trial from the Swedish Lumbar Spine Study Group. Spine (Phila Pa 1976). 2001;26(23):2521–2532; discussion 2532-4.
2. Mannion AF, Brox JI, Fairbank JC. Comparison of spinal fusion and nonoperative treatment in patients with chronic low back pain: long-term follow-up of three randomized controlled trials. Spine J. 2013;13(11):1438–48. https://doi.org/10.1016/j.spinee.2013.06.101.
3. Kim KT, Lee SH, Lee YH, Bae SC, Suk KS. Clinical outcomes of 3 fusion methods through the posterior approach in the lumbar spine. Spine (Phila Pa 1976). 2006;31(12):1351–7. discussion 1358
4. Chamoli U, Chen AS, Diwan AD. Interpedicular kinematics in an in vitro biomechanical assessment of a bilateral lumbar spondylolytic defect. Clin Biomech (Bristol, Avon). 2014;29(10):1108–15. https://doi.org/10.1016/j.clinbiomech.2014.10.002.
5. Verma K, Gandhi SD, Maltenfort M, Albert TJ, Hilibrand AS, Vaccaro AR,

Radcliff KE. Rate of adjacent segment disease in cervical disc arthroplasty versus single-level fusion: meta-analysis of prospective studies. Spine (Phila Pa 1976). 2013;38(26):2253–7. https://doi.org/10.1097/BRS.0000000000000052.

6. Javedan SP, Dickman CA. Cause of adjacent-segment disease after spinal fusion. Lancet. 1999;354(9178):530–1.

7. Mannion AF, Leivseth G, Brox JI, Fritzell P, Hägg O, Fairbank JC. ISSLS Prize winner: long-term follow-up suggests spinal fusion is associated with increased adjacent segment disc degeneration but without influence on clinical outcome: results of a combined follow-up from 4 randomized controlled trials. Spine (Phila Pa 1976). 2014;39(17):1373–83. https://doi.org/10.1097/BRS.0000000000000437.

8. Park P, Garton HJ, Gala VC, Hoff JT, McGillicuddy JE. Adjacent segment disease after lumbar or lumbosacral fusion: review of the literature. Spine (Phila Pa 1976). 2004;29(17):1938–44.

9. Moreau PE, Ferrero E, Riouallon G, Lenoir T, Guigui P. Radiologic adjacent segment degeneration 2 years after lumbar fusion for degenerative spondylolisthesis. Orthop Traumatol Surg Res. 2016;102(6):759–63. https://doi.org/10.1016/j.otsr.2016.03.012.

10. Chen BL, Wei FX, Ueyama K, Xie DH, Sannohe A, Liu SY. Adjacent segment degeneration after single-segment PLIF: the risk factor for degeneration and its impact on clinical outcomes. Eur Spine J. 2011;20(11):1946–50. https://doi.org/10.1007/s00586-011-1888-1.

11. Mageswaran P, Techy F, Colbrunn RW, Bonner TF, McLain RF. Hybrid dynamic stabilization: a biomechanical assessment of adjacent and supraadjacent levels of the lumbar spine. J Neurosurg Spine. 2012;17(3):232–42. https://doi.org/10.3171/2012.6.SPINE111054.

12. Khoueir P, Kim KA, Wang MY. Classification of posterior dynamic stabilization devices. Neurosurg Focus. 2007;22(1):E3.

13. Pfirrmann CW, Metzdorf A, Zanetti M, Hodler J, Boos N. Magnetic resonance classification of lumbar intervertebral disc degeneration. Spine (Phila Pa 1976). 2001;26(17):1873–8.

14. Siewe J, Bredow J, Oppermann J, Koy T, Delank S, Knoell P, Eysel P, Sobottke R, Zarghooni K, Röllinghoff M. Evaluation of efficacy of a new hybrid fusion device: a randomized, two-centre controlled trial. BMC Musculoskelet Disord. 2014;15:294. https://doi.org/10.1186/1471-2474-15-294.

15. Modic M, Masaryk T, Ross J, Carter J. Imaging of degenerative disk disease. Radiology. 1988;168(1):177–86.

16. Weiner DK, Distell B, Studenski S, Martinez S, Lomasney L, Bongiorni D. Does radiographic osteoarthritis correlate with flexibility of the lumbar spine? J Am Geriatr Soc. 1994;42(3):257–63.

17. Rohlmann A, Burra NK, Zander T, Bergmann G. Comparison of the effects of bilateral posterior dynamic and rigid fixation devices on the loads in the lumbar spine: a finite element analysis. Eur Spine J. 2007;16(8):1223–31.

18. Greiner-Perth R, Sellhast N, Perler G, Dietrich D, Staub LP, Röder C. Dynamic posterior stabilization for degenerative lumbar spine disease: a large consecutive case series with long-term follow-up by additional postal survey. Eur Spine J. 2016;25(8):2563–70. https://doi.org/10.1007/s00586-016-4532-2.

19. Reyes-Sánchez A, Zárate-Kalfópulos B, Ramírez-Mora I, Rosales-Olivarez LM, Alpizar-Aguirre A, Sánchez-Bringas G. Posterior dynamic stabilization of the lumbar spine with the Accuflex rod system as a stand-alone device: experience in 20 patients with 2-year follow-up. Eur Spine J. 2010;19(12):2164–70. https://doi.org/10.1007/s00586-010-1417-7.

20. Hoppe S, Schwarzenbach O, Aghayev E, Bonel H, Berlemann U. Long-term outcome after monosegmental L4/5 stabilization for degenerative spondylolisthesis with the Dynesys device. Clin Spine Surg. 2016;29(2):72–7. https://doi.org/10.1097/BSD.0b013e318277ca7a.

21. Zhang Y, Shan JL, Liu XM, Li F, Guan K, Sun TS. Comparison of the Dynesys dynamic stabilization system and posterior lumbar interbody fusion for lumbar degenerative disease. PLoS One. 2016;11(1):e0148071. https://doi.org/10.1371/journal.pone.0148071.

22. Putzier M, Hoff E, Tohtz S, Gross C, Perka C, Strube P. Dynamic stabilization adjacent to single-level fusion: part II. No clinical benefit for asymptomatic, initially degenerated adjacent segments after 6 years follow-up. Eur Spine J. 2010;19(12):2181–9. https://doi.org/10.1007/s00586-010-1517-4.

23. Cheng BC, Gordon J, Cheng J, Welch WC. Immediate biomechanical effects of lumbar posterior dynamic stabilization above a circumferential fusion. Spine (Phila Pa 1976). 2007;32(23):2551–7.

24. Cakir B, Carazzo C, Schmidt R, Mattes T, Reichel H, Käfer W. Adjacent segment mobility after rigid and semirigid instrumentation of the lumbar spine. Spine (Phila Pa 1976). 2009;34(12):1287–91. https://doi.org/10.1097/BRS.0b013e3181a136ab.

25. Herren C, Beckmann A, Meyer S, Pishnamaz M, Mundt M, Sobottke R, Prescher A, Stoffel M, Markert B, Kobbe P, Pape HC, Eysel P, Siewe J. Biomechanical testing of a PEEK-based dynamic instrumentation device in a lumbar spine model. Clin Biomech (Bristol, Avon). 2017;44:67–74. https://doi.org/10.1016/j.clinbiomech.2017.03.009.

26. Strube P, Tohtz S, Hoff E, Gross C, Perka C, Putzier M. Dynamic stabilization adjacent to single-level fusion: part I. Biomechanical effects on lumbar spinal motion. Eur Spine J. 2010;19(12):2171–80. https://doi.org/10.1007/s00586-010-1549-9.

27. Schnake KJ, Schaeren S, Jeanneret B. Dynamic stabilization in addition to decompression for lumbar spinal stenosis with degenerative spondylolisthesis. Spine (Phila Pa 1976). 2006;31(4):442–9.

28. Stoll TM, Dubois G, Schwarzenbach O. The dynamic neutralization system for the spine: a multi-center study of a novel non-fusion system. Eur Spine J. 2002;11(2):S170–8.

29. Schmoelz W, Huber JF, Nydegger T, Dipl-Ing CL, Wilke HJ. Dynamic stabilization of the lumbar spine and its effects on adjacent segments: an in vitro experiment. J Spinal Disord Tech. 2003;16(4):418–23.

30. Baioni A, Di Silvestre M, Greggi T, Vommaro F, Lolli F, Scarale A. Does hybrid fixation prevent junctional disease after posterior fusion for degenerative lumbar disorders? A minimum 5-year follow-up study. Eur Spine J. 2015;24(7):855–64. https://doi.org/10.1007/s00586-015-4269-3.

31. Maserati MB, Tormenti MJ, Bonfield CM, Gerszten PC. The use of a hybrid dynamic stabilization and fusion system in the lumbar spine: preliminary experience. Neurosurg Focus. 2010;28(6):E2. https://doi.org/10.3171/2010.3.FOCUS1055.

32. Hoff E, Strube P, Rohlmann A, Gross C, Putzier M. Which radiographic parameters are linked to failure of a dynamic spinal implant? Clin Orthop Relat Res. 2012;470(7):1834–46. https://doi.org/10.1007/s11999-011-2200-8.

6

Meta-analysis of the potential role of extracorporeal shockwave therapy in osteonecrosis of the femoral head

Yangquan Hao[1*†], Hao Guo[1†], Zhaochen Xu[1], Handeng Qi[2], Yugui Wang[2], Chao Lu[1], Jie Liu[2] and Puwei Yuan[2*]

Abstract

Background: We aimed to evaluate the role of extracorporeal shockwave therapy (ESWT) in improving osteonecrosis of the femoral head (ONFH).

Methods: We searched studies focusing on the role of ESWT in ONFH using PubMed, Embase, the Cochrane Library, WanFang, VIP, and CNKI databases updated up to July 28, 2017, without language restriction. Standardized mean difference (SMD) values and 95% confidence intervals (95% CIs) were pooled to compare the pain score and Harris hip score for ESWT treatment and other treatment strategies.

Results: Four articles, including 230 ONFH patients, were eligible for the meta-analysis. No significant differences were found in the pain score (SMD = − 1.0104; 95% CI − 2.3279–0.3071) and Harris hip score (SMD = 0.3717; 95% CI − 0.3125–1.0559) between the two groups before treatment. After treatment, significant differences were found between the experimental and control groups in the pain score (SMD = − 2.1148; 95% CI − 3.2332–0.9965) and Harris hip score (SMD = 2.1377; 95% CI 1.2875–2.9880). There were no significant differences in pain score before and after treatment between the two groups (SMD = − 0.7353; 95% CI − 2.1272–0.6566), but significant differences were found in the Harris hip score (SMD = 1.2969; 95% CI 0.7171–1.8767).

Conclusion: For patients at an early stage, ESWT may be safe and effective for relief of pain and improvement of motor function.

Keywords: Osteonecrosis of the femoral head, Extracorporeal shockwave therapy, Pain score, Harris hip score, Meta-analysis

Background

Osteonecrosis of the femoral head (ONFH) is a pathological process that follows ischemic insult [1]. High morbidity occurs in both young and old worldwide [2]. In China, 8.12 million patients have been diagnosed with ONFH as of 2017 [3, 4], and the average annual number of new cases in Korea was 14,103 [5]. The occurrence of osteonecrosis is associated with various risk factors including trauma, hip surgery, corticosteroid use, alcoholism, and coagulopathy [6]. The treatment of ONFH

remains a challenge, and a standardized and improved treatment strategy for ONFH is urgently needed.

"Joint-preserving" treatments, including both surgical (such as core decompression, trochanteric rotational osteotomy, and vascularized bone grafts) and conservative approaches [extracorporeal shock wave therapy (ESWT) and pulsed electromagnetic field] have been developed to prevent progression of ONFH [7, 8]. ESWT is used in physical therapy, orthopedics, urology, and cardiology, and a previous study demonstrated that the technology can successfully treat ONFH [9]. However, the efficacy of ESWT compared with other treatments remains unclear [10, 11]. For example, no significant difference in efficacy was found between ESWT and core decompression in a study by Wang et al. [10]. A study by Chen and colleagues demonstrated better outcomes with ESWT than with physical

* Correspondence: yangquanhaop17@21cn.com; spine_surgeon@163.com
†Yangquan Hao and Hao Guo contributed equally to this work.
[1]Department of Osteonecrosis and Joint Reconstruction, Honghui Hospital Xi'an Jiao Tong University Health Science Center, No. 555 Youyi East Road, Xi'an, Shaanxi 710054, People's Republic of China
[2]Shaanxi University of Chinese Medicine, Shiji Ave, New Economic Zone, Xi'an-Xianyang, Shaanxi 712046, People's Republic of China

therapy [12]. Although the effect of ESWT in the treatment of ONFH has been investigated by previous researchers, there is no consistent conclusion about its efficacy when compared with other treatments.

This meta-analysis was performed to evaluate the role of ESWT in improving ONFH. Standardized mean difference (SMD) values and 95% confidence intervals (95% CIs) were pooled to compare the pain score and Harris hip score for ESWT treatment and other treatment strategies.

Methods
Study selection
Studies were selected using PubMed (http://www.ncbi.nlm.nih.gov/pubmed), Embase (http://www.embase.com), the Cochrane Library (http://www.cochranelibrary.com), WanFang, VIP, and CNKI databases updated to July 28, 2017, without language restriction. A combination of Medical Subject Headings (MeSH) terms and free-text keywords were used for study selection: ("ESWT" OR "Extracorporeal shock wave") AND ("osteonecrosis" OR "Osteonecrosis" OR "femoral head necrosis" OR "ONFH" OR "Osteonecrosis of the Femoral Head" OR "avascular necrosis of femoral head" OR "necrosis of the femoral head" OR "avascular necrosis of bone" OR "Kienbock disease" OR "Aseptic necrosis of bone").

Selection criteria
Literature focusing on the efficacy of ESWT in patients with femoral head necrosis were included in the meta-analysis. Studies were included in the meta-analysis if they met the following criteria: (1) published Chinese or English language literature focusing on the efficacy of ESWT in patients with ONFH, in which the experimental group was treated with ESWT and the control group received a different treatment strategy; (2) reported outcomes included the pain score and Harris hip score at baseline and corresponding scores after a period of treatment; and (3) research designed as an interventional study.

Exclusion criteria were as follows: (1) incomplete data or data that could not be used for statistical analysis and (2) reviews, letters, and comments. In addition, if studies duplicated published literature or data for the same population, only the latest research with the most comprehensive information was included.

Data extraction and quality evaluation
The authors independently extracted the following data from the included literature: the first author's name, year of publication, study period, stage of ONFH (according to Association Research Circulation Osseous), type of study, follow-up duration, baseline characteristics of enrolled patients (e.g., sex ratio, age composition), baseline pain and Harris hip scores, and corresponding scores after treatment, sample sizes, and general demographic data.

The quality of randomized controlled trials was evaluated using Cochrane Collaboration recommendations [13]. Disagreements were resolved by discussion or by consultation with a third reviewer.

Statistical analysis
Meta-analysis was performed using R 3.12 software (R Foundation for Statistical Computing, "meta" package, Beijing, China). The SMD values and 95% CIs were pooled to compare the pain score and Harris hip score for ESWT treatment and other treatment strategies. For $P < 0.05$ or $I^2 > 50\%$, the random effects model was used to calculate the combined effect value. Otherwise, the fixed effects model was chosen to combine data [14]. Publication bias was assessed using Egger's method. Finally, sensitivity analysis was performed by omitting one study at a time to determine the effect on the overall SMD value.

Results
The general characteristics of included studies
The flow chart used for study selection is shown in Fig. 1. Of 482 articles initially reviewed, 48 were from PubMed, 91 from Embase, 4 from the Cochrane Library, 61 from WanFang, 46 from VIP, and 232 from CNKI. After excluding duplicated literature, 295 articles were left. Then, the title and abstract were reviewed, and 221 articles obviously inconsistent with the inclusion criteria excluded. Subsequently, a total of 74 articles were fully reviewed, and 52 articles were excluded including 9 letters, 14 reviews, 10 case series/reports, and 19 animal studies. Moreover, another 18 articles including 9 articles without relevant data, 6 descriptive studies, and 3 reduplicative studies were excluded. Finally, 4 articles were included in the meta-analysis [10, 12, 14, 15].

A total of 230 patients (185 men and 45 women, a significant difference) with ONFH were enrolled in this study, including 120 in the experimental group and 110 in the control group. The general characteristics of the selected literature are shown in Table 1. The publication year ranged from 2008 to 2015. Patients with ONFH were mainly in stages I–III. Only one randomized controlled study was included. No significant difference in sex or age distribution was found in individual studies. Follow-up time in three studies was more than 1 year. Figure 2 shows that the quality of the included literature was relatively poor.

Meta-analysis of pain score and Harris hip score
The pain and Harris hip scores before and after treatment in the experimental and control groups were analyzed. The main results are shown in Table 2 and Fig. 3. No significant differences were found between the two groups in the baseline pain score (SMD = − 1.0104;95% CI − 2.3279–0.3071) and baseline Harris hip score

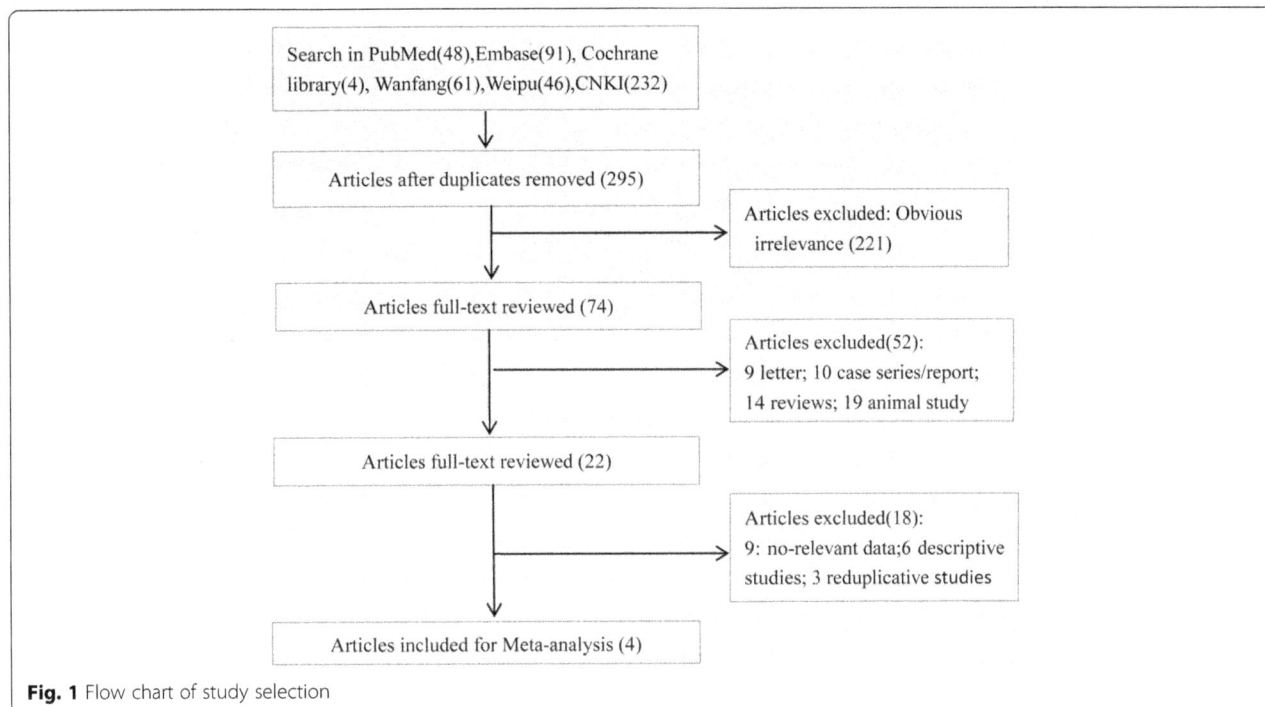

Fig. 1 Flow chart of study selection

(SMD = 0.3717; 95% CI – 0.3125–1.0559). After a period of treatment, significant differences were found between the experimental and control groups in the pain score (SMD = – 2.1148; 95% CI – 3.2332–0.9965) and Harris hip score (SMD = 2.1377; 95% CI 1.2875–2.9880). No significant differences in pain score were found before and after treatment (SMD = – 0.7353; 95% CI – 2.1272–0.6566), but significant differences were found in the Harris hip score (SMD = 1.2969; 95% CI 0.7171–1.8767).

Publication bias

Significant bias was found among individual studies in the comparison of Harris hip scores ($t = 3.5824$, $P = 0.0231$), but no publication bias was found in the change before and after treatment ($t = 0.9755$, $P = 0.3846$) in the baseline pain score and Harris hip score ($t = 1.9243$, $P = 0.1267$).

Sensitivity analysis

Sensitivity analysis of pain scores demonstrated that the results were unstable, but sensitivity analysis of Harris hip scores demonstrated that the results were stable.

Discussion

In the present study, we evaluated the role of ESWT in improving ONFH. A total of 230 patients with ONFH were included in the study. No significant difference was found between the two groups in the pain score and Harris hip score before treatment. After treatment, significant differences were found between the experimental and control groups in the pain score and Harris hip score. No significant differences in pain score were found before and after treatment, but significant differences were found in the Harris hip score.

Table 1 The baseline characteristics of included studies

Study	Year	Study year	ONFH stage	Study style	Group	Number/hips	Gender (M/F)	Age (year)	Duration (month)
Wang CJ	2012	2001–2001	Stages I, II, early III	Non-RCT	ESWT	23/29	20/3	39.8 ± 12.1	25.2 ± 3.7
					Surgical group	25/28	22/3	39.9 ± 9.3	25.8 ± 4.6
Chen JM	2009	1999.7–2006.1	Stages I–III	Non-RCT	ESWT	17/17	14/3	42.9 ± 9.3	11.3 ± 3.4
			Stages I–IV		THA	17/17	14/3	42.9 ± 9.3	14.7 ± 0.93
Zhang HJ	2015	2009.1–2012.12	Stages I–II	RCT	BMSC+ESWT	20/29	15/5	36.1 ± 6.2	24
					BMSC	20/27	14/6	35.5 ± 5.7	24
Zhai L	2008	1998.1–2007.6	Stages I–III	Non-RCT	CD + ESWT	50/50	41/9	20.9(18–25)	6.4(3–18)
					CD	58/58	45/13	20.5(18–25)	7.3(3–20)

ESWT extracorporeal shock wave treatment, *THA* total hip arthroplasty, *CD* core decompression, *M/F* males/females, *RCT* randomized controlled trail, *ONFH* osteonecrosis of the femoral head, *THA* total hip, *BMSC* bone marrow stem cells

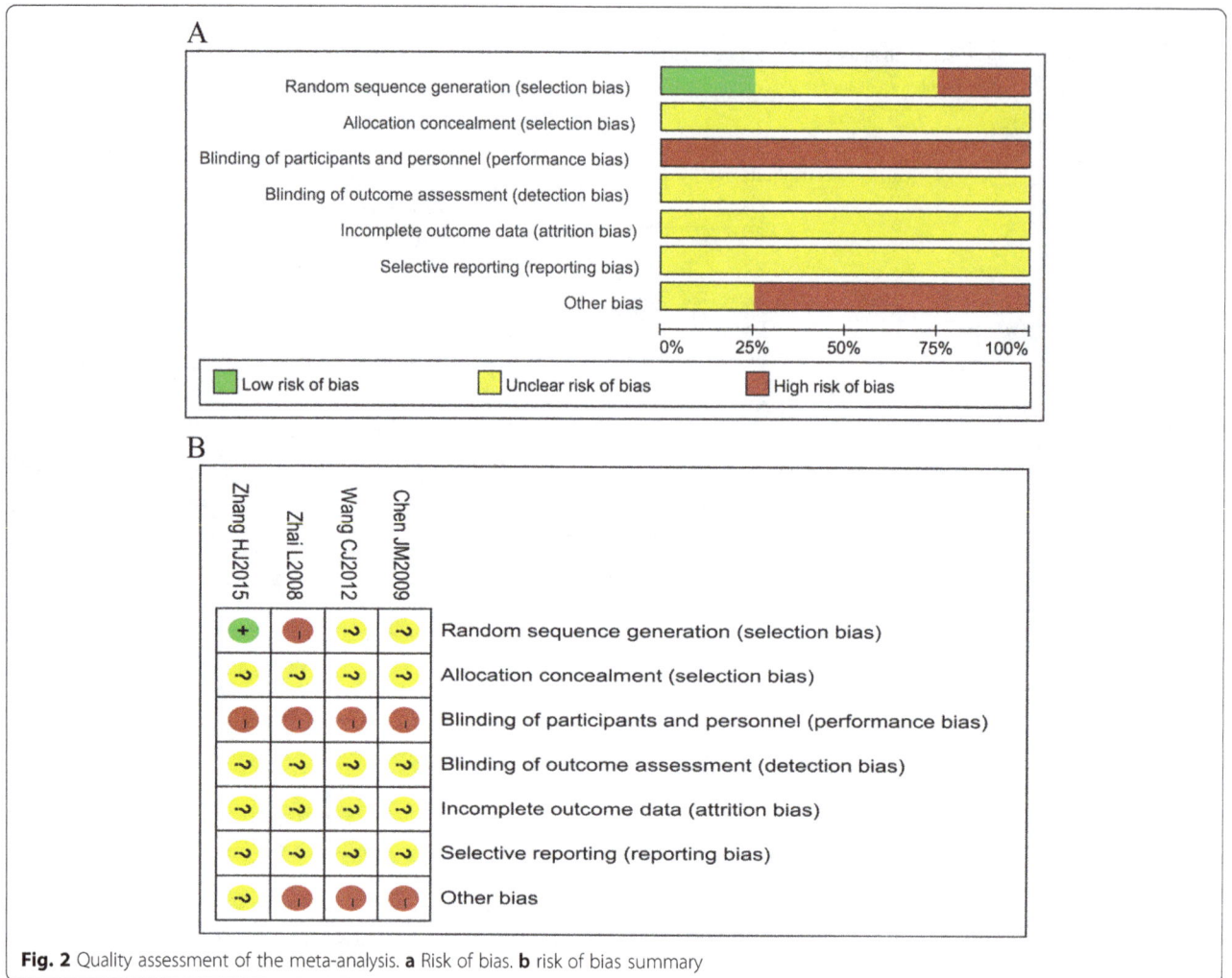

Fig. 2 Quality assessment of the meta-analysis. **a** Risk of bias. **b** risk of bias summary

Physical therapy can improve bone oxygenation, reduce edema, reduce bone pressure, improve bone circulation, prevent ischemia, restore blood supply in hypoxic tissue, and promote necrotic bone repair [16]. Wang et al. demonstrated greater improvement with ESWT compared with core decompression and nonvascularized fibular grafting in patients with early-stage ONFH [17].

A previous study demonstrated that ESWT could increase the expression of angiogenic factors, reduce vessel wall stenosis, and improve limb perfusion [18]. The effect of ESWT might be related to stress-induced piezoelectricity, cavitation and osteogenesis, and metabolic activation. These effects promote healing of femoral head necrosis by inducing improved blood circulation,

Table 2 Meta-analysis results for pain score and Harris hip score

Variable	Group	Sample size			Test of association			Model	Test of heterogeneity[a, b]			Egger's test[c]	
		K	ESWT	Control	SMD (95% CI)	Z	P		Q	P	I^2 (%)	t	P
Pain score	Base	2	46	45	−1.0104 [− 2.3279; 0.3071]	1.5032	0.1328	Random	6.61	0.0058	86.9	–	–
	Post	2	46	45	− 2.1148 [− 3.2332; − 0.9965]	3.7063	0.0002	Random	4.42	0.0035	77.4	–	–
	Change	2	46	46	− 0.7353 [− 2.1272; 0.6566]	1.0354	0.3005	Random	9.81	0.0017	89.8	–	–
Harris hip score	Base	4	125	130	0.3717 [− 0.3125; 1.0559]	1.0647	0.287	Random	34.06	< 0.001	85.3	1.9243	0.1267
	Post	4	125	130	2.1377 [1.2875; 2.9880]	4.9281	< 0.001	Random	35.77	< 0.001	86.0	3.5824	0.0231
	Change	4	125	125	1.2969 [0.7171; 1.8767]	4.3839	< 0.001	Random	20.72	0.001	75.9	0.9755	0.3846

OR odds ratio, *CI* confidence interval, *K* number of studies combined

[a]Random-effects model was used when the *P* for heterogeneity test < 0.05; otherwise, the fixed-effect model was used

[b]*P* < 0.05 is considered statistically significant for Q statistics

[c]Egger's test to evaluate publication bias, *P* < 0.05 is considered statistically significant

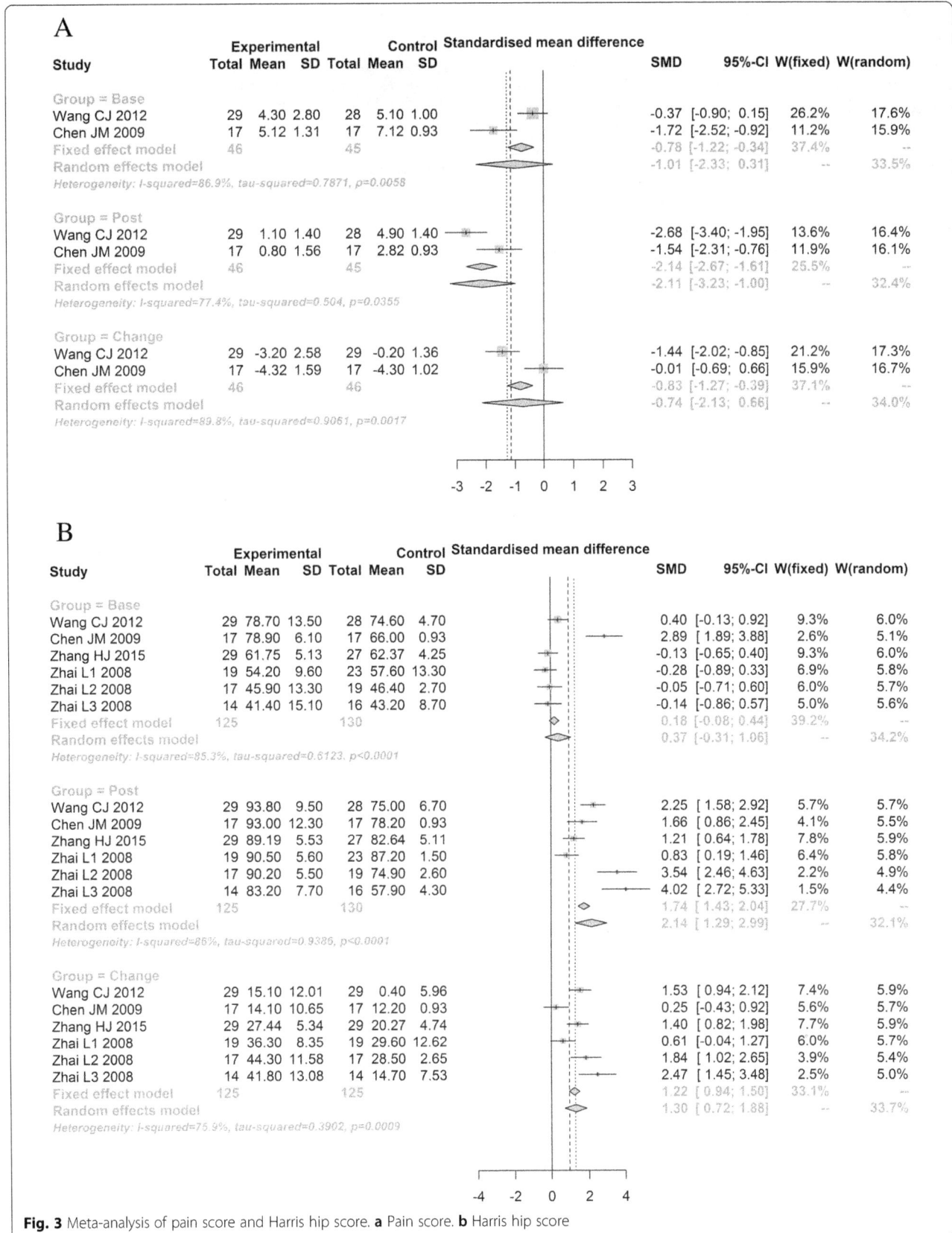

Fig. 3 Meta-analysis of pain score and Harris hip score. **a** Pain score. **b** Harris hip score

mitigating a hypercoagulable state, and enhancing osteoblast and blood vessel activity [18, 19]. Similar to previous reports, the present study suggested that ESWT might be a safe and effective method to improve motor function and relieve pain, especially at an early stage of ONFH. Significant heterogeneity was observed in the study. Heterogeneity might be introduced by different combined treatment strategies. For example, patients in experimental groups underwent ESWT in two studies [12], while patients in experimental groups in two other studies underwent combined treatment [15, 20]. Although the age difference between groups in individual studies was not significant, the age in the four studies ranged from 20.9 to 40.9 years. Bone density, structure, and strength are correlated with age [21, 22]. Thus, efficacy should be confirmed with further studies after adjusting for background factors that can affect ESWT treatment.

Some limitations should be noted. First, the small sample size introduced more obvious heterogeneity between individual studies [23]. Additionally, the included populations were small and the baseline characteristics of included studies were not complete. Thus, subgroup analysis based on age and sex distribution could not be performed. Second, the quality of the included studies was poor, limiting the strength of the conclusion. Third, publication bias for the Harris hip score after treatment might affect the results. Fourth, only two studies reported pain scores, and further research with larger sample sizes is needed to validate the conclusions.

Conclusion

For patients at an early stage, ESWT may be a safe and effective way to relieve pain and improve motor function. Nevertheless, due to the low quality of the included publications, the conclusion should be confirmed with further research using a larger sample size. The long-term follow-up studies are favorable to the use of ESWT in ONFH in future.

Abbreviations
CI: Confidence interval; ESWT: Extracorporeal shockwave therapy; ONFH: Osteonecrosis of the femoral head; SMD: Standardized mean difference

Acknowledgements
This work was supported by the key scientific and technological innovation team of Shaanxi province (grant number: 2013KCT-26).

Funding
This work was supported by key scientific and technological innovation team of Shaanxi province (grant number: 2013KCT-26).

Authors' contributions
YH and PY conceived and designed the research. JL acquired the data. YW analyzed and interpreted the data. CL and HG performed the statistical analyses. PY obtained the funding. ZX and HQ drafted the manuscript. YH and PY revised the manuscript for important intellectual content. All authors read and approved the final manuscript.

Competing interests
The authors declare that they have no competing interests.

References
1. Nakai T, Masuhara K, Nakase T, Sugano N, Ohzono K, Ochi T. Pathology of femoral head collapse following transtrochanteric rotational osteotomy for osteonecrosis. Arch Orthop Trauma Surg. 2000;120(9):489–92.
2. Leclerc C, Néant I, Moreau M. The calcium: an early signal that initiates the formation of the nervous system during embryogenesis. Jorgchem. 2012; 36(18):2720–1.
3. Pascart T, Falgayrac G, Migaud H, Quinchon JF, Norberciak L, Budzik JF, et al. Region specific Raman spectroscopy analysis of the femoral head reveals that trabecular bone is unlikely to contribute to non-traumatic osteonecrosis. Sci Rep. 2017;7(1):017–00162.
4. Zhao DW, Yu M, Hu K, Wang W, Yang L, Wang BJ, et al. Prevalence of nontraumatic osteonecrosis of the femoral head and its associated risk factors in the Chinese population: results from a nationally representative survey. Chin Med J. 2015;128(21):2843–50.
5. Kang JS, Park S, Song JH, Jung YY, Cho MR, Rhyu KH. Prevalence of osteonecrosis of the femoral head: a nationwide epidemiologic analysis in Korea. J Arthroplasty. 2009;24(8):1178–83.
6. Qiang H, Liu H, Ling M, Wang K, Zhang C. Early steroid-induced osteonecrosis of rabbit femoral head and Panax notoginseng saponins: mechanism and protective effects. Evid Based Complement Alternat Med. 2015;2015:719370. https://doi.org/10.1155/2015/719370.
7. Sadile F, Bernasconi A, Russo S, Maffulli N. Core decompression versus other joint preserving treatments for osteonecrosis of the femoral head: a meta-analysis. Br Med Bull. 2016;118(1):33–49.
8. Kuroda Y, Matsuda S, Akiyama H. Joint-preserving regenerative therapy for patients with early-stage osteonecrosis of the femoral head. Inflamm Regen. 2016;36(4):016–0002.
9. Lin PC, Wang CJ, Yang KD, Wang FS, Ko JY, Huang CC. Extracorporeal shockwave treatment of osteonecrosis of the femoral head in systemic lupus erythematosis. J Arthroplast. 2006;21(6):911–5.
10. Wang CJ, Huang CC, Wang JW, Wong T, Yang YJ. Long-term results of extracorporeal shockwave therapy and core decompression in osteonecrosis of the femoral head with eight- to nine-year follow-up. Biom J. 2012;35(6):481–5.
11. Zhang Q, Liu L, Sun W, Gao F, Cheng L, Li Z. Extracorporeal shockwave therapy in osteonecrosis of femoral head: a systematic review of now available clinical evidences. Medicine. 2017;96(4):e5897.
12. Chen JMHS, Wong T, Chou WY, Wang CJ, Wang FS. Functional outcomes of bilateral hip necrosis: total hip arthroplasty versus extracorporeal shockwave. Arch Orthop Trauma Surg. 2009;129:837–41.
13. Higgins JP, Green S. Cochrane handbook for systematic reviews of interventions version 5.1.0: The Cochrane Collaboration; 2011. Available from http://handbook.cochrane.org.
14. Feng R-N, Zhao C, Sun C-H, Li Y. Meta-analysis of TNF 308 G/A polymorphism and type 2 diabetes mellitus. PLoS One. 2011;6(4):e18480.
15. Lei ZGX, Chuan J, Bing L, Zhe Z, Xuming W. Therapeutic effects of extracorporeal shock waves combined with drilling decompression for the treatment of femoral head ischemic necrosis due to training in servicemen. Med J Chin PLA. 2008;33:348–50.
16. Neumayr LD, Aguilar C, Earles AN, Jergesen HE, Haberkern CM, Kammen BF, et al. Physical therapy alone compared with core decompression and physical therapy for femoral head osteonecrosis in sickle cell disease. Results of a multicenter study at a mean of three years after treatment. J Bone Joint Surg Am. 2006;88(12):2573–82.
17. Wang CJ, Wang FS, Huang CC, Yang KD, Weng LH, Huang HY. Treatment for osteonecrosis of the femoral head: comparison of extracorporeal shock

waves with core decompression and bone-grafting. J Bone Joint Surg Am. 2005;87(11):2380–7.

18. Raza A, Harwood A, Totty J, Smith G, Chetter I. Extracorporeal shockwave therapy for peripheral arterial disease: a review of the potential mechanisms of action. Ann Vasc Surg. 2017;45:294–8.

19. Korakakis V, Whiteley R, Tzavara A, Malliaropoulos N. The effectiveness of extracorporeal shockwave therapy in common lower limb conditions: a systematic review including quantification of patient-rated pain reduction. Br J Sports Med. 2018;52(6):387–407.

20. Hongjun ZSW, Kejie F, Shaohui W, Yanzhao Z. Extracorporeal shock wave therapy combined with autologous bone marrow stem cells transplantation for treating early-stage osteonecrosis of the femoral head. Chin J Phys Med Rehabil. 2015;37:287–90.

21. Alvarenga JC, Fuller H, Pasoto SG, Pereira RM. Age-related reference curves of volumetric bone density, structure, and biomechanical parameters adjusted for weight and height in a population of healthy women: an HR-pQCT study. Osteoporos Int. 2017;28(4):1335–46.

22. Zura R, Braid-Forbes MJ, Jeray K, Mehta S, Einhorn TA, Watson JT, et al. Bone fracture nonunion rate decreases with increasing age: a prospective inception cohort study. Bone. 2017;95:26–32.

23. IntHout J, Ioannidis JP, Borm GF, Goeman JJ. Small studies are more heterogeneous than large ones: a meta-meta-analysis. J Clin Epidemiol. 2015;68(8):860–9.

7

A novel revision surgery for treatment of cervical ossification of the posterior longitudinal ligament after initial posterior surgery: preliminary clinical investigation of anterior controllable antidisplacement and fusion

Hai-Dong Li[1]* ![ORCID], Qiang-Hua Zhang[1], Shi-Tong Xing[1], Ji-Kang Min[1], Jian-Gang Shi[2] and Xiong-Sheng Chen[2]

Abstract

Background: Cervical ossification of the posterior longitudinal ligament (OPLL) is a progressive disease. Posterior decompression surgery is reported to be an effective and comparatively safe procedure with few complications for treatment of patients with myelopathy caused by OPLL. However, some patients require revision surgery because of late neurological deterioration due to OPLL progression or kyphotic changes in cervical alignment. This study reports preliminary clinical results of anterior controllable antidisplacement and fusion (ACAF), a novel revision surgery after initial posterior surgery for OPLL.

Methods: From January 2017 to June 2018, ten patients with cervical OPLL who underwent ACAF revision surgery after initial posterior surgery were included in this study. The mean age was 62.1 ± 8.0 years (52–78), and the mean interval between initial posterior surgery and revision was 78.0 ± 48.2 months (5–180). The Japanese Orthopaedic Association (JOA) scales, Neck Disability Index (NDI), visual analog scale (VAS), and surgical complications were recorded.

Results: The mean surgery time was 179.3 ± 41.8 min (120–240), and the mean blood loss was 432.5 ± 198.3 ml (225–850). The patients were followed up for at least 12 months. The JOA scores improved from 8.7 ± 2.8 to 13.4 ± 2.4; the mean improvement rate was $59.9\% \pm 16.1\%$. Postoperative NDI and VAS scores were 13.3 ± 3.7 and 2.0 ± 1.6, respectively, and were significantly improved compared to those before the procedure ($P < 0.05$). Cervical lordosis improved from $3.8 \pm 4.3°$ to $17 \pm 4.6°$ after revision surgery. There was only one instance of cerebrospinal fluid (CSF) leakage; no instances of postoperative hematoma, C5 root palsy, or hoarseness occurred.

Conclusions: The present study demonstrates that excellent postoperative outcomes can be achieved with the ACAF technique for revision treatment of OPLL. Though further study is required to confirm the conclusion, this novel technique has the potential to serve as an alternative surgical technique for revision treatment of OPLL.

Keywords: Cervical, Ossification of the posterior longitudinal ligament, Revision, Antidisplacement

---

* Correspondence: hd_lee2008@163.com
[1]Department of Spine Surgery, First People's Hospital affiliated to the Huzhou University Medical College, 158# GuangChang Hou Road, Huzhou, Zhejiang Province, China
Full list of author information is available at the end of the article

Background

Ossification of the posterior longitudinal ligament (OPLL) is frequently related to cervical myelopathy [1]. Minimally symptomatic patients can be treated conservatively; however, patients with progressive myelopathy require surgical treatment [2, 3]. Several options for treating cervical OPLL have been established involving anterior and posterior surgery. Anterior decompression surgery can directly decompress the cervical spinal cord by removing the ossified ligament and always results in better outcomes and neurological improvement [4, 5]. However, it is considered technically demanding and is associated with serious complications, such as intraoperative neural injury, symptomatic cerebrospinal fluid leakage (CSF), graft dislodgment, and adjacent segment disease [6, 7].

The two typical posterior methods, laminoplasty and laminectomy, are reported as comparatively safe procedures with few complications for the treatment of OPLL [8, 9]. They decompress the spinal cord indirectly, depending on the backward shift of the cervical spinal cord [10]. Long-term outcomes of posterior surgery seem to be favorable, although it is criticized for C5 nerve root palsy, progression of OPLL, and poor cervical lordosis [11, 12]. In cases with poor cervical lordosis or progressive OPLL lesion, neurological improvement is always diminished [8, 13]. Therefore, after cervical posterior surgery, some patients require revision surgery due to late neurological deterioration [14]. Revision surgery is challenging, perhaps because of a combination of progressive kyphosis, segmental instability, massive progressive OPLL, and dural ossification [15].

Sun et al. first described the anterior controllable antidisplacement and fusion (ACAF) technique for the treatment of multilevel severe ossification of the posterior longitudinal ligament with myelopathy [16]. The goal of ACAF is to isolate and "actively transport" residual osteophytes or ossification to restore the space of the spinal canal and thus achieve direct decompression of the neural elements with their location unchanged. The purpose of this study was to investigate the clinical results of ACAF as a revision surgery for cervical OPLL after initial posterior surgery.

Methods

Patient population

We conducted a retrospective study of ACAF as a revision surgery performed after initial posterior surgery for cervical myelopathy due to OPLL. From January 2017 to June 2018, ten patients who underwent ACAF revision surgery were identified and included in this study. Follow-up was conducted in all patients for at least 12 months. Patients with severe osteoporosis (WHO criteria), pre-existing spinal deformity, cervical spine trauma, spinal infection, or chronic systemic illness were excluded from the study. This study was approved by the Ethics Committee of the authors' affiliated institutions, and all the patients signed an informed consent document.

Radiographic assessment

Based on preoperative radiographic findings, OPLL of the cervical spine was classified into three types: continuous, segmental, or mixed [15]. The K-line connects the midpoints of the spinal canal at C2 and C7 on neutral lateral radiographs. When anterior compression of the OPLL exceeds this line, the K-line is defined as negative [16]. Cervical lordosis was measured as the angle between a line parallel to the posterior aspect of the C2 vertebral body and that of the C7 body. Patients were also evaluated radiographically with plain and dynamic cervical spinal radiographs at 3 and 6 months postoperatively and every 6 months thereafter. Pseudarthrosis was defined as an interspinous motion of > 1 mm on dynamic flexion-extension images.

Clinical assessment

The Japanese Orthopaedic Association (JOA) scores, visual analog score (VAS), and Neck Disability Index (NDI) were used to measure neck pain, arm pain, and the degree of disability. The improvement rate (IR) of neurologic function was calculated as IR = (postoperative JOA score – preoperative JOA score/17 – preoperative JOA score)/100%. The surgical outcome was defined using the IR as follows: excellent (IR ≥ 75%), good (75% > IR ≥ 50%), fair (50% > IR ≥ 25%), and poor (IR < 25%).

Surgical technique

After general endotracheal anesthesia, the patient was placed in a supine position appropriately padded under the shoulders and neck. Neurophysiologic monitoring, such as somatosensory-evoked potentials (SSEPs), was utilized to predict the neurologic deficit during the operation. The exposure was obtained through a Smith–Robinson approach on the right side. First, discectomies of the involved levels were performed. In the cephalad and caudal levels, the posterior longitudinal ligament was resected to facilitate later hoisting of the vertebrae-OPLL complex (VOC). Then, resection of the anterior vertebral bodies of the VOC was performed using a high-speed burr; third, the intervertebral cages and anterior cervical plate were installed. Fourth, bilateral troughs were created along the widest edge of the OPLL. We used a 2-mm high-speed burr to thin the corticocancellous bone first and 1-mm Kerrison rongeurs to remove the posterior vertebral wall on the bottom of the troughs. Finally, the VOC was hoisted by gradually tightening with screws. An illustration of the procedure is shown in Fig. 1. Autogenous bone pieces were grafted

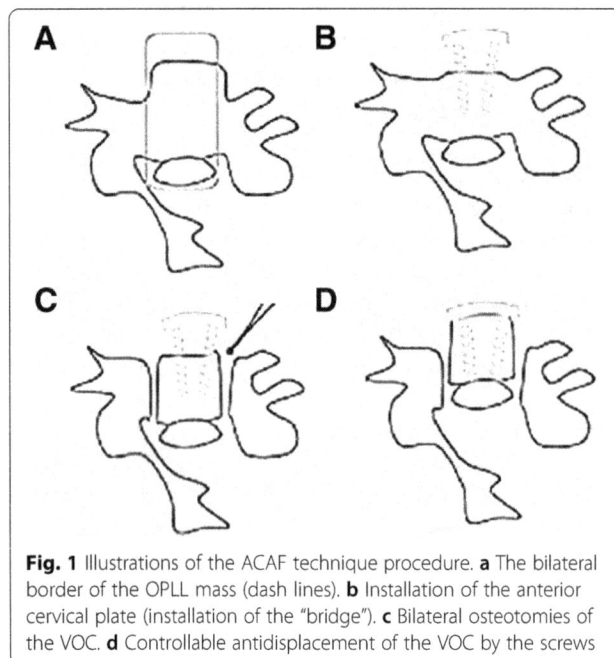

Fig. 1 Illustrations of the ACAF technique procedure. **a** The bilateral border of the OPLL mass (dash lines). **b** Installation of the anterior cervical plate (installation of the "bridge"). **c** Bilateral osteotomies of the VOC. **d** Controllable antidisplacement of the VOC by the screws

Table 1 Summary of patient demographics and the results of revision ACAF after initial posterior surgery for cervical OPLL

Variable	Value
Sex	
Male	6
Female	4
Age	62.1 ± 8.0 (52–78)
Previous pst op	
Laminectomy	4
Laminoplasty	4
Decompression	2
Mean interval btwn initial op and revision, months	78.0 ± 48.2 (5–180)
Type of the ossification	
Continuous	4
Segmental	3
Mixed	3
K-line	
Minus	6
Plus	4
Mean op time, min	179.3 ± 41.8 (120–240)
Mean blood loss, ml	432.5 ± 198.3 (225–850)
Complications, number of patients	
CSF leakage	1
C5 palsy	0
Postoperative hematoma	0
Implant complication	0

Pst posterior, *op* operation, *btwn* between
Values are expressed as the mean ± SD (range)

into the bilateral troughs to obtain further fusion. A hard cervical brace was routinely used postoperatively for 3 months.

Statistical analysis

Statistical analysis was performed using SPSS 16.0. Preoperative and postoperative data such as JOA, VAS, and NDI scores were compared using paired t tests. The level of significance was set at $P < 0.05$.

Results

The patient demographic data are shown in Table 1. According to physical and radiological findings just before revision surgery, we considered the major reasons for neurological deterioration to be anterior spinal cord compression due to residual OPLL progression and local kyphosis.

Clinical and radiographic results

The mean operative time in this group was 179 min (range 120–240 min). The mean intraoperative blood loss was 432 ml (range 225–850 ml). The mean JOA score was 8.7 ± 2.8 (range 5–14) preoperatively and 13.4 ± 2.4 (range 9–16) after the ACAF surgery ($P < 0.05$). The average IR was 59.9 ± 16.1%. Two (20%) patients were graded as excellent, six (60%) as good, and two (20%) as fair. The mean VAS score decreased from 4.5 ± 1.6 (range 2–7) preoperatively to 2.0 ± 1.6 (range 0–5) ($P < 0.05$). The NDI decreased from 24.4 ± 10.0 (range 10–40) at the preoperative assessment to 13.3 ± 3.7 (range 8–20) ($P < 0.05$). The postoperative cervical lordosis was 17 ± 4.6°, which was much better than it was

before. No patients demonstrated a progression of kyphotic deformity at subsequent follow-ups (all results are shown in Table 2). Images of typical cases are shown in Figs. 2 and 3.

Complication

There was only one case of intraoperative CSF leakage. The leakage happened when the posterior longitudinal ligament of the cephalad level was resected. Fortunately, it was a small hole and was healed using a sponge and elastic bandage. There were no occurrences of postoperative hematoma or C5 root palsy. No instrument failure was observed during the follow-up.

Discussion

The gold standard surgical treatment for cervical myelopathy caused by OPLL remains controversial. The choice of surgical method for initial or revision surgery should depend on the location of spinal cord compression, the sagittal alignment of the cervical spine, and the general health status of the patient [17, 18].

Table 2 Clinical and radiological results of patients

Item	Value
JOA	
Before surgery	8.7 ± 2.8 (5–14)
After surgery	13.4 ± 2.4 (9–16)*
NDI	
Before surgery	24.4 ± 10.0 (10–40)
After surgery	13.3 ± 3.7 (8–20)*
VAS	
Before surgery	4.5 ± 1.6 (2–7)
After surgery	2.0 ± 1.6 (0–5)*
Cervical lordosis (°)	
Before surgery	3.8 ± 4.3 (− 7.6 to − 15)
After surgery	17 ± 4.6 (16 to 27)*

JOA Japanese Orthopaedic Association scores, VAS visual analog score, NDI Neck Disability Index
Values are expressed as the mean ± SD (range)
*$P < 0.05$, compared with the data before surgery

The posterior procedure is relatively simple and with low complication rates, and it has been widely used as an initial surgery for cervical OPLL [15]. Though the results of the posterior surgery depend on the backward shift of the cervical spinal cord [5], it has been shown to have the same excellent results as anterior decompression surgery [19, 20]. Relief of symptoms or prevention of symptom progression has been achieved in most patients after surgical decompression of cervical OPLL. However, some patients need revision surgery because of late neurological deterioration [21, 22]. There are two explanations for late deterioration. First, the loss of cervical lordosis or even development of kyphosis is not uncommon after posterior surgery [23, 24]. Second, OPLL tends to progress more often after cervical laminoplasty or laminectomy than it does after anterior decompression surgery [22, 25]. The frequency of OPLL progression has been reported to be as high as 70% [26]. And the mean annual rate of lesion increase was reported as about 3.33% [27].

When considering revision surgery for patients who have already received posterior decompression surgery, it is impossible to again perform decompression from the posterior aspect. Anterior cervical corpectomy and fusion may be a good choice; however, it is considered technically demanding and is associated with serious complications, such as intraoperative spinal cord injury, symptomatic CSF leakage, adjacent segment disease, and graft dislodgment [5]. Macdonald et al. reported that multilevel anterior cervical corpectomy and fusion carries an approximately 22% risk of surgical mortality and morbidity, including pneumonia, deep vein thrombosis,

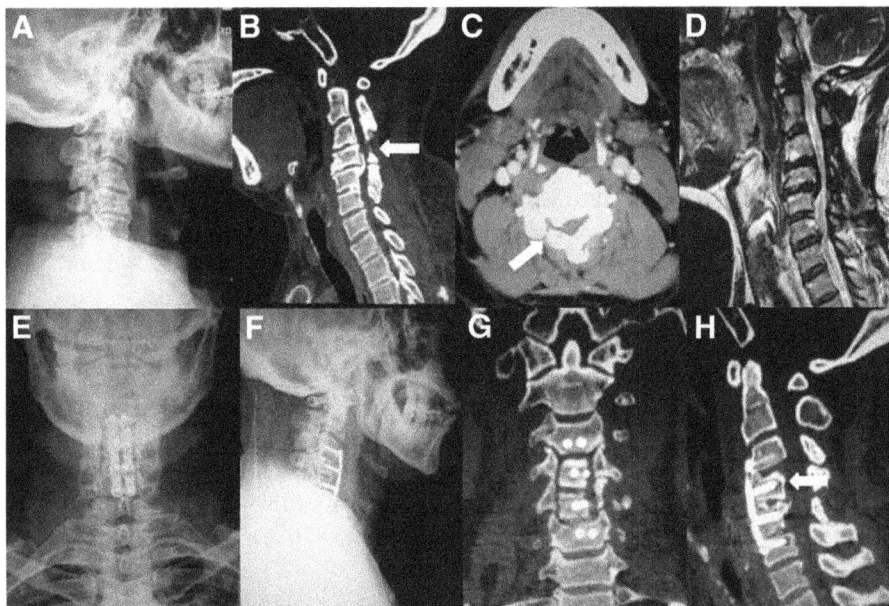

Fig. 2 A revision case of a 59-year-old man 5 years after initial posterior decompression surgery. **a** The lateral image showed that cervical kyphosis occurred after the initial posterior surgery. **b, c** The CT scan showed that there was only a window decompressing without fixation in the initial posterior surgery (arrows). **d** The MRI showed that the cervical spinal cord of C4–5 was compressed by the OPLL. **e, f** The postoperative anterior–posterior and lateral images showed good device positioning and persistent poor cervical lordosis. **g, h** The postoperative CT scan showed that the bilateral troughs were created along the widest edge of the OPLL, and we hoisted the VOC by the screws (arrows). We usually used a 2-mm high-speed cutting burr and 1-mm Kerrison rongeurs to remove the posterior vertebral wall on the bottom of the troughs

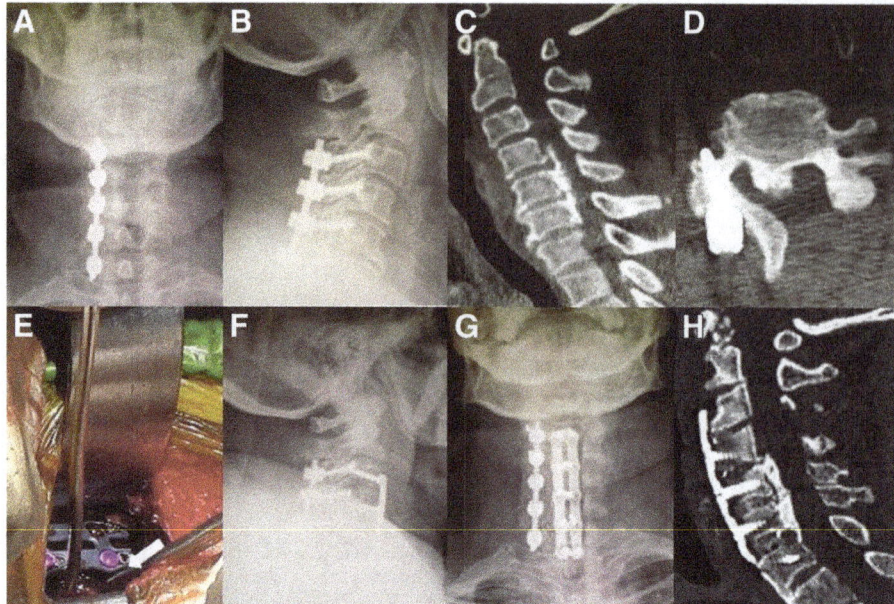

Fig. 3 A revision case of a 61-year-old man 12 months after initial posterior laminectomy. **a, b** The anterior–posterior and lateral images showed the loss of cervical lordosis after the initial laminectomy. **c, d** The CT scan showed that there was a continuous type of OPLL, and only a semilaminectomy with one-sided lateral mass fixation was done in the initial surgery. **e** The intraoperative photo showed that after installation of the intervertebral cages and anterior cervical plate, we used 1-mm Kerrison rongeurs to remove the posterior vertebral wall on the bottom of the troughs for isolation of the VOC (arrows). **f, g** The postoperative anterior–posterior and lateral images showed good internal fixation position and improved cervical lordosis. **h** The CT scan showed that the VOC was hoisted forward, and the cervical spinal canal was obviously wider than it was before

and death [28]. Odate et al. suggested that the use of anterior compression revision surgery for OPLL must be limited due to the high probability of intraoperative CSF leakage and extremely low improvement rate [15]. In their study, surgery-related complications occurred in 63% of patients, the main complication being intraoperative CSF leakage (42%), and the mean improvement rate of the JOA score was only 18%. To minimize the surgical risk of CSF leakage, hemorrhage, and spinal cord injury, Yamaura et al. reported the floating method for the treatment of cervical myelopathy due to OPLL [29]. However, the anterior migration of the OPLL in the floating method is not controlled by the surgeon and owes much to the pressure of the CSF, and approximately 14% of the cases showed inadequate decompression of the spinal canal due to residual ossification with or without postoperative progression of OPLL.

In our study, we used a novel technique called ACAF as the revision surgery for OPLL. It can isolate and actively transport the OPLL ventrally to restore the space of the spinal canal and thus achieve direct decompression of the neural elements with their location unchanged. In contrast to the floating method, the antidisplacement of the OPLL is achieved by the gradual hoisting force of the anterior plate and screws, with immediate feedback. The anatomical basis for the clinical effect of these cases lies in the direct decompression of

the spinal cord and nerve roots. Bilateral osteotomies of the vertebrae with a width of 18 mm give enough decompression to the bilateral nerve roots. In this study, the mean improvement rate of the JOA scores was 59.9%. There was only one surgery-related complication (10%) in the study patients. In that case, there was severe adhesion between the dura mater and the ossified posterior longitudinal ligament, and the CSF leak happened when resecting the posterior longitudinal ligament of the cephalad level. Fortunately, it was healed by a sponge and elastic bandage.

Limitation

This study was only a retrospective study with a small sample size to explore a new revision method for multilevel cervical OPLL after initial posterior surgery. Prospective multiple-center studies, long-term data, and a control group are needed to confirm the result.

Conclusion

The present study demonstrates that excellent postoperative outcomes can be achieved with the use of ACAF. Though further study is required to confirm the conclusion, this novel technique has the potential to serve as an alternative revision technique for cervical OPLL after initial posterior surgery.

Acknowledgements

We express deep thanks to Dr. Jian-Gang Shi and Xiong-Sheng Chen for their technical support.

Authors' contributions

HDL had full access to all of the data in the study and took responsibility for the integrity of the data and the accuracy of the data analysis. All authors meet all three of the requirements for authorship. QHZ, STX, and JKM were highly involved in the planning and execution of this study. Furthermore, JGS and XSC were highly involved in the acquisition of data and in the process of data interpretation. All authors read and approved the final manuscript.

Competing interests

The authors declare that they have no competing interests.

Author details

[1]Department of Spine Surgery, First People's Hospital affiliated to the Huzhou University Medical College, 158# GuangChang Hou Road, Huzhou, Zhejiang Province, China. [2]Department of Spine Surgery, Changzheng Hospital, 415# Fengyang Road, Huangpu District, Shanghai, China.

References

1. Matsunaga S, Sakou T. Ossification of the posterior longitudinal ligament of the cervical spine: etiology and natural history. Spine. 2012;37:E309–14.
2. Iwasaki M, Okuda S, Miyauchi A, Sakaura H, Mukai Y, Younenobu K, Yoshikawa H. Surgical strategy for cervical myelopathy due to ossification of the posterior longitudinal ligament: part I: clinical results and limitations of laminoplasty. Spine (Phila Pa 1976). 2007;32:647–53.
3. Iwasaki M, Okuda S, Miyauchi A, Sakaura H, Mukai Y, Younenobu K, Yoshikawa H. Surgical strategy for cervical myelopathy due to ossification of the posterior longitudinal ligament. Part 2: advantages of anterior decompression and fusion over laminoplasty. Spine (Phila Pa 1976). 2007;32:654–60.
4. Kim B, Yoon DH, Shin HC, Kim KN, Yi S, Shin DA, Ha Y. Surgical outcome and prognostic factors of anterior decompression and fusion for cervical compressive myelopathy due to ossification of the posterior longitudinal ligament. Spine J. 2015;15:875–84.
5. Wang S, Xiang Y, Wang X, Li H, Hou Y, Zhao H, Pan X. Anterior corpectomy comparing to posterior decompression surgery for the treatment of multilevel ossification of posterior longitudinal ligament: a meta-analysis. Int J Surg. 2017;40:91–6.
6. Tani T, Ushida T, Ishida K, Iai H, Noguchi T, Yamamoto H. Relative safety of anterior microsurgical decompression versus laminoplasty for cervical myelopathy with a massive ossified posterior longitudinal ligament. Spine (Phila Pa 1976). 2002;27:2491–8.
7. Liu T, Xu W, Chen T, Yang HL. Anterior versus posterior surgery for multilevel cervical myelopathy, which one is better? A systematic review. Eur Spine J. 2011;20:224–35.
8. Iwasaki M, Kawaguchi Y, Kimura T, Yonenobu K. Long-term results of expansive laminoplasty for ossification of the posterior longitudinal ligament of the cervical spine: more than 10 years follow up. J Neurosurg. 2002;96(2 Suppl):180–9.
9. Lee SE, Chung CK, Jahng TA, Kim HJ. Long-term outcome of laminectomy for cervical ossification of the posterior longitudinal ligament. J Neurosurg Spine. 2013;18:465–71.
10. Quinn JC, Kiely PD, Lebl DR, Hughes AP. Anterior surgical treatment of cervical spondylotic myelopathy: review article. HSS J. 2015;11:15–25.
11. Chen Y, Chen D, Wang X, Guo Y, He Z. C5 palsy after laminectomy and posterior cervical fixation for ossification of posterior longitudinal ligament. J Spinal Disord Tech. 2007;20:533–5.
12. Lee CK, Shin DA, Yi S, Kim KN, Shin HC, Yoon DH, Ha Y. Correlation between cervical spine sagittal alignment and clinical outcome after cervical laminoplasty for ossification of posterior longitudinal ligament. J Neurosurg Spine. 2016;24:100–7.
13. Hirabayashi M, Watanabe K, Wakano K, Suzuki N, Satomi K, Ishii Y. Expansive open-door laminoplasty for cervical spinal stenotic myelopathy. Spine (Phila Pa 1976). 1983;8:693–9.
14. Tokuhashi Y, Ajiro Y, Umezawa N. A patient with two re-surgeries for delayed myelopathy due to progression of ossification of the posterior longitudinal ligaments after cervical laminoplasty. Spine (Phila Pa 1976). 2009;34:E101–5.
15. Odate S, Shikata J, Soeda S, Yamamura S, Kawaguchi S. Surgical results and complications of anterior decompression and fusion as a revision surgery after initial posterior surgery for cervical myelopathy due to ossification of the posterior longitudinal ligament. J Neurosurg Spine. 2017;26:466–73.
16. Sun J, Shi J, Xu X, Yang Y, Wang Y, Kong Q, Yang H, Guo Y, Han D, Jiang J, Shi G, Yuan W, Jia L. Anterior controllable antidisplacement and fusion surgery for the treatment of multilevel severe ossification of the posterior longitudinal ligament with myelopathy: preliminary clinical results of a novel technique. Eur Spine J. 2018;27(6):1469–78.
17. Fujimori T, Iwasaki M, Okuda S, Takenaka S, Kashii M, Kaito T, Yoshikawa H. Long-term results of cervical myelopathy due to ossification of the posterior longitudinal ligament with an occupying ratio of 60% or more. Spine (Phila Pa 1976). 2014;39:58–67.
18. Fujimori T, Le H, Ziewacz JE, Chou D, Mummaneni PV. Is there a difference in range of motion, neck, and outcomes in patients with ossification of posterior longitudinal ligament versus those with cervical spondylosis, treated with plated laminoplasty? Neurosurg Focus. 2013;35:E9.
19. Katsumi K, Izumi T, Ito T, Hirano T, Watanabe H, Ohashi M. Posterior instrumented fusion suppressed the progression of ossification of the posterior longitudinal ligament: a comparison of laminoplasty with and without instrumented fusion by three-dimensional analysis. Eur Spine J. 2016;25:1634–40.
20. Chiba K, Ogawa Y, Ishii K, Takaishi H, Nakamura M, Maruiwa H, Matsumoto M, Toyama Y. Long-term results of expansive open-door laminectomy for cervical myelopathy-average 14-year follow-up study. Spine (Phila Pa 1976). 2006;31:2998–3005.
21. Matsumoto M, Chiba K, Toyama Y. Surgical treatment of ossification of posterior longitudinal ligament and its outcomes: posterior surgery by laminoplasty. Spine (Phila Pa 1976). 2012;37:E303–8.
22. Sakai K, Okawa A, Takahashi M, Arai Y, Kawabata S, Enomoto M, Kato T, Hirai T, Shinomiya K. Five-year follow-up evaluation of surgical treatment for cervical myelopathy caused by ossification of posterior longitudinal ligament: a prospective comparative study of anterior decompression and fusion with floating method versus laminoplasty. Spine (Phila Pa 1976). 2012;37:367–76.
23. Liu H, Li Y, Chen Y, Wu W, Zou D. Cervical curvature, spinal cord MRIT2 signal, and occupying ratio impact surgical approach selection in patients with ossification of the posterior longitudinal ligament. Eur Spine J. 2013;22:1480–8.
24. Lee CH, Jahng TA, Hyun SJ, Kim KJ, Kim HJ. Expansive laminoplasty versus laminectomy alone versus laminectomy and fusion for cervical ossification of the posterior longitudinal ligament: is there a difference in the clinical outcome and sagittal alignment? Clin Spine Surg. 2016; 29:E9–E15.
25. Lee CH, Sohn MJ, Lee CH, Choi CY, Han SR, Choi BW. Are there differences in the progression of ossification of the posterior longitudinal ligament following laminoplasty versus fusion?: a meta-analysis. Spine (Phila Pa 1976). 2017;42:887–94.
26. Kalb S, Martirosyan NL, Perez-Orribo L, Kalani MY, Theodore N. Analysis of demographic, risk factor, presentation, and surgical treatment modalities for ossified posterior longitudinal ligament. Neurosurg Focus. 2011;30:E11.
27. Izumi T, Hirano T, Watanabe K, Sano A, Ito T, Endo N. Three-dimensional evaluation of volume change in ossification of the posterior longitudinal ligament of the cervical spine using computed tomography. Eur Spine J. 2013;22:2569–74.
28. Macdonald RL, Fehlings MG, Tator CH, Lozano A, Fleming JR, Gentili F, Berstein M, Wallace MC, Tasker RR. Multilevel anterior cervical corpectomy and fibular allograft fusion for cervical myelopathy. J Neurosurg. 1997;86:990–7.
29. Yamaura I, Kurosa Y, Matuoka T, Shido S. Anterior floating method for cervical myelopathy caused by ossification of the posterior longitudinal ligament. Clin Orthop Related Res. 1999:27–34.

8

Five-year outcomes of posterior affected-vertebrae fixation in lumbar tuberculosis patients

Qiang Liang[1†], Qian Wang[2†], Guangwei Sun[1], Wenxin Ma[1], Jiandang Shi[1], Weidong Jin[1], Shiyuan Shi[3*] and Zili Wang[1,2*]

Abstract

Background: Posterior instrumentation after deformity correction is an important method for reconstruction of spinal stability in the management of lumbar tuberculosis (TB). However, the commonly used methods include both long- and short-segment fixation of normal motor units. There has been no report regarding affected-vertebrae fixation of lumbar TB.

Methods: Data from 135 patients with lumbar TB who underwent posterior instrumentation and either affected-vertebrae fixation or short-segment fixation using a combined posterior and anterior approach were retrospectively reviewed. Among these patients, 71 cases were treated with affected-vertebrae fixation, and 64 cases were treated with short-segment fixation. Debridement, bone grafting, deformity correction, and decompression were performed within all affected segments. Operative times, intra-operative blood loss, TB cure rates, bone graft fusion rates, degree of deformity correction, neurological function, pain recovery, and complications were analyzed.

Results: Comparing affected-vertebrae fixation vs. short-segment fixation groups, respectively, the number of the affected segments was 107 vs. 98; average number of affected segments was 1.51 vs. 1.53; total number of fixed segments was 107 vs. 226; average number of fixed segments was 1.51 vs. 3.53; average blood loss was 726.2 ml vs. 948.5 ml; average operative time was 210.4 min vs. 270.3 min; and average hospitalization costs were 29,000 RMB vs. 42,000 RMB (all p values < 0.05). In the affected-vertebrae fixation vs. short-segment fixation groups, respectively, TB cure rates were 82.61% vs. 84.62% at 6 months after operation and 97.83% vs. 97.44% at 5 years after operation; bone fusion rates were 86.96% vs. 87.18% at 6 months after operation and 97.83% vs. 97.66% at 5 years after operation; average number of degrees of Cobb's angle correction were 13.1° vs. 13.7°; average correction losses were 1.9° vs. 1.4°; and complication rates were 12.04% vs. 12.97% (all p values > 0.05).

Conclusion: Under strict surgical indications, posterior instrumentation on affected-vertebrae is a safe, effective, and feasible fixation method in the treatment of lumber TB.

Keywords: Lumbar spinal tuberculosis, Affected-vertebrae fixation, Combined posterior and anterior approach

* Correspondence: ssyif@sina.com; wangzlnx@126.com
†Qiang Liang and Qian Wang contributed equally to this work.
[3]Department of Orthopedics, Hospital of Integrated Traditional Chinese and Western Medicine in Zhejiang Province, Hangzhou 310003, Zhejiang, China
[1]Department of Spinal Surgery, General Hospital of Ningxia Medical University, 804 Shengli Street, Yinchuan 750004, China
Full list of author information is available at the end of the article

Background

Lumbar tuberculosis (TB) accounts for approximately 50% of spinal TB. Since spinal TB can lead to deformity and neurological dysfunction in serious cases, surgery is necessary for these patients [1, 2]. Internal fixation using instrumentation is an important method of reconstructing the stability of the spine in the surgical management of spinal TB [3, 4]. Common internal fixation methods include long-segment fixation (involving two or more normal motor units superior to the affected vertebrae and two or more normal units inferior to it) and short-segment fixation (involving one normal motor unit superior to the affected vertebrae and one motor unit inferior to it) [5–7]. Although both long-segment and short-segment can restore the normal structure of the spine and maintain the correction effectively, the relatively long stretch of the fixed segments not only causes the normal motor units to lose motor function resulting in stiffness of the related segments, but also accelerates degeneration of adjacent segments [8].

In order to solve this problem, instrumentation of the affected vertebrae was proposed, which means that complete debridement [9] was performed within the affected motor units; the screws were placed into the pedicle and centrum of the affected vertebrae, the strut bone graft placed in the interval between the affected vertebrae, and decompression and deformity correction were being carried out within the interval between the affected vertebrae. The above-mentioned surgical procedure (termed affected-vertebra fixation) is performed within the affected motor units while the normal motor units are not involved, which maximally preserves motor function of the spine. However, there has been no report concerning the treatment of lumbar TB using this procedure.

A retrospective study comparing affected-vertebra fixation vs. short-segment fixation in the treatment of lumbar TB was performed with the aim to explore the feasibility of affected-vertebrae fixation and to summarize its technical points.

Methods

Patient data

The study protocol was approved by the Ethics Committee of the General Hospital of Ningxia Medical University and written informed consent was obtained from every subject. The present study included 135 patients with lumbar TB who underwent affected-vertebra fixation or short-segment fixation in our department between March 2007 and March 2013. Patients were selected if the three dimensional CT showed the upper and lower end plates of the affected vertebrae are intact, so as could provide a reliable host bed for the strut bone graft. Patients were excluded if they had severe kyphosis deformity (> 60°) and

could not be corrected by changing the patient's position using manual techniques and instrument application, the pedicle of vertebra had been invaded by TB, or the patients had severe osteoporosis.

Surgical indications were as follows: (1) patients with neurological dysfunction caused by spinal cord or cauda equina compression; (2) patients with spinal instability and kyphosis; (3) patients with a relatively large abscess, sequestrum, or prolonged healing of a sinus tract; and (4) patients cannot tolerate the pain caused by the lesions of lumbar tuberculosis. Patients were diagnosed with instability preoperatively when the patients meet one or more of these criterions: (1) the vertebral body was invaded by tuberculosis and the height of vertebral destruction was more than one third of the original vertebral body height; (2) vertebral spatial displacement > 3 mm; (3) lumbar kyphosis angle $> 10°$; (4) rotational displacement: L1,2; L2,3; L3,4 $> 15°$; L4,5 $> 20°$; L5, S1 $> 25°$.

All patients underwent complete debridement, bone grafting and fusion, decompression, and deformity correction within the affected segments. According to the various fixation methods, patients were divided into two groups: (1) the affected-vertebrae fixation group ($n = 71$), in which internal fixation was carried out within the affected motor units; and (2) the short-segment fixation group ($n = 64$), in which the fixation included the affected vertebrae together with one normal motor unit superior to the affected vertebrae and one inferior to it. Patient demographic and baseline variables are shown in Table 1.

In this article, the application situations of the two internal fixation methods were very similar. According to the inclusive and exclusive criteria, all cases included in this study (either of the affected-vertebrae fixation group or of the short-segment fixation group) can be treated with affected-vertebrae fixation. For patients who must undergo short-segment fixation, they were excluded according to the inclusion and exclusion criteria. Because the theory and technology of affected-vertebrae fixation were not quite developed before 2010 (during the early stage of the study), we performed short-segment fixation on some patients, even though they could have met the indications of affected-vertebrae fixation. In this article, we included these cases in short-segment fixation group as a control group to evaluate the efficacy of affected-vertebrae fixation. After we have confirmed that the affected-vertebrae fixation was a safe, effective, and feasible surgical procedure through our earlier research, the affected-vertebrae fixation was implemented more often in the latter period of the study (after 2010).

Preoperative preparation

After admission, patients were placed on strict bed rest and supportive treatment was performed. For preoperative anti-tuberculosis treatment, isoniazid (INH, H, 5 mg/kg/d),

Table 1 Preoperative patient characteristics in the two groups

Items	Affected-vertebrae fixation group	Short-segment fixation group	p values
Patients	71	64	
Gender m/f	32/39	31/33	p = 0.695
Age ($\bar{x}\pm s$, years)	41.7 ± 21.7	43.5 ± 19.6	p = 0.738
Disease duration ($\bar{x}\pm s$, months)	8.3 ± 4.1	7.6 ± 4.7	p = 0.257
Clinical manifestations			
Back pain	63	58	p = 0.719
Low-grade fever	52	46	p = 0.859
Night sweating	61	53	p = 0.619
Weakness	55	48	p = 0.737
Formation of cold abscess	32	29	p = 0.977
Lesion location			
L1–2	6	8	p = 0.880
L2–3	11	13	
L3–4	13	10	
L4–5	18	16	
L1–3	9	4	
L2–4	2	3	
L3–5	6	4	
L1–4	1	2	
L2–5	3	1	
L1–2 + L4–5	2	3	
Number of the affected segments			
Single segment	54	47	p = 0.903
Double segments	13	14	
Triple segments	4	3	
Cobb's angle ($\bar{x}\pm s$, °)	24.8 ± 15.2	26.2 ± 14.1	p = 0.735
CRP ($\bar{x}\pm s$, mg/l)	27.0 ± 24.9	25.8 ± 22.3	p = 0.718
ESR ($\bar{x}\pm s$, mm/h)	36.5 ± 22.5	40.4 ± 20.1	p = 0.349

rifampicin (RFP, R, 10 mg/kg/d), pyrazinamide (PZA, Z, 20 mg/kg/d), and streptomycin (SM, S, 20 mg/kg/d) were administered for 2–4 weeks (average, 2.3 weeks). Liver function and kidney function were monitored, including liver and kidney damage being managed promptly. After the patient's general condition had improved, surgery was carried out. A feasible surgical plan was developed for each patient according to the imaging data from CT, MRI, and ultrasonography.

Surgical procedures

All patients underwent combined posterior-anterior surgery. Posterior pedicle screw fixation, deformity correction, and posterolateral bone grafting were carried out first and then complete anterior debridement, decompression, and strut bone grafting were performed.

Surgical procedure in the affected-vertebrae fixation group

In affected-vertebrae fixation, after general anesthesia, the posterior midline approach was applied. The posterior structures of the affected segments (of the spine) were exposed by dissecting the erector spinae. Pedicle screws were placed into the pedicle of the affected vertebrae, and deformity correction was carried out using the patient's position, manual technique, and instrument application. The principle of affected-vertebrae fixation was as follows: routine pedicle screws were placed in the affected vertebrae if the residual heights of the affected vertebrae were more than one third after debridement; short pedicle screws 25–35 mm in length were inserted if the destruction of the affected vertebrae was severe; and residual heights of the affected vertebrae were less than one third after debridement, because routine pedicle screws could not be placed. A cross bar was used for all patients to increase stability. After internal fixation, posterolateral autogenous bone grafting and fusion was applied. The posterior incision was closed after surgery via the posterior approach. Thereafter, an anterior kidney incision or a "V" incision was made use to expose the affected vertebrae via the retroperitoneal approach, and complete debridement, autologous iliac bone grafting, and anterolateral decompression were carried out. The anterior and posterior surgeries were performed at the same time or separately according to the patient's condition (Fig. 1). In the present study, 59 out of 71 patients underwent one-stage surgery, and 12 patients underwent two-stage surgery.

Surgical procedure in the short-segment fixation group

The surgical approach and basic steps of short-segment fixation were the same as those of the affected-vertebrae fixation. The only difference between the two procedures involved is the placement of the pedicle screws, which were not only placed in the affected vertebrae, but also inserted in the normal motor units (superior and inferior to the affected vertebrae, one for each side) in short-segment fixation. A cross bar was also used for all patients to increase stability. However, posterolateral bone grafting and anterior strut bone grafting were the same as those of affected-vertebrae fixation (Fig. 2). In the short-segment fixation group, 45 out of 64 patients underwent one-stage surgery, and 19 patients underwent two-stage surgery.

Postoperative treatment and follow-up

A drainage tube was placed in the surgical wound under negative pressure, and the tube was removed when the volume of drainage was < 20 ml per day. The patient was placed on bed rest for 2–3 weeks after surgery and then ambulating with orthosis was started. Waist flexion, overextension, lateral bending, and rotation were avoided

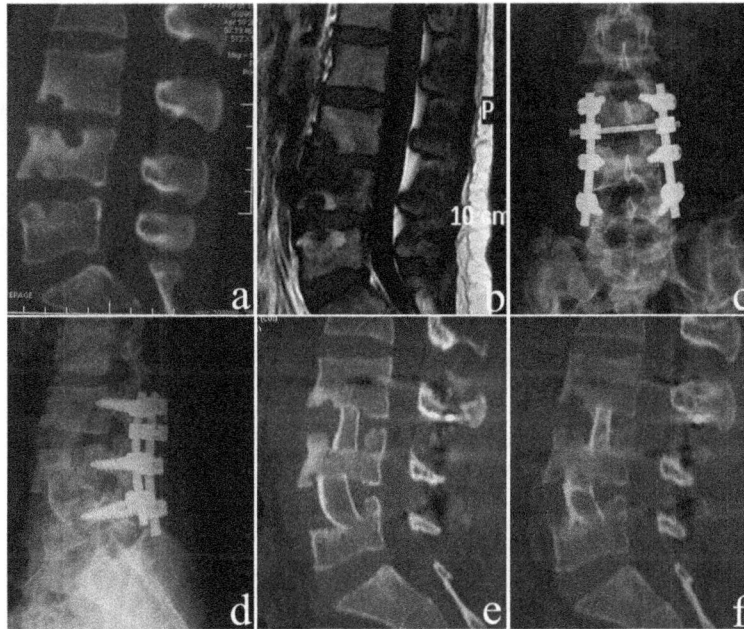

Fig. 1 A 34-year-old female patient underwent anterior-posterior surgery and affected-vertebrae fixation. **a** The preoperative sagittal CT reconstruction image shows destruction of L3, L4, and L5 vertebrae and narrowing of the L3-L4 intervertebral space. **b** The preoperative sagittal contrast-enhanced MRI shows destruction of L3, L4, and L5 vertebrae and destruction of the L3-L4 and L4-L5 intervertebral disks. **c, d** One month after surgery, the anteroposterior and lateral X-ray images show that the fixation of the affected vertebrae is excellent. L3 and L4 vertebras are fixed with short pedicle screws. **e** Three months after surgery, the sagittal CT reconstruction shows that the lesion in the L3, L4, and L5 vertebrae has debrided completely, and the iliac bone grafts are firm. **f** Five years after surgery, the sagittal CT reconstruction shows that the L3–5 tuberculosis lesions are cured, and the bone graft fusion is solid

before bone graft fusion. A 2HRZS/2-xHRZ regimen was used for chemotherapy; the duration of intensive chemotherapy was 2 months and that of consolidation chemotherapy was 2–7 months [10, 11]. Both the patient's follow-up and chemotherapy management were performed by a specifically assigned doctor. For the 6 months after surgery, each patient visited our hospital once every month, and from 6 months to 5 years after surgery, the patient visited the hospital once a year. Follow-up included medical history and physical exam, erythrocyte sedimentation rate (ESR), C-reactive protein level, liver function panel, renal function panel, X-rays, CT reconstruction, MRI, and ultrasonography. When these indicators normalized, the healing of the lesion was determined based on the imaging findings, and a decision regarding drug withdrawal was made.

We used the Cobb's angle to evaluate the sagittal deformity of spinal tuberculosis. The Cobb's angle was measured by drawing lines along the uppermost and lowermost endplate of the affected segment in lateral radiograph. An initial halo sign (radiolucent line around the implant > 1 mm wide) followed by a double halo sign on later radiographs or CT scans was defined as screw loosening. Bone graft fusion was determined based on a three-dimensional CT reconstruction using the following parameters: no displacement or tilting of the bone graft, no absorption or hardening of the boundary

between the bone graft and the host bed, the bone graft was in close contact with the graft bed, and there was trabecular bone formation, bone bridge connection, and reshaping in the blurred boundary. Standards used to determine the healing of spinal TB included an excellent general condition of the patient, lack of local pain or tenderness, no cold abscess or sinus formation, ESR and CRP levels which were continuously normal, and imaging which the data showed complete bone graft fusion without new TB lesions.

Statistical analysis

Statistical analysis was performed using the SPSS 22.0 (SPSS, USA) statistical software package. Differences in age, follow-up time, VAS (visual analogue scale) score, volume of blood loss, operative time, hospitalization cost, CRP, ESR, and Cobb's angle between the two groups were compared using the Student's t test (data conformed to normal distribution by Shapiro-Wilk test) or non-parametric test (data not conformed to normal distribution by Shapiro-Wilk test). Gender, clinical symptoms, the number of affected segments, the number of fixed segments, bone graft fusion rate, the rate of TB healing, and the incidence of complications were compared by χ^2 test. A statistical significance level of 0.05 was adopted.

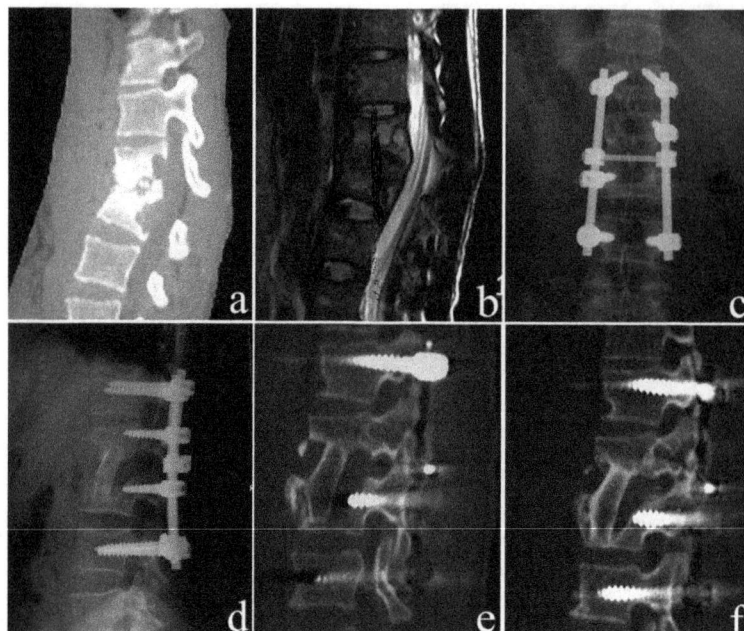

Fig. 2 A 25-year-old male who underwent anterior-posterior surgery and short-segment fixation. **a** Preoperative sagittal CT reconstruction shows destruction of L2 and L3 vertebrae and narrowing of the L2-L3 intervertebral space. **b**. The preoperative sagittal contrast-enhanced MRI shows confounding signals in L2 and L3 vertebrae, destruction of the L2-L3 intervertebral space, and nerve compression. **c**, **d** Postoperative X-ray anteroposterior image shows that the strut bone is located firmly between the affected vertebrae, the short-segment fixation is excellent, and the L2 and L3 vertebrae are fixed with short pedicle screws. **e** Three months after surgery, the sagittal CT reconstruction shows that the lesion of L2 and L3 vertebrae is removed completely, and the strut bone is located firmly. **f** Five years after surgery, the sagittal CT reconstruction shows healing of L2 and L3 tuberculosis lesions and bone graft fusion

Results

All patients were followed up for more than 5 years. The average intraoperative blood loss of the affected-vertebrae fixation group vs. short-segment fixation group, respectively, was 726.2 ml vs. 948.5 ml ($t = -18.57$, $p = 0.000$), average operative time was 210.4 min vs. 270.3 min ($t = -7.94$, $p = 0.000$), and average hospitalization cost was 29,000 RMB vs. 42,000 RMB ($t = -2.65$, $p = 0.009$) (Table 2).

In the affected-vertebrae fixation group vs. short-segment fixation group, respectively, the total number of affected segments was 107 vs. 98, average number of affected segments was 1.51 vs. 1.53, total number of fixed segments was 107 vs. 226, and average number of fixed segments was 1.51 vs. 3.53 in each case. The fixed segments of the affected-vertebrae fixation group were 2.02 segments less than those of the short-segment fixation group in each case. In the affected-vertebrae fixation group vs. short-segment fixation group, respectively, the average number of degrees of Cobb's angle correction was 13.1° vs. 13.3°, while the mean correction loss was 1.9° vs. 1.4°, ($p > 0.05$) (Table 3). At the last follow-up, the TB healing rates and bone graft fusion rates were > 98% in the two groups (Table 4), and the differences were not significant. Six months after surgery, ESR and CRP were reduced to normal levels in both groups (Table 5).

In the affected-vertebrae fixation group vs. short-segment fixation group, respectively, average preoperative VAS score (visual analogue scale pain score) was 7 (range, 6–8) vs. 6.5 (range, 5–8), while the average score at the last follow-up was 1 (range, 0–2) vs. 1.5 (range, 1–3). The neural function of both groups improved significantly after surgery, and the outcomes were satisfactory (Table 6). In the affected-vertebrae fixation group vs. short-segment fixation group, respectively, the preoperative JOA (JOA = Japanese Orthopedic Association)

Table 2 Operative time, intraoperative blood loss, and hospitalization cost in the affected-vertebrae fixation group and short-segment fixation group ($\bar{x}\pm s$)

Groups	Number of patients	Operation time (min)	Intraoperative blood loss (ml)	Hospitalization cost (10,000 RMB)
Affected-vertebrae fixation group	71	210.4 ± 36.8	726.2 ± 60.3	2.9 ± 2.6
95% CI		201.8 to 219.0	712.2 to 740.2	2.3 to 3.5
Short-segment fixation group	64	270.3 ± 50.4	948.5 ± 78.4	4.2 ± 3.1
95% CI		257.9 to 282.7	929.3 to 967.7	3.4 to 5.0
p value		0.000	0.000	0.006

Table 3 Postoperative recovery of Cobb's angle in the affected-vertebrae fixation group and short-segment fixation group ($\bar{x}\pm s$)

Groups	No. of patients	Before operation (°)	After operation (°)	Last follow-up (°)	Correction (°)	Loss (°)
Affected-vertebrae fixation group	71	24.8 ± 15.2	8.9 ± 3.5	10.8 ± 3.8	15.9 ± 10.2	1.9 ± 0.6
95% CI		21.3 to 28.3	8.1 to 9.7	9.9 to 11.7	13.5 to 18.3	1.8 to 2.0
Short-segment fixation group	64	26.2 ± 14.1	9.5 ± 4.1	11.1 ± 4.3	17.7 ± 9.5	1.6 ± 1.7
95% CI		22.7 to 29.7	8.5 to 10.5	10.0 to 12.2	15.4 to 20.0	1.2 to 2.0
p value		0.735	0.361	0.668	0.326	0.174

score was 14.43 vs. 14.25 ($t = 0.520$, $p = 0.405$), the postoperative JOA score was 27.93 and 27.74 ($t = 1.086$, $p = 0.415$), and the improvement rate was 92.66% vs. 91.46% ($\chi^2 = 0.098$, $p = 0.754$).

No damage occurred to the spinal cord, cauda equina, nerve roots, large blood vessels, or important organs in any of these patients. In four cases, fat liquefaction occurred at the anterior incisions, which healed after 3 weeks of dressing. In two cases (one in each group) debridement was incomplete, and TB was not cured. After 2 months, a psoas muscle abscess appeared, and secondary surgery was performed. Both patients were treated successfully. In two cases (one in each group), the loosening of internal fixation occurred at 3 months and 5 months after surgery, and they quickly underwent revision surgery. In three cases (two cases in the affected-vertebrae fixation group and one case in the short-segment fixation group), the strut bone graft was tilted, and both time of immobilization and duration of anti-TB treatment were prolonged. Bone graft fusion was achieved thereafter.

Discussion

Lumbar TB has the highest incidence of spinal TB, and surgical intervention combined with anti-TB chemotherapy can ensure good outcomes and treat paralysis [12–14]. Internal fixation is a necessary method for reconstruction of spinal stability. At present, short- and long-segment fixations are commonly used for internal fixation during surgical treatment of spinal TB [15, 16]. These methods not only provide strong fixation, but also have a certain impact on the structure and motor function of the spine.

The range of movement in each normal motor unit of the lumbar spine includes 10–15° of flexion and extension, 6–8° of lateral bending, and 2° of axial rotation, while the short-segment and long-segment fixations restrict at least

two normal motor units. In addition, if the range of fixation is too long, degenerative changes may easily occur in adjacent segments. Biomechanical studies and clinical observations suggest that the longer the fixed fusion segment, the greater the activity of the adjacent segments and the greater the pressure on the intervertebral disc, the more likely the chances that degeneration will occur in the adjacent segments [17, 18]. Affected-vertebrae fixation can carry out debridement, decompression, deformity correction, bone grafting, and internal fixation within the affected motor units without involving adjacent normal motor units, thus, maximizing the retention of spinal motion function and reducing adjacent segmental degeneration.

The results of this study show that compared with the short-segment fixation group, the affected-vertebrae group had shorter operative times, less intraoperative blood loss, and because fixation was limited to the affected motor units, as well as the average number of fixation segments being reduced by 2.02. However, there was no significant difference between the two groups with regards to the VAS score, ASIA impairment scale, ESR, CRP, lesion cure rate, bone graft healing rate, or incidence of complications. In addition, there was no significant difference between the two groups with regards to deformity correction, average postoperative correction in Cobb's angle, and loss of correction at 5 years after surgery. The degree of correction in Cobb's angle and loss of correction in the affected-vertebrae group were similar to the results of Wang et al. [19] and Mukhtar et al. [20], who studied long-segment vs. short-segment fixation and reported a loss of correction of < 3°. Therefore, affected-vertebrae fixation, used in the treatment of lumbar TB, can safely and effectively reconstruct spinal stability and maintain the correction of deformity for long periods.

Table 4 Disease healing and bone graft fusion in the affected-vertebrae fixation group and short-segment fixation group

Groups	Cases	Lesion cured (cases)			Bone graft fusion (cases)		
		6 months after surgery	1 year after surgery	5 years after surgery	6 months after surgery	1 year after surgery	5 years after surgery
Affected-vertebrae fixation group	71	57	69	71	54	68	71
Short-segment fixation group	64	52	61	64	44	57	64
p value		0.887	0.566	–	0.342	0.137	–

Table 5 Preoperative and postoperative ESR and CRP in the affected-vertebrae fixation group and short-segment fixation group ($\bar{x}\pm s$)

Groups	Cases	Before surgery		6 months after surgery		5 years after surgery	
		ESR (mm/h)	CRP (mg/l)	ESR (mm/h)	CRP (mg/l)	ESR (mm/h)	CRP (mg/l)
Affected-vertebrae fixation group	71	36.5 ± 22.5	27.0 ± 24.9	16.6 ± 4.2	2.2 ± 1.7	9.3 ± 2.4	1.4 ± 1.1
95% CI		31.3 to 41.7	21.3 to 32.7	15.6 to 17.6	1.8 to 2.6	8.7 to 9.9	1.1 to 1.7
Short-segment fixation group	64	40.4 ± 20.1	25.8 ± 22.3	17.4 ± 3.7	2.4 ± 2.3	8.6 ± 3.5	1.1 ± 1.5
95% CI		35.5 to 45.3	20.3 to 31.3	16.5 to 18.3	1.8 to 3.0	7.7 to 9.5	0.7 to 1.5
p value		0.349	0.718	0.245	0.498	0.174	0.164

The normal range for ESR: male 0–15 mm/h, female 0–20 mm/h; the normal range for CRP 0–2.87 mg/l
CRP C-reactive protein, *ESR* erythrocyte sedimentation rate

During an earlier study, we produced a reconstruction model with iliac strutting in the anterior and mid column, affected-vertebrae fixation in calf spine. The ranges of motion (ROM) of intact spines were tested as control. The ROM in axial compression, lateral bending, flexion-extension, and rotation were tested. No statistical difference of the ROM was found between affected-vertebrae fixation group and control group ($p > 0.05$). So we concluded that with iliac strutting in the anterior and mid column, affected-vertebrae fixation can provide instant stability [21]. The above-mentioned biomechanical study provides a strong theoretical basis for clinical implementation of affected-vertebrae fixation. In clinical studies, Xu et al. [22] and Liu et al. [23] treated thoracolumbar fractures with single-segment fixation and obtained satisfactory outcomes without complications such as internal fixation breakage or loosening. These studies provide the biomechanical and clinical bases for affected-vertebrae fixation in the treatment of spinal TB.

Although the mechanical properties of affected-vertebrae fixation are less rigid than those of short-segment fixation and long-segment fixation, we found that an appropriate technique can meet the requirement of rigid fixation. Therefore, it is very important to define strict indications for surgery. We summarized the indications and contraindications of affected-vertebrae fixation as follows. The indications of affected-vertebrae fixation are as follows: (1) the upper and lower end plates of the affected vertebrae were intact showed by preoperative computer tomography (CT) scan and three-dimensional (3D) CT imaging

reconstruction, so as to provide a reliable host bed for the strut bone graft; (2) the kyphosis deformity was not serious (< 60°) and could be corrected by changing the patient's position using manual techniques and instrument application; (3) the pedicle should be relatively intact without TB invasion. The contraindications of affected-vertebrae fixation are as follows: (1) patients with severe osteoporosis; and (2) bony-diseases cured or bony-stationary of spinal tuberculosis need to be treated with corrective osteotomy. The affected-vertebrae fixation will be implemented once the patient meets the criteria for affected-vertebrae fixation, as it is less invasive and the cost is lower. For those patients with (1) the pedicle of the affected vertebrae was invaded by TB, (2) the kyphosis deformity was serious (> 60°), (3) severe osteoporosis, and (4) bony-diseases cured or bony-stationary of spinal tuberculosis, we will consider to give them a short-segment fixation in our clinic work now.

Affected-vertebrae fixation is one component of affected-vertebrae surgery, which requires removal of the lesion, decompression, deformity correction, bone grafting, and fixation within the affected vertebrae. The application of posterior affected-vertebrae fixation can stabilize the posterior column, but there is a relatively large bone defect in the anterior and middle columns after anterior debridement, which results in instability in the anterior and middle columns. Therefore, strut bone grafting should be carried out to support the anterior and middle columns for successful fixation of the affected vertebrae. Strut bone grafting can reduce the load

Table 6 Preoperative and postoperative ASIA grade in the affected-vertebrae fixation group and short-segment fixation group

Grades	Affected-vertebrae fixation group (n = 71)						Short-segment fixation group (n = 64)					
	Before surgery	After surgery					Before surgery	After surgery				
		A	B	C	D	E		A	B	C	D	E
A	0						0					
B	2			1	1		3			1	1	
C	5				2	3	6				2	4
D	36				2	34	34				1	33
E	28					28	21					21

ASIA grade American Spinal Injury Association grade

of posterior fixation devices in the corresponding segments, reduce stress, and protect internal fixation devices [24]. After debridement, the host bed for bone grafting should be trimmed evenly to produce an adequate condition for the survival of the bone graft. The strut bone should be placed perpendicular to the upper and lower end plates and placed as close to the center as possible to avoid loss of correction and difficulty in bone fusion due to uneven loads. Moreover, our previous biomechanical study showed that the crosslink could increase the anti-torsion ability of the screw-rod system, reduce stress on the posterior articular process, and enhance axial stability of the spine. Therefore, it should not be disregarded in the process of posterior affected-vertebrae fixation.

Conclusion

In conclusion, based on chemotherapy requirements and using strict surgical indications, posterior affected-vertebrae fixation (together with anterior debridement and bone grafting) is a safe, effective, and feasible surgical procedure in the treatment of lumbar TB. In addition, it is less invasive, and the cost is lower. However, the present study is a single-center study, and the sample size is relatively small. Therefore, multicenter, large-sample, prospective randomized controlled studies should be carried out in the future to improve the level of evidence-based medicine and support our findings.

Abbreviations
ASIA: American Spinal Injury Association; CRP: C-reactive protein; CT: Computed tomography; ESR: Erythrocyte sedimentation rate; HRZS: Isoniazid (H), rifampicin (R), pyrazinamide (Z), chain toxin (S); MRI: Magnetic resonance imaging; TB: Tuberculosis; VAS: Visual analogue scale

Funding
This work was supported by the National Natural Science Foundation of China (item number: 81660370) and the Key Program of Ningxia Province (item number: 2016–25).

Authors' contributions
LQ, SSY, and WZL designed the study. JWD and WZL obtained the funding. LQ, SGW, and MWX collected the data. SJD and SGW analyzed the data. MWX, and JWD interpreted the data. LQ and WQ composed the article. All authors read and approved the final manuscript.

Competing interests
The authors declare that they have no competing interests.

Author details
¹Department of Spinal Surgery, General Hospital of Ningxia Medical University, 804 Shengli Street, Yinchuan 750004, China. ²Hillsborough Community College, Tampa, USA. ³Department of Orthopedics, Hospital of Integrated Traditional Chinese and Western Medicine in Zhejiang Province, Hangzhou 310003, Zhejiang, China.

References
1. Gao Y, Ou Y, Deng Q, He B, Du X, Li J, et al. Comparison between titanium mesh and autogenous iliac bone graft to restore vertebral height through posterior approach for the treatment of thoracic and lumbar spinal tuberculosis. PLoS One. 2017;12:e0175567.
2. Kandwal P, G V, Jayaswal A. Management of tuberculous infection of the spine. Asian Spine J. 2016;10:792–800.
3. Hassan K, Elmorshidy E. Anterior versus posterior approach in surgical treatment of tuberculous spondylodiscitis of thoracic and lumbar spine. Eur Spine J. 2016;25:1056–63.
4. Huang Y, Lin J, Chen X, Lin J, Lin Y, Zhang H. A posterior versus anterior debridement in combination with bone graft and internal fixation for lumbar and thoracic tuberculosis. J Orthop Surg Res. 2017;12:150–6.
5. Pang X, Wu P, Shen X, Li D, Luo C, Wang X. One-stage posterior transforaminal lumbar debridement, 360° interbody fusion, and posterior instrumentation in treating lumbosacral spinal tuberculosis. Arch Orthop Trauma Surg. 2013;133:1033–9.
6. Wang Y, Zhang H, Tang M, Guo C, Deng A, Wu J, et al. One-stage posterior focus debridement, interbody grafts, and posterior instrumentation and fusion in the surgical treatment of thoracolumbar spinal tuberculosis with kyphosis in children: a preliminary report. Childs Nerv Syst. 2016;32:1–8.
7. Zeng H, Wang X, Zhang P, Peng W, Liu Z, Zhang Y. Single-stage posterior transforaminal lumbar interbody fusion, debridement, limited decompression, 3-column reconstruction, and posterior instrumentation in surgical treatment for single-segment lumbar spinal tuberculosis. Acta Orthop Traumatol Turc. 2015;49:513–21.
8. Wang H, Ma L, Yang D, Wang T, Liu S, Yang S, et al. Incidence and risk factors of adjacent segment disease following posterior decompression and instrumented fusion for degenerative lumbar disorders. Medicine (Baltimore). 2017;96:e6032–40.
9. Shi J, Wang Q, Wang Z. Primary issues in the selection of surgical procedures for thoracic and lumbar spinal tuberculosis. Orthop Surg. 2014;6:259–68.
10. Wang Z, Ge Z, Jin W, Qiao Y, Ding H, Zhao H, et al. Treatment of spinal tuberculosis with ultrashort-course chemotherapy in conjunction with partial excision of pathologic vertebrae. Spine J. 2007;7:671–81.
11. Wang Z, Shi J, Geng G, Qiu H. Ultra-short-course chemotherapy for spinal tuberculosis: five years of observation. Eur Spine J. 2013;22:274–81.
12. Rajasekaran S, Kanna RM, Shetty AP. History of spine surgery for tuberculous spondylodiscitis. Unfallchirurg. 2015;118:19–27.
13. Jin W, Wang Q, Wang Z, Geng G. Complete debridement for treatment of thoracolumbar spinal tuberculosis: a clinical curative effect observation. Spine J. 2014;14:964–70.
14. Jiang T, Zhao J, He M, Wang K, Fowdur M, Wu Y. Outcomes and treatment of lumbosacral spinal tuberculosis: a retrospective study of 53 patients. PLoS One. 2015;10:e0130185.
15. Alam MS, Phan K, Karim R, Jonayed SA, Munir HK, Chakraborty S, et al. Surgery for spinal tuberculosis: a multi-center experience of 582 cases. J Spine Surg. 2015;1:65–71.
16. Gong K, Wang Z, Luo Z. Single-stage posterior debridement and transforaminal lumbar interbody fusion with autogenous bone grafting and posterior instrumentation in the surgical management of lumbar tuberculosis. Arch Orthop Trauma Surg. 2011;131:217–23.
17. Park P, Garton HJ, Gala VC, Hoff JT, McGillicuddy JE. Adjacent segment disease after lumbar or lumbosacral fusion: review of the literature. Spine (Phila Pa 1976). 2004;29:1938–44.
18. Virk SS, Niedermeier S, Yu E, Khan SN. Adjacent segment disease. Orthopedics. 2014;37:547–55.
19. Wang X, Pang X, Wu P, Luo C, Shen X. One-stage anterior debridement, bone grafting and posterior instrumentation vs. single posterior

debridement, bone grafting, and instrumentation for the treatment of thoracic and lumbar spinal tuberculosis. Eur Spine J. 2014;23:830–7.

20. Mukhtar AM, Farghaly MM, Ahmed SH. Surgical treatment of thoracic and lumbar tuberculosis by anterior interbody fusion and posterior instrumentation. Med Princ Pract. 2003;12:92–6.

21. Wu QJ, Wang ZL, Ge CH. Biomechanical test of interbody bone graft in spinal tuberculosis constructed by monosegment fixation. NingXia Med J. 2010;32:131–3.

22. Xu G, Fu X, Du C, Ma J, Li Z, Tian P, et al. Biomechanical comparison of mono-segment transpedicular fixation with short-segment fixation for treatment of thoracolumbar fractures: a finite element analysis. Proc Inst Mech Eng H. 2014;228:1005–13.

23. Liu L, Gan Y, Zhou Q, Wang H, Dai F, Luo F, et al. Improved monosegment pedicle instrumentation for treatment of thoracolumbar incomplete burst fractures. Biomed Res Int. 2015;2015:1–7.

24. Talu U, Gogus A, Ozturk C, Hamzaoglu A, Domanic U. The role of posterior instrumentation and fusion after anterior radical debridement and fusion in the surgical treatment of spinal tuberculosis: experience of 127 cases. J Spinal Disord Tech. 2006;19:554–9.

9

Comparison of tourniquet application only during cementation and long-duration tourniquet application in total knee arthroplasty: a meta-analysis

Cong Wang[†], Chenhe Zhou[†], Hao Qu, Shigui Yan and Zhijun Pan[*]

Abstract

Background: Tourniquet is widely used by orthopedic surgeons in total knee arthroplasty (TKA). However, there are still controversies on the optimal timing of tourniquet application. The aim of this meta-analysis was to compare the effect and safety of tourniquet application only during cementation with long-duration tourniquet application in TKA.

Methods: An electronic literature search of PubMed, the Cochrane library, Embase, and Web of Science was conducted in July 2017. All randomized controlled trials (RCTs) comparing tourniquet application only during cementation with long-duration tourniquet application in TKA were included. RevMan 5.3 software was selected to perform the meta-analysis.

Results: Seven studies involving 440 TKAs were included for meta-analysis. The results suggested that although significant less intraoperative and total blood loss were observed with long-duration tourniquet application, tourniquet application only during cementation would not increase the number of transfusion and operation time. Tourniquet application only during cementation results in less knee pain on post-operative day 1 (POD 1), less time needed to achieve straight-leg raise, and less minor complications following TKA.

Conclusions: Tourniquet application only during cementation might reduce the rate of minor complications and have faster functional recovery during the early rehabilitation period following TKA, but it could not limit intraoperative and total blood loss. No definitive conclusions can be drawn based on the current evidences. Further, large well-designed RCTs with extensive follow-up are still needed to validate this research.

Keywords: Tourniquet, Total knee arthroplasty (TKA), Cementation, Meta-analysis

Background

Total knee arthroplasty (TKA) is a successful procedure for reducing pain and restoring function in patients with end-stage osteoarthritis. TKA has been reported to be associated with a significant amount of blood loss, sometimes necessitating blood transfusion [1]. Although the application of tourniquet is still highly controversial [2], considering the fact of providing clearer surgical visualization, less intraoperative blood loss, thus ensuring better cementation, it has become a common practice and is widely used by orthopedic surgeons during TKA.

However, tourniquet's use may also be associated with several complications, including thigh pain, limb swelling, nerve palsy, vascular injuries, subcutaneous thigh fat necrosis, postoperative stiffness, delayed recovery of quadriceps strength, wound complications, and deep vein thrombosis (DVT) [3–8].

There are still controversies on the optimal timing of tourniquet application, which may have vital influence on clinical outcomes following TKA. It is widely accepted that the prolonged duration of tourniquet application might be a crucial factor for complications [6, 8, 9], which suggests longer ischemic time for tissues. Hence, it is

* Correspondence: zrpzj@zju.edu.cn
Cong Wang and Chenhe Zhou are co-first authors.
Cong Wang and Chenhe Zhou are equal contributors.
Department of Orthopaedic Surgery, The Second Affiliated Hospital, Zhejiang University School of Medicine, No. 88 Jiefang Road, Hangzhou 310009, China

important to minimize the tourniquet time. Some investigators begin to focus on whether the limited application of tourniquet (tourniquet application only during the cementation) in TKA could reduce the complications and facilitate functional recovery. Fan et al. [10] demonstrated that limited use of a tourniquet in TKA provides the benefit of decreased limb swelling and knee joint pain while not compromising the operation time or blood loss and recovery. Meanwhile, Wang et al. [11] showed tourniquet application only during cementation would reduce postoperative and hidden blood losses without increasing the allogeneic blood transfusion rate. In addition, short-duration tourniquet use would result in faster recovery and less pain during the early rehabilitation period following TKA. In contrast, Mittal et al. [12] reported restricting tourniquet application to the period of cementing is associated with a significantly higher risk of transfusion, and indicated the approach is impractical if it is not offset by gains in functional recovery. Thus, this has to be balanced against the increased blood loss and risk of transfusion when using the tourniquet only during the cementation.

Therefore, whether tourniquet application only during cementation in TKA is beneficial remains debatable. And there has been no meta-analysis evaluating tourniquet application only during cementation compared with the long-duration tourniquet application in TKA. Accordingly, we systematically reviewed the current randomized controlled trials (RCTs) to investigate which tourniquet application strategy is better. Our hypothesis is that tourniquet application only during cementation may result in less knee pain, faster functional recovery during the early rehabilitation, and less complications, but may increase intraoperative and total blood loss.

Methods
Search strategy
This meta-analysis was preformed according to the Preferred Reporting Items for Systematic Reviews and Meta-Analyses guidelines (the PRISMA statement) [13]. The electronic databases of PubMed, the Cochrane library, Embase, and Web of Science were systematically searched for relevant academic clinical trials comparing tourniquet application only during cementation to long-duration tourniquet application in TKA from inception to July 2017. The following search terms were used to maximize scope of the search: tourniquet and (total knee arthroplasty or total knee replacement). Furthermore, the reference lists of the identified articles were reviewed to search for additional studies of interest that potentially met the study criteria, and no restriction was made on the language of the publication.

Inclusion and exclusion criteria
We identified literature that met the following inclusion criteria: (1) patients underwent primary TKA, (2) randomized controlled trials, (3) comparison of tourniquet application only during cementation and long-duration tourniquet application in total knee arthroplasty. The tourniquet inflated before skin incision and deflated following the completion of cementation or the wound closure was considered as long-duration tourniquet application. (4) Outcome measurements should include at least one of these parameters (tourniquet time, surgery time, calculated blood loss, total measured blood loss, intraoperative blood loss, postoperative blood loss, number of transfusion, knee pain, time needed to achieve straight-leg raise and complications).

Exclusion criteria were (1) non-randomized controlled trials, (2) unpublished data, (3) proceedings of meetings, (4) revision TKA, (5) different tourniquet application strategy.

Data extraction
Two researchers independently extracted the data from the individual study using the same format, after which the data were checked by a third author and any disagreement was resolved by consensus. Whenever necessary, we contacted the authors of the studies for the missing data and additional information. Relevant data extracted included publication information; demographic characteristic; tourniquet time; operative time; blood loss measures, including the intraoperative blood loss, postoperative blood loss, total measured blood loss, and calculated blood loss; number of transfusion; time needed to achieve straight-leg raise; knee pain scores; complications (including minor complications and major complications). Total measured blood loss was defined as the sum of intraoperative and measured postoperative blood loss, the calculated blood loss was estimated with formulas [14]. The complication was distinguished as a minor or major one according to whether a second operation was needed. We defined minor complications as wound complications such as oozing, erythema, marginal necrosis, superficial infection, slight knee stiffness, significant leg swelling, and DVT, which could be healed through conservative treatment and did not need another operation. We defined major complications as vessel injuries, infections, wound dehiscence, active hemorrhage and hematomas that required drainage or debridement or revision, and serious knee stiffness which need manipulation with the patient under anesthesia.

Quality assessment
Two authors independently assessed the risk of bias of included studies, with the following items: randomization, allocation concealment, blinding of participants, blinding of outcome assessment, incomplete outcome data,

selective outcome reporting, and other bias [15]. Based on the information provided from included studies, each item was recorded by "low," "high," or "unclear". Low indicates low risk of bias, high indicates high risk of bias, unclear indicates lack of information or unknown risk of bias.

Statistical analysis

The software of RevMan 5.3 was used to perform meta-analysis. Odds ratios (OR) with 95% confidence interval (95% CI) was calculated for dichotomous outcomes, and mean difference (MD) with 95% CI were used for continuous outcomes. p values less than 0.05 were considered statistically significant ($p < 0.05$). Heterogeneity among studies was tested using I^2 statistic and substantial heterogeneity was represented by an I^2 value greater than 50%. If significant heterogeneity was found in the meta-analysis, we used a random effect model; otherwise, we used a fixed effect model.

Results

Study selection

A flow chart of literature screening is shown in Fig. 1. From the initial database search, a total of 2250 relevant trials were yielded. After removing 1402 duplicates, 848 studies were reserved for title or abstract reviewing according to the inclusion criteria. The remaining 25 articles were subjected to full-text screen. Finally, seven studies were considered to be eligible for meta-analysis [10–12, 16–19].

Study characteristics

The characteristics of the included studies are showed in Table 1. The studies were published between 1997 and 2016. A total of 440 TKAs were performed in 377 adult patients. The mean age ranged from 63.27–72.5, and the mean body mass index (BMI) ranged from 26.26–32.6. The patients' parameters (age, BMI, preoperative knee function) were reported similar between groups. The results of the quality assessment are summarized in Table 2. Regarding the risk of bias, the overall quality of the included studies was considered adequate.

Blood loss

Two studies [11, 19] including 129 knees were included for analysis of the intraoperative blood loss and demonstrated significant more blood loss in the group with tourniquet application only during cementation (MD = 161.63; 95% CI 37.96 to 285.31; $p = 0.01$) (Fig. 2a). In two studies [11, 19], postoperative blood loss showed no significant difference between the groups (MD = – 46.50; 95% CI – 104.19 to 11.18; $p = 0.11$) (Fig. 2b). In addition, a total of four studies [11, 12, 17, 18] addressed the calculated blood loss, the pooled results showed tourniquet application only during cementation significantly increased the blood loss compared to that of long-duration tourniquet application (MD = 251.20; 95% CI 3.67 to 498.73; $p = 0.05$) (Fig. 2c). Two studies [11, 19] in which the total measured blood loss was measured also showed significant

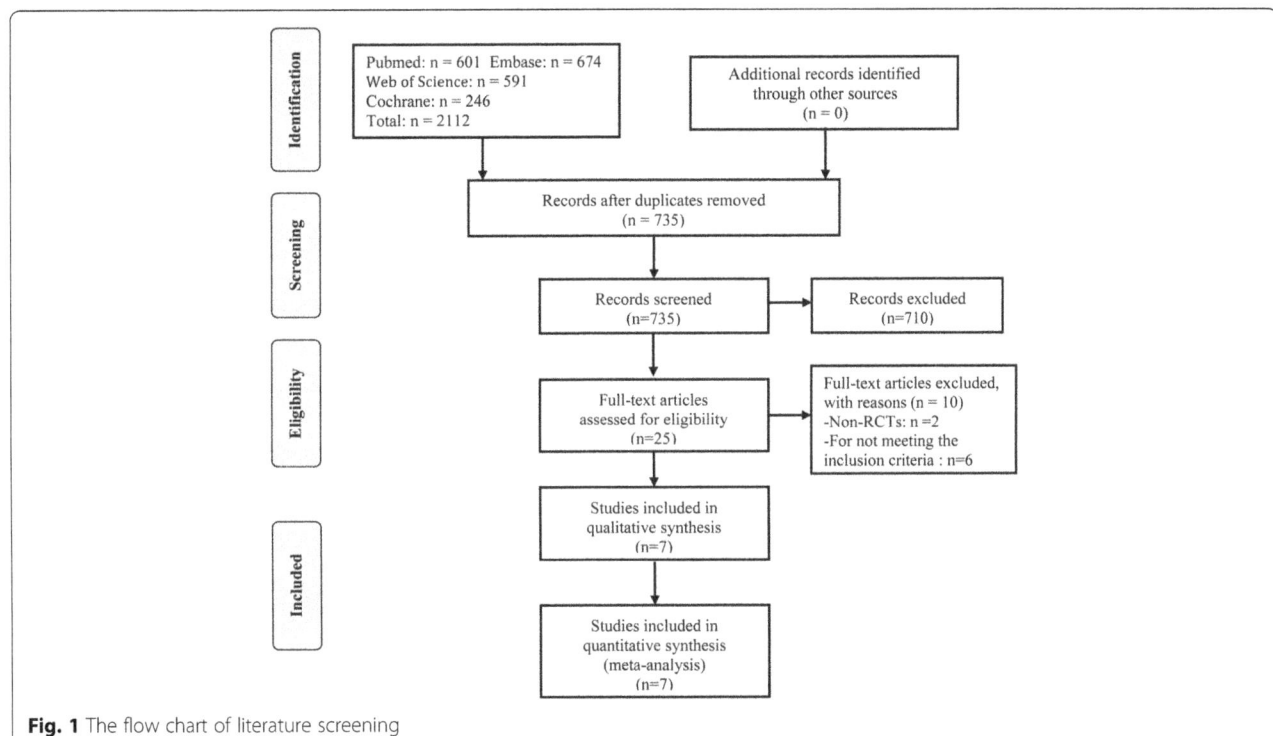

Fig. 1 The flow chart of literature screening

Table 1 Characteristics of included studies

Author/year	Patients	Knees		Gender (male/female)		Mean age (years)		BMI		Operative time (min)		Tourniquet time (min)	
		Cementation	Long	Cementation	Long	Cementation	Long	Cementation	Long	Cementation	Long	Cementation	Long
Fan 2014	60	30	30	9/21	7/23	63.27 ± 7.39	65.37 ± 7.11	26.26 ± 1.52	27.24 ± 2.69	111.25 ± 20.04	120.81 ± 8.12	23.20 ± 5.30	75.03 ± 133.99
Hakkalamani 2015	55	30	30	13/17	17/13	66.7 ± 8.5	69 ± 8.5	31.9 ± 6.2	31.5 ± 5.5	73.5 ± 13	76.7 ± 19	14 ± 4	76.7 ± 19
Harvey 1997	52	16	36	NA	NA	72.4	68.3	NA	NA	NA	NA	NA	NA
Kvederas 2013	24	12	12	3/9	1/11	67.3 ± 6.4	72.9 ± 4.5	31.1 ± 4.8	31.8 ± 4.1	59.8 ± 5.0	60.6 ± 8.7	11	60
Mittal 2012	65	31	34	6/25	9/25	67.5 ± 8.9	66.6 ± 8.4	32.5 ± 5.6	32.6 ± 5.6	105 ± 18.4	103 ± 16.6	22.5 ± 14.4	76.4 ± 15.1
Tarwala 2014	71	40	39	13/22	14/22	64.6 ± 9.3	66.1 ± 9.8	31.4 ± 6.4	29.9 ± 5.3	90 ± 23	86 ± 22	9(7–14)	43(24–62)
Wang 2016	50	25	25	4/21	5/20	72.5 ± 6.8	72.3 ± 7.1	29.1 ± 6.6	28.8 ± 6.2	93.8 ± 22.7	84.7 ± 12.4	10.9 ± 1.8	54.8 ± 6.7

NA, not available

Table 2 Risk of bias in included studies

Author/year	Randomization	Allocation concealment	Blinding of participants	Blinding of outcome assessment	Incomplete outcome data	Selective outcome reporting	Other bias
Fan 2014	Low	Unclear	Low	Low	Low	Low	Unclear
Hakkalamani 2015	Low	Low	Low	Low	Low	Low	Unclear
Harvey 1997	Unclear	Unclear	Low	Low	Low	Low	Unclear
Kvederas 2013	Low	Low	Low	Low	Low	Low	Unclear
Mittal 2012	Low	Low	Low	Low	Low	Low	Unclear
Tarwala 2014	Low	Unclear	Low	Low	Low	Low	Unclear
Wang 2016	Low	Low	Low	Low	Low	Low	Unclear

difference between the two groups (MD = 126.60; 95% CI 76.69 to 176.52; $p < 0.00001$) (Fig. 2d).

Number of transfusion

Three included studies [11, 12, 17] investigated the number of transfusion after TKA. The combined data

showed no significant difference between the groups (OR = 1.00; 95% CI 0.45 to 2.22; $p = 1.00$) (Fig. 3).

Operation time

Six studies [10–12, 16, 18, 19] involving the operation time during TKA showed no difference between the

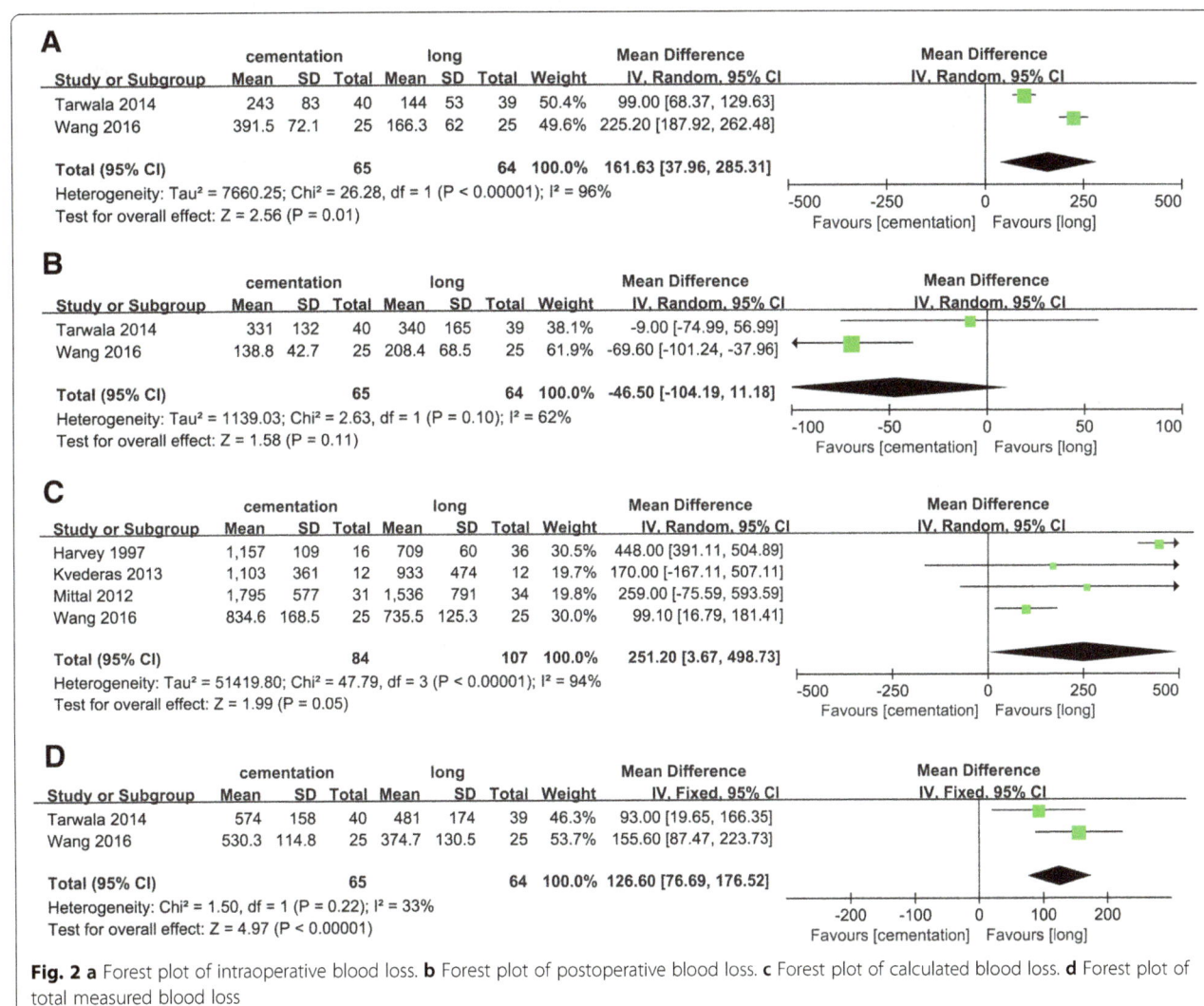

Fig. 2 a Forest plot of intraoperative blood loss. **b** Forest plot of postoperative blood loss. **c** Forest plot of calculated blood loss. **d** Forest plot of total measured blood loss

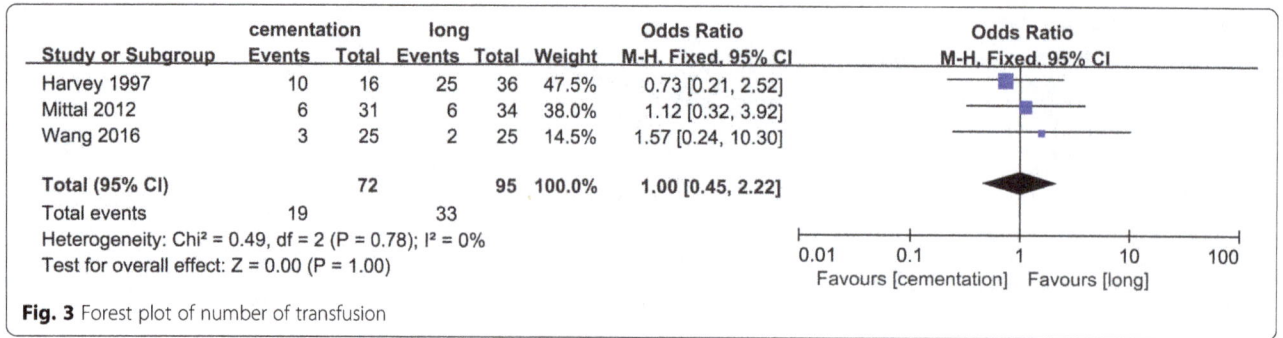

Fig. 3 Forest plot of number of transfusion

groups (MD = – 0.34; 95% CI – 5.10 to 4.43; $p = 0.89$) (Fig. 4).

Tourniquet time

Six studies [10–12, 16, 18, 19] providing the tourniquet time indicated that it was significantly shorter in the group with tourniquet use only during cementation (MD = – 48.91; 95% CI – 56.71 to – 41.11; $p < 0.00001$) (Fig. 5).

Knee pain

Three included studies [11, 16, 19] investigated visual analogue scale (VAS) knee pain scores on post-operative day 1 (POD 1). The pooled results showed less knee pain scores in the group tourniquet application only during cementation (MD = – 0.66; 95% CI – 1.16 to – 0.15; $p = 0.01$) (Fig. 6a). Of these seven RCTs, two studies [11, 19] reported the VAS knee pain scores on POD 2. Analysis of two studies showed no difference (MD = – 0.28; 95% CI – 1.94 to 1.39; $p = 0.74$) (Fig. 6b). Only two studies [10, 19] investigated VAS knee pain score on POD 3. There was no difference between the groups (MD = – 0.75; 95% CI – 2.32 to 0.81; $p = 0.35$) (Fig. 6c).

Straight-leg raise

Two studies [11, 16] assessed the time needed to achieve straight-leg raise after TKA, and the results showed that the group tourniquet application only during cementation was associated with significant less time needed to achieve straight-leg raise compared to long-duration tourniquet

application group (MD = – 0.89; 95% CI – 1.48 to – 0.31; $p = 0.003$) (Fig. 7).

Complications

Six studies [11, 12, 16, 17, 19] reported complications including minor complications and major complications. From Fig. 8a, we could draw the conclusion that tourniquet application only during cementation significantly decreased the risk of minor complications (OR = 0.40; 95% CI 0.19 to 0.87; $p = 0.02$). With regard to DVT, a subgroup analysis was conducted and the result indicated no significant difference between the two groups (OR = 0.54; 95% CI 0.23 to 1.31; $p = 0.17$) (Fig. 8b). Only one study reported major complications which could not be pooled in meta-analysis [19].`

Discussion

To our knowledge, this is the first meta-analysis of RCTs comparing the effect and safety of tourniquet application only during cementation with long-duration tourniquet application in TKA. The most important finding of the meta-analysis was that although significant less intraoperative and total blood loss were observed with long-duration tourniquet application, tourniquet application only during cementation would not increase the number of transfusion and operation time. Besides, tourniquet application only during cementation result in less knee pain, less time needed to achieve straight-leg raise, and less minor complications following TKA.

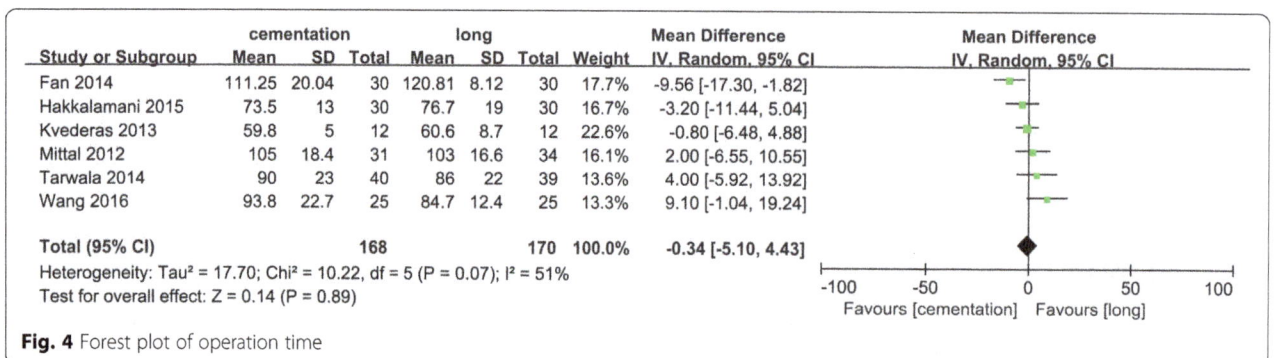

Fig. 4 Forest plot of operation time

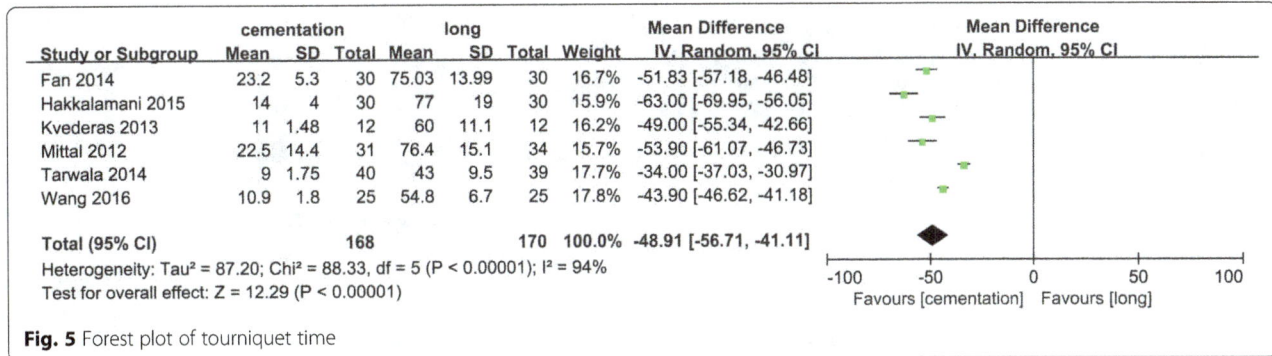

Study or Subgroup	cementation Mean	SD	Total	long Mean	SD	Total	Weight	Mean Difference IV, Random, 95% CI
Fan 2014	23.2	5.3	30	75.03	13.99	30	16.7%	-51.83 [-57.18, -46.48]
Hakkalamani 2015	14	4	30	77	19	30	15.9%	-63.00 [-69.95, -56.05]
Kvederas 2013	11	1.48	12	60	11.1	12	16.2%	-49.00 [-55.34, -42.66]
Mittal 2012	22.5	14.4	31	76.4	15.1	34	15.7%	-53.90 [-61.07, -46.73]
Tarwala 2014	9	1.75	40	43	9.5	39	17.7%	-34.00 [-37.03, -30.97]
Wang 2016	10.9	1.8	25	54.8	6.7	25	17.8%	-43.90 [-46.62, -41.18]
Total (95% CI)			168			170	100.0%	-48.91 [-56.71, -41.11]

Heterogeneity: Tau² = 87.20; Chi² = 88.33, df = 5 (P < 0.00001); I² = 94%
Test for overall effect: Z = 12.29 (P < 0.00001)

Fig. 5 Forest plot of tourniquet time

For blood loss, the result demonstrates that long-duration tourniquet application significantly reduced the intraoperative blood loss, calculated blood loss, and total measured blood loss, which were consistent with some previous studies [20–23]. Deflating the tourniquet after the cementation theoretically allows a better control of wound bleeding and patients would have better hemostasis, thus leading to less blood loss. However, rapid reactive hyperemia and increase in fibrinolytic activity have been demonstrated to occur in the first period after tourniquet releasing, leading to excessive bleeding [24–27]. The higher perioperative blood loss caused by fibrinolytic activity can probably be controlled by a closed wound and pressure dressing [28]. Releasing tourniquet after cementation provides a window of time to the activation of

fibrinolytic leading to increasing bleeding [29]. Based on this, tourniquet application only during cementation theoretically would result in more perioperative blood loss.

No significant difference was found in the incidence of transfusion between these two groups. However, differences were obviously detected between the groups in perioperative blood loss. Theoretically, the transfusion is supposed to be associated with the loss of blood. Moráis et al. [30] reported perioperative transfusion rate had no significant relevance with application time of tourniquet in TKA but was relevant with preoperative hemoglobin level and body mass index. Moreover, no difference in transfusion rate between the groups also may result from the variability in the criteria for transfusion.

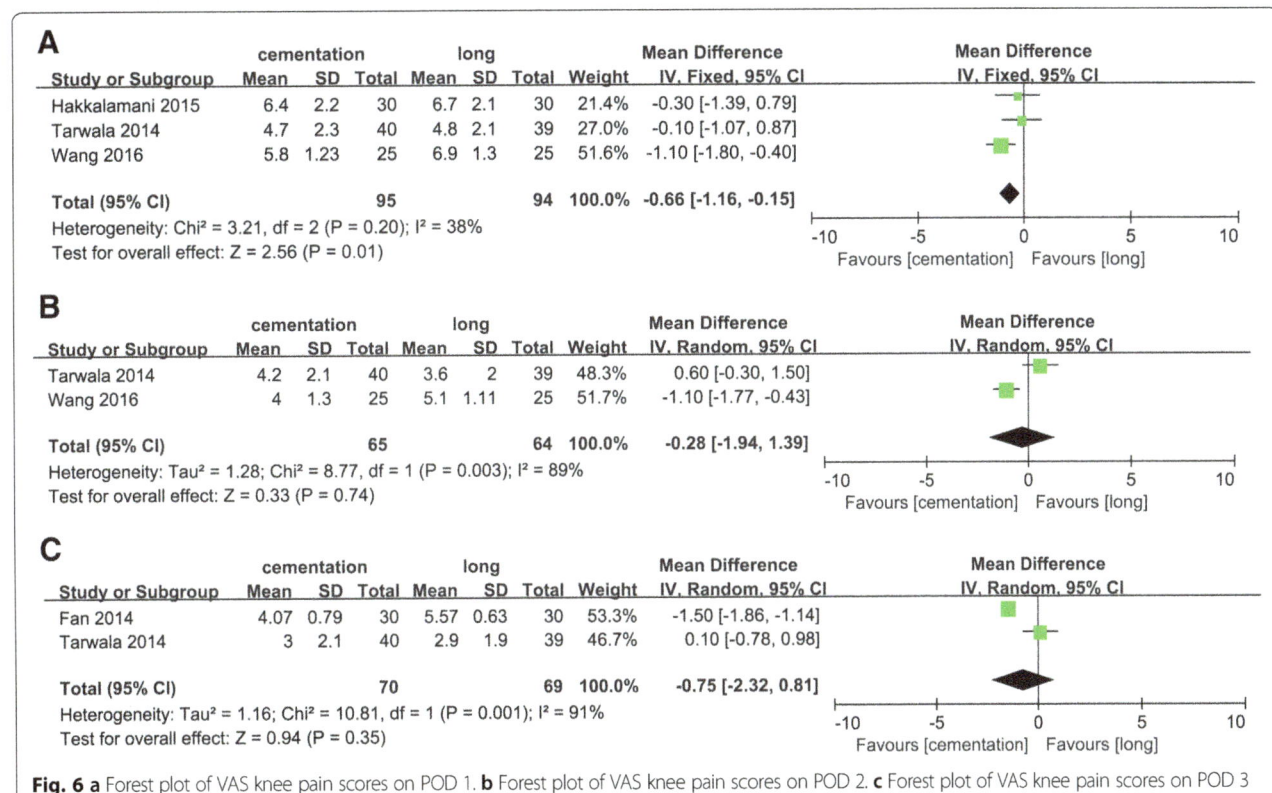

A

Study or Subgroup	cementation Mean	SD	Total	long Mean	SD	Total	Weight	Mean Difference IV, Fixed, 95% CI
Hakkalamani 2015	6.4	2.2	30	6.7	2.1	30	21.4%	-0.30 [-1.39, 0.79]
Tarwala 2014	4.7	2.3	40	4.8	2.1	39	27.0%	-0.10 [-1.07, 0.87]
Wang 2016	5.8	1.23	25	6.9	1.3	25	51.6%	-1.10 [-1.80, -0.40]
Total (95% CI)			95			94	100.0%	-0.66 [-1.16, -0.15]

Heterogeneity: Chi² = 3.21, df = 2 (P = 0.20); I² = 38%
Test for overall effect: Z = 2.56 (P = 0.01)

B

Study or Subgroup	cementation Mean	SD	Total	long Mean	SD	Total	Weight	Mean Difference IV, Random, 95% CI
Tarwala 2014	4.2	2.1	40	3.6	2	39	48.3%	0.60 [-0.30, 1.50]
Wang 2016	4	1.3	25	5.1	1.11	25	51.7%	-1.10 [-1.77, -0.43]
Total (95% CI)			65			64	100.0%	-0.28 [-1.94, 1.39]

Heterogeneity: Tau² = 1.28; Chi² = 8.77, df = 1 (P = 0.003); I² = 89%
Test for overall effect: Z = 0.33 (P = 0.74)

C

Study or Subgroup	cementation Mean	SD	Total	long Mean	SD	Total	Weight	Mean Difference IV, Random, 95% CI
Fan 2014	4.07	0.79	30	5.57	0.63	30	53.3%	-1.50 [-1.86, -1.14]
Tarwala 2014	3	2.1	40	2.9	1.9	39	46.7%	0.10 [-0.78, 0.98]
Total (95% CI)			70			69	100.0%	-0.75 [-2.32, 0.81]

Heterogeneity: Tau² = 1.16; Chi² = 10.81, df = 1 (P = 0.001); I² = 91%
Test for overall effect: Z = 0.94 (P = 0.35)

Fig. 6 a Forest plot of VAS knee pain scores on POD 1. **b** Forest plot of VAS knee pain scores on POD 2. **c** Forest plot of VAS knee pain scores on POD 3

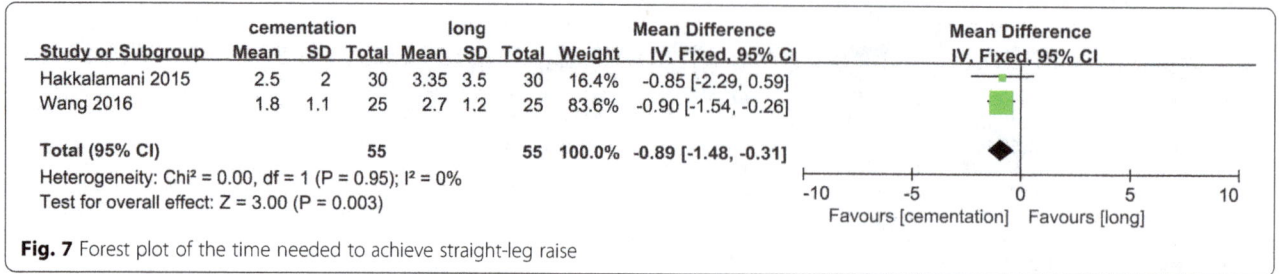

Fig. 7 Forest plot of the time needed to achieve straight-leg raise

Postoperative functional recovery for TKA is particularly important. The current study showed that tourniquet application only during cementation significantly reduced VAS knee pain and the time needed to achieve straight-leg raise following TKA. Fan et al. [10] also discovered the limited use of a tourniquet in TKA provides the benefit of decreased limb swelling and better active knee flexion while not compromising the operation time or blood loss and recovery. The possible reason is the direct damage of the tourniquet and reperfusion injury might increase pain that would hamper patients' postoperative rehabilitation [31]. And additional limb swelling in the long-duration tourniquet group after TKA might cause an increased weight in the affected limb sufficient to require more muscle strength for performing straight-leg raise. Furthermore, Dennis et al. [32] indicated that patients who underwent TKA using a tourniquet had diminished quadriceps strength during the first 3 months after TKA. Early mobilization after TKA may

be delayed in the patients with quadriceps weakness. It therefore seems to be highly desirable to keep the duration of tourniquet to a minimum [33–36]. The tourniquet application only during cementation may be considered superior since it hardly influences the functional recovery after TKA.

As for complications, this study shows that tourniquet application only during cementation reduced the risks of minor complication. With respect to major complication, only one study reported one patient suffered a compartment syndrome in the long-duration tourniquet application group [19]. Previous studies have showed that the prolonged duration of tourniquet application might be a crucial factor for complications [6, 8, 9, 37]. In our included studies, the most common minor complications were wound complications. It is well known that oxygen supply in the soft tissue around the incision is one of the key elements for sound incision healing. Clarke et al. [38] indicated that tourniquet sharply

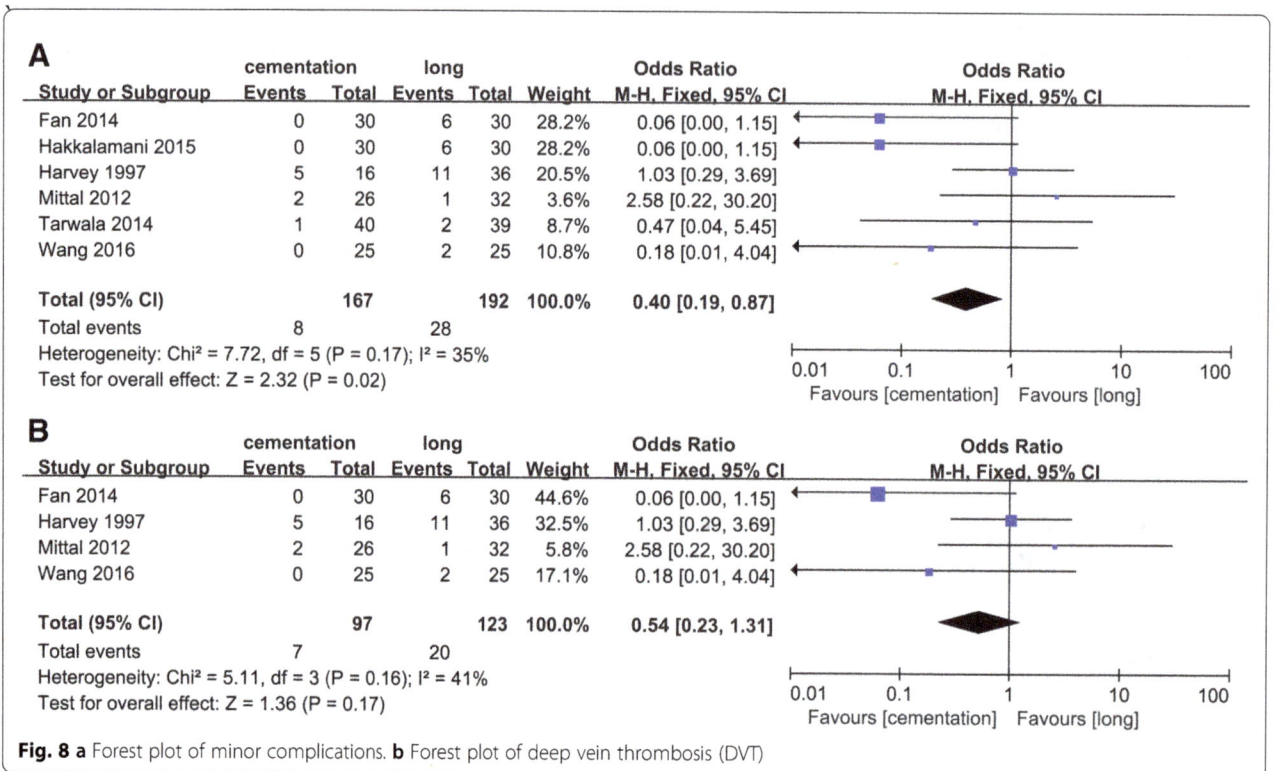

Fig. 8 a Forest plot of minor complications. **b** Forest plot of deep vein thrombosis (DVT)

decreased the oxygen content in the soft tissue around the incision for ischemia-reperfusion injuries in TKA. Longer tourniquet application would further aggravate the soft tissue hypoxia around the incision, cause more excessive inflammation and muscle damage, and consequently increase the risk of wound complications. It was also reported that every additional 10 min of tourniquet time was associated with an increased risk for complications [39]. Therefore, it is important to shorten the duration of tourniquet time to minimize the potential complications.

Thromboembolism is one of the most common complications after TKA. Clinically, the application of the tourniquet is considered to be one of the most important risk factors for thromboembolism [40, 41]. Separated from the other complications, DVT was evaluated individually in this study, and there were no significant differences between the groups. Olivecrona et al. [39] demonstrated that using a tourniquet for more than 100 min in TKA would increase the incidence of DVT. The durations of tourniquet application were all less than 100 min in the included studies, and no difference was found in operative time between the groups. With increasing concerns about the negative effects related to DVT after TKA, perioperative DVT prophylaxis is now routinely applied. Thus, low incidence nature of this complication and the small sample size involved for comparison may partially account for the similar incidence of DVT in the two groups.

In the present meta-analysis, several important limitations should be recognized. First, the major limitation of this analysis is the small sample size of the included studies, and only seven RCTs were included, which may have caused imprecise outcomes. Second, some confounding factors such as the tourniquet pressure, method of thromboembolic prophylaxis, the type of anesthesia, analgesic methods, whether use drainage might influence the outcomes. Third, although some outcomes were reported in the included study, for the insufficient data and varied reporting of outcomes, some data were not sufficiently provided to perform meta-analysis, such as limb swelling. Finally, the follow-up period in most studies was relatively short, which might overlook the long-term outcomes, such as prosthetic fixation quality and joint function recovery.

Conclusions

In conclusion, tourniquet application only during cementation increases intraoperative and total blood loss, while not increasing the number of transfusion and operation time. In addition, compared to long-duration tourniquet application, the limited use of a tourniquet results in less knee pain, less time needed to achieve straight-leg raise, and less minor complications following TKA, and

functional recovery seems to be faster during the early rehabilitation period. Considering the relatively small sample size, no definitive conclusions can be drawn based on the current evidences. We hope our meta-analysis presented here will enable orthopedic surgeons to make an informed decision as to choose an appropriate tourniquet application strategy. Further large well-designed RCTs with extensive follow-up are still needed to validate this research.

Abbreviations
BMI: Body mass index; CI: Confidence interval; DVT: Deep vein thrombosis; MD: Mean difference; OR: Odds ratios; POD 1: Post-operative day 1; RCTs: Randomized controlled trials; TKA: Total knee arthroplasty; VAS: Visual analogue score

Acknowledgements
The authors thank all patients and clinical researchers involved in the RCTs that included in our study.

Authors' contributions
CW and ZP participated in the design of the study. CZ and HQ participated in the literature search, study selection, data extraction, and quality assessment. CW and CZ performed the statistical analysis and drafted the manuscript. SY and ZP revised the manuscript. All authors read and approved the final manuscript.

Competing interests
The authors declare that they have no competing interests.

References
1. Noticewala MS, Nyce JD, Wang W, Geller JA, Macaulay W. Predicting need for allogeneic transfusion after total knee arthroplasty. J Arthroplast. 2012;27:961–7.
2. Alcelik I, Pollock RD, Sukeik M, et al. A comparison of outcomes with and without a tourniquet in total knee arthroplasty: a systematic review and meta-analysis of randomized controlled trials. J Arthroplasty. 2012;27(3):331–40.
3. Ochoa J, Fowler TJ, Gilliatt RW. Anatomical changes in peripheral nerves compressed by a pneumatic tourniquet. J Anat. 1972;113:433–55.
4. Naresh Kumar S, Chapman J, Rawlins I. Vascular injuries in total knee arthroplasty: a review of the problem with special reference to the possible effects of the tourniquet. J Arthroplasty. 1998;13:211–6.
5. Tamvakopoulos GS, Toms AP, Glasgow M. Subcutaneous thigh fat necrosis as a result of tourniquet control during total knee arthroplasty. Ann R Coll Surg Engl. 2005;87(5):W11–3.
6. Saunders KC, Louis DL, Weingarden SI, Waylonis GW. Effect of tourniquet time on postoperative quadriceps function. Clin Orthop Relat Res. 1979;143:194–9.
7. Kageyama K, Nakajima Y, Shibasaki M, Hashimoto S, Mizobe T. Increased platelet, leukocyte, and endothelial cell activity are associated with increased coagulability in patients after total knee arthroplasty. J Thromb Haemost. 2007;5:738–45.
8. Horlocker TT, Hebl JR, Gali B, et al. Anesthetic, patient, and surgical risk factors for neurologic complications after prolonged total tourniquet time during total knee arthroplasty. Anesth Analg. 2006;102(3):950–5.
9. Christodoulou AG, Ploumis AL, Terzidis IP, Chantzidis P, Metsovitis SR, Nikiforos DG. The role of timing of tourniquet release and cementing on perioperative blood loss in total knee replacement. Knee. 2004;11(4):313–7.
10. Fan Y, Jin J, Sun Z, Li W, Lin J, Weng X, Qiu G. The limited use of a tourniquet during total knee arthroplasty: a randomized controlled trial. Knee. 2014;21(6):1263–8.

11. Wang K, Ni S, Li Z, Zhong Q, Li R, Li H, Ke Y, Lin J. The effects of tourniquet use in total knee arthroplasty: a randomized, controlled trial. Knee Surg Sports Traumatol Arthrosc. 2017;25(9):2849–57. https://doi.org/10.1007/s00167-015-3964-2.

12. Mittal R, Ko V, Adie S, Naylor J, Dave J, Dave C, et al. Tourniquet application only during cement fixation in total knee arthroplasty: a double-blind, randomized controlled trial. ANZ J Surg. 2012;82(6):428–33.

13. Moher D, Liberati A, Tetzlaff J, Altman DG, Group P. Preferred reporting items for systematic reviews and meta-analyses: the PRISMA statement. J Clin Epidemiol. 2009;10:1006–12.

14. Gross JB. Estimating allowable blood loss: corrected for dilution. Anesthesiology. 1983;58(3):277–80.

15. Higgins JPT, Green S. Cochrane handbook for systematic reviews of interventions version 5.1.0. In: The cochrane collaboration; 2011. http://www.handbook.cochrane.org. Accessed 15 Nov 2016.

16. Hakkalamani S, Clark V, Pradhan N. Short versus standard duration tourniquet use during Total Knee Replacement: A pilot study. Acta Orthop Belg. 2015;81(1):52–6.

17. Harvey EJ, Leclerc J, Brooks CE, Burke DL. Effect of tourniquet use on blood loss and incidence of deep vein thrombosis in total knee arthroplasty. J Arthroplast. 1997;12(3):291–6.

18. Kvederas G, Porvaneckas N, Andrijauskas A, Svensen CH, et al. A randomized double-blind clinical trial of tourniquet application strategies for total knee arthroplasty. Knee Surg Sports Traumatol Arthrosc. 2013;21(12):2790–9.

19. Tarwala R, Dorr LD, Gilbert PK, Wan Z, Long WT. Tourniquet use during cementation only during total knee arthroplasty: a randomized trial. Clin Orthop Relat Res. 2014;472(1):169–74.

20. Yi S, Tan J, Chen C, Chen H, Huang W. The use of pneumatic tourniquet in total knee arthroplasty: a meta-analysis. Arch Orthop Trauma Surg. 2014;134(10):1469–76.

21. Zan PF, Yang Y, Fu D, Yu X, Li GD. Releasing of tourniquet before wound closure or not in total knee arthroplasty: a meta-analysis of randomized controlled trials. J Arthroplast. 2015;30(1):31–7.

22. Tai TW, Chang CW, Lai KA, Lin CJ, Yang CY. Effects of tourniquet use on blood loss and soft-tissue damage in total knee arthroplasty: a randomized controlled trial. J Bone Joint Surg Am. 2012;94(24):2209–15.

23. Vandenbussche E, Duranthon LD, Couturier M, Pidhorz L, Augereau B. The effect of tourniquet use in total knee arthroplasty. Int Orthop. 2002;26(5):306–9.

24. Silver R, de la Garza J, Rang M, Koreska J. Limb swelling after release of a tourniquet. Clin Orthop Relat Res. 1986;206:86–9.

25. Aglietti P, Baldini A, Vena LM, Abbate R, Fedi S, Falciani M. Effect of tourniquet use on activation of coagulation in total knee replacement. Clin Orthop Relat Res. 2000;371:169–77.

26. Klenerman L, Chakrabarti R, Mackie I, Brozovic M, Stirling Y. Changes in haemostatic system after application of a tourniquet. Lancet. 1977;1(8019):970–2.

27. Fahmy NR, Patel DG. Hemostatic changes and postoperative deep-vein thrombosis associated with use of a pneumatic tourniquet. J Bone Joint Surg Am. 1981;63(3):461–5.

28. Chang C, Lan S, Tai T, Lai K, Yang C. An effective method to reduce ischemia time during total knee arthroplasty. J Formos Med Assoc. 2012;111(1):19–23.

29. Risberg B. The response of the fibrinolytic system in trauma. Acta Chir Scand Suppl. 1984;522:245.

30. Moráis S, Ortega-Andreu M, Rodríguez- Merchán EC, et al. Blood transfusion after primary total knee arthroplasty can be significantly minimised through a multimodal blood-loss prevention approach. Int Orthop. 2014;38(2):347–54.

31. Ledin H, Aspenberg P, Good L. Tourniquet use in total knee replacement does not improve fixation, but appears to reduce final range of motion. Acta Orthop. 2012;83(5):499–503.

32. Dennis DA, Kittelson AJ, Yang CC, Miner TM, Kim RH, Stevens-Lapsley JE. Does tourniquet use in TKA affect recovery of lower extremity strength and function? A randomized trial. Clin Orthop Relat Res. 2016;474(1):69–77.

33. Klenerman L, Biswas M, Hulands GH, Rhodes AM. Systemic and local effects of the application of a tourniquet. J Bone Joint Surg. Br. 1980;62:385–8.

34. Patterson S, Klenerman L. The effect of pneumatic tourniquets on the ultrastructure of skeletal muscle. J Bone Joint Surg Br. 1979;61-B:178–83.

35. Erskine JG, Fraser C, Simpson R, Protheroe K, Walker ID. Blood loss with knee joint replacement. J R Coll Surg Edinb. 1981;26(5):295–7.

36. Pedowitz RA, Gershuni DH, Schmidt AH, Friden J, Rydevik BL, Hargens AR. Muscle injury induced beneath and distal to a pneumatic tourniquet: a quantitative animal study of effects of tourniquet pressure and duration. J Hand Surg Am. 1991;16:610–21.

37. Abbas K, Raza H, Umer M, Hafeez K. Effect of early release of tourniquet in total knee arthroplasty. J Coll Physicians Surg Pak. 2013;23(8):562–5.

38. Clarke MT, Longstaff L, Edwards D, Rushton N. Tourniquet-induced wound hypoxia after total knee replacement. J Bone Joint Surg Br. 2001;83(1):40–4.

39. Olivecrona C, Lapidus LJ, Benson L, Blomfeldt R. Tourniquet time affects postoperative complications after knee arthroplasty. Int Orthop. 2013;37(5):827–32.

40. Katsumata S, Nagashima M, Kato K, Tachihara A, Wauke K, Saito S, Jin E, Kawanami O, Ogawa R, Yoshino S. Changes in coagulation-fibrinolysis marker and neutrophil elastase following the use of tourniquet during total knee arthroplasty and the influence of neutrophil elastase on thromboembolism. Acta Anaesthesiol Scand. 2005;49(4):510–6.

41. Wauke K, Nagashima M, Kato N, Ogawa R, Yoshino S. Comparative study between thromboembolism and total knee arthroplasty with or without tourniquet in rheumatoid arthritis patients. Arch Orthop Trauma Surg. 2002;122(8):442–6.

10

The efficacy and safety of platelet-rich fibrin for rotator cuff tears: a meta-analysis

Xiu-hua Mao[1] and Ye-jun Zhan[2*]

Abstract

Background: The aim of this meta-analysis was to evaluate the efficacy and safety of platelet-rich fibrin (PRF) in improving clinical outcomes in rotator cuff tears.

Methods: We searched the following databases: Pubmed, Embase, and Cochrane library databases from inception to April 2018. Studies that compared platelet-rich fibrin versus placebo for rotator cuff tears were included in this meta-analysis. Risk ratio (RR) with 95% confidence interval (CI) was pooled for discontinuous outcome, and weighted mean difference (WMD) with 95% CI was pooled for continuous outcome. Stata 12.0 was used for meta-analysis.

Results: A total of eight studies with 219 patients were finally included in this meta-analysis. Compared with the control group, PRF has a negative role in reducing the re-tear rate (RR = 1.30, 95% CI = 0.97 to 1.75; $P = 0.082$). Subgroup analysis of re-tear rate was consistent in all subgroup analyses (single row or double row, volume, and risk of bias). There was no significant difference between the American Shoulder and Elbow Surgeons scale, University of California at Los Angeles scale, Constant score, and side effect ($P > 0.05$).

Conclusion: In conclusion, our meta-analysis suggests that the PRF does not have better effect on improving the overall clinical outcomes and re-tear rate in the arthroscopic repair of rotator cuff tears.

Keywords: Rotator cuff tears, Platelet-rich fibrin, Meta-analysis

Introduction

Rotator cuff tears are one of the most common disorders of the shoulder with 250,000 to 300,000 rotator cuff repairs being performed annually in the USA [1]. Rotator cuff tears have a significant effect on daily life due to shoulder pain, range of motion decreased, and function loss [2]. Arthroscopic rotator cuff repair has become popular for orthopedic surgeons to improve patient outcomes and quality of life. However, a high re-tear rate was still a concern for extensively clinical use.

The reason for re-tear was that at the repair site, inferior fibrovascular tissue rather than native fibrocartilage tissue was formed, and thus, the repair site was exposing the insertion site to high stresses and increasing the risk of re-tear [3, 4]. In the past decades, some strategies, like the "transosseous-equivalent" suture-bridge technique, have been investigated for the treatment of rotator cuff tears to promote healing, but the outcomes were not promising enough.

Nowadays, the repair of rotator cuff tendon to bone is raising more and more interest. Lately, many growth factors were reported to be effective on the proliferation and collagen secretion of tenocytes in vitro. These growth factors could increase the biomechanical strength and promoted the tendon-to-bone healing in vivo. Many growth factors such as bone morphogenetic proteins (BMPs), basic fibroblast growth factor (bFGF), platelet-derived growth factor (PDGF), vascular endothelial growth factor (VEGF), insulin-like growth factor 1 (IGF-1), and transforming growth factor-b (TGF-b) have shown to be promising agents for rotator cuff tears in vivo and in vitro [5, 6].

Platelet-rich plasma (PRP) is a whole-blood fraction containing high platelet concentrations, which can release various growth factors mentioned above to promote healing [7]. Studies have reported that PRP can be used in the management of tendinopathy [8, 9]. But of legal restrictions on blood handling, a new family of platelet concentrate appears in France, which is called platelet-rich fibrin (PRF) [10]. PRF, unlike other platelet concentrates, can progressively release cytokines during fibrin matrix remodeling.

* Correspondence: 3035822669@qq.com
[2]Physical Health and Sports, College of Education, Lishui University, 1. No, Xueyuan Road, Liandu District, Lishui City 323000, Zhejiang, China
Full list of author information is available at the end of the article

Therefore, applying growth factor mixtures through platelet-rich fibrin maps a promising future for tendon-bone insertion regeneration like rotator cuff repair. In fact, these technologies have been applied on treating chronic tendinopathy [11], bone healing [12], acute ligament repair [13], and tendon repair [14].

Additionally, these products were approved by the US Food and Drug Administration (FDA) for clinical use. Although approved, these products have not been required by the FDA to show efficacy. Nevertheless, to our best knowledge, none of the previous studies, which involved a large number of patients, has been performed to investigate the efficacy of rotator cuff repair with or without PRF by analyzing clinical and radiological outcomes.

The aim of the present meta-analysis was to assess whether administration with PRF has a beneficial role in improving clinical outcomes and side effect during the arthroscopic repair of rotator cuff tears.

Methods
Search strategies
Two reviewers searched the Pubmed, Embase, Web of Science, and Cochrane library independently (Xiu-hua Mao and Ye-jun Zhan) from inception to April 2018. The following keywords and Mesh terms were used for searching: "rotator cuff," "rotator cuff tears," "Rotator Cuff Injuries"[Mesh] "platelet rich fibrin," "platelet rich," "PRF," "platelet rich fibril matrix," "PRFM," and "Platelet-Rich Fibrin"[Mesh]. Publication language was restricted to English. Reference list in systematic review or meta-analysis was also manually searched to avoid omitting any relevant studies.

Inclusion criteria
The inclusion criteria were as follows:

Participant (P): arthroscopic rotator cuff repair as regards the age and sex.

Intervention (I): administration with PRF as the intervention group.

Comparison (C): placebo or saline as the control group.

Outcomes (O): re-tear rate, American Shoulder and Elbow Surgeons scale (ASES), University of California at Los Angeles scale (UCLA), Constant score, and adverse effect.

Study (S): only RCTs were included in this meta-analysis.

Data extraction and quality assessment
Two readers (Xiu-hua Mao and Ye-jun Zhan) independently extracted all the data as follows: general characteristics (no. of patients, mean age, country, intervention, follow-up, and outcomes). The methodological quality of the trials was assessed using the *Cochrane Handbook for Systematic Reviews of Interventions 5.3*. A total of seven items were included to assess the quality of study:

random sequence generation, allocation concealment, blinding to the participant, blinding to outcome assessment, incomplete outcome, selective reporting, and other potential bias. Each item was assessed as "low," "unclear," and "high."

Statistical analysis
We used Review Stata 12.0 to perform statistical analysis. For continuous variables, we used the weighted mean difference, whereas for those categorical dichotomous, we used relative risks (RR) to analyze, and 95% confidence intervals (CI) were reported in analysis of both continuous and dichotomous variables. P value beneath 0.05 was considered to be statistically significant. Homogeneity was tested by the Q statistic (significance level at $P = 0.10$) and the I^2 statistic (significance level at $I^2 = 50\%$). A random-effects model was used if the Q or I^2 statistic was significant; otherwise, a fixed-effects model was used. Subgroup analysis were performed in the analysis of re-tear rate according to the operative technique (single row or double row), risk of bias (low or unclear/high), volume of PRP (< 5 or ≥ 5 ml), follow-up duration (< 15 or ≥ 15 months), and size of rotator cuff tears (small-medium or large-massive). Sensitivity analysis was performed based on omitting one study in turn to investigate the influence of a single study on the overall RR estimates. Publication bias was not performed because the included studies were less than ten.

Results
Search results
Details of study identification, screening, and selection are given in Fig. 1. Firstly, we retrieved 320 relevant reports from electronic databases. And 114 papers were removed by Endnote software for duplications. Thus, 206 papers were screened for the next step. Then, according to the inclusion criteria, 198 records were excluded. Finally, eight RCTs [15–22] involving 364 patients (PRF = 177, control = 187) finally met the predetermined inclusion criteria and were included for final analysis.

Demographic characteristics
We summarized the general characteristics of all the included studies and listed in Table 1. All of the included studies were published from the year 2011. Three studies were originated from the USA, two from Spain, two from Italy, and one from France. Only one study did not report the tear size, and the rest of the studies all reported the tear size. Mean age of the included patients ranged from 55.2 to 66. Sample size ranged from 14 to 43 with a total of 364 patients. Follow-up duration ranged from 12 to 27.2 months.

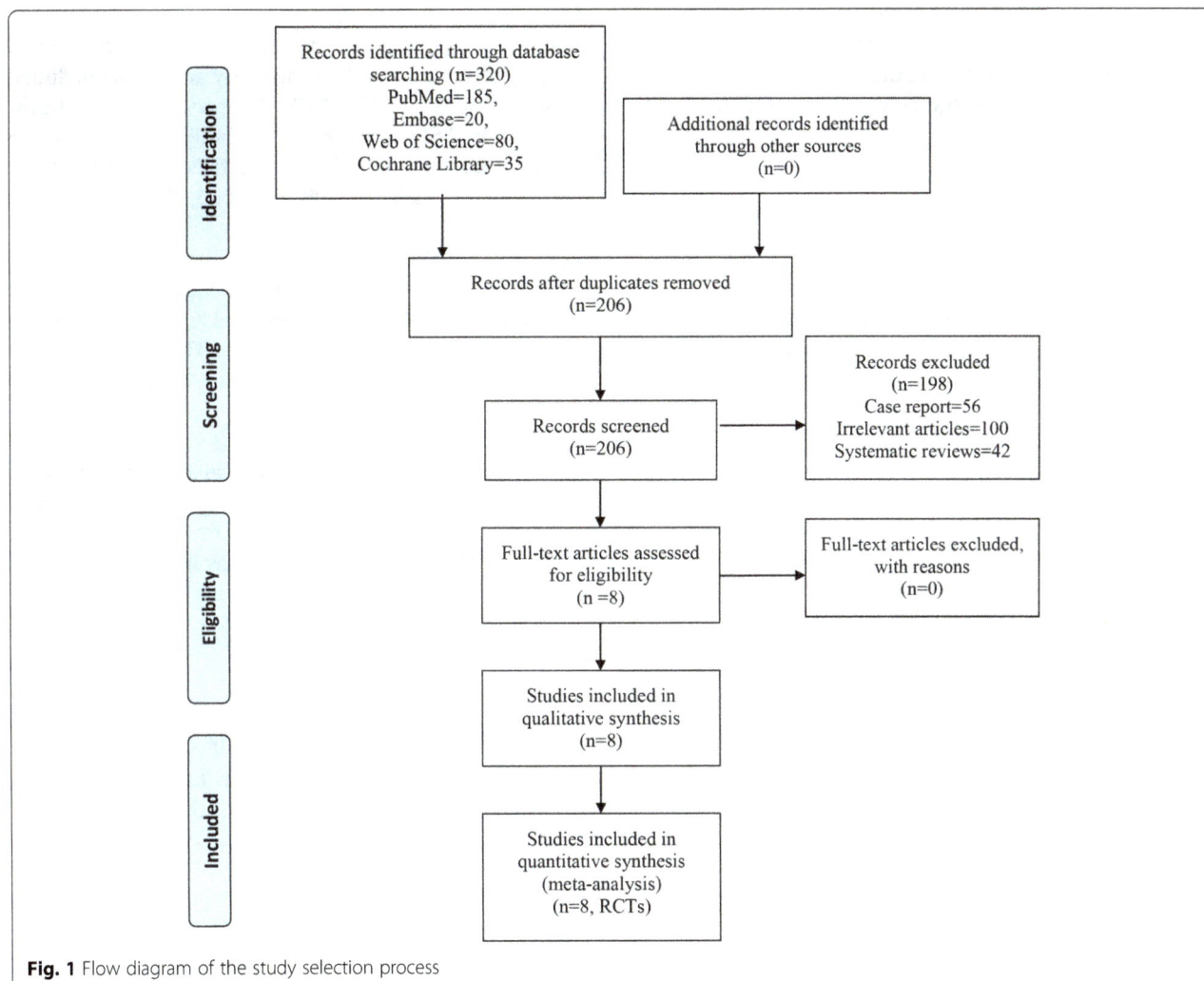

Fig. 1 Flow diagram of the study selection process

Table 1 General characteristics of the included studies. 1, re-tear rate; 2, ASES; 3, UCLA; 4, Constant score; 5, adverse event

Study	Country	Participants	Surgical procedure	Mean age		No. of patients		Follow-up (months)	Outcomes
				PRF	Control	PRF	Control		
Antuna 2013	Spain	Massive full-thickness rotator cuff tears	Double-row techniques	NS	NS	14	14	24	1, 4
Bergeson 2012	USA	Full-thickness rotator cuff tears	Single- or double-row techniques	65	65	16	21	27	1, 2, 3, 5
Rodeo 2012	USA	Full-thickness rotator cuff tears	Single or double-row techniques	58.9	57.2	19	22	19	1, 2, 5
Weber 2013	USA	Full-thickness rotator cuff tears	Single-row techniques	59.7	64.5	29	30	12	1, 2, 3, 4, 5
Castricini 2011	Italy	NS	Double-row technique	55.5	55.2	43	45	20.2	1, 5
Gumina 2012	Italy	Large full-thickness posterosuperior rotator cuff tear	Single-row technique	60	63	39	37	13	4, 5
Márquez 2011	Spain	Massive rotator cuff tear of at least 5 cm and including 2 tendons	Single-row technique	65	NS	14	14	12	1, 2, 4
Zumstein 2016	France	Full-thickness rotator cuff tears	Single- or double-row techniques	65	66	17	18	12	1, 5

Figures 2 and 3 present the risk of bias summary and risk of graph respectively. Six studies reported the random sequence generation and one with high risk of bias. Five studies were with low risk of bias, and two were with unclear risk of bias.

Meta-analysis results
Re-tear rate
Seven studies [15–19, 21, 22] perform available data for postoperative re-tear rate. There was no heterogeneity across the included studies (I^2 = 0.0%, P = 0.614). Compared with the control group, PRF group was not associated with a reduction of the re-tear rate (RR = 1.30, 95% CI = 0.97 to 1.75; P = 0.082, Fig. 4). Table 2 presents the results of subgroup analyses. The findings of re-tear rate were consistent in all subgroup analyses.

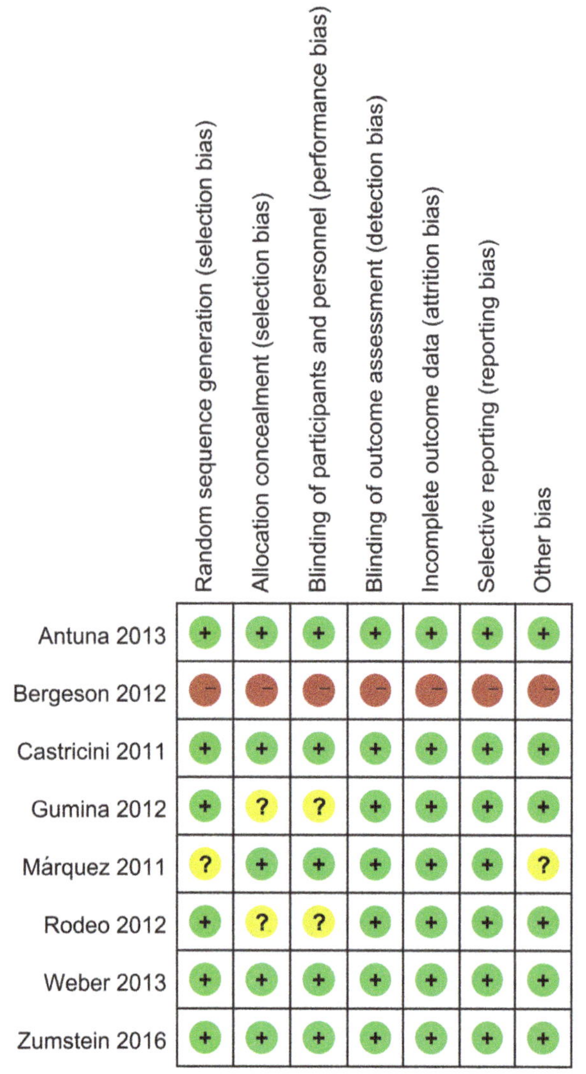

ASES
Four studies [16–18, 21] reported postoperative ASES scores. There was little heterogeneity across the included studies (I^2 = 15.0%, P = 0.317). There was no significant difference in ASES score between the PRF group and the control group (weighted mean difference (WMD) = – 1.25, 95% CI = – 2.58 to 0.08; P = 0.066, Fig. 5).

UCLA
Two studies [16, 18] reported postoperative UCLA scores. There was no significant difference in UCLA score between the PRF group and the control group. The MD was – 0.96 (WMD = – 0.97, 95% CI = – 2.56 to 0.62; P = 0.230, Fig. 6).

Constant score
Four studies [15, 19–21] perform available data for postoperative constant score. There was no heterogeneity across the included studies (I^2 = 0.0%, P = 0.967). Compared with the control group, PRF group was not associated with a reduction of the constant score (WMD = 0.73, 95% CI = – 1.30 to 2.77; P = 0.481, Fig. 7).

Side effect
A total of seven studies [15–20, 22] reported postoperative complication. The pooled result showed that there was no significant difference in the side effect between the PRF group and the control group (RR = 1.26; 95% CI = 0.28, 5.67; P = 0.767; Fig. 8).

Discussion
Main findings
Our meta-analysis comprehensively and systematically reviewed the current available literature and found that (1) PRF compared with placebo did not significantly reduced re-tear rate for rotator cuff tear patients; the evidence of the re-tear rate was consistent in most subgroup analyses and was confirmed by TSA; (2) PRF has no benefit on the shoulder function at the final follow-up when compared with placebo; (3) PRF was not associated with an increase of the complications than the control group.

Comparison with other meta-analyses
Only one relevant meta-analysis on the topic has been published [23]. Several differences between ours and the previous ones should be noted. First, the previous ones mixed PRP and PRF in the same intervention group and thus cause large heterogeneity across the studies. Second, two studies were not included in the previous meta-analysis and the publication bias was inevitable. Andia et al. [24] conducted a review about the PRP therapy for tendinopathy, plantar fasciopathy, and muscle injuries. Results showed that PRP therapies were useless. Meanwhile, Andia et al. [25] revealed that PRP has no effects on muscle injury and tendinopathy.

Fig. 2 Risk of bias summary

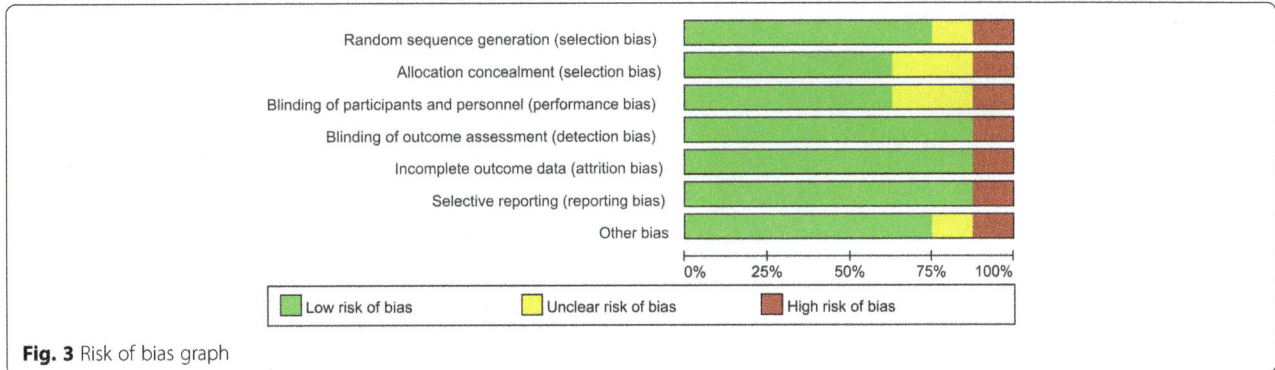

Fig. 3 Risk of bias graph

The current meta-analysis systematically scanned all of the available studies and has given a relative credible evidence for the clinical effects of PRF on rotator cuff tear patients. In this meta-analysis, we identified re-tear rate as the primary outcome. Results showed that PRF has a negative effect on the overall incidence of re-tear at the final follow-up. Previous meta-analysis did not pool this important outcome [23]. Re-tear could make the patients dissatisfied and increase additional costs. Subgroup analysis indicated that PRF has a positive role in reducing the incidence of re-tear rate than the control group. However, long-term effects of PRF were extremely important for clinical administration.

Hueley et al. [23] conducted a meta-analysis, and the pooled result was similar with our meta-analysis. PRF is considered as one kind of platelet concentrates, and its molecular structure with low thrombin concentration is an optimal matrix for migration of endothelial cells and fibroblasts, which can progressively release several cytokines to help fibrin matrix remodeling.

In an animal experiment, we found that PRF has a beneficial role in tissue regeneration whereas there was a negative role in a clinical experiment [19]. Randelli et al. [26] reported that autologous PRP reduced pain in the first postoperative months and affected cuff rotator healing for both grade 1 and 2 tears. Furthermore, Andia et al. [27] revealed that PRP, as an autologous biotechnology product, has a positive effect on experimental tendon healing.

The reason for the failure of PRF to fulfill its promise remains unclear. There are some possible interpretations for this phenomenon. On the one hand, patients all received autologous source PRF and the growth factors contained in PRF vary from person to person, for which there were much more difficulty for experimentally bias control. To be specific, there is a chance that the patient's blood plasma contains excessive TGF-β, and its potential effect on exuberant fibrosis may affect the therapeutic effect of PRF. Nevertheless, some patients' plasma may contain abundant inflammatory mediators, which could adversely affect healing process. More importantly, none of us has enough data to determine the best clinical usage of PRF

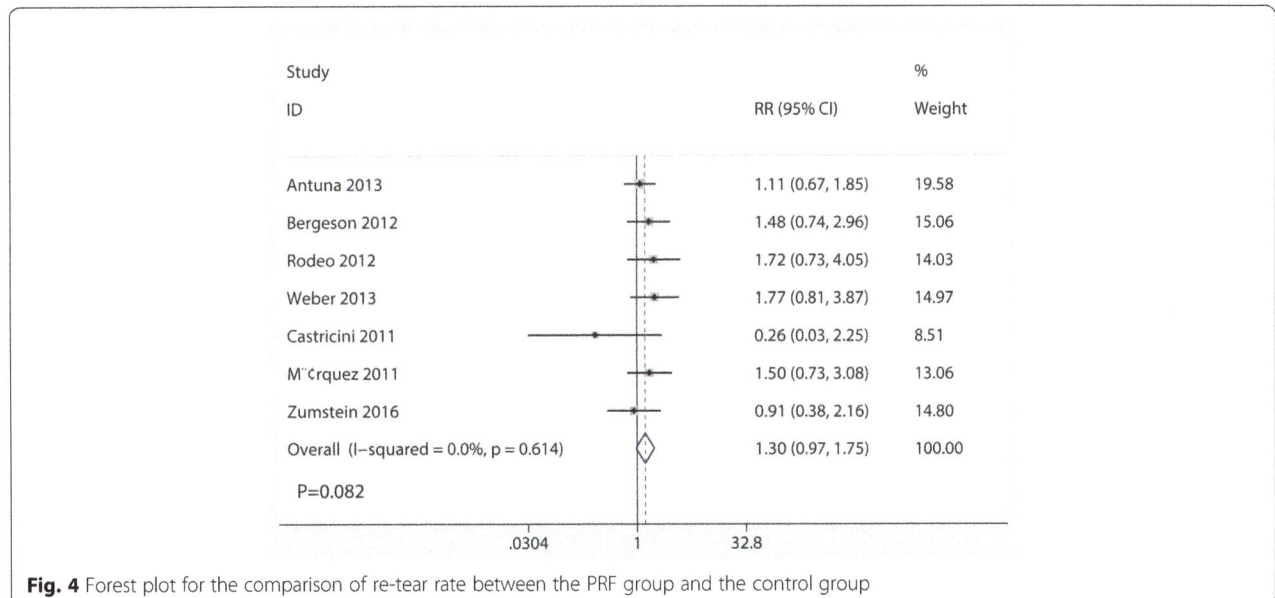

Fig. 4 Forest plot for the comparison of re-tear rate between the PRF group and the control group

Table 2 Subgroup analysis for the re-tear rate

Subgroup	No. trials	Relative risk (95% CI)	P value	I^2 (%)	Test of interaction, P
Total	7	1.30 (0.97, 1.75)	0.082	0.0	
Operative technique					
Single row	2	1.65 (0.82, 2.77)	0.069	0.0	0.106
Double row	2	0.87 (0.55, 1.39)	0.566	3.3	
Single or double row	3	1.60 (0.92, 2.77)	0.097	0.0	
Risk of bias					
Low	3	1.49 (0.99, 2.25)	0.058	0.0	0.098
Unclear/high	4	1.12 (0.73, 1.71)	0.607	7.1	
Volume					
< 5 ml	1	1.77 (0.81, 3.87)	0.150	–	0.152
≥ 5 ml	3	1.40 (0.94, 2.10)	0.097	0.0	
Unclear	3	0.99 (0.59, 1.67)	0.963	28.2	
Follow-up					
< 15 months	4	1.95 (0.87, 4.37)	0.103	0.0	0.105
≥ 15 months	3	1.37 (0.60, 3.10)	0.449	0.0	
Size of rotator cuff tears					
Small-medium	3	0.77 (0.31, 1.86)	0.271	0.0	0.226
Large-massive	4	1.72 (0.64, 4.28)	0.582	0.0	

products. And there were some prior articles that noticed this problem [27]. On the other hand, platelet-rich products may also influence the effect.

For example, recent studies showed that not all separation systems yield a similar product, because there are many factors that can influence the separation, including the volume of blood, single- versus double-spin cycles, centrifuge rates, the need for an activator, white blood cell concentrations, and the final platelet and growth factor concentrations. In other words, different products can have varied platelet concentrations, and therefore, platelet-derived growth factor concentrations may differ between various systems [28]. Additionally, it is also possible that the clot may occupy the space between the tendon and bone, resulting in a gap. Once the material dissolves, they may inhibit the healing process.

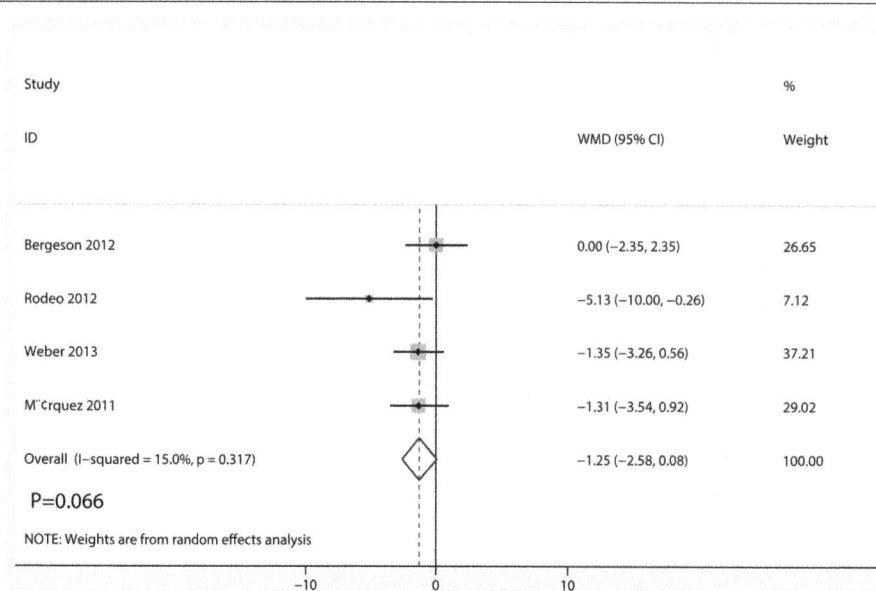

Fig. 5 Forest plot for the comparison of ASES between the PRF group and the control group

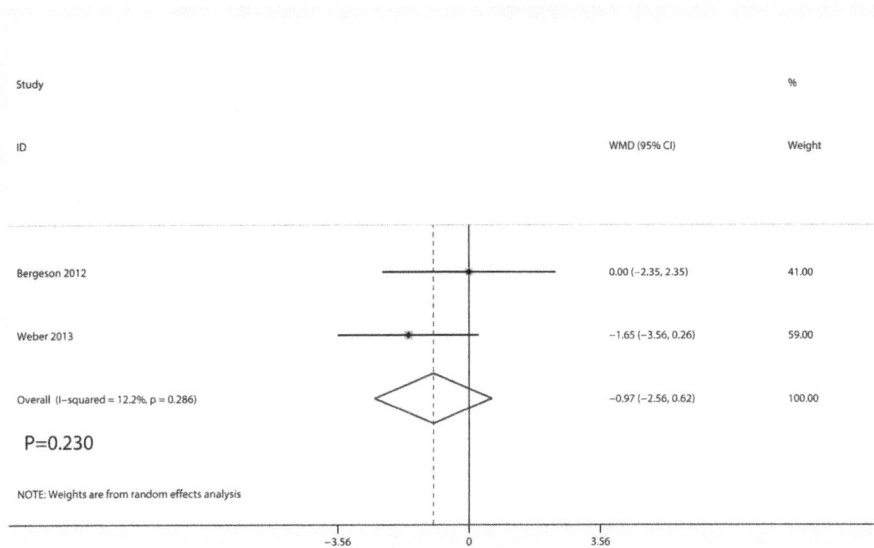

Fig. 6 Forest plot for the comparison of UCLA between the PRF group and the control group

Moreover, although patients all received autologous source PRF, these procedures are not absolutely safe. Some postoperative complications seem to be related with PRF. The most common one is infection. Even though it is performed with aseptic techniques, the PRF group has a higher infection rate than the control group [29]. The cause of infection is unclear, but multiple steps obliged to prepare PRFM require additional interactions between sterile and non-sterile fields and introduce variables, increasing infection risk. However, we did not find a significant difference in postoperative complication between the two groups in our meta-analysis.

Several limitations also existed in this meta-analysis: (1) initial tear size was not compared between the PRF and control group; (2) PRF volume, platelet concentration, and activating agent were different in the included studies, and thus, clinical heterogeneity was large in the outcomes; (3) the follow-up period varied among included studies, and thus, clinical effects of PRF in the same follow-up period need to be further confirmed; (4) sample size was relatively small in the included studies, and thus, high quality with large-scale sample RCTs were needed.

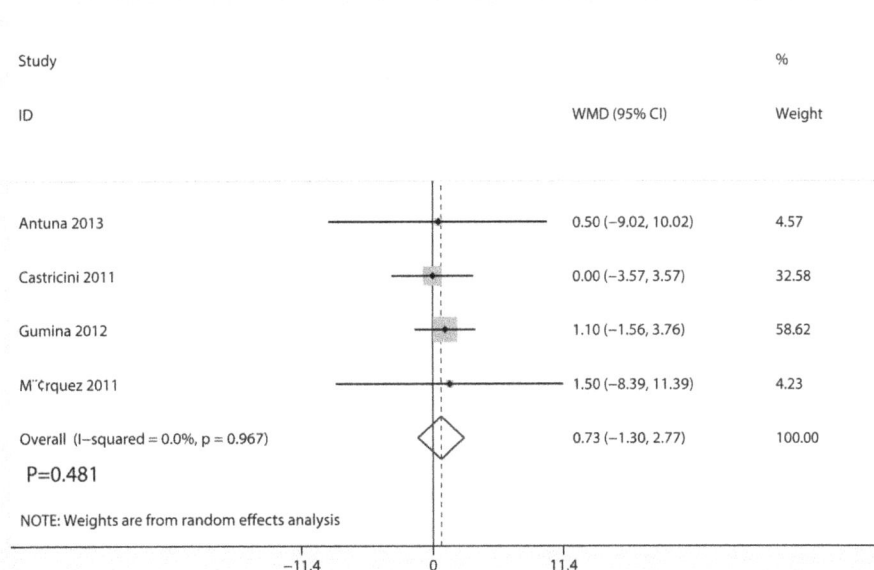

Fig. 7 Forest plot for the comparison of Constant score between the PRF group and the control group

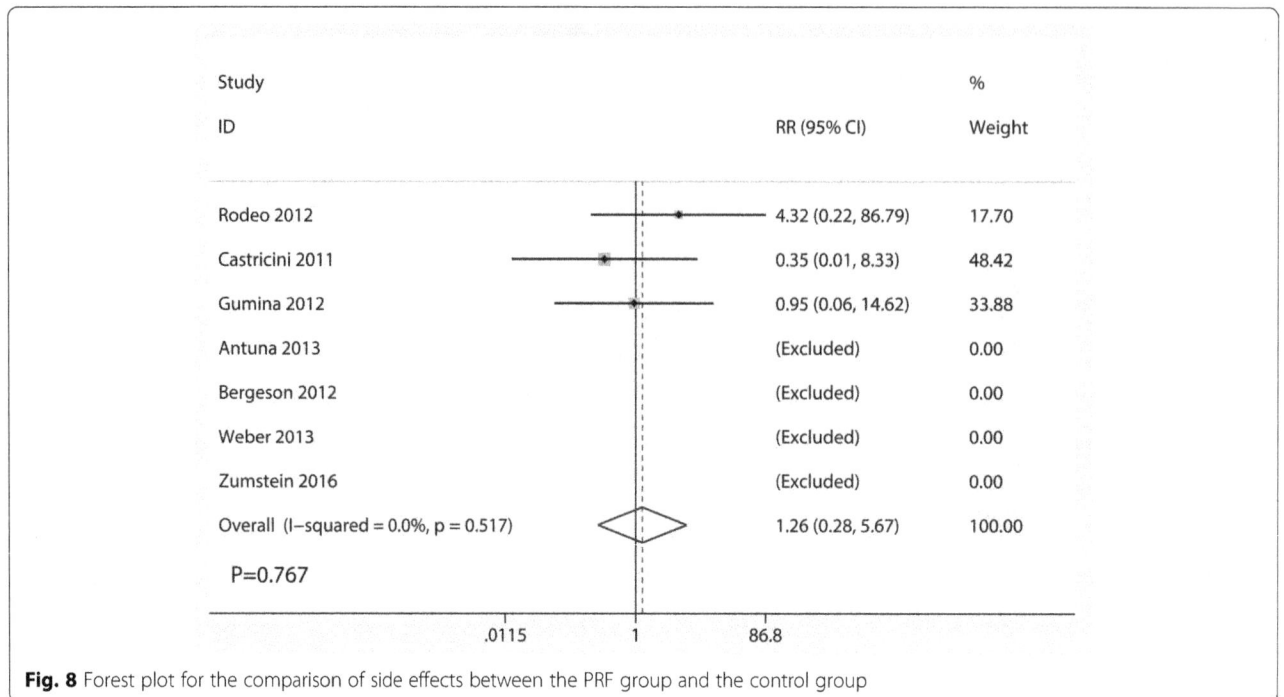

Study ID	RR (95% CI)	% Weight
Rodeo 2012	4.32 (0.22, 86.79)	17.70
Castricini 2011	0.35 (0.01, 8.33)	48.42
Gumina 2012	0.95 (0.06, 14.62)	33.88
Antuna 2013	(Excluded)	0.00
Bergeson 2012	(Excluded)	0.00
Weber 2013	(Excluded)	0.00
Zumstein 2016	(Excluded)	0.00
Overall (I–squared = 0.0%, p = 0.517)	1.26 (0.28, 5.67)	100.00

P=0.767

.0115   1   86.8

Fig. 8 Forest plot for the comparison of side effects between the PRF group and the control group

Conclusion

In conclusion, this meta-analysis suggests that the PRF has no benefits on the overall clinical outcomes and re-tear rate for the arthroscopic repair of full-thickness rotator cuff tears. But, given all the shortness that this meta-analysis has, further research and analysis are required to make a more reliable conclusion.

Abbreviations

ASES: American Shoulder and Elbow Surgeons scale; bFGF: Basic fibroblast growth factor; BMPs: Bone morphogenetic proteins; IGF-1: Insulin-like growth factor 1; PDGF: Platelet-derived growth factor; PRF: Platelet-rich fibrin; PRP: Platelet-rich plasma; TGF-b: Transforming growth factor-b; UCLA: University of California at Los Angeles scale; VEGF: Vascular endothelial growth factor

Acknowledgements

We are grateful to all the patients and surgeons of the included studies.

Authors' contributions

XHM and YJZ conceived of the design of this meta-analysis. XHM and YJZ performed the literature retrieval and article writing. XHM and YJZ contributed to the data extraction, and YJZ revised the manuscript. All authors read and approved the final manuscript.

Competing interests

The authors declare that they have no competing interests.

Author details

[1]Department of Pain Treatment, Ningbo No.2 Hospital, Ningbo 315000, Zhejiang, China. [2]Physical Health and Sports, College of Education, Lishui University, 1. No, Xueyuan Road, Liandu District, Lishui City 323000, Zhejiang, China.

References

1. Yamaguchi K, Ditsios K, Middleton WD, Hildebolt CF, Galatz LM, Teefey SA. The demographic and morphological features of rotator cuff disease: a comparison of asymptomatic and symptomatic shoulders. J Bone Joint Surg Am. 2006;88:1699–704.
2. Liu CT, Ge HA, Hu R, et al. Arthroscopic knotless single-row repair preserving full footprint versus tear completion repair for partial articular-sided rotator cuff tear. J Orthop Surg (Hong Kong). 2018;26:2309499018770897.
3. Galatz LM, Rothermich SY, Zaegel M, Silva MJ, Havlioglu N, Thomopoulos S. Delayed repair of tendon to bone injuries leads to decreased biomechanical properties and bone loss. J Orthop Res. 2005;23:1441–7.
4. Newsham-West R, Nicholson H, Walton M, Milburn P. Long-term morphology of a healing bone-tendon interface: a histological observation in the sheep model. J Anat. 2007;210:318–27.
5. Pauly S, Klatte F, Strobel C, et al. BMP-2 and BMP-7 affect human rotator cuff tendon cells in vitro. J Shoulder Elb Surg. 2012;21:464–73.
6. Seeherman HJ, Archambault JM, Rodeo SA, et al. rhBMP-12 accelerates healing of rotator cuff repairs in a sheep model. J Bone Joint Surg Am. 2008;90:2206–19.
7. Kim SJ, Kim EK, Kim SJ, Song DH. Effects of bone marrow aspirate concentrate and platelet-rich plasma on patients with partial tear of the rotator cuff tendon. J Orthop Surg Res. 2018;13:1.
8. Andia I, Martin JI, Maffulli N. Advances with platelet rich plasma therapies for tendon regeneration. Expert Opin Biol Ther. 2018;18:389–98.
9. Andia I, Maffulli N. Biological therapies in regenerative sports medicine. Sports Med. 2017;47:807–28.
10. Natto ZS, Green MS. A leukocyte- and platelet-rich fibrin showed a regenerative potential in intrabony defects and furcation defects but not in periodontal plastic surgery. J Evid Based Dent Pract. 2017;17:408–10.
11. Mishra A, Pavelko T. Treatment of chronic elbow tendinosis with buffered platelet-rich plasma. Am J Sports Med. 2006;34:1774–8.
12. Giovanini AF, Grossi JR, Gonzaga CC, et al. Leukocyte-platelet-rich plasma (L-PRP) induces an abnormal histophenotype in craniofacial bone repair

associated with changes in the immunopositivity of the hematopoietic clusters of differentiation, osteoproteins, and TGF-beta1. Clin Implant Dent Relat Res. 2014;16:259–72.

13. Orrego M, Larrain C, Rosales J, et al. Effects of platelet concentrate and a bone plug on the healing of hamstring tendons in a bone tunnel. Arthroscopy. 2008;24:1373–80.

14. Jo CH, Kim JE, Yoon KS, et al. Does platelet-rich plasma accelerate recovery after rotator cuff repair? A prospective cohort study. Am J Sports Med. 2011; 39:2082–90.

15. Antuna S, Barco R, Martinez Diez JM, Sanchez Marquez JM. Platelet-rich fibrin in arthroscopic repair of massive rotator cuff tears: a prospective randomized pilot clinical trial. Acta Orthop Belg. 2013;79:25–30.

16. Bergeson AG, Tashjian RZ, Greis PE, Crim J, Stoddard GJ, Burks RT. Effects of platelet-rich fibrin matrix on repair integrity of at-risk rotator cuff tears. Am J Sports Med. 2012;40:286–93.

17. Rodeo SA, Delos D, Williams RJ, Adler RS, Pearle A, Warren RF. The effect of platelet-rich fibrin matrix on rotator cuff tendon healing: a prospective, randomized clinical study. Am J Sports Med. 2012;40:1234–41.

18. Weber SC, Kauffman JI, Parise C, Weber SJ, Katz SD. Platelet-rich fibrin matrix in the management of arthroscopic repair of the rotator cuff: a prospective, randomized, double-blinded study. Am J Sports Med. 2013;41:263–70.

19. Castricini R, Longo UG, De Benedetto M, et al. Platelet-rich plasma augmentation for arthroscopic rotator cuff repair: a randomized controlled trial. Am J Sports Med. 2011;39:258–65.

20. Gumina S, Campagna V, Ferrazza G, et al. Use of platelet-leukocyte membrane in arthroscopic repair of large rotator cuff tears: a prospective randomized study. J Bone Joint Surg Am. 2012;94:1345–52.

21. Márquez JMS, Díez JMM, Barco R, Antuña S. Functional results after arthroscopic repair of massive rotator cuff tears; influence of the application platelet-rich plasma combined with fibrin. Rev Esp Cir Ortop Traumatol. 2011;55:282–7.

22. Zumstein MA, Rumian A, Thelu CE, et al. Use of platelet- and leucocyte-rich fibrin (L-PRF) does not affect late rotator cuff tendon healing: a prospective randomized controlled study. J Shoulder Elb Surg. 2016;25:2–11.

23. Hurley ET, Lim Fat D, Moran CJ, Mullett H. The efficacy of platelet-rich plasma and platelet-rich fibrin in arthroscopic rotator cuff repair: a meta-analysis of randomized controlled trials. Am J Sports Med. 2018. [Epub ahead of print].

24. Andia I, Maffulli N. Muscle and tendon injuries: the role of biological interventions to promote and assist healing and recovery. Arthroscopy. 2015;31:999–1015.

25. Andia I, Maffulli N. Platelet-rich plasma for muscle injury and tendinopathy. Sports Med Arthrosc Rev. 2013;21:191–8.

26. Randelli P, Arrigoni P, Ragone V, Aliprandi A, Cabitza P. Platelet rich plasma in arthroscopic rotator cuff repair: a prospective RCT study, 2-year follow-up. J Shoulder Elb Surg. 2011;20:518–28.

27. Andia I, Sanchez M, Maffulli N. Tendon healing and platelet-rich plasma therapies. Expert Opin Biol Ther. 2010;10:1415–26.

28. Castillo TN, Pouliot MA, Kim HJ, Dragoo JL. Comparison of growth factor and platelet concentration from commercial platelet-rich plasma separation systems. Am J Sports Med. 2011;39:266–71.

29. Randelli PS, Arrigoni P, Cabitza P, Volpi P, Maffulli N. Autologous platelet rich plasma for arthroscopic rotator cuff repair. A pilot study. Disabil Rehabil. 2008;30:1584–9.

11

Exploring the key genes and pathways of side population cells in human osteosarcoma using gene expression array analysis

Yi-Ming Ren[t], Yuan-Hui Duan[t], Yun-Bo Sun[t], Tao Yang, Wen-Jun Zhao, Dong-Liang Zhang, Zheng-Wei Tian and Meng-Qiang Tian[*]

Abstract

Background: Human osteosarcoma (OS) is one of the most common primary bone sarcoma, because of early metastasis and few treatment strategies. It has been reported that the tumorigenicity and self-renewal capacity of side population (SP) cells play roles in human OS via regulating of target genes. This study aims to complement the differentially expressed genes (DEGs) that regulated between the SP cells and the non-SP cells from primary human OS and identify their functions and molecular pathways associated with OS.

Methods: The gene expression profile GSE63390 was downloaded, and bioinformatics analysis was made.

Results: One hundred forty-one DEGs totally were identified. Among them, 72 DEGs (51.06%) were overexpressed, and the remaining 69 DEGs (48.94%) were underexpressed. Gene ontology (GO) and pathway enrichment analysis of target genes were performed. We furthermore identified some relevant core genes using gene–gene interaction network analysis such as EIF4E, FAU, HSPD1, IL-6, and KISS1, which may have a relationship with the development process of OS. We also discovered that EIF4E/mTOR signaling pathway could be a potential research target for therapy and tumorigenesis of OS.

Conclusion: This analysis provides a comprehensive understanding of the roles of DEGs coming from SP cells in the development of OS. However, these predictions need further experimental validation in future studies.

Keywords: Osteosarcoma, Side population cells, Differentially expressed genes, Bioinformatics analysis

Background

Osteosarcoma (OS), which is produced by mesenchymal cells, is the most common primary malignant tumor originating from bone tissues. OS occurs mainly in children and adolescents and accounts for 8.9% of cancer-related diseases which lead to death [1, 2]. Although new therapies of neoadjuvant chemotherapy and surgery have contributed greatly to OS treatment, the 5-year survival rate of OS is difficult to exceed 60–65% [3, 4]. To sum up, the early diagnosis and effective treatment of OS are the breakthrough point of OS research and clinical application, and exploring the pathogenesis, development, and metastasis of OS is the key. Although a large number of studies have been made on OS at molecular and cellular levels, the mechanisms of OS formation and metastasis have not been fully elucidated.

Side population (SP) cells are a group of special cells, which were found when Hoechst and flow cytometry are used to separate hematopoietic stem cells and progenitor cells. SP cells are widely distributed in a variety of adult tissues, embryos, and some tumor cell lines [5]. They not only have self-renewal and multipotential differentiation potential, but also have unique phenotypic markers and biological characteristics of stem cells, whose

---

* Correspondence: tmqjoint@126.com
[t]Yi-Ming Ren, Yuan-Hui Duan and Yun-Bo Sun contributed equally to this work.
Department of Joint and Sport Medicine, Tianjin Union Medical Center, Jieyuan Road 190, Hongqiao District, Tianjin 300121, People's Republic of China

characteristics are very similar to those of tumor stem cells [6, 7]. SP cells help maintain the tumorigenic potential of some tumor cell lines [8–10]. Ho et al. reported that SP cells were enriched in tumor-initiating capability compared with non-SP cells by nonobese diabetic/severe combined immunodeficiency xenograft experiments. Matrigel invasion assay showed that SP cells also have higher potential for invasiveness. Human telomerase reverse transcriptase expression was higher in the SP cells, suggesting that this fraction may represent a reservoir with unlimited proliferative potential for generating cancer cells [11]. Chiba et al. hold that a minority population of SP cells detected in hepatocellular carcinoma cells possessed extreme tumorigenic potential and provided heterogeneity to the cancer stem cell system characterized by distinct hierarchy [12]. Wang et al. observed a strong tumorigenesis ability of SP cells from HeLa cell line following in vivo transplantation into 5- to 6-week-old female Balb/c mice [13]. These findings indicate that SP cells is an enriched source of tumor-initiating cells with stem cell properties and may be an important target for effective therapy and a useful tool to investigate the tumorigenic process.

Interestingly, SP cells are present in primary mesenchymal neoplasms, including primary OS [14]. Here, we downloaded the gene expression profile GSE63390 from the Gene Expression Omnibus (GEO) database and made bioinformatics analysis to investigate differentially expressed genes (DEGs) that regulated between the SP cells and the non-SP cells from primary human OS. By doing this, we hope that the key target genes and pathways involved in the carcinogenesis and progression of human OS could be identified and existing molecular mechanisms could be revealed.

Methods

Gene expression microarray data

The gene expression profile GSE63390 was downloaded from the Gene Expression Omnibus (GEO, www.ncbi.nlm.nih.gov/geo/). GSE63390 was based on Illumina Human HT-12 V4.0 expression beadchip GPL10558 platform. The GSE63390 dataset contained three samples, including three SP cell samples and three non-SP cell samples.

DEGs in SP cells and non-SP cells

The raw data files used for the analysis included TXT files (Illumina platform). The analysis was carried out using GEO2R, which can perform comparisons on original submitter-supplied processed data tables using the GEO query and limma R packages from Bioconductor project. The P value < 0.05 and log fold change (FC) > 1.0 or log FC < − 1.0 were used as the cut-off criteria. The DEGs with statistical significance between the SP cells and non-SP cells were selected and identified.

GO and KEGG analysis of DEGs

Target genes list were submitted to the Cytoscape software version 3.4.0 (www.cytoscape.org) and ClueGO version 2.33 to identify overrepresented GO categories and pathway categories. Gene Ontology (GO) analysis was used to predict the potential functions of the DEGs in biological process (BP), molecular function (MF), and cellular component (CC). The Kyoto Encyclopedia of Genes and Genomes (KEGG, http://www.genome.jp/) is a knowledge base for systematic analysis of gene functions, linking genomic information with higher-level systemic functions. Finally, the overrepresented pathway categories with a P value < 0.05 were considered statistically significant using KEGG pathway enrichment analysis.

Gene interaction network construction

A large number of DEGs we obtained may be human OS-associated genes, and it is suggested that these DEGs in SP cells may participate in the progression of human OS. Firstly, DEGs list was submitted to the Search Tool for the Retrieval of Interacting Genes (STRING) database (http://www.string-db.org/) and an interaction network chart with a combined score > 0.4 was saved and exported. Subsequently, the interaction regulatory network of human OS-associated genes was visualized using Cytoscape software version 3.4.0. The distribution of core genes in the interaction network was made by NetworkAnalyzer in Cytoscape. Then, the plugin Molecular Complex Detection (MCODE) was applied to screen the modules of the gene interaction network in Cytoscape.

Results

Identification of DEGs

The gene expression profile GSE63390 was downloaded from the GEO, and the GEO2R method was used to identify DEGs in SP cells compared with non-SP cells. P value < 0.05, log FC > 1.0, or log FC < − 1.0 were used as the cut-off criteria. After analyzing, differentially expression gene profiles were obtained. Totally, 141 DEGs were identified including 72 upregulated DEGs and 69 downregulated DEGs screened in SP cells of human OS compared with non-SP cells. Parts of DEGs were listed in Table 1.

GO term enrichment analysis of DEGs

Functional annotation of the 141 DEGs was clarified using the Cytoscape software online tool. GO analysis indicated that these DEGs were significantly enriched in cellular amide metabolic process, peptide metabolic process, translation, translational initiation, selenium compound metabolic process, cellular modified amino acid metabolic process, aromatic compound catabolic process, cellular nitrogen compound catabolic process,

Table 1 The top 10 regulated DEGs in OS SP cells with P value < 0.05

ID	P value	logFC	Gene symbol
Upregulated			
ILMN_2184250	6.45E−05	3.0817572	SERPINB9
ILMN_1713706	4.08E−02	3.08089766	ZNF786
ILMN_2260756	4.98E−02	2.76569527	GSDMB
ILMN_2189870	3.65E−03	2.52175439	FCF1
ILMN_2078724	2.68E−02	2.46037207	APOPT1
ILMN_1681490	3.27E−02	2.34502196	ZNF568
ILMN_1809957	1.68E−03	2.32352121	AP2S1
ILMN_1812392	1.46E−02	2.28124068	TMSB10
ILMN_2246548	3.62E−02	2.24405561	GSTTP2
ILMN_2053178	0.96444	2.21210244	ACTG1
Downregulated			
ILMN_1789196	2.84E−03	− 2.95354379	TPM2
ILMN_1672496	2.45E−04	− 2.53681489	DNAJA1
ILMN_1755733	7.92E−03	− 2.32101519	RPLP2
ILMN_1690494	3.37E−03	− 2.30094686	RPL6
ILMN_1686367	1.42E−02	− 2.28782734	HSPA8
ILMN_1728870	6.65E−03	− 2.24915587	DDX3X
ILMN_2230624	2.93E−03	− 2.22730708	RPL18
ILMN_1666385	5.79E−03	− 2.18496943	CALM3
ILMN_2378868	3.56E−02	− 2.17417408	SRSF5
ILMN_2139943	3.81E−03	− 2.15657539	RPS3A

OS osteosarcoma, *DEGs* differentially expressed genes, *SP* side population, *FC* fold change

heterocycle catabolic process, organic cyclic compound catabolic process, nucleobase-containing compound catabolic process, RNA catabolic process, viral transcription, establishment of protein, localization to endoplasmic reticulum, alpha-amino acid metabolic process, translational elongation, mRNA catabolic process, translational termination, serine family amino acid metabolic process, SRP-dependent cotranslational protein targeting to membrane, nuclear-transcribed mRNA catabolic process, nonsense-mediated decay, and other biological processes (Fig. 1). For MF, the DEGs were enriched in RNA binding, mRNA binding, mRNA 5′-UTR binding and others. In addition, GO CC analysis also showed that the DEGs were significantly enriched in intracellular ribonucleoprotein complex, adherens junction, focal adhesion, ribosome, ribosomal subunit, cytosolic part, large ribosomal subunit, cytosolic large ribosomal subunit, cytosolic small ribosomal subunit, and others.

KEGG pathway analysis of DEGs

The result of KEGG pathway analysis revealed that target genes were enriched in estrogen signaling pathway, hippo signaling pathway, adherens junction, NOD-like receptor signaling pathway, apelin signaling pathway, ECM−receptor interaction, Toll-like receptor signaling pathway, mTOR signaling pathway, FoxO signaling pathway, cell adhesion molecules (CAMs) and hedgehog signaling pathway, and others. These key pathways were showed in Fig. 2. Fifty-five nodes and 163 edges could be discovered in this network. FoxO signaling pathway and mTOR signaling pathway clustered together. Estrogen signaling pathway and hippo signaling pathway clustered together. Besides, these core pathways and their associated genes found were summarized in Table 2. The first-ranking estrogen signaling pathway had the 6.12% associated genes, which included CALM3, CALML4, HSPA1L, HSPA8, ITPR3, and MAPK3. The second-placed hippo signaling pathway had the 5.84% associated genes, which included ACTG1, APC2, BIRC2, BMP2, FRMD6, LLGL2, RASSF6, SOX2, and WNT8A.

Interaction network of DEGs and core genes in the interaction network

Based on the information in the STRING database, the gene interaction network contained 542 nodes and 1163 edges. The nodes indicated the DEGs, and the edges indicated the interactions between the DEGs. NetworkAnalyzer in Cytoscape software was used to analysis these genes, and core genes were ranked according to the predicted scores. The top 10 high-degree hub nodes included glyceraldehyde-3-phosphate dehydrogenase (GAPDH), phosphoribosylglycinamide formyltransferase, phosphoribosylglycinamide synthetase, phosphoribosylaminoimidazole synthetase (GART), ubiquitin-like and ribosomal protein S30 fusion (FAU), heat shock protein family A member 8 (HSPA8), eukaryotic translation elongation factor 1 alpha 1 (EEF1A1), ribosomal protein S3A (RPS3A), eukaryotic translation initiation factor 4E (EIF4E), mitogen-activated protein kinase 3 (MAPK3), interleukin 6 (IL6), and ribosomal protein L6 (RPL6). Among these genes, GAPDH showed the highest node degree, which was 56. The core genes and their corresponding degree were shown in Table 3. The distribution of core genes in the interaction network was revealed in Fig. 3. The correlation between the data points and corresponding points on the line is approximately 0.932. The R-squared value is 0.846, giving a relatively high confidence that the underlying model is indeed linear. Then, we used MCODE to screen the modules of the gene interaction network, and 10 modules were showed in Fig. 4.

The score of top 1 module including FAU and EIF4E was 19.81, which had 22 nodes and 208 edges. The score of top 2 module including GAPDH and GART was 6.824, which had 18 nodes and 58 edges. The score of top 3 module including FBXO10, RNF213, SIAH1, TRIM50, and TRIP12 was 5, which had 5 nodes and 10 edges. Lastly, the interaction network of the top 10

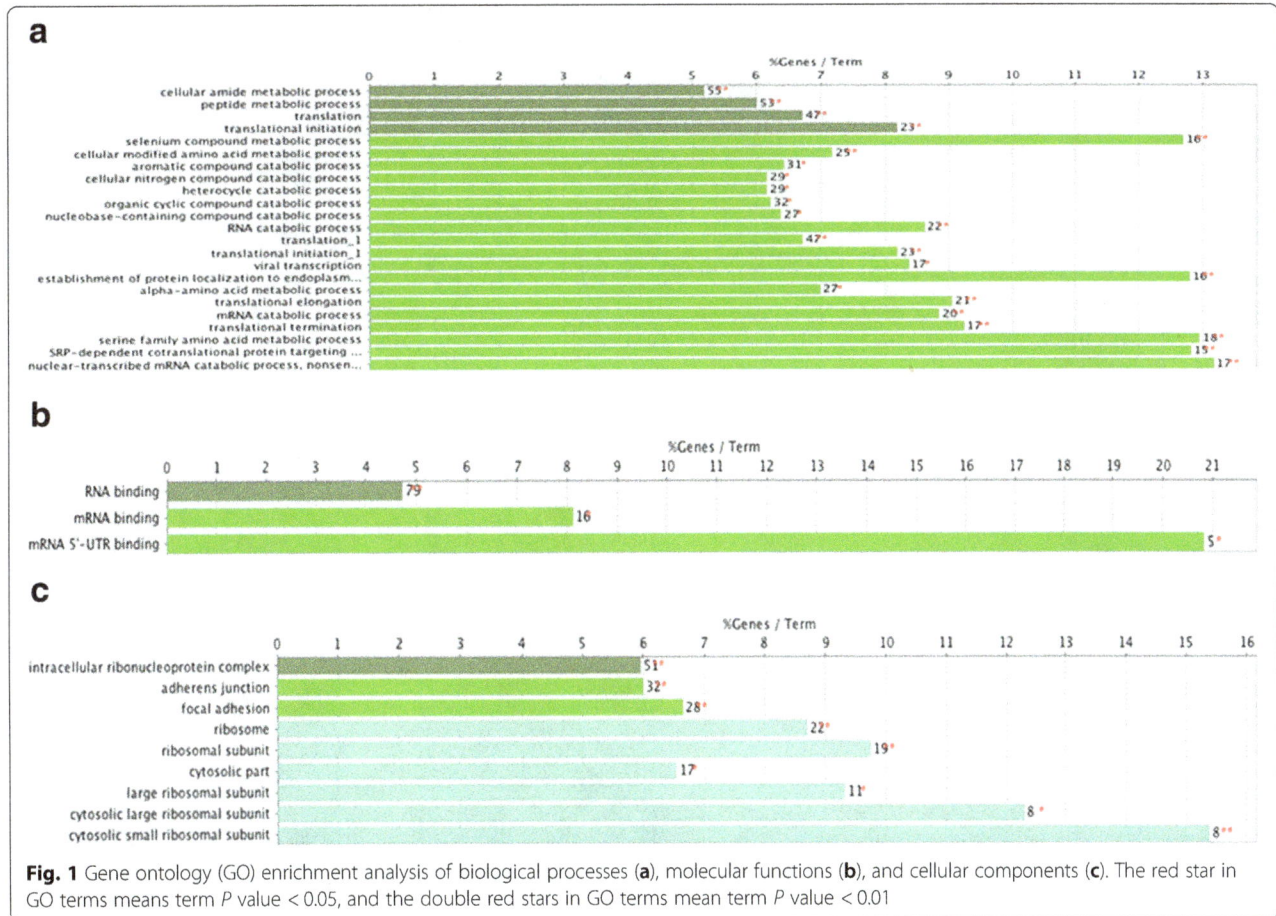

Fig. 1 Gene ontology (GO) enrichment analysis of biological processes (**a**), molecular functions (**b**), and cellular components (**c**). The red star in GO terms means term *P* value < 0.05, and the double red stars in GO terms mean term *P* value < 0.01

high-degree hub nodes (core genes) was made by STRING database in Fig. 5. GAPDH, GART, FAU, HSPA8, EEF1A1, RPS3A, EIF4E, MAPK3, IL6, and RPL6, which regulate 8, 4, 5, 6, 6, 6, 5, 3, 2, and 4 targets, respectively, showed the good connectivity.

Discussion

OS is the most common primary bone sarcoma [15–19]. Previous studies discovered that sarcomas contain a small subpopulation of tumor-propagating cells (TPCs) such as SP cells, characterized by enhanced tumorigenicity and self-renewal capacity [20–22]. Self-renewal is a defining characteristic of these cells and is associated with tumor recurrence [23, 24]. The inhibition of self-renewal in OS SP cells may offer valuable targets of therapy and tumorigenesis mechanisms. In the present study, the gene expression profile of GSE63390 was downloaded and a bioinformatics analysis was performed. The results showed that there were 141 DEGs in SP cells compared with non-SP cells of human OS. Furthermore, GO and KEGG pathway and gene–gene interaction network analysis were performed to obtain the biomarkers or the major genes related to cytogenetic pathways to OS tumorigenesis.

In order to disclose the underlying molecular mechanisms between SP cells and human OS, we characterized the possible GO functional terms and signaling pathways of DEGs. Considering the results of GO function analysis, we linked the DEGs with mRNA catabolic process and cellular modified amino acid metabolic process, which are probably very important for the development process of human OS. As previous articles reported, our KEGG pathway analysis showed that hippo signaling pathway, mTOR signaling pathway, hedgehog signaling pathway, and others were among the most relevant pathways for OS. Zhou et al. found that the correlation between the mTOR/p70S6K signal transduction pathway in human OS and patients' prognosis, and the overexpression of mTOR and p70S6K, is well correlated with tumor metastasis pattern, which might be an important mechanism responsible for the survival and proliferation of OS cells [25]. Wang et al. identified that hippo/YAP signaling pathway not only is involved in tumorigenesis, but also hippo/YAP signaling pathway induces OS chemoresistance [26]. Chai et al. deemed that the oncogenic activities in OS are mediated by TED1 through hippo–YAP1 signaling [27]. Cheng et al. highlighted a new discovery that CNOT1–LMNA–Hedgehog signaling pathway axis exerts an oncogenic role in OS

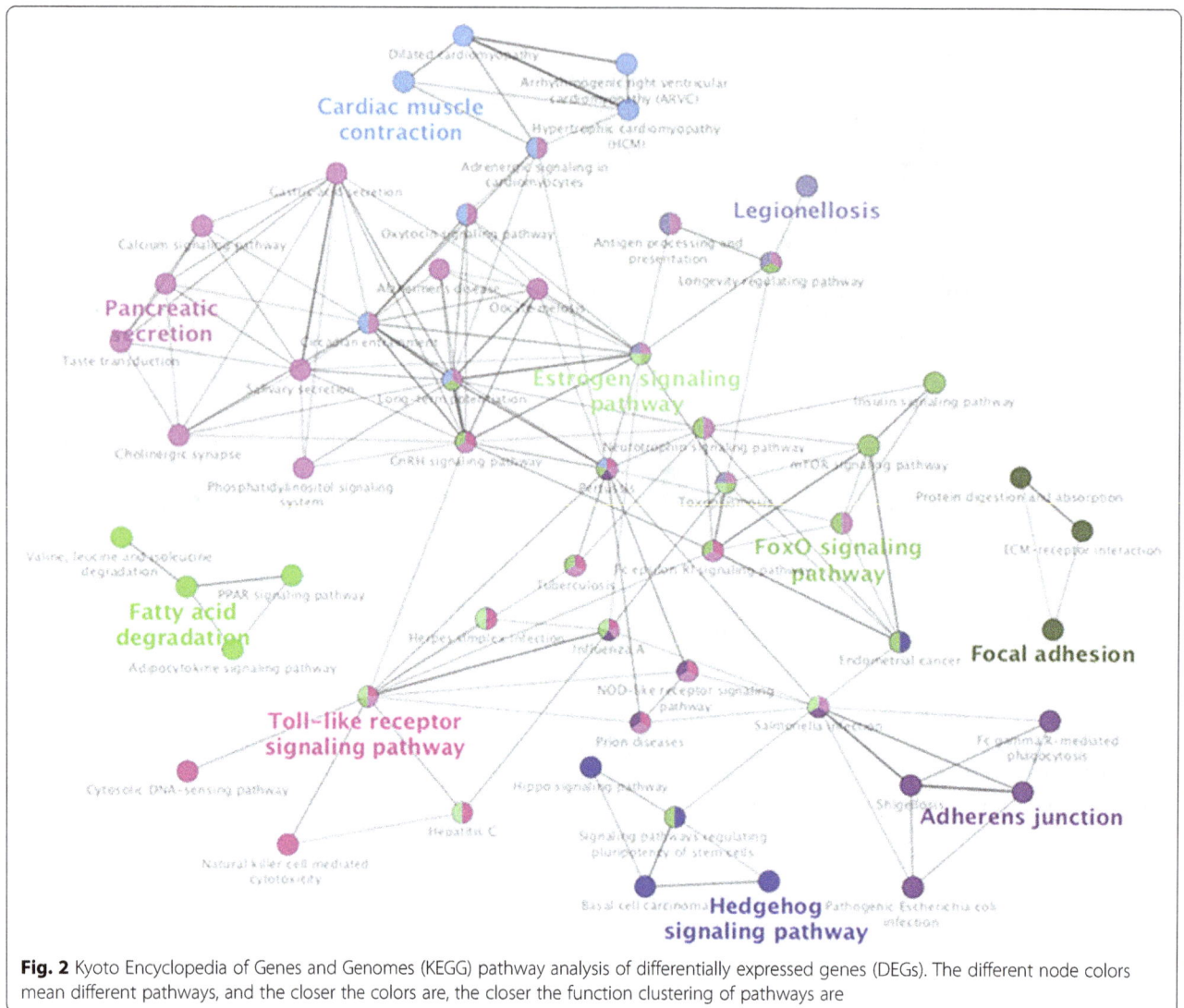

Fig. 2 Kyoto Encyclopedia of Genes and Genomes (KEGG) pathway analysis of differentially expressed genes (DEGs). The different node colors mean different pathways, and the closer the colors are, the closer the function clustering of pathways are

progression, which could be a potential target for gene therapy [28]. Emerging data suggested that interference with hedgehog signaling signal transduction by inhibitors may reduce OS cell proliferation and tumor growth, thereby preventing osteosarcomagenesis [29]. All these signaling pathways may play important roles in molecular mechanism of development process between SP cells and human OS.

Also of note is that there were numerous evidences for our DEGs of SP cells, which have proven to play important roles during OS tumorigenesis. The STRING database revealed top 20 high-degree hub nodes of DEGs including GAPDH, GART, FAU, HSPA8, EEF1A1, RPS3A, EIF4E, MAPK3, IL6, RPL6, eukaryotic translation initiation factor 3 beta (EIF3b), DEAD-box helicase 5 (DDX5), heat shock protein family D member 1 (HSPD1), ribosomal protein S29 (RPS29), ribosomal protein L18a (RPL18A), ribosomal protein L18 (RPL18), calmodulin 3 (CALM3), actin gamma

1 (ACTG1), ribosomal protein S27 (RPS27), and ribosomal protein L32 (RPL32). Furthermore, we analyzed the gene interaction network and top 10 modules using MCODE and found that ACTG1, eukaryotic translation initiation factor 3 subunit E (EIF3E), EIF4E, FAU, HSPD1, IL-6, KiSS-1 metastasis-suppressor (KISS1), PRIM1, pituitary tumor-transforming 1 (PTTG1), PRL32, S100 calcium-binding protein A8 (S100A8), S100 calcium-binding protein A9 (S100A9), serine hydroxymethyltransferase 1 (SHMT1), and TNF receptor-associated protein 1 (TRAP1) were the core interaction genes, which may be potential therapeutic targets for OS. Parts of them were in accord with STRING database results. Ajiro et al. found that serine/arginine-rich splicing factor 3 (SRSF3) regulates the expression of DDX5 in human OS U2OS cells [30]. By participating in the transcriptional regulation of ribosomal protein L34 (RPL34) which plays an important role

Table 2 Core pathways and their associated genes found

GOID	GOTerm	Term P value	% associated genes	Associated genes found
GO:0004915	Estrogen signaling pathway	130.0E−3	6.12	[CALM3, CALML4, HSPA1L, HSPA8, ITPR3, MAPK3]
GO:0004390	Hippo signaling pathway	62.0E−3	5.84	[ACTG1, APC2, BIRC2, BMP2, FRMD6, LLGL2, RASSF6, SOX2, WNT8A]
GO:0004520	Adherens junction	290.0E−3	5.56	[ACTG1, MAPK3, PTPRM, WAS]
GO:0004657	IL-17 signaling pathway	220.0E−3	5.38	[IL6, MAPK15, MAPK3, S100A8, S100A9]
GO:0004621	NOD-like receptor signaling pathway	110.0E−3	5.29	[BIRC2, ERBIN, IFNA1, IFNAR2, IL6, ITPR3, MAPK3, RNASEL, TP53BP1]
GO:0004210	Apoptosis	210.0E−3	5.07	[ACTG1, BIRC2, ITPR3, LMNA, MAPK3, PDPK1, TUBA3D]
GO:0004371	Apelin signaling pathway	210.0E−3	5.07	[CALM3, CALML4, GNG11, ITPR3, MAPK3, PRKAG2, RYR2]
GO:0004722	Neurotrophin signaling pathway	270.0E−3	5.04	[CALM3, CALML4, IRAK2, MAGED1, MAPK3, PDPK1]
GO:0004020	Calcium signaling pathway	190.0E−3	4.95	[CALM3, CALML4, CHRM3, ITPR3, P2RX2, PTGER3, RYR2, SLC25A4, STIM2]
GO:0004512	ECM−receptor interaction	330.0E−3	4.88	[COL1A2, COL2A1, COL6A1, HSPG2]
GO:0004620	Toll-like receptor signaling pathway	380.0E−3	4.81	[IFNA1, IFNAR2, IL6, MAP2K3, MAPK3]
GO:0004150	mTOR signaling pathway	340.0E−3	4.61	[ATP6V1B2, DEPDC5, EIF4E, MAPK3, PDPK1, PRR5, WNT8A]
GO:0004068	FoxO signaling pathway	310.0E−3	4.55	[BCL6, CCNG2, IL6, MAPK3, PDPK1, PRKAG2]
GO:0004510	Focal adhesion	290.0E−3	4.52	[ACTG1, BCAR1, BIRC2, COL1A2, COL2A1, COL6A1, MAPK3, PARVB, PDPK1]
GO:0004514	Cell adhesion molecules (CAMs)	460.0E−3	4.14	[CADM1, CLDN5, NCAM2, PTPRC, PTPRM, SELP]

in the proliferation of OS cells, MYC interacts with the subunits of EIF3 and probably involves the translational control of growth-promoting proteins [31]. EIF3, a multi-subunit complex, plays a critical role in translation initiation. Expression levels of EIF3 subunits are elevated or decreased in various cancers, suggesting a role for EIF3 in tumorigenesis [32]. Choi et al. confirmed that EIF3b silencing could completely suppress cell growth in multiple OS cell lines [33]. Osborne et al. also discovered that EIF4E is uniformly expressed in OS patient samples and it could be a relevant protein biomarker in OS [34]. Rossman et al. found that overexpressing FAU itself is able to transform human osteogenic sarcoma cells to anchorage independence and make them easy to proliferate [35]. Liang et al. proved that the expression of HSPD1 was high in OS tissues and cells; moreover, targeted inhibition of this gene could inhibit the proliferation of the tumor [36]. Zhang et al. indicated that the decreased expression of KISS1 is correlated with distant metastasis of OS, and KISS1

may function as a tumor suppressor in OS cells through inhibition of the MAPK pathway [37]. EEF1A1 is overexpressed in OS cell lines, and siRNA treatment against EEF1A1 produces a chemosensitization toward methotrexate, which showed that this gene is a potential therapeutic target of OS [38]. Through ASK1/p38/AP-1 signal pathway, IL-6 occurs, which in turn results in the activations of vascular endothelial growth factor (VEGF) expression and contributing the angiogenesis of human OS cells [39]. In addition, the ILK/Akt/AP-1 pathway is activated after IL-6 treatment, and IL-6 induces expression of ICAM-1 and migration activity of human OS cells [40]. Yotov et al. proposed that PRIM1 is a major target of 12q13 amplifications, playing an essential role in tumorigenesis of human OS [41]. PTTG1 siRNA markedly downregulates the expression of PTTGl protein in OS cells, leading to obvious inhibition of cell proliferation, alters cell cycle distribution, and reduces ability of invasion of OS cells [42]. Tsai et al. deemed that expression stability of RPL32 is high in OS samples, and this gene could be a potential target [43]. In Montesano's study, the anti-apoptotic role of TRAP1 is confirmed in Saos-2 OS cells, which suggested that increased expression of this gene could make diethylmaleate-adapted and chemoresistant cells evade toxic effects of oxidants and anticancer drugs [44]. Endo-Munoz et al. proved downregulation of S100A8 between chemo-naive OS biopsies and non-malignant bone biopsies, highlighting their

Table 3 The core genes and their corresponding degree

Gene	Degree	Gene	Degree	Gene	Degree	Gene	Degree
GAPDH	56	RPS3A	32	EIF3b	28	RPL18	25
GART	41	EIF4E	31	DDX5	28	CALM3	25
FAU	39	MAPK3	31	HSPD1	28	ACTG1	25
HSPA8	38	IL6	29	RPS29	26	RPS27	24
EEF1A1	36	RPL6	28	RPL18A	26	RPL32	24

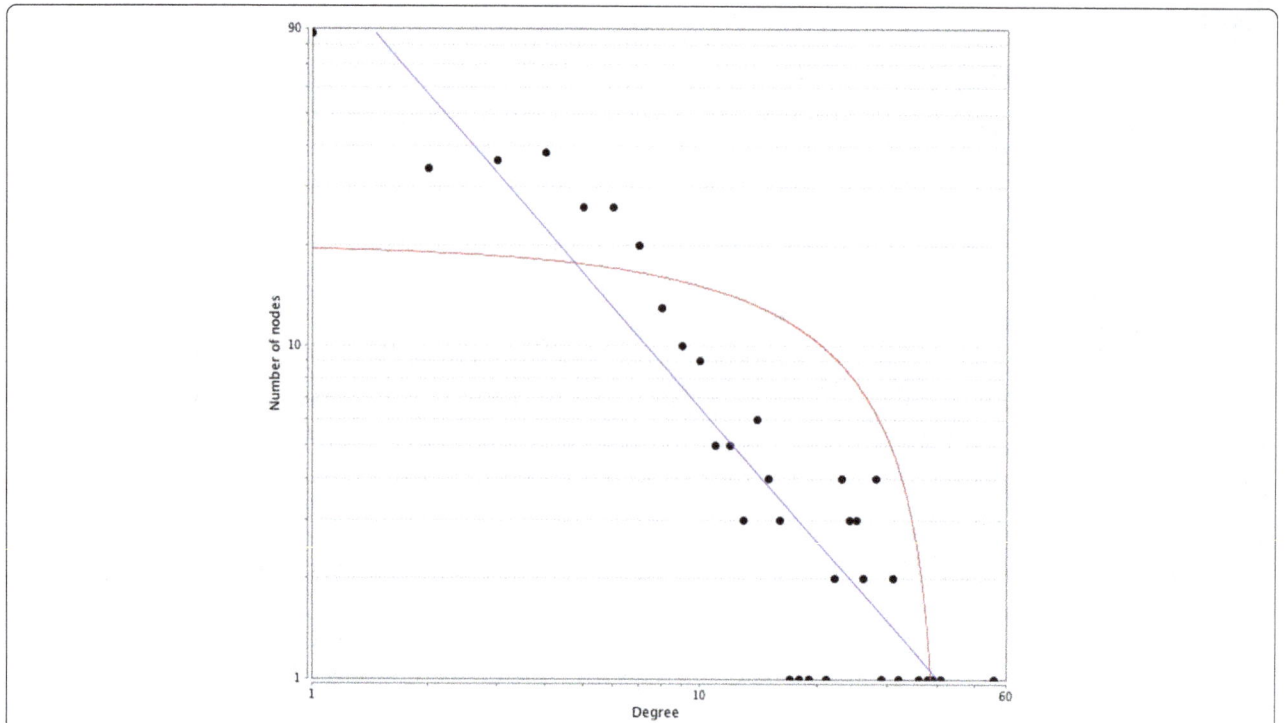

Fig. 3 The distribution of core genes in the interaction network. The black node means the core gene. The red line means the fitted line, and the blue line means the power law. The correlation between the data points and corresponding points on the line is approximately 0.932. The R-squared value is 0.846, giving a relatively high confidence that the underlying model is indeed linear

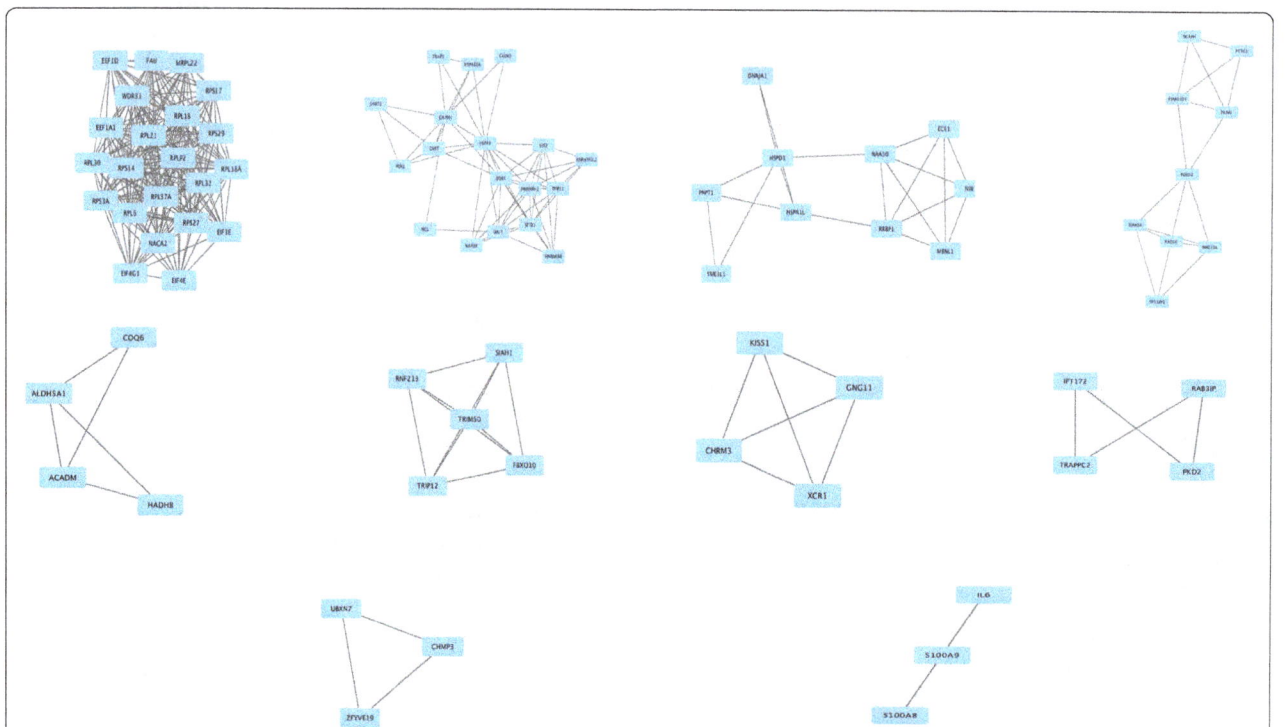

Fig. 4 The top 10 modules from the gene–gene interaction network. The squares represent the differentially expressed genes (DEGs) in modules, and the lines show the interaction between the DEGs

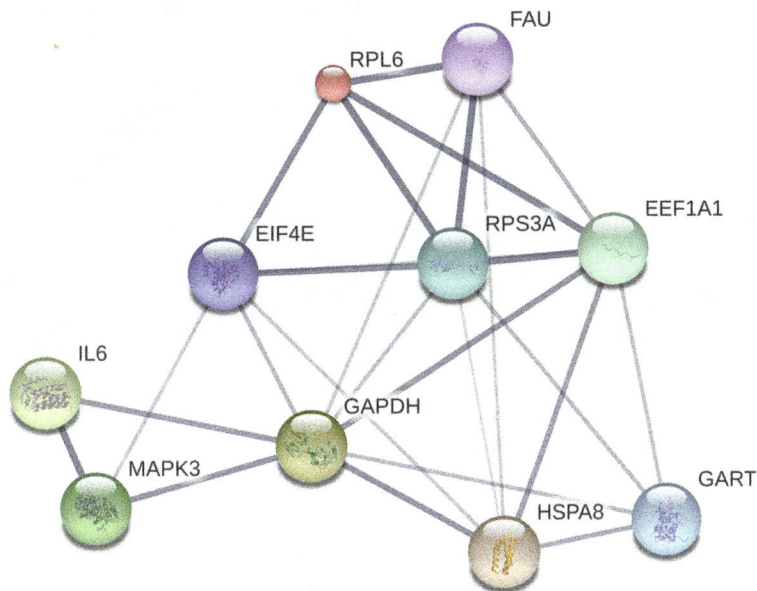

Fig. 5 The interaction network of the top 10 core genes. The nodes indicated the top core genes, and the edges indicated the interactions between the core genes

potential as therapeutic targets for OS [45]. Cheng et al. confirmed that through inactivating MAPK and NF-κB signaling pathways, downregulation of S100A9 could inhibit OS cell growth [46]. Besides, Both et al. concluded that some genes, including SHMT1, are candidate oncogenes in 17p11.2–p12 of importance in OS tumorigenesis [47]. Taken together, all these core genes discovered in OS SP cells by bioinformatics enrichment analysis and gene interaction network analysis may increase or decrease tumorigenicity and self-renewal capacity of OS SP cells; further, these changed SP cells could result in development process of human OS.

Some gene and pathway interaction relationship predicted in our study has been reported in previous researches. Oncogenic activation of mTOR signaling significantly contributes to the progression of different types of cancers including OS. EIF4E is one of the downstream effectors of mTOR. Activated mTOR contributes to OS cellular transformation and poor cancer prognosis via targeting the downstream effectors such as EIF4E [48]. In addition, our results of core pathways and their associated genes found also confirmed the relationship of EIF4E and mTOR signaling pathway. Therefore, EIF4E/mTOR signaling pathway could be a potential research target for therapy and tumorigenesis of OS.

Lastly, there are several limitations of this study. It is acknowledged that predicting key genes merely by means of bioinformatics is not sufficient, and further molecular biological experiments such as the use of gene transfection/knockdown and quantitative real-time polymerase chain reaction are needed to confirm these results.

Conclusion

In summary, 141 DEGs were identified including 72 upregulated DEGs and 69 downregulated DEGs screened in SP cells compared with non-SP cells. GO and KEGG pathway analysis provided a series of related key genes and pathways to contribute to the understanding of the molecular mechanisms between SP cells and human OS, thus yielding clues to speculate the EIF4E/mTOR signaling pathway is highly correlated with the development process of OS. Furthermore, these predictions need further experimental validation in future studies.

Abbreviations
ACTG1: Actin gamma 1; BP: Biological process; CALM3: Calmodulin 3; CAMs: Cell adhesion molecules; CC: Cellular component; DDX5: DEAD-box helicase 5; DEG: Differentially expressed gene; EEF: Eukaryotic translation elongation factor; EIF3b: Eukaryotic translation initiation factor 3 beta; FAU: Ubiquitin-like and ribosomal protein S30 fusion; FC: Fold change; GAPDH: Glyceraldehyde-3-phosphate dehydrogenase; GART: Phosphoribosylglycinamide formyltransferase, phosphoribosylglycinamide synthetase, phosphoribosylaminoimidazole synthetase; GEO: Gene Expression Omnibus database; GO: Gene Ontology; HSPA8: Heat shock protein family A member 8; HSPD1: Heat shock protein family D member 1; IL6: Interleukin 6; KEGG: Kyoto Encyclopedia of Genes and Genomes; KISS1: KiSS-1 metastasis-suppressor; MAPK3: Mitogen-activated protein kinase 3; MCODE: Molecular complex detection; MF: Molecular function; OS: Osteosarcoma; PTTG1: Pituitary tumor-transforming 1; RPL6: Ribosomal protein L6; RPS: Ribosomal protein; S100A8: S100 calcium-binding protein A8; SHMT1: Serine hydroxymethyltransferase 1; SP: Side population; SRSF3: Serine/arginine-rich splicing factor 3; STRING: Search Tool for the Retrieval of Interacting Genes; TPC: Tumor-propagating cell; TRAP1: TNF receptor associated protein 1; VEGF: Vascular endothelial growth factor

Acknowledgements

Yi-Ming Ren wants to thank, in particular, the continued supports received from Fiona Xue over 8 years.

Authors' contributions

YMR, YHD, and YBS conceived the design of the study. TY, WJZ, DLZ, and ZWT performed and collected the data and contributed to the design of the study. TY and WJZ analyzed the data. YMR and MQT prepared and revised the manuscript. All authors read and approved the final content of the manuscript.

Competing interests

The authors declare that they have no competing interests.

References

1. Mirabello L, Troisi RJ, Savage SA. Osteosarcoma incidence and survival rates from 1973 to 2004: data from the surveillance, epidemiology, and end results program. Cancer. 2009;115(7):1531–43.
2. Damron T, Ward WA. Osteosarcoma, chondrosarcoma, and Ewing's sarcoma: National Cancer Data Base Report. Clin Orthop Related Res. 2007;459(459): 40.
3. Ottaviani G, Jaffe N. The epidemiology of osteosarcoma. Pediatr Adolesc Osteosarcoma. 2009;152:3–13.
4. Marina N, Gebhardt M, Teot L, et al. Biology and therapeutic advances for pediatric osteosarcoma. Oncologist. 2004;9(4):422.
5. Folio C, Zalacain M, Zandueta C, et al. Cortactin (CTTN) overexpression in osteosarcoma correlates with advanced stage and reduced survival. Cancer Biomarkers. 2011;10(1):35.
6. Wu C, Alman BA. Side population cells in human cancers. Cancer Lett. 2008; 268(1):1–9.
7. Patrawala L, Calhoun T, Schneiderbroussard R, et al. Side population is enriched in tumorigenic, stem-like cancer cells, whereas ABCG2+ and ABCG2– cancer cells are similarly tumorigenic. Cancer Res. 2005;65(14):6207.
8. Mitsutake N, Iwao A, Nagai K, et al. Characterization of side population in thyroid cancer cell lines: cancer stemlike cells are enriched partly but not exclusively. Endocrinology. 2007;148(4):1797–803.
9. Kondo T, Setoguchi T, Taga T, Kondo T, Setoguchi T. Taga TPersistence of a small subpopulation of cancer stem-like cells in the C6 glioma cell line. Proc Natl Acad Sci U S A. 2004;101(3):781–6.
10. Haraguchi N, Utsunomiya T, Inoue H, et al. Characterization of a side population of cancer cells from human gastrointestinal system. Stem Cells. 2006;24(3):506.
11. Ho MM, Ng AV, Lam S, et al. Side population in human lung cancer cell lines and tumors is enriched with stem-like cancer cells. Cancer Res. 2007; 67(10):4827–33.
12. Chiba T, Kita K, Zheng YW, et al. Side population purified from hepatocellular carcinoma cells harbors cancer stem cell-like properties. Hepatology. 2006;44(1):240–51.
13. Wang K, Zeng J, Luo L, et al. Identification of cancer stem cell-like side population cells in human cervical carcinoma cell line HeLa[C]// The Tenth National Conference on obstetrics and Gynecology of China Medical Association, 2012.
14. Hirschmann-Jax C, et al. A distinct "side population" of cells with high drug efflux capacity in human tumor cells. Proc Natl Acad Sci U S A. 2004;101(39):14228–33.
15. Zhou W, Hao M, Du X, et al. Advances in targeted therapy for osteosarcoma. Discov Med. 2014;17(96):301.
16. Li S, Dong Y, Ke W, et al. Transcriptomic analyses reveal the underlying pro-malignant functions of PTHR1 for osteosarcoma via activation of Wnt and angiogenesis pathways. J Orthop Surg Res. 2017;12(1):168.
17. Fei Z, Hao P. LncRNA-ANCR regulates the cell growth of osteosarcoma by interacting with EZH2 and affecting the expression of p21 and p27. J Orthop Surg Res. 2017;12(1):103.
18. Feng J, Lan R, Cai G, et al. Verification ofTREX1as a promising indicator of judging the prognosis of osteosarcoma. J Orthop Surg Res. 2016;11(1):150.
19. Yang XR, Xiong Y, Duan H, et al. Identification of genes associated with methotrexate resistance in methotrexate-resistant osteosarcoma cell lines. J Orthop Surg Res. 2015;10(1):136.
20. Wang CY, Wei Q, Han I, et al. Hedgehog and notch signaling regulate self-renewal of undifferentiated pleomorphic sarcomas. Cancer Res. 2012;72(4):1013–22.
21. Dela CFS. Cancer stem cells in pediatric sarcomas. Front Oncol. 2013;3:168.
22. Wu C, Wei Q, Utomo V, et al. Side population cells isolated from mesenchymal neoplasms have tumor initiating potential. Cancer Res. 2007;67(17):8216–22.
23. Kreso A, Van GP, Pedley NM, et al. Self-renewal as a therapeutic target in human colorectal cancer. Nat Med. 2014;20(1):29–36.
24. Zhu Z, Khan MA, Weiler M, et al. Targeting self-renewal in high-grade brain tumors leads to loss of brain tumor stem cells and prolonged survival. Cell Stem Cell. 2014;15(2):185–98.
25. Zhou Q, Deng Z, Zhu Y, et al. mTOR/p70S6K signal transduction pathway contributes to osteosarcoma progression and patients' prognosis. Med Oncol. 2010;27(4):1239–45.
26. Wang DY, Wu YN, Huang JQ, et al. Hippo/YAP signaling pathway is involved in osteosarcoma chemoresistance. Chin J Cancer. 2016;35(7):366–73.
27. Chai J, Xu S, Guo F. TEAD1 mediates the oncogenic activities of hippo-YAP1 signaling in osteosarcoma. Biochem Biophys Res Commun. 2017; 488(2):297–302.
28. Cheng DD, Li J, Li SJ, et al. CNOT1 cooperates with LMNA to aggravate osteosarcoma tumorigenesis through the hedgehog signaling pathway. Mol Oncol. 2017;11(4):388–404.
29. Kumar RM, Fuchs B. Hedgehog signaling inhibitors as anti-cancer agents in osteosarcoma. Cancers. 2015;7(2):784–94.
30. Ajiro M, Jia R, Yang Y, et al. A genome landscape of SRSF3-regulated splicing events and gene expression in human osteosarcoma U2OS cells. Nucleic Acids Res. 2016;44(4):1854.
31. Luo S, Zhao J, Fowdur M, et al. Highly expressed ribosomal protein L34 indicates poor prognosis in osteosarcoma and its knockdown suppresses osteosarcoma proliferation probably through translational control. Sci Rep. 2016;6:37690.
32. Mamane Y, Petroulakis E, Rong L, et al. eIF4E from translation to transformation. Oncogene. 2004;23(18):3172–9.
33. Choi YJ, Lee YS, Lee HW, et al. Silencing of translation initiation factor eIF3b promotes apoptosis in osteosarcoma cells. Bone Joint Res. 2017:186–93.
34. Osborne TS, Ren L, Healey JH, et al. Evaluation of eIF4E expression in an osteosarcoma-specific tissue microarray. J Pediatr Hematol Oncol. 2011; 33(7):524–8.
35. Rossman TG, Visalli MA, Komissarova EV. Fau and its ubiquitin-like domain (FUBI) transforms human osteogenic sarcoma (HOS) cells to anchorage-independence. Oncogene. 2003;22(12):1817.
36. Liang W, Yang C, Peng J, et al. The expression of HSPD1, SCUBE3, CXCL14 and its relations with the prognosis in osteosarcoma. Cell Biochem Biophys. 2015;73(3):763–8.
37. Zhang Y, Tang YJ, Li ZH, et al. KISS1 inhibits growth and invasion of osteosarcoma cells through inhibition of the MAPK pathway. Eur J Histochem Ejh. 2013;57(4):199–204.
38. Selga E, Oleaga C, Ramírez S, et al. Networking of differentially expressed genes in human cancer cells resistant to methotrexate. Genome Med. 2009;1(9):83.
39. Tzeng HE, Tsai CH, Chang ZL, et al. Interleukin-6 induces vascular endothelial growth factor expression and promotes angiogenesis through apoptosis signal-regulating kinase 1 in human osteosarcoma. Biochem Pharmacol. 2013;85(4):531–40.
40. Lin YM, Chang ZL, Liao YY, et al. IL-6 promotes ICAM-1 expression and cell motility in human osteosarcoma. Cancer Lett. 2013;328(1):135–43.
41. Yotov WV, Hamel H, Rivard GE, et al. Amplifications of DNA primase 1 (PRIM1) in human osteosarcoma. Genes Chromosomes Cancer. 1999;26(1):62.
42. Wu D, Xia Y, Xu H, et al. Impact of PTTG1 downregulation on cell proliferation, cell cycle and cell invasion of osteosarcoma and related molecular mechanisms. Zhonghua Bing Li Xue Za Zhi. 2014;43(10):695.

43. Tsai PC, Breen M. Array-based comparative genomic hybridization-guided identification of reference genes for normalization of real-time quantitative polymerase chain reaction assay data for lymphomas, histiocytic sarcomas, and osteosarcomas of dogs. Am J Vet Res. 2012;73(9):1335.

44. Montesano GN, Chirico G, Pirozzi G, et al. Tumor necrosis factor-associated protein 1 (TRAP-1) protects cells from oxidative stress and apoptosis. Stress-Int J Biol Stress. 2007;10(4):342–50.

45. Endo-Munoz L, Cumming A, Sommerville S, et al. Osteosarcoma is characterised by reduced expression of markers of osteoclastogenesis and antigen presentation compared with normal bone. Br J Cancer. 2010;103(1):73–81.

46. Cheng S, Zhang X, Huang N, et al. Down-regulation of S100A9 inhibits osteosarcoma cell growth through inactivating MAPK and NF-κB signaling pathways. BMC Cancer. 2016;16(1):1–12.

47. Both J, et al. Identification of novel candidate oncogenes in chromosome region 17p11.2-p12 in human osteosarcoma. PLoS One. 2012;7(1):e30907.

48. Hu K, Dai HB, Qiu ZL. mTOR signaling in osteosarcoma: oncogenesis and therapeutic aspects (review). Oncol Rep. 2016;36(3):1219.

12

A systematic review and meta-analysis of direct anterior approach versus posterior approach in total hip arthroplasty

Zhao Wang, Jing-zhao Hou, Can-hua Wu, Yue-jiang Zhou, Xiao-ming Gu, Hai-hong Wang, Wu Feng, Yan-xiao Cheng, Xia Sheng and Hong-wei Bao*

Abstract

Background: This meta-analysis aimed to evaluate the postoperative clinical outcomes and safety of the direct anterior approach (DAA) versus posterior approach (PA) in total hip arthroplasty (THA).

Methods: We searched PubMed, Embase, Web of Science, the Cochrane Library, and Google databases from inception to June 2018 to select studies that compared the DAA and PA for THA. Only randomized controlled trials (RCTs) were included. Outcomes included Harris hip score at 2 weeks, 6 weeks, 12 weeks, and 1 year; VAS at 24 h, 48 h, and 72 h; incision length, operation time, postoperative blood loss, length of hospital stay, and complications (intraoperative fracture, postoperative dislocation, heterotopic ossification (HO), and groin pain).

Results: Nine RCTs totaling 754 THAs (DAA group = 377, PA group = 377) met the criteria to be included in this meta-analysis. The present meta-analysis indicated that, compared with PA group, DAA group was associated with an increase of the Harris hip score at the 2-week and 4-week time points. No significant difference was found between DAA and PA groups of the Harris hip scores at 12 weeks, 1 year length of hospital stay ($p > 0.05$). DAA group was associated with a reduction of the VAS at 24 h, 48 h, and 72 h with statistical significance ($p < 0.05$). What is more, DAA was associated with a reduction of the incision length and postoperative blood loss ($p < 0.05$). There was no significant difference between the operation time and complications (intraoperative fracture, postoperative dislocation, HO, and groin pain).

Conclusion: In THA patients, compared with PA, DAA was associated with an early functional recovery and less pain scores. What is more, DAA was associated with shorter incision length and blood loss.

Keywords: Direct anterior approach, Posterior approach, Total hip arthroplasty, Meta-analysis

Introduction

Total hip arthroplasty (THA) is an effective surgery alternative for patients with hip osteoarthritis (OA) or femoral head necrosis [1, 2]. Kurtz et al. [3] reported a 50% increase in the prevalence of THA from 1990 to 2002 and estimated nearly 572,000 THAs in 2030. Most THA patients experience pain relief, improved function, and restoration of quality of life [4]. However, nearly 7–15% patients were dissatisfied with THA due to the postoperative pain and functional recovery [5, 6]. The potential causes of postoperative pain include failure of fixation and

damage of soft tissues [7]. Among the causes of damage of soft tissues, surgical approach was one of the influential factors [8, 9]. Choosing the optimal surgical approach could minimize pain severity, improve hip function, and thus increase patients' satisfaction.

Currently, there are two common surgical approaches; direct anterior approach (DAA) and posterior approach (PA) are utilized in THA's [10, 11]. Several reports have shown that the DAA was superior to the PA in terms of the postoperative blood loss and faster rehabilitation. The reason may be that DAA results in less soft tissue damage due to the fact that DAA relies on an intermuscular plane for insertion of the components [9]. For the above reasons, DAA has gained popularity in recent

* Correspondence: zhangxuening09@qq.com
From the department of orthopaedics, Jingjiang People's Hospital, 28 No, Zhongzhou Road, Jingjiang, Taizhou City 214500, Jiangsu Province, China

years [12]. However, some studies reported that DAA has more complications (femoral neck fracture, femoral perforation) than other approaches. Additionally, the learning curve of DAA has been reported to be relatively longer than other approaches [13, 14]. Two relevant meta-analyses [11, 15] that compare DAA with other approaches were published. However, shortcoming of these two meta-analyses should be noted. Higgins et al. [11] included retrospective studies and found that there was no significant difference between DAA and PA groups in the functional outcomes. Miller et al. [15] conducted a meta-analysis that compares DAA and PA for THA patients. However, they mixed the different follow-up outcomes for analysis and thus the heterogeneity was large. Another limitation was that they also included retrospective studies and thus selection bias could not be avoided.

Therefore, we conducted a meta-analysis based only on randomized controlled trials (RCTs) to compare the clinical outcomes of DAA versus PA in THA. We hypothesized that DAA is superior to PA in terms of the clinical outcomes in THA.

Methods

This systematic review fully adhered to the preferred reporting items for systematic reviews and meta-analyses (PRISMA) guidelines [16].

Search strategy

We manually searched PubMed, Embase, Web of Science, the Cochrane Library, and Google databases from inception to June 2018. There was no language restriction for all of the publications. The search terms included key words and Medical Subject Headings (MeSH) terms related to ""Arthroplasty, Replacement, Hip"[Mesh]"; total hip arthroplasty; total hip replacement; THA, THR, direct anterior approach, DAA, posterior approach, and PA. The reference lists of included studies or meta-analysis were also manually examined for potential missing records. This meta-analysis did not involve direct contact with individual patients; therefore, no ethics approval was needed.

Inclusion criteria and exclusion criteria

(1) Participants: patients prepared for THA.
(2) Interventions: the intervention group received the DAA for THA.
(3) Comparisons: the control group received PA for THA.
(4) Outcomes: Harris hip score at 2 weeks, 6 weeks, 12 weeks, and 1 year; VAS at 24 h, 48 h, and 72 h; incision length, operation time, postoperative blood loss, length of hospital stay, and complications

(intraoperative fracture, postoperative dislocation, heterotopic ossification (HO), and groin pain).
(5) Study design: RCTs were regarded as eligible in the study.

Non-RCTs, letters, and editorial comments were excluded in this meta-analysis.

Study selection

According to the formulated search strategy, all papers were guided into Endnote X7 (Thompson Reuters, CA, USA). Two reviewers (Zhao Wang and Hong-wei Bao) independently scanned the titles and abstracts of the potential studies. If there was a controversy between the reviewers, we asked a senior reviewer to make a decision.

Date extraction

Two reviewers (Zhao Wang and Jing-zhao Hou) independently extract the following information: first author name and publication year, country, patients' general characteristic (no. of patients, age, proportion of female patients, BMI), outcomes, study, and follow-up duration. The primary outcomes were Harris hip score at 2 weeks, 6 weeks, 12 weeks and 1 year, VAS at 24 h, 48 h, and 72 h; incision length, operation time, postoperative blood loss, length of hospital stay, and complications (intraoperative fracture, postoperative dislocation, heterotopic ossification (HO), and groin pain).

Outcome measures and statistical analysis

Continuous outcomes (Harris hip score at 2 weeks, 6 weeks, 12 weeks, and 1 year; VAS at 24 h, 48 h, and 72 h; incision length, operation time, postoperative blood loss, and length of hospital stay) were expressed as the weighted mean differences (WMD) with 95% confidence intervals (CIs). Complications (intraoperative fracture, postoperative dislocation, HO, and groin pain) were expressed as risk ratio (RR) with 95% CIs. $p < 0.05$ was considered statistically significant difference. Statistical analysis was performed using Stata software, version 12.0 (Stata Corp., College Station, TX, USA). To assess the heterogeneity, the I^2 index and corresponding p value were calculated. When I^2 was less than 50%, there was low heterogeneity; otherwise, there was a high heterogeneity. Publication bias was visually assessed using funnel plots (effect size was symmetry = no publication bias) and was quantitatively assessed using Begg's test ($p > 0.05$ = no publication bias).

Results
Search results and general characteristic

Figure 1 shows the flowchart for selection of studies. First, a total of 285 studies were identified from the electronic databases (PubMed = 147, Embase = 56, Web of

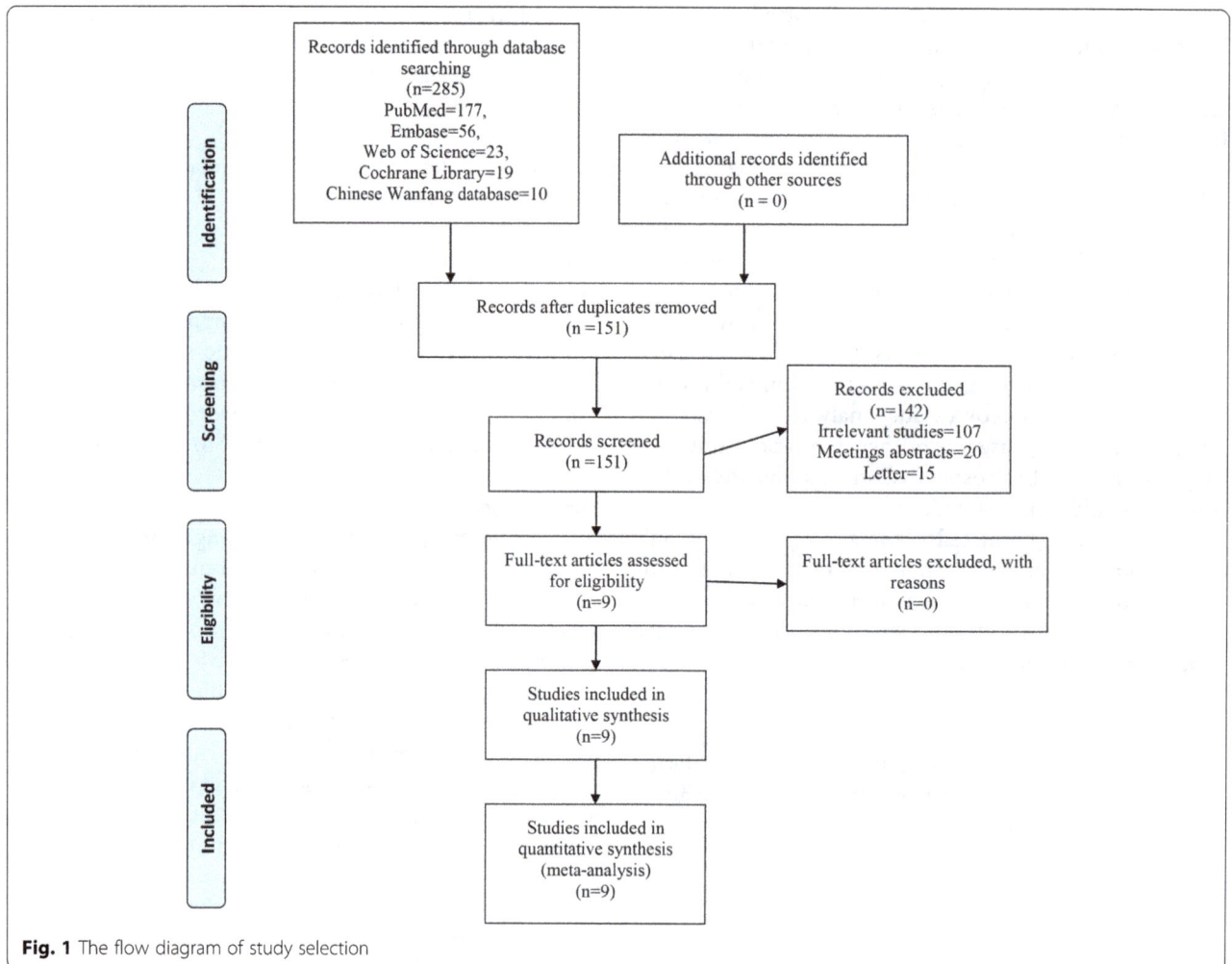

Fig. 1 The flow diagram of study selection

Science = 23, Cochrane Library = 19, Google database = 30). Then, all papers were input into Endnote X7 (Thomson Reuters Corp., USA) software for the removal of duplicate papers. A total of 151 papers were reviewed, and 142 papers were removed according to the inclusion criteria at abstract and title levels. Additionally, one study was a duplicate publication so we only included the most recently published paper. Ultimately, 9 clinical studies with 754 patients (DAA group = 377, PA group = 377) were involved in the meta-analysis [17–25]. The general characteristic of the included studies can be seen in Table 1. Publication years ranged from 2006 to 2018. Number of patients ranged from 27 to 60, and mean age ranged from 59 to 65. Follow-up duration ranged from 1 month to 1 year.

Quality assessment

The risk of bias graph and risk of bias summary is summarized in Figs. 2 and 3 respectively. Random sequence generation procedure (selection bias) was low and unclear in two and five of the included studies respectively.

Allocation concealment was low in four studies and high in two studies. Blinding of participant was with high risk of bias in all of the included studies. Attrition bias was unclear in six studies. Other bias was high in one study and two were with unclear risk of bias, the rest were all with low risk of bias.

Results of meta-analysis

Harris hip score at 2 weeks, 6 weeks, 12 weeks, and 1 year
Data on 661 primary THAs (including 329 with DAA and 322 with PA) were pooled from 5 trials analyzing the Harris hip score at 2 weeks. The DAA group was associated with an increase of the Harris hip at 2 weeks and 6 weeks (2 weeks, WMD = 7.41, 95%CI 4.91 to 9.92, $p = 0.000$; Fig. 4; 6 weeks, WMD = 6.80, 95%CI 0.64 to 12.95, $p = 0.030$, Fig. 5). The DAA and PA groups were not statistically significantly different with regard to pain at 12 weeks and 1 year (12 weeks, WMD = 2.56, 95%CI -0.40 to 5.51, $p = 0.090$, Fig. 6; 1 year, WMD = 0.36, 95%CI -1.51 to 2.23, $p = 0.709$, Fig. 7).

Table 1 General characteristic of the included studies

Author	No. of patients	Mean age (years)	Female (%)	BMI	Outcomes	Study	Follow-up
Barrett 2013[1,2,3,5,7]	43/44	61/63	33/57	31/29		RCT	3 months
Bergin 2011[2,4,8,9,10,11,12]	29/28	69/65	68/50	26/28		RCT	1 month
Christensen 2015[1,5,8,9,]	28/23	64/65	54/52	31/30		RCT	42 days
Rodriguez 2014[2,3,5,6]	60/60	59/60	34/32	28/24		RCT	1 year
Taunton 2014[1,3,4,8,10]	27/27	62/66	56/52	28/29		RCT	42 days
Cheng 2017[2,3,4,10,11,12]	35/27	59/63	57/53	28/28		RCT	84 days
Zhang 2006[1,2,5,8,10,12]	60/60	61/63	58/53	NS		RCT	3 months
Zhao 2017[2,3,5,6,8,9,11]	60/60	65/62	60/56	24/26		RCT	3 months
Zhang 2018[1,2,4,5,6,7,]	35/48	NS	NS	26/25		RCT	6 months

NS, not stated; RCT, randomized controlled trials; 1 Harris hip score at 2 weeks, 2, Harris hip score at 6 weeks, 3, Harris hip score at 12 weeks, 4 Harris hip score at 1 year, 5, VAS at 24 h, 6, VAS at 48 h, 7, VAS at 72 h, 8 incision length, 9, operation time, 10. postoperative blood loss, 11 length of hospital stay, 12 complications (intraoperative fracture, postoperative dislocation, heterotopic ossification (HO) and groin pain)

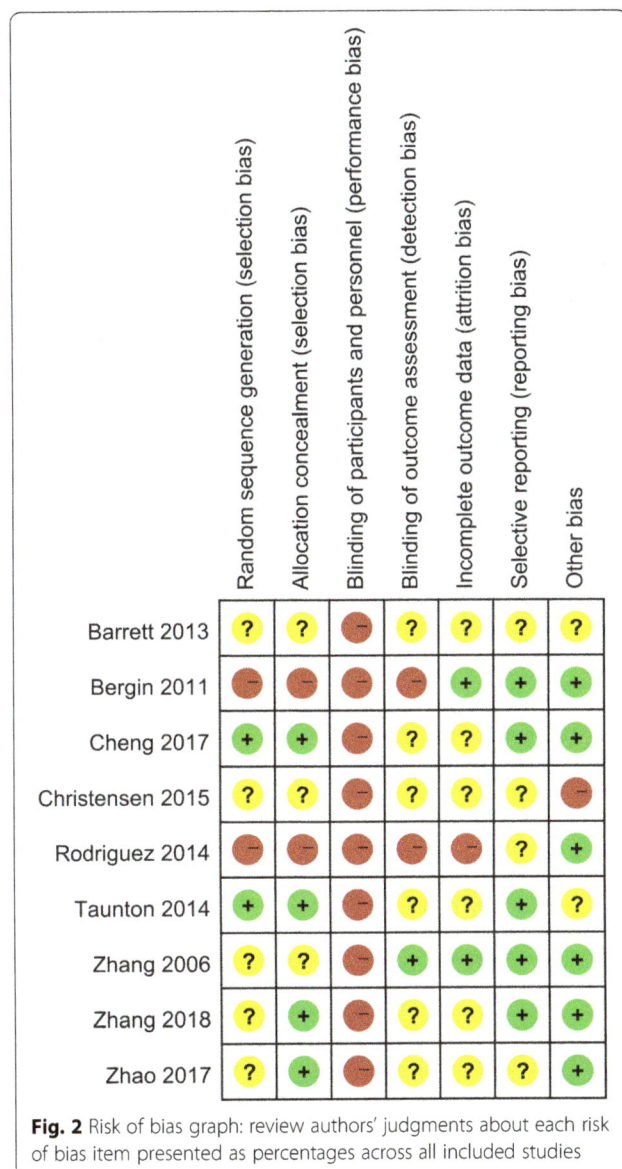

Fig. 2 Risk of bias graph: review authors' judgments about each risk of bias item presented as percentages across all included studies

VAS at 24 h, 48 h, and 72 h

Compared with PA group, the DAA group was associated with a decrease of the VAS at each time point (24 h, WMD = -0.71, 95%CI -0.90 to -0.51, $p = 0.000$; 48 h, WMD = -1.55, 95%CI -2.24 to -0.86, $p = 0.000$; 72 h, WMD = -1.56, 95%CI -2.64 to -0.48, $p = 0.005$, Fig. 8).

Incision length

Data on 359 primary THAs (including 184 with DAA and 175 with PA) were pooled from 4 trials analyzing the incision length. Compared with PA, DAA group was associated with a reduction of the incision length by 3.51 cm (WMD = -3.51, 95%CI -4.15 to -2.86, $p = 0.000$, Fig. 9).

Operation time

Data on 446 primary THAs (including 227 with DAA and 219 with PA) were pooled from 5 trials analyzing the operation time. Compared with PA, DAA group was not associated with an increase of the operation time (WMD = 3.83, 95%CI -14.39 to 22.06, $p = 0.680$, Fig. 10).

Postoperative blood loss

Data on 380 primary THAs (including 184 with DAA and 196 with PA) were pooled from 4 trials analyzing the postoperative blood loss. Compared with PA, DAA group was associated with a reduction of the postoperative blood loss (WMD = -67.02, 95%CI -131.46 to -2.58, $p = 0.041$, Fig. 11).

Length of hospital stay

Four studies totaling 290 THAs (DAA = 152, PA = 138) analyzing the length of hospital stay. There was no significant difference between the DAA group and PA group in terms of the length of hospital stay (WMD = -0.26, 95%CI -0.58 to 0.06, $p = 0.118$, Fig. 12).

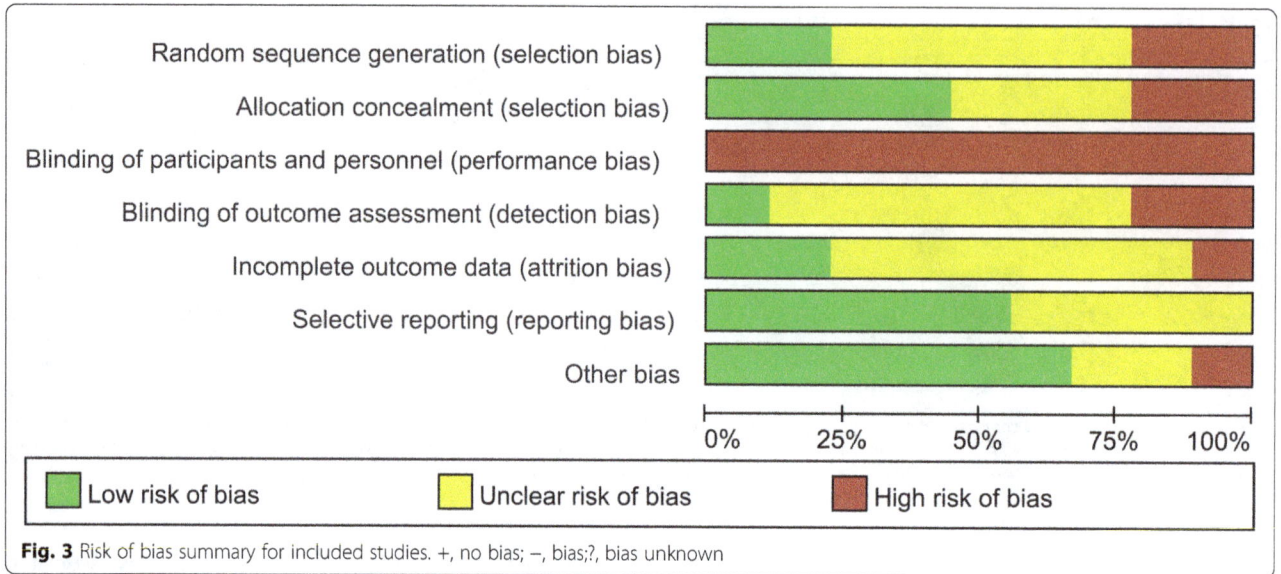

Fig. 3 Risk of bias summary for included studies. +, no bias; –, bias;?, bias unknown

Complications

There was no significant difference between DAA group and PA group in terms of the intraoperative fracture (RR = 1.62, 95%CI 1.62 to 4.46, *p* = 0.350, Fig. 13); postoperative dislocation (RR = 0.52, 95%CI 0.10 to 2.27, *p* = 0.441, Fig. 13), HO (RR = 1.57, 95%CI 0.49 to 5.09, *p* = 0.450, Fig. 13), and groin pain (RR = 2.62, 95%CI 0.63 to 10.94, *p* = 0.191, Fig. 13).

Discussion
Main findings

Our meta-analysis indicated that DAA has a positive role in reducing acute pain intensity, improving postoperative rehabilitation, and decreasing the length of incision and blood loss. We used sensitivity analysis to further confirm the reliability of our conclusion. Most of our analyses were low- to middle-quality evidence.

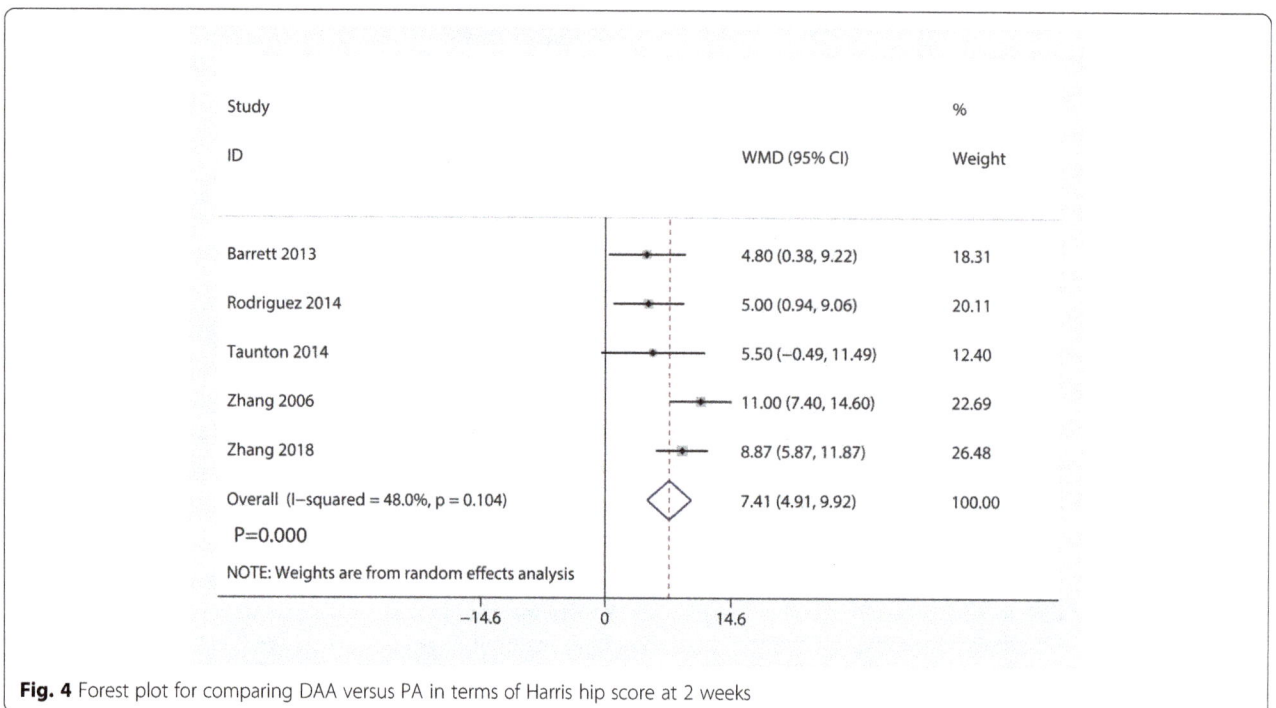

Fig. 4 Forest plot for comparing DAA versus PA in terms of Harris hip score at 2 weeks

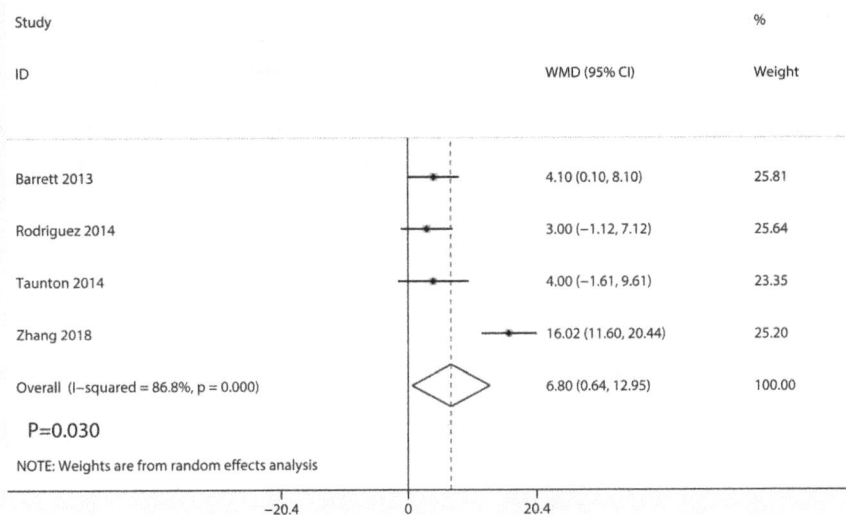

Fig. 5 Forest plot for comparing DAA versus PA in terms of Harris hip score at 6 weeks

New knowledge of this meta-analysis

A major strength of our current meta-analysis is that we limited the inclusion criteria to RCTs. Another new knowledge of this meta-analysis is that we performed a comprehensive analysis (postoperative hip function at same duration follow-up, postoperative pain intensity, blood loss, length of incision, and the length of hospital stay). As far as we know, this meta-analysis is the most comprehensive one to date to compare DAA versus PA for THA.

Implications for clinical practice

We found statistically significant differences between DAA and PA with regards to Harris hip score at 2 weeks and 4 weeks post op. Putananon et al. [26] performed a network meta-analysis that compares DAA, lateral, PA,

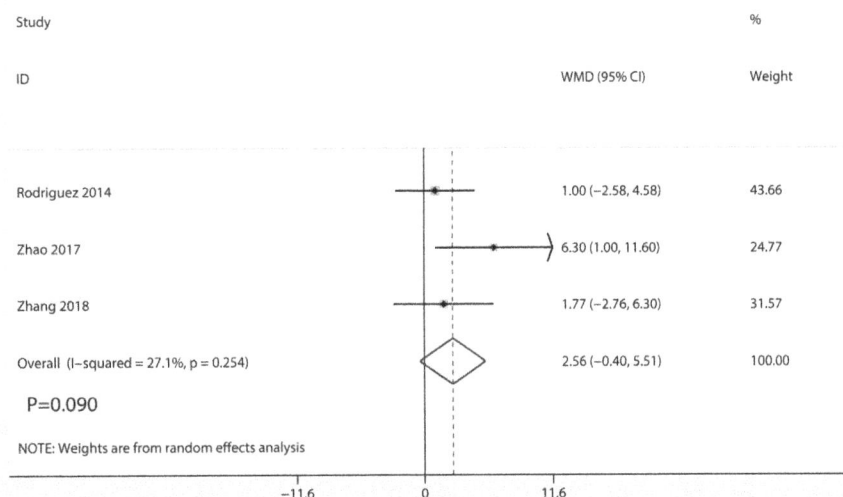

Fig. 6 Forest plot for comparing DAA versus PA in terms of Harris hip score at 12 weeks

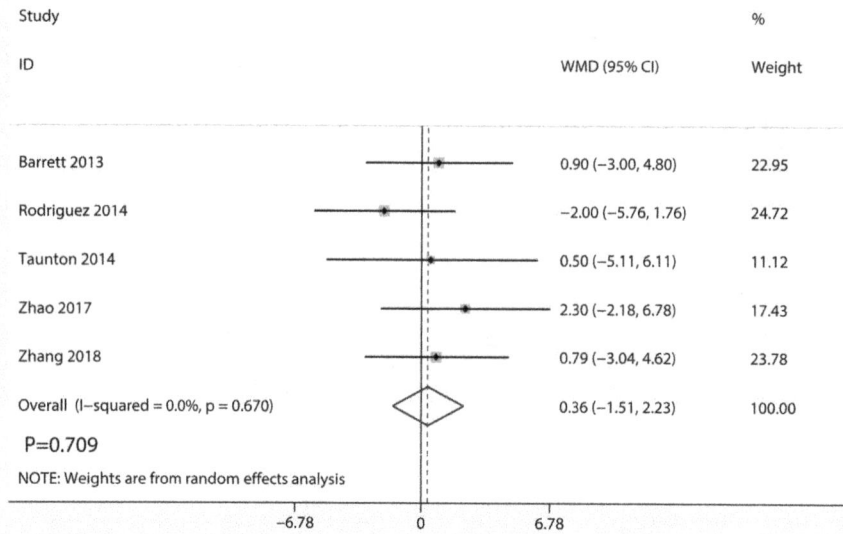

Fig. 7 Forest plot for comparing DAA versus PA in terms of Harris hip score at 1 year

and posterior approaches in THA. Those results showed that DAA for THA gave the best postoperative VAS and Harris hip score. However, they only compared the VAS and Harris hip scores at final follow-up. In our current meta-analysis, we categorized the VAS and Harris hip score at multiple time intervals post-operatively. Our results showed that DAA was superior to PA in terms of the Harris hip score at 2 weeks and 6 weeks. There was no significant difference between the DAA and PA groups in terms of the Harris hip score at 12 weeks and

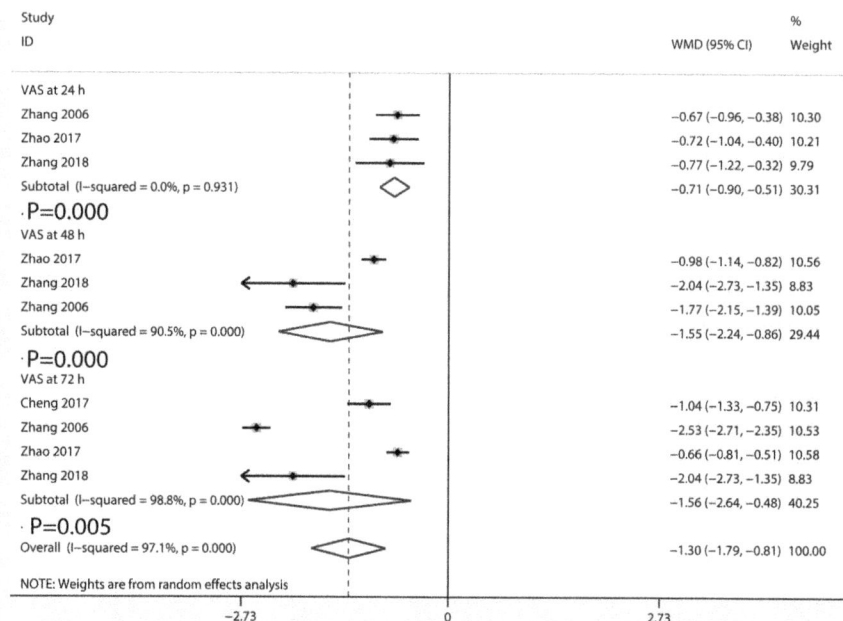

Fig. 8 Forest plot for comparing DAA versus PA in terms of VAS at 24 h, 48 h, and 72 h

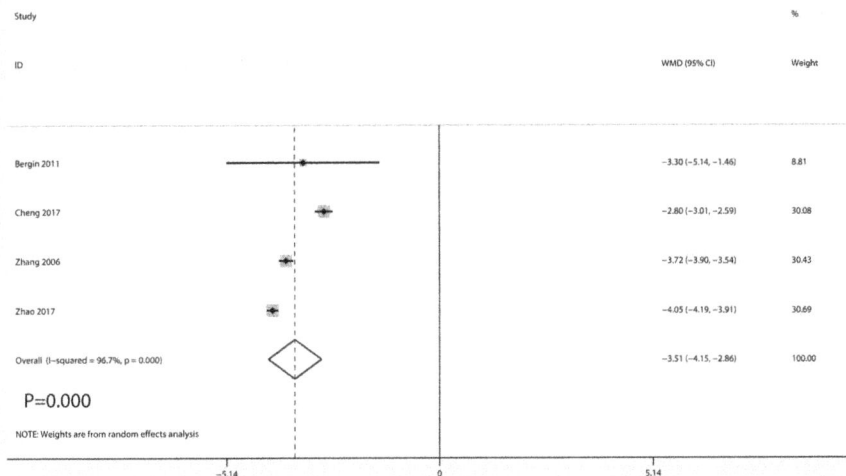

Fig. 9 Forest plot for comparing DAA versus PA in terms of incision length

1 year follow-up. Zhao et al. [24] found that DAA group was associated with a better functional recovery than PA group at 3 months. However, there was no significant difference between DAA and PA groups at 6 month follow-up.

We also found that the DAA group was associated with a reduction of pain intensity at 24 h, 48 h, and 72 h compared to the PA group. One possible rationale for improving Harris hip score and decreasing pain intensity

was the avoidance of muscle splitting and reduced soft tissue damage in DAA group than that of PA group. We found two RCTs that use C-reactive protein (CRP) level to support our hypothesis [24]. Zhao et al. [24] found that, for postoperative day 1 to 4, the level of CRP, IL-6, and ESR was significantly lower in DAA group than that in PA group.

We compared four complications (intraoperative fracture, postoperative dislocation, HO, and groin pain)

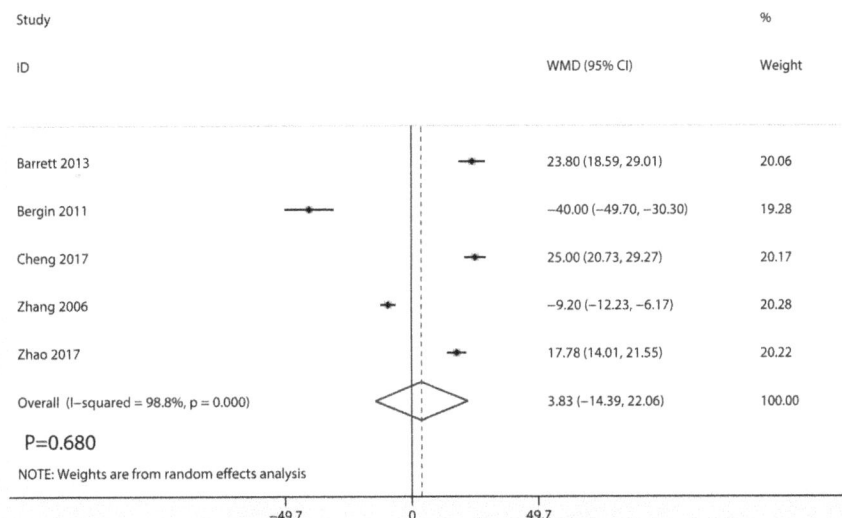

Fig. 10 Forest plot for comparing DAA versus PA in terms of operation time

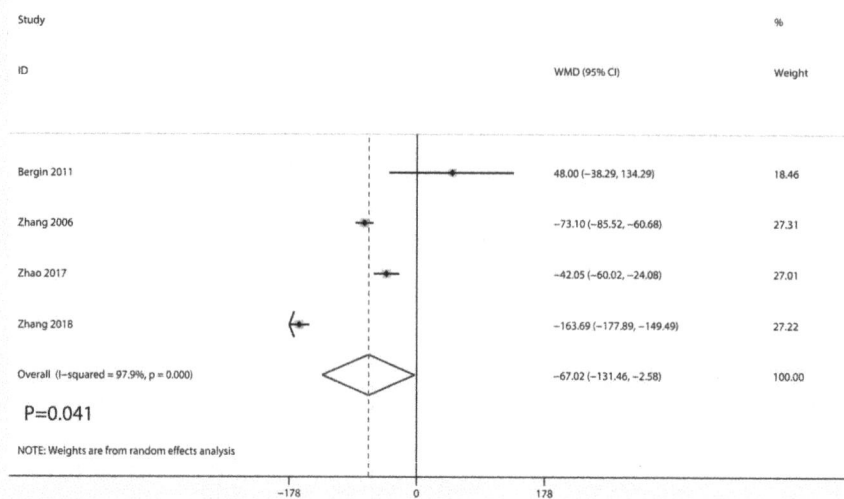

Fig. 11 Forest plot for comparing DAA versus PA in terms of postoperative blood loss

between DAA group and PA group. Results showed that there was no significant difference between these complications ($p > 0.05$). Theoretically speaking, DAA has also been suggested to have an advantage in terms of dislocation risk over PA THA. Current meta-analysis found no significant difference between DAA and PA groups in terms of the postoperative dislocation. Two studies [20, 24] initiated after performance of 150 or 100 THAs via the direct anterior approach and thus could

minimize the influence of a learning curve. The revision rate and risk of revision was comparable in DAA group and PA group in THA [27].

Several limitations in this meta-analysis should be noted. First, the follow-up duration of VAS was relatively short, and long-term follow-up is necessary to identify the long-term effects of DAA. Second, learning curve of the DAA and PA were not reported in the included studies and thus we cannot comment on the learning

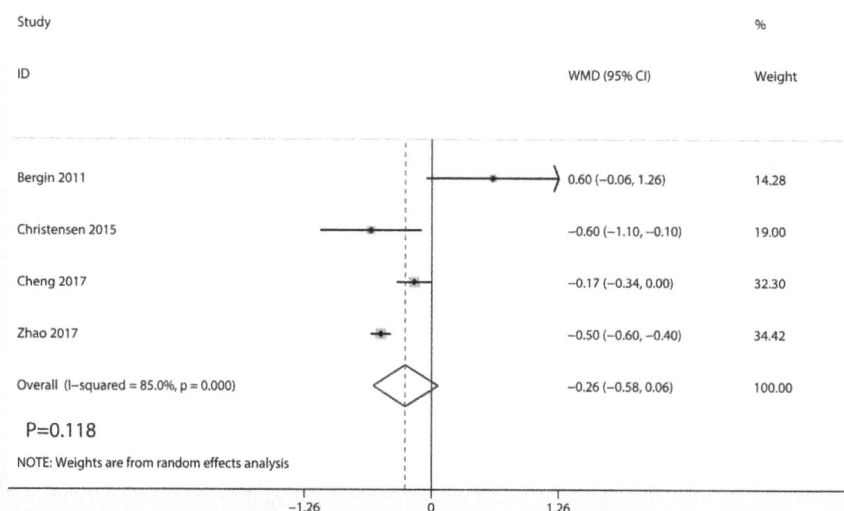

Fig. 12 Forest plot for comparing DAA versus PA in terms of the length of hospital stay

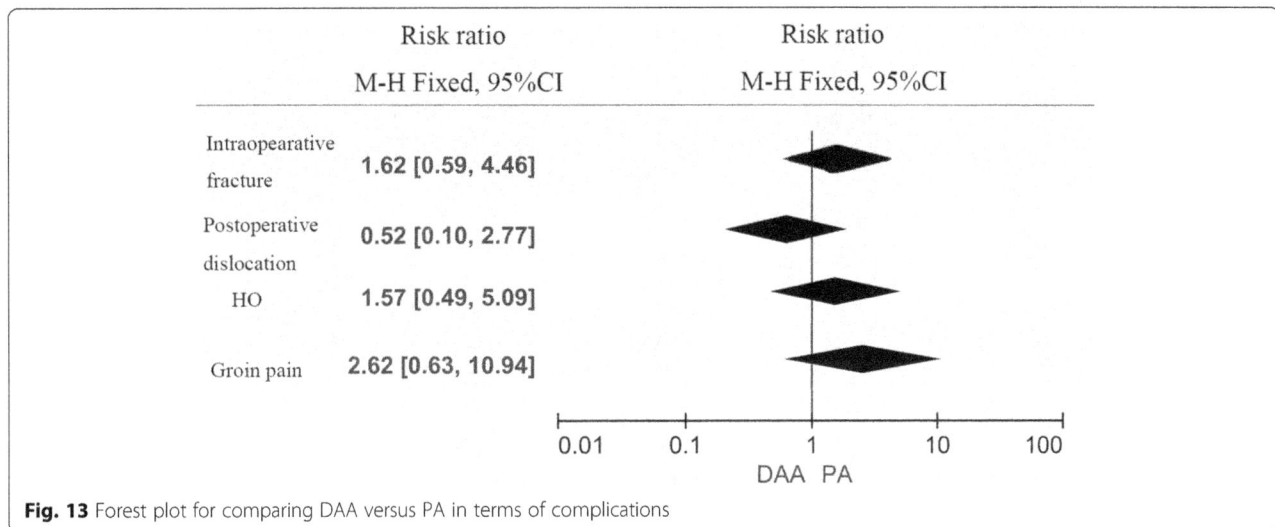

Fig. 13 Forest plot for comparing DAA versus PA in terms of complications

curve regarding either approach. Third, postoperative rehabilitation program was different and thus may cause heterogeneity for the final outcome. Lastly, the blinding of the participant was high in all of the studies, and this high bias affects the final outcomes.

Conclusion

In THA patients, compared with PA, DAA was associated with an early functional recovery and lower pain scores. What's more, DAA was associated with shorter incision length and blood loss. There was no significant difference in complication rated between the DAA and PA groups. Considering the limitation of this meta-analysis, more high quality RCTs are needed to further identify the effects of DAA in THA patients.

Abbreviations

CIs: Confidence intervals; CRP: C-reactive protein; DAA: Direct anterior approach; HO: Heterotopic ossification; MeSH: Medical Subject Headings; OA: Osteoarthritis; PA: Posterior approach; PRISMA: preferred reporting items for systematic reviews and meta-analyses; RCT: Randomized controlled trials; RR: Risk ratio; THA: Total hip arthroplasty; WMD: Weighted mean difference

Authors' contributions

ZW designed the study and developed the retrieve strategy. JZH, CHW, and YJZ searched and screened the summaries and titles. XMG, HHW, YXC, XS, HWB, and WF drafted the article. All authors read and approved the final draft.

Competing interests

The authors declare that they have no competing interests.

References

1. Chen X, Xiong J, Wang P, et al. Robotic-assisted compared with conventional total hip arthroplasty: systematic review and meta-analysis. Postgrad Med J. 2018;94:335–41.
2. Yang Q, Zhang Z, Xin W, Li A. Preoperative intravenous glucocorticoids can decrease acute pain and postoperative nausea and vomiting after total hip arthroplasty: a PRISMA-compliant meta-analysis. Medicine (Baltimore). 2017; 96:e8804.
3. Kurtz S, Ong K, Lau E, Mowat F, Halpern M. Projections of primary and revision hip and knee arthroplasty in the United States from 2005 to 2030. J Bone Joint Surg Am. 2007;89:780–5.
4. Zhao Z, Ma X, Ma J, Sun X, Li F, Lv J. A systematic review and meta-analysis of the topical administration of fibrin sealant in total hip arthroplasty. Sci Rep. 2018;8:78.
5. Anakwe RE, Jenkins PJ, Moran M. Predicting dissatisfaction after total hip arthroplasty: a study of 850 patients. J Arthroplast. 2011;26:209–13.
6. Jones CA, Beaupre LA, Johnston DW, Suarez-Almazor ME. Total joint arthroplasties: current concepts of patient outcomes after surgery. Rheum Dis Clin N Am. 2007;33:71–86.
7. Zomar BO, Bryant D, Hunter S, Howard JL, Vasarhelyi EM, Lanting BA. A randomised trial comparing spatio-temporal gait parameters after total hip arthroplasty between the direct anterior and direct lateral surgical approaches. Hip Int. 2018; https://doi.org/10.1177/1120700018760262.
8. Sutphen SA, Berend KR, Morris MJ, Lombardi AV Jr. Direct anterior approach has lower deep infection frequency than less invasive direct lateral approach in primary total hip arthroplasty. J Surg Orthop Adv. 2018;27:21–4.
9. Graves SC, Dropkin BM, Keeney BJ, Lurie JD, Tomek IM. Does surgical approach affect patient-reported function after primary THA? Clin Orthop Relat Res. 2016;474:971–81.
10. Bernard J, Razanabola F, Beldame J, et al. Electromyographic study of hip muscles involved in total hip arthroplasty: surprising results using the direct anterior minimally invasive approach. Orthop Traumatol Surg Res. 2018. [Epub ahead of print].
11. Higgins BT, Barlow DR, Heagerty NE, Lin TJ. Anterior vs. posterior approach for total hip arthroplasty, a systematic review and meta-analysis. J Arthroplast. 2015;30:419–34.
12. Post ZD, Orozco F, Diaz-Ledezma C, Hozack WJ, Ong A. Direct anterior approach for total hip arthroplasty: indications, technique, and results. J Am Acad Orthop Surg. 2014;22:595–603.
13. Stone A, Sibia U, Atkinson R, Turner T, King P. Evaluation of the learning curve when transitioning from posterolateral to direct anterior hip arthroplasty: a consecutive series of 1000 cases. J Arthroplast. 2018; [epub ahead of print]

14. Ponzio D, Poultsides L, Salvatore A, Lee Y, Memtsoudis S, Alexiades M. In-hospital morbidity and postoperative revisions after direct anterior vs posterior total hip arthroplasty. J Arthroplast. 2018;33:1421–5.

15. Miller LE, Gondusky JS, Bhattacharyya S, Kamath AF, Boettner F, Wright J. Does surgical approach affect outcomes in total hip arthroplasty through 90 days of follow-up? A systematic review with meta-analysis. J Arthroplast. 2018;33:1296–302.

16. Liberati A, Altman DG, Tetzlaff J, et al. The PRISMA statement for reporting systematic reviews and meta-analyses of studies that evaluate healthcare interventions: explanation and elaboration. BMJ. 2009;339:b2700.

17. Barrett WP, Turner SE, Leopold JP. Prospective randomized study of direct anterior vs postero-lateral approach for total hip arthroplasty. J Arthroplast. 2013;28:1634–8.

18. Bergin PF, Doppelt JD, Kephart CJ, et al. Comparison of minimally invasive direct anterior versus posterior total hip arthroplasty based on inflammation and muscle damage markers. J Bone Joint Surg Am. 2011;93:1392–8.

19. Christensen CP, Jacobs CA. Comparison of patient function during the first six weeks after direct anterior or posterior total hip arthroplasty (THA): a randomized study. J Arthroplast. 2015;30:94–7.

20. Rodriguez JA, Deshmukh AJ, Rathod PA, et al. Does the direct anterior approach in THA offer faster rehabilitation and comparable safety to the posterior approach? Clin Orthop Relat Res. 2014;472:455–63.

21. Taunton MJ, Mason JB, Odum SM, Springer BD. Direct anterior total hip arthroplasty yields more rapid voluntary cessation of all walking aids: a prospective, randomized clinical trial. J Arthroplast. 2014;29:169–72.

22. Cheng TE, Wallis JA, Taylor NF, et al. A prospective randomized clinical trial in total hip arthroplasty-comparing early results between the direct anterior approach and the posterior approach. J Arthroplast. 2017;32:883–90.

23. Zhang XL, Wang Q, Jiang Y, Zeng BF. Minimally invasive total hip arthroplasty with anterior incision. Zhonghua Wai Ke Za Zhi. 2006;44:512–5.

24. Zhao HY, Kang PD, Xia YY, Shi XJ, Nie Y, Pei FX. Comparison of early functional recovery after total hip arthroplasty using a direct anterior or posterolateral approach: a randomized controlled trial. J Arthroplast. 2017;32:3421–8.

25. Zhang Z, Wang C, Yang P, Dang X, Wang K. Comparison of early rehabilitation effects of total hip arthroplasty with direct anterior approach versus posterior approach. Zhongguo Xiu Fu Chong Jian Wai Ke Za Zhi. 2018;32:329–33.

26. Putananon C, Tuchinda H, Arirachakaran A, Wongsak S, Narinsorasak T, Kongtharvonskul J. Comparison of direct anterior, lateral, posterior and posterior-2 approaches in total hip arthroplasty: network meta-analysis. Eur J Orthop Surg Traumatol. 2018;28:255–67.

27. Mjaaland KE, Svenningsen S, Fenstad AM, Havelin LI, Furnes O, Nordsletten L. Implant survival after minimally invasive anterior or anterolateral vs. conventional posterior or direct lateral approach: an analysis of 21,860 Total hip arthroplasties from the Norwegian Arthroplasty Register (2008 to 2013). J Bone Joint Surg Am. 2017;99:840–7.

13

A novel ultrasound scanning approach for evaluating femoral cartilage defects of the knee: comparison with routine magnetic resonance imaging

Junyan Cao[1†], Bowen Zheng[1†], Xiaochun Meng[2], Yan Lv[1], Huading Lu[3], Kun Wang[3], Dongmei Huang[1] and Jie Ren[1*]

Abstract

Background: This study aimed to assess a novel ultrasound (US) scanning approach in evaluating knee femoral cartilaginous defects, compared with magnetic resonance imaging (MRI, commonly used for knee imaging) and arthroscopy (gold standard).

Methods: Sixty-four consecutive patients (65 knees) were prospectively evaluated between April 2010 and July 2011.

Results: The overall sensitivity (62.2 and 69.4%), specificity (92.9 and 90.5%), accuracy (75.4 and 78.5%), and adjusted positive (88.7 and 90.4%) and negative predictive (69.5 and 73.3%) were similar for both radiologists (weighted $\kappa = 0.76$). Furthermore, agreement between grading by US and MRI was substantial (weighted $\kappa = 0.61$).

Conclusions: In conclusion, the novel US scanning approach allows similar diagnostic performance compared to routine MRI for knee cartilage defects. US is more accessible, easier to perform, and less expensive than MRI, with potential advantages of easier initial screening and assessment of cartilage defects.

Keywords: Cartilage disease, Ultrasound, Magnetic resonance imaging, Diagnostic performance, Arthroscopy, Sensitivity, Specificity

Background

Progressive articular cartilage defects in the knee are a major cause of pain, disability, and medical expenses in the general population and particularly in the elderly [1]. Precise assessment of cartilaginous abnormality is important to determine the appropriate treatments, e.g., osteotomy, mosaicplasty, drugs, and autologous chondrocyte transplantation [2]. Ultrasound (US) is widely available and relatively inexpensive and has proven to be a useful modality for the routine clinical assessment of joint diseases [3]. US is radiation-free and non-invasive and allows dynamic assessment of moving structures [4].

Previous studies evaluated the feasibility and diagnostic value of US for detecting cartilaginous defects [5–15]. Previous studies reported associations of US with histologic and arthroscopic classifications of cartilage defects [11, 13], and with an acceptable diagnostic performance [14], suggesting that knee US is a promising technique for screening degenerative changes of articular cartilage in patients with osteoarthritis (OA) [14]. Nevertheless, the correlations observed in previous studies were low, with coefficients of 0.262–0.655 [13, 14] and could be due to the selection of the indicators, the selection of US systems, and the experience of the raters. In addition, negative predictive values (NPV) remained low (23.8–45.8%), implying that a negative finding using US does not rule out cartilage degenerative changes [14]. Although a positive finding in US is a strong indicator of arthroscopic degenerative changes of cartilage [14], the

* Correspondence: renjieguangzhou@126.com
Junyan Cao and Bowen Zheng share the first authorship.
†Junyan Cao and Bowen Zheng contributed equally to this work.
[1]Department of Medical Ultrasonics, The Third Affiliated Hospital of Sun Yat-sen University, 600 Tianhe Road, Guangzhou 510630, People's Republic of China
Full list of author information is available at the end of the article

technique still needs improvements before routine clinical use.

Previous assessments were performed with a transducer capable of the highest frequency available for routine clinical use, already resulting in the highest sensitivity possible [13, 14]. The diagnostic accuracy of US is often dependent upon the scanning approach in different US indications [16–18]. Therefore, we hypothesized that improvement of the scanning technique could enhance US diagnostic value. Indeed, previous studies used a fixed flexed knee (e.g., 120°) with transverse scanning only [13, 14], but the knee flexion angle influences the correlation between US and histologic classification of cartilage defects, although the optimal angle remains unknown [13]. In addition, since only transverse scanning was applied, it remains unclear whether longitudinal scanning could offer more benefits, especially when depicting the condyle [14].

Therefore, this study aimed to assess a novel US scanning approach in evaluating knee femoral cartilaginous defects, compared with magnetic resonance imaging (MRI, commonly used for knee imaging) and arthroscopy (gold standard).

Methods

Study design and patients

In this prospective study, 64 consecutive patients (65 knees) scheduled for knee arthroscopy between April 2010 and July 2011 were prospectively evaluated by US and MRI at our hospital. The study was approved by the research ethics committee of the Third Affiliated Hospital of Sun Yat-sen University. All patients signed an informed consent prior to participation in the study.

Patients with a chief complaint of knee pain or disability and scheduled for arthroscopy were enrolled in this study. The patients underwent arthroscopy of the knee because of suspicion of internal derangement. Patients with prior knee surgery (e.g., total knee arthroplasty) and contraindications to MRI were excluded.

US examination

US examination of the knee joint was conducted a week before arthroscopy using a LOGIQ 700 (GE Medical Systems, Milwaukee, WI, USA) with a 7–9-MHz high-resolution linear transducer. A novel US scanning approach based on the functional anatomy of the knee (Fig. 1) [15] was proposed, considering articular motions and both transverse and longitudinal scanning (Fig. 2). (1) In the supine position with a fully extended knee (0°), transverse and longitudinal scanning of bilateral sides of the patella for the anterior portions of both condyles was carried out (Fig. 2a). (2) In the prone position, longitudinal and transverse scanning of the popliteal fossa for the posterior portions of both condyles was

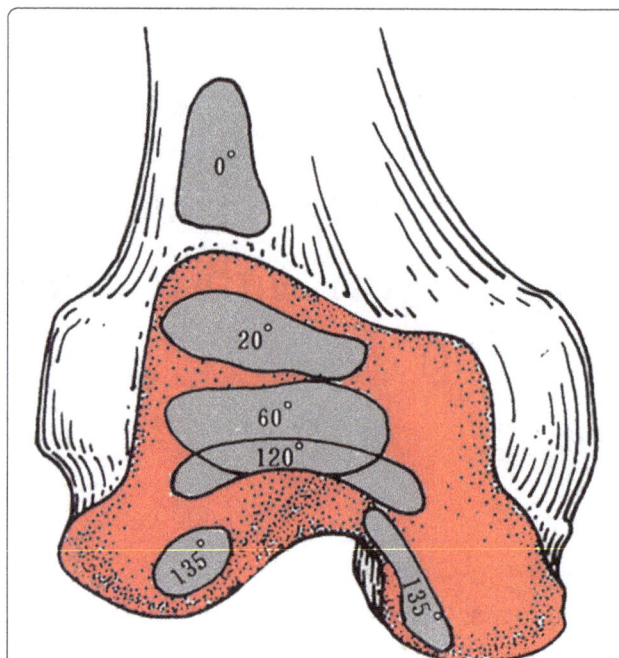

Fig. 1 Contact areas of the patellofemoral articulation during different arcs of motion, adapted from Shahriaree's O'Connor's Textbook of Arthroscopic Surgery [15]. Red area, femoral cartilage; gray areas, contact areas of the femoral cartilage of the patellofemoral articulation during different arcs of motion

performed (Fig. 2b). (3) In the supine position with maximum knee flexion, transverse and longitudinal scanning of the suprapatellar recess for the trochlear surface was undertaken (Fig. 2c). (4) Finally, in the same position, transverse and longitudinal scanning of bilateral sides of the patella was performed again, for the weight-bearing portion of the condyles (Fig. 2c). The US beam was always kept perpendicular to the femur surface. Maximum flexion angle of each patient was recorded, and an angle > 135° was considered good flexion. This angle was confirmed using a lateral photography and the Angler app (an iOS app for angle measurement which was available only on Apple Store China but is unfortunately no longer available). The patient was in the supine position with maximum knee flexion, then a lateral photography was taken and the flexion angle was measured by this app.

A US grading system for knee femoral cartilage defects, based on the International Cartilage Repair Society (ICRS) classification [5, 7, 19, 20], was used: grade 0, normal cartilage; grade 1, nearly normal cartilage with blurred margin or partial lack of clarity without thickness change; grade 2, abnormal cartilage with blurring or obliteration of the margin, lack of clarity, and overt local thinning of the cartilage (< 50% of cartilage depth); grade 3, severely abnormal cartilage with blurring and obliteration of the margin and obvious focal thinning for

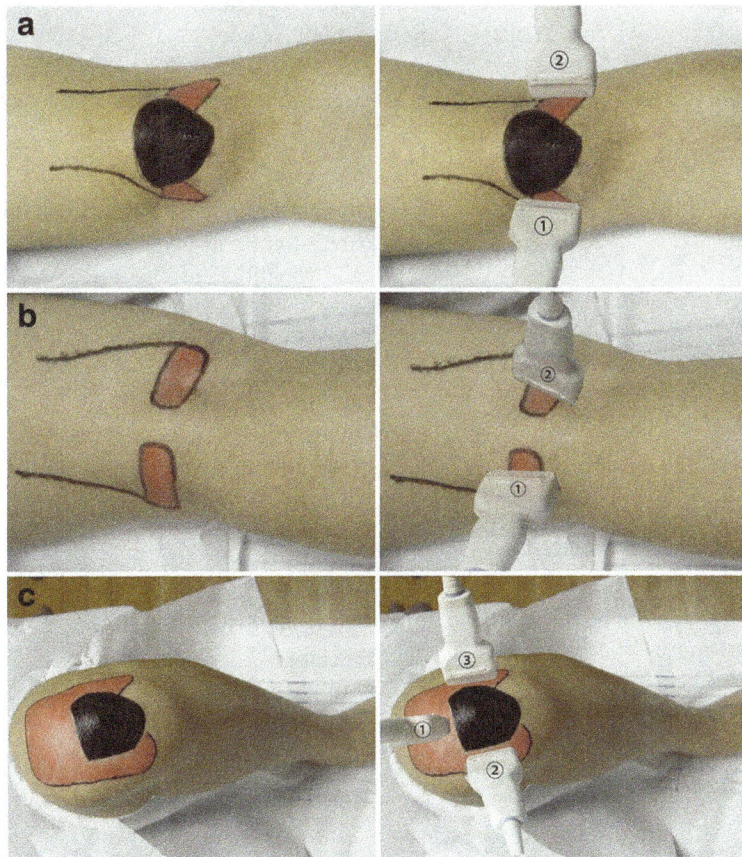

Fig. 2 Novel ultrasound (US) scanning approach for the detection of femoral cartilage. **a** With fully extended knee (0°), transverse and longitudinal scanning of bilateral sides of the patella for cartilage of the anterior portion of medial (1) and lateral (2) condyles with the patient in the supine position. **b** Transverse and longitudinal scanning of the popliteal fossa for the posterior portion of medial (1) and lateral (2) condyles with the patient in a prone position with a fully extended knee. **c** With maximum knee flexion in the supine position, transverse and longitudinal scanning of the trochlear surface (1) and weight-bearing portion of medial (2) and lateral (3) condyles. Red area, surface projection of the femoral cartilage; black area, surface projection of the patella

> 50% of the cartilage depth but intact cartilage-bone interface; and grade 4, severely abnormal cartilage with complete loss of cartilage and coarse or irregular cartilage-bone interface.

Two musculoskeletal radiologists (JYC and JR, with 5 and 15 years of clinical experience, respectively) were trained for 2 months to perform the novel examination method before the present study. This training involved ten volunteers. The radiologists repeatedly scanned those volunteers, alone and together, and compared their results. In this study, the radiologists scanned each patient immediately one after another (according to their availability, without a predefined order) and made assessments independently during real-time scanning, based on individual findings. A form with a schematic drawing of the articular surfaces of the femoral cartilage [19] was used. The trochlear surface and lateral and medial femoral condyles were evaluated separately. In the presence of

multiple cartilaginous defects on the same articular surface, the worst score was attributed.

MRI evaluation

MRI examinations were performed within 1 week before arthroscopy on a Signa Excite 1.5 Tesla MR System (GE Medical Systems, Milwaukee, WI, USA), using a phased array knee coil. Patients were placed in the supine position with the knee fully extended. All MRI examinations consisted of sagittal T1- and T2-weighted, sagittal fat-saturated (fs) proton density (PD)-weighted, coronal fs PD-weighted, and axial fs PD-weighted fast spin echo (FSE) sequences. The imaging parameters are presented in Additional file 1: Table S1.

All MRI images were interpreted by one radiologist (XCM) with over 15 years of experience in musculoskeletal imaging. The radiologist was blinded to the clinical history and US findings. The cartilage was morphologically graded according to a modified ICRS classification system [19]: grade 0, normal cartilage; grade 1, cartilage with intact surface and no tissue loss, but fibrillation and superficial fissures; grade 2, deep defects, but < 50%; grade 3, lesions representing > 50% of the cartilage thickness; and grade 4, defects extending into the subchondral bone. The same schematic drawing of articular surfaces of the femoral cartilage was used to mark defect locations and degrees. The trochlear surface and lateral and medial femoral condyles were evaluated separately. In the presence of multiple cartilaginous defects on the same articular surface, the worst score was attributed.

Arthroscopy

Two orthopedic surgeons (HDL and KW, with 15 and 25 years of clinical experience, respectively) were involved in this study. They were blinded to the US and MRI findings. Knee arthroscopy with fluid irrigation was performed using the standard anterolateral and anteromedial portals to assess the articular cartilage defects and potential comorbidities. The surgeons were free to flex and extend the patients' knees. For cartilage evaluation by arthroscopy, the same schematic drawing of the femoral cartilage surfaces of the knee was used. The surgeons performed their assessment in consensus. The trochlear surface and lateral and medial femoral condyles were evaluated separately. The cartilage lesions were graded analogously to the US and MRI using the ICRS classification [19]. In the presence of multiple cartilaginous defects on the same articular surface, the worst score was attributed. Arthroscopic grading served as the gold standard.

Statistical analysis

With arthroscopic findings as a reference, sensitivity, specificity, and accuracy of US and MRI for femoral cartilage defects were assessed. In addition, positive predictive value (PPV) and NPV were calculated and adjusted for the prevalence of femoral cartilage lesions documented in arthroscopy at our institution (51.9%), based on previous recommendations [21]. The threshold of femoral cartilage abnormality was set between grade 0 as negative and grades 1–4 as positive. Furthermore, detection rates of each grade of cartilage defects and proportion of cartilage lesions graded identically and within one grade in arthroscopy and imaging modalities were calculated. The McNemar chi-square test was used to compare the groups.

Weighted κ statistics for the level of agreement among different methods and between radiologists (US) were used [22]. The Student t test was used to compare the κ values between grades assigned by arthroscopy and US or MRI. Error analysis was performed for the first blinded US evaluation by the same radiologists after the revelation of arthroscopic findings. All false-positive or false-negative results were analyzed, and the most likely reason for the diagnostic error was recorded.

All statistical analyses were performed with SPSS 17.0 (IBM, Armonk, NY, USA) and STATA 11 (StataCorp LP, College Station, TX, USA). Two-sided P values < 0.05 were considered significantly significant.

Results

Patient baseline characteristics and arthroscopy data

Sixty-four consecutive patients (65 knees) with various abnormalities of the knee were assessed, including 21 men and 43 women, with a mean age of 42 years (range, 18–75). Final diagnoses included OA (25 knees), meniscus injury (11 knees), traumatic arthritis (11 knees), chondromalacia patella (7 knees), anterior cruciate ligament tears (6 knees), dislocation of the patella (3 knees), and meniscus cyst (2 knees). Among the 65 knees, 90.8% (59/65) had a good flexion. Altogether, 195 knee femoral cartilage surfaces, including the trochlear surface (TS), lateral femoral condyles (LC), and medial femoral condyles (MC), were evaluated by US, MRI, and arthroscopy. Arthroscopy revealed that 84, 20, 30, 38, and 23 surfaces had grades 0, 1, 2, 3, and 4 defects, respectively (Table 1). The distribution of cartilage defects identified by arthroscopy is shown in Table 1.

Overall diagnosis performances of US and MR

Table 2 shows the overall sensitivity, specificity, accuracy, and crude and adjusted PPV and NPV for US and MRI in detecting knee femoral cartilage defects, using arthroscopy as the gold standard. Figures 3 presents typical cases of each grade of cartilage defects. The sensitivity (62.2 and 69.4%), specificity (92.9 and 90.5%), and accuracy (75.4 and 78.5%) were similar between two independent radiologists performing the US. Interobserver agreement was obtained between the two radiologists, as indicated by a weighted κ value of 0.76. Considering the prevalence of cartilage lesions of 51.9% at our institution, obtained based on the analysis of 832 knee arthroscopies from January 2002 to December 2011, adjusted PPV was 88.7–90.4% (false PPV = 9.6–11.3%), and adjusted NPV was 69.5–73.3% (false NPV = 26.7–30.5%). Only a lower sensitivity of US was observed for radiologist 1 (JYC, 5 years of clinical experience) compared with MRI (P = 0.042). Other parameters showed non-significant

Table 1 Location and grades of cartilaginous defects in 65 knees by arthroscopy

Surface	Grade 0	Grade 1	Grade 2	Grade 3	Grade 4
TS	27 (13.9)	7 (3.6)	11 (5.6)	13 (6.7)	7 (3.6)
MC	25 (12.8)	7 (3.6)	11 (5.6)	14 (7.2)	8 (4.1)
LC	32 (16.4)	6 (3.1)	8 (4.1)	11 (5.6)	8 (4.1)
Total	84 (43.1)	20 (10.3)	30 (15.3)	38 (19.5)	23 (11.8)

Data are the numbers of surfaces. Values in parentheses are percentages
TS trochlear surface, *MC* medial condyles, *LC* lateral condyles

Table 2 Overall diagnostic performance and predictive value of US and MRI in evaluating cartilaginous defects

		TP#	TN#	FP#	FN#	Sensitivity (95%CI) (%)	Specificity (95%CI) (%)	Accuracy (95%CI) (%)	Crude predictive value (95%CI) (%)		Adjusted predictive value (%)		AUC (95% CI)
									PPV	NPV	PPV	NPV	
US	Radiologist 1	69	78	6	42	62.2 (53.1–71.2) (0.042)	92.9 (87.3–98.4) (1.000)	75.4 (69.3–81.4) (0.060)	92.0 (85.9–98.1) (0.756)	65.0 (56.5–73.5) (0.148)	90.4	69.5	0.775 (0.722–0.828)
	Radiologist 2	77	76	8	34	69.4 (60.8–77.9) (0.367)	90.5 (84.2–96.8) (0.565)	78.5 (72.7–84.2) (0.245)	90.6 (84.4–96.8) (0.397)	69.1 (60.5–77.7) (0.450)	88.7	73.3	0.799 (0.746–0.853)
MRI		84	79	5	27	75.7 (67.7–83.7)	94.0 (89.0–99.1)	83.6 (78.4–88.8)	94.4 (89.6–99.2)	74.5 (66.2–82.8)	93.2	78.2	0.849 (0.801–0.896)

Numbers in parentheses are the P values compared with MRI data
TP true positive, *TN* true negative, *FP* false positive, *FN* false negative
#Data are the surface numbers

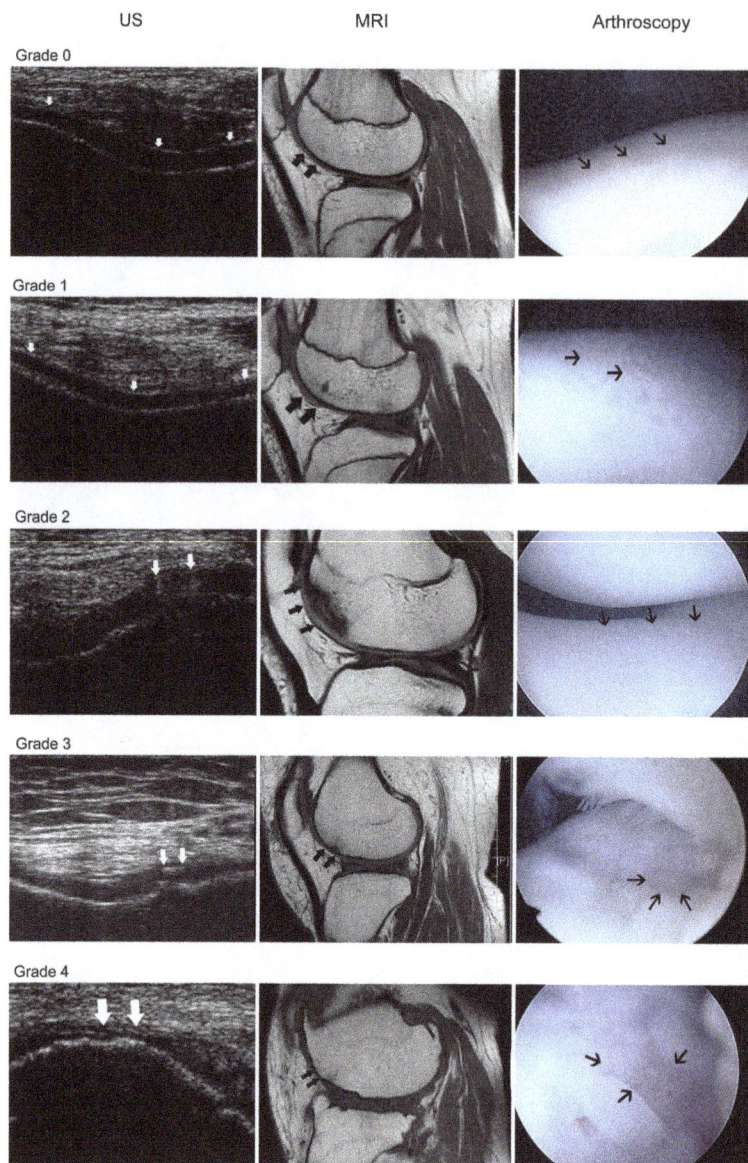

US   MRI   Arthroscopy

Grade 0

Grade 1

Grade 2

Grade 3

Grade 4

Fig. 3 Typical cases of each grade of cartilage defects at the trochlear surface. Defects are shown as white arrows for US, bold black arrows for MRI, and thin black arrows for AS

differences between US and MRI ($P = 0.060$ to 1.000), as shown in Table 2.

US and MR diagnosis performance comparisons for different surfaces

For all cartilage defect grades on each articular surface, some differences were seen between US and MRI for specific surfaces (Table 3), but there were differences between the two radiologists.

US and MR diagnosis performance comparisons for different defect grades

The respective detection rates and comparisons between US and MRI for cartilage defects of each grade are shown

in Tables 4 and 5. Generally, compared with MRI, no significant differences were obtained in detecting grades 0, 2, 3, and 4 defects ($P = 0.083$ to 0.317), but a lower detection rate with US for grade 1 defects was obtained for both radiologists ($P = 0.025$). Indeed, for radiologist 1, ten lesions were diagnosed as grade 0, eight as grade 2, and two as grade 3. For radiologist 2, eight lesions were diagnosed as grade 0, six as grade 2, and six as grade 3. The proportions of cartilage defects graded identically and matched within one grade of arthroscopic values using US by the two radiologists were 80.0 and 80.5%, respectively, with no significant difference between both radiologists ($P = 0.179$ and $P = 0.224$, respectively). A moderate agreement between arthroscopy and US for grade assignment (weighted $\kappa =$

Table 3 Diagnostic performance of US and MRI for evaluating cartilaginous defects on different surfaces

Surface	TP#	TN#	FP#	FN#	Sensitivity (95%CI) (%)	Specificity (95%CI) (%)	Accuracy (95%CI) (%)	Crude predictive value (95%CI) (%)		Adjusted predictive value (%)		AUC (95%CI)
								PPV	NPV	PPV	NPV	
US Radiologist 1												
TS	31	25	2	7	81.6 (69.3–93.9) (0.317)	92.6 (82.7–102) (1.000)	86.2 (77.8–94.6) (1.000)	93.9 (85.5–102) (1.000)	78.1 (63.8–92.4) (1.000)	92.2	82.3	0.871 (0.791–0.951)
MC	20	22	3	20	50.0 (34.5–65.5) (0.005)	88.0 (75.3–101) (0.046)	64.6 (53.0–76.2) (0.046)	87.0 (73.2–100) (0.310)	52.4 (37.3–67.5) (0.251)	81.8	62.0	0.690 (0.588–0.792)
LC	18	31	1	15	54.5 (37.6–71.5) (0.083)	96.9 (90.8–103) (0.317)	75.4 (64.9–85.9) (0.046)	94.7 (84.7–105) (1.000)	67.4 (53.8–80.9) (0.818)	95.0	66.4	0.757 (0.666–0.849)
US Radiologist 2												
TS	35	24	3	3	92.1 (83.5–101) (0.025)	88.9 (77.0–101) (0.317)	90.8 (83.7–97.8) (0.424)	92.1 (83.5–101) (1.000)	88.9 (77.0–101) (0.315)	90.0	91.3	0.905 (0.831–0.979)
MC	22	22	3	18	55.0 (39.6–70.4) (0.248)	88.0 (75.3–101) (0.014)	67.7 (56.3–79.1) (0.157)	88.0 (75.3–101) (0.424)	55.0 (39.6–70.4) (0.352)	83.2	64.4	0.715 (0.613–0.817)
LC	20	30	2	13	60.6 (43.9–77.3) (1.000)	93.8 (85.4–102) (1.000)	76.9 (66.7–87.2) (1.000)	90.9 (78.9–103) (0.424)	69.8 (56.0–83.5) (1.000)	91.3	68.8	0.772 (0.677–0.867)
MRI												
TS	30	25	2	8	78.9 (66.0–91.9)	92.6 (82.7–102)	84.6 (75.8–93.4)	93.8 (85.4–102)	75.8 (61.1–90.4)	92.0	80.3	0.858 (0.775–0.940)
MC	28	24	1	12	70.0 (55.8–84.2)	96.0 (88.3–104)	80.0 (70.3–89.7)	96.6 (89.9–103)	66.7 (51.3–82.1)	95.0	74.8	0.830 (0.748–0.712)
LC	21	30	2	12	63.6 (47.2–80.0)	93.8 (85.4–102)	78.5 (68.5–88.5)	91.3 (79.8–103)	71.4 (57.8–85.1)	91.7	70.5	0.787 (0.693–0.881)

Numbers in parentheses are the P values compared to MRI data (McNemar test)

TS trochlear surface, *MC* medial condyles, *LC* lateral condyles, *TP* true positive, *TN* true negative, *FP* false positive, *FN* false negative

#Data are the surface numbers

Table 4 Results of US and MR imaging for detecting knee cartilage defects of each grade

Grade	US		MRI
	Radiologist 1	Radiologist 2	
0	92.9 (78/84) (0.317)	90.5 (76/84) (0.083)	94.0 (79/84)
1	0.0 (0/20) (0.025)	0.0 (0/20) (0.025)	25.0 (5/20)
2	33.3 (10/30) (0.083)	40.0 (12/30) (0.317)	43.3 (13/30)
3	55.3 (21/38) (0.014)	65.8 (25/38) (0.157)	71.1 (27/38)
4	73.9 (17/23) (0.083)	82.6 (19/23) (0.317)	87.0 (20/23)

Data are the percentages, followed by the raw data; numbers in parentheses are the P values in comparison with MRI (McNemar test)

Table 6 Error analysis: reasons for false positive and false negative diagnoses

Surface	False-negative finding[#]			False-positive finding[#]	
	Particular sites	Partial volume effect	Small or superficial lesion	Thin cartilage	Partial volume effect
TS	0/0	3/3	4/3	0/0	2/3
MC	9/7	5/4	6/5	1/1	2/3
LC	11/9	4/3	0/0	0/0	1/1
Total	20/16	12/10	10/8	1/1	5/7

TS trochlear surface, MC medial condyles, LC lateral condyles
[#]Data are the surface numbers for radiologist 1/radiologist 2

0.60, 95% CI 0.50–0.71, and 0.63, 95% CI 0.52–0.74, for the two radiologists) was obtained, with no significant difference ($P = 0.57$ and $P = 0.11$, respectively) in comparison with MRI data (weighted $\kappa = 0.73$, 95% CI 0.62–0.84). In addition, substantial agreement was found between grades assigned using US and MRI (weighted $\kappa = 0.61$, 95% CI 0.50–0.72).

Reasons for false-positive and false-negative diagnoses

Error analysis was carried out to determine the reasons for false-positive and false-negative diagnoses by US, and the results are shown in Table 6. The majority of false negatives were due to the lesions being located at certain sites, including the femoral condyles near the intercondyloid fossa, where no defects were detected by US (Fig. 4). The majority of false positives were attributed to the partial volume effect (Fig. 5).

Discussion

In this study, we aimed to improve the diagnostic accuracy of US for the diagnosis of knee lesions with the intention of improving the accessibility and decreasing the costs of knee examination associated with MRI and arthroscopy, particularly for outpatients. Nevertheless, MRI and arthroscopy are still necessary. Therefore, this study assessed the diagnostic value of a novel US scanning approach in evaluating knee femoral cartilaginous defects and found that it allows a similar diagnostic

Table 5 Comparison of aberrations between US and MRI grades and surgical grades

	Modality	US radiologist 1	US radiologist 2	MRI
Undergrading	2–4 grades	29 (14.9)	14 (7.2)	19 (9.8)
	1 grade	18 (9.2)	12 (6.1)	14 (7.2)
Identical grading	–	126 (64.6)	132 (67.7)	144 (73.8)
Overgrading	1 grade	12 (6.2)	13 (6.7)	9 (4.6)
	2–4 grades	10 (5.1)	24 (12.3)	9 (4.6)

Data are the number of defects. Values in parentheses are percentages

performance as routine MRI, but with improved NPV compared with previous US scanning approach, which is of clinical significance. Different articular surfaces of the femur can be accessible with an external US probe by varying the angle range of knee flexion [23–25]. Interestingly, the novel scanning approach had similar sensitivity, specificity, and accuracy compared with MRI for detecting lesions on the whole femoral cartilage and individual articular surfaces. In addition, moderate agreement was obtained between grades assigned by arthroscopy and US.

In the present study, a substantial interobserver agreement was observed, while similar PPVs and higher NPVs were obtained in comparison with recent reports [13, 14]. The improved NPV (i.e., decreased false-negative rate) could be a consequence of more visibility of the femoral cartilage in the novel scanning approach. The fairly low NPV reported by Saarakkala et al. [14] is probably not related to an intrinsic limitation of the US itself or a need for higher resolution imaging but rather a lack of thorough observation of the overall femoral cartilage. An available acoustic window is the most important factor for US examination. The difficulty in visualizing the whole femoral cartilage due to the shadow of the patella and tibia is a major disadvantage. By using multiple knee angles, the novel approach markedly decreased false-negative femoral cartilage defect diagnoses.

In full extension (0°), the patella rests over the supratrochlear fat pad and is almost completely proximal to the superior border of the femoral articular cartilage [22, 23]. In this position, US can show the cartilage of the anterior and posterior femoral condyles but not the trochlear surface and weight-bearing femoral condyles due to the interference of the patella and tibia. In 10°–20° flexion, the patella first hugs the femoral shaft closely then slips distally and always remains in contact with the trochlear surface of the femur [22, 23], which may lead to poor visibility of most parts of the femoral articular surfaces. At approximately 135° of flexion, the patella reaches as far as the intercondylar notch [23]. At this time, good exposure

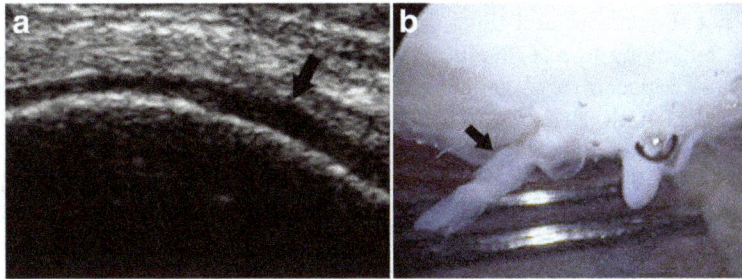

Fig. 4 A grade 2 lesion at the lateral femoral condyles near the intercondyloid fossa, missed by US. **a** On the US, the diagnosis was normal (grade 0), but on arthroscopy **b**, the diagnosis was grade 2 (black arrow) cartilage defect, presenting as a velvet-like formation with intact cartilage surface, located at the lateral femoral condyles near the intercondyloid fossa

of the entire trochlear surface and most parts of the lateral and medial condyles can be achieved. Therefore, scanning on minimum (0°) and maximum (≥ 135°) angles of the knee flexion may provide a more thorough scan of the femoral cartilage than those using only a fixed flexed knee (e.g., 120°).

MRI is considered a method of choice for thorough evaluation of cartilage morphology, but its routine use in all symptomatic patients with clinical suspicion of knee cartilage defects is limited due to unavailability in many district and community hospitals in China and high costs (in terms of money and time) [26]. Therefore, the application of the simple, widely available, and inexpensive US technique as the initial screening method for femoral cartilage lesions could be more appropriate. The novel US approach proposed here may satisfy the above requirements and can be used as an initial screening modality to provide a morphological assessment of the femoral articular cartilage in outpatient clinics.

As a non-invasive imaging modality, the novel approach needed further clinical validation. Therefore, the novel approach was compared with MRI, which is probably the most important method for cartilage imaging [26]. Previous comparative studies [27, 28] between US and MRI mainly focused on the thickness measurement of femoral cartilage, an important defect indicator, and showed a significant correlation (coefficients = 0.44–0.84). Comparison of US and MRI was further assessed in the present study; although a relatively lower detection rate of grade 1 defects was observed, the novel approach showed similar diagnostic ability for the detection and classification of cartilage defects compared with routine 2D FSE MRI, with a significant agreement for grading lesions.

The first major problem is that although the novel approach allows a significant decrease of false-negative diagnoses, it should be highlighted that the risk of false negatives was still as high as 26.7–30.5%, representing the majority of erroneous diagnoses. This likely results from the inability to visualize the lateral and medial condyles near the intercondylar notch, even at the maximum angle (e.g., 135°) of the knee flexion, due to their continuous articulation with the lateral and odd facet of the patella [15]. Thus, defects in these locations were the major cause of false negatives, as none of them was detected. Therefore, the blind areas of US have been improved by using varying flexion (0–135°) rather than a fixed flexion (120°), but the novel approach still needs to be improved. Patients suspected to be with cartilage defects should undergo additional diagnostic modalities, e.g., MRI, even with a negative US finding to verify the cartilage status.

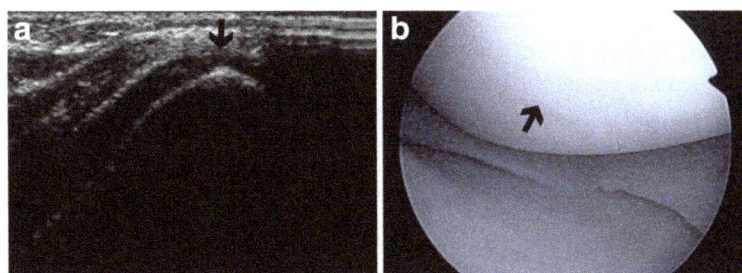

Fig. 5 Example of a false-positive case. **a** The case was diagnosed as grade 3 cartilage defect on the trochlear surface (black arrow), presenting as blurred margin, lack of clarity, and overt local thinning (> 50% of cartilage depth). **b** On AS, the diagnosis was grade 0, i.e., normal cartilage (black arrow)

The second major problem is that only femoral surfaces can be seen by US, not the patellar and tibial surfaces, which precludes the technique from providing an overall assessment of the knee articular cartilage. Nevertheless, strong correlations (Pearson's correlation coefficients = 0.75–0.77) between volume changes in femoral cartilage and that in tibial cartilage in OA patients have been reported [29], indicating that evaluating one of the two features should be adequate. Therefore, US findings from the femoral cartilage might be reliable for evaluating arthritic cartilage changes of the tibial cartilage in clinical practice.

The US systems and technique are possible sources of error in US, as well as the operator. Although similar diagnostic accuracy between the novel approach and MRI was presented here, a substantial number of patients with small or superficial lesions (grade 1 defects) were misdiagnosed or missed by the US. Indeed, the US equipment available for routine clinical use can only assess conspicuous morphological changes of cartilage, not determining its internal characteristics, while MRI can. Therefore, subtle morphological changes in the early stage of cartilage defects might explain the misdiagnoses. More advanced equipment and techniques (e.g., a 50-MHz transducer, which can detect layers in immature cartilage [30]) may provide a solution. Further studies are necessary to verify this hypothesis. Another issue is operator dependency, a known problem in US examination [31]. As shown above, the difference in overall sensitivity was obtained between the two radiologists participating in this study. Therefore, a standardized training to learn the correct scanning approach and associated diagnoses is essential to avoid misdiagnoses or missed diagnoses.

There were some limitations to this study. First, although routine 2D FSE MRI sequences were performed as previously described [32–34], it may be argued that this study underestimated the actual diagnostic ability of MRI, as it is not optimal for cartilage evaluation due to anisotropic voxels, section gaps, and partial volume effects [26]. In addition, several MRI techniques are available to facilitate the assessment of the femoral cartilage for changes of morphology [35–37] and even biochemical composition [38, 39]. The results of MRI achieved in such sequences may be more favorable than those reported here. Nevertheless, since the cause of pain or disability of the knee is frequently multifactorial or unknown, 2D FSE sequences are most commonly applied in the clinical setting for initial examinations. In this study, we simulated a hypothetical situation of the first-time examination, which optimized the likelihood of screening cartilage defects.

Another limitation is that the same cartilage lesion could be attributed to different sites between US and MRI or arthroscopy. To minimize such discrepancies,

the same standard schematic drawing of the femoral cartilage surfaces was used for all techniques. Nevertheless, a lesion located on the very edge of three articular surfaces would be likely assigned to different surfaces in various examination methods. Therefore, an overall assessment of the femoral cartilage from all three sites is necessary before the diagnosis and subsequent treatment of cartilage lesion; this is not affected by the possible misplacement. Further studies regarding treatment evaluation are required to target the precise lesion localization of cartilage.

In addition, the correlation between US findings and other assessment tools was not established. Indeed, in this initial study, we prioritized the associations of US with arthroscopy (gold standard) and MRI (most important imaging modality of cartilage). In the future, the correlation between the novel US scanning approach and clinical assessment should be evaluated for its recommendation in routine clinical use, including evaluation of degenerative changes and therapeutic effects.

The aim of the present study was to investigate the value of US as a screening tool for cartilage defects in patients with a chief complaint of knee pain (without any previous examination and diagnosis). It is indeed possible that some patients were not definitely diagnosed with OA. On the other hand, cartilage degeneration caused by OA may also present as cartilage defect. Therefore, it could be hypothesized that OA will not directly affect the capability of the US detection of cartilage defects, but this specific point will have to be examined in the future.

Conclusions

The novel US scanning approach taking knee articular motion into consideration is more valid in a clinical setting to significantly decrease false-negative diagnoses compared with fixed-angle (120°) transverse scanning. It also has similar diagnostic performance, PPV, and agreement as routine MRI approaches for evaluating the knee cartilage defects in patients with a broad spectrum of knee diseases, but the NPV was higher than the previous US scanning approach. As a non-invasive, fast, inexpensive, and radiation-free imaging modality, US has a potential to be used for initial screening assessments of cartilage defects in first-visit patients with a chief complaint of knee pain and/or disability.

Abbreviations
fs: Fat-saturated; LC: Lateral femoral condyles; MC: Medial femoral condyles; MRI: Magnetic resonance imaging; NPV: Negative predictive values; OA: Osteoarthritis; PD: Proton density; PPV: Positive predictive value; TS: Trochlear surface; US: Ultrasound

Acknowledgements
The authors acknowledge the invaluable participation of the patients as well as the help from the Radiology and Orthopedics Departments of the Third Affiliated Hospital of Sun Yat-Sen University and Dr. Jibin Liu of Department of Radiology, Thomas Jefferson University Hospital.

Authors' contributions
JYC, BWZ, and JR contributed to the conception and design; JYC, BWZ, XCM, YL, HDL, KW, DMH, and JR contributed to the acquisition of data or analysis and interpretation of data; JYC, BWZ, XCM, YL, HDL, KW, DMH, and JR have been involved in the drafting of the manuscript and revised it critically for important intellectual content; all authors have given final approval of the version to be published.

Competing interests
The authors declare that they have no competing interests.

Author details
[1]Department of Medical Ultrasonics, The Third Affiliated Hospital of Sun Yat-sen University, 600 Tianhe Road, Guangzhou 510630, People's Republic of China. [2]Department of Radiology, The Third Affiliated Hospital of Sun Yat-sen University, 600 Tianhe Road, Guangzhou 510630, People's Republic of China. [3]Department of Orthopedics, The Third Affiliated Hospital of Sun Yat-sen University, 600 Tianhe Road, Guangzhou 510630, People's Republic of China.

References
1. Urwin M, Symmons D, Allison T, Brammah T, Busby H, Roxby M, et al. Estimating the burden of musculoskeletal disorders in the community: the comparative prevalence of symptoms at different anatomical sites, and the relation to social deprivation. Ann Rheum Dis. 1998;57:649–55.
2. Buckwalter JA, Mankin HJ. Articular cartilage repair and transplantation. Arthritis Rheum. 1998;41:1331–42.
3. Qvistgaard E, Kristoffersen H, Terslev L, Danneskiold-Samsoe B, Torp-Pedersen S, Bliddal H. Guidance by ultrasound of intra-articular injections in the knee and hip joints. Osteoarthr Cartil. 2001;9:512–7.
4. Wakefield RJ, Gibbon WW, Emery P. The current status of ultrasonography in rheumatology. Rheumatology (Oxford). 1999;38:195–8.
5. McCune WJ, Dedrick DK, Aisen AM, MacGuire A. Sonographic evaluation of osteoarthritic femoral condylar cartilage. Correlation with operative findings. Clin Orthop Relat Res. 1990;254:230–5.
6. Iagnocco A, Coari G, Zoppini A. Sonographic evaluation of femoral condylar cartilage in osteoarthritis and rheumatoid arthritis. Scand J Rheumatol. 1992; 21:201–3.
7. Grassi W, Lamanna G, Farina A, Cervini C. Sonographic imaging of normal and osteoarthritic cartilage. Semin Arthritis Rheum. 1999;28:398–403.
8. Batalov AZ, Kuzmanova SI, Penev DP. Ultrasonographic evaluation of knee joint cartilage in rheumatoid arthritis patients. Folia Med (Plovdiv). 2000;42:23–6.
9. Disler DG, Raymond E, May DA, Wayne JS, McCauley TR. Articular cartilage defects: in vitro evaluation of accuracy and interobserver reliability for detection and grading with US. Radiology. 2000;215:846–51.
10. Mathiesen O, Konradsen L, Torp-Pedersen S, Jorgensen U. Ultrasonography and articular cartilage defects in the knee: an in vitro evaluation of the accuracy of cartilage thickness and defect size assessment. Knee Surg Sports Traumatol Arthrosc. 2004;12:440–3.
11. Tsai CY, Lee CL, Chai CY, Chen CH, Su JY, Huang HT, et al. The validity of in vitro ultrasonographic grading of osteoarthritic femoral condylar cartilage—a comparison with histologic grading. Osteoarthr Cartil. 2007;15:245–50.
12. Yoon CH, Kim HS, Ju JH, Jee WH, Park SH, Kim HY. Validity of the sonographic longitudinal sagittal image for assessment of the cartilage thickness in the knee osteoarthritis. Clin Rheumatol. 2008;27:1507–16.
13. Lee CL, Huang MH, Chai CY, Chen CH, Su JY, Tien YC. The validity of in vivo ultrasonographic grading of osteoarthritic femoral condylar cartilage: a comparison with in vitro ultrasonographic and histologic gradings. Osteoarthr Cartil. 2008;16:352–8.
14. Saarakkala S, Waris P, Waris V, Tarkiainen I, Karvanen E, Aarnio J, et al. Diagnostic performance of knee ultrasonography for detecting degenerative changes of articular cartilage. Osteoarthr Cartil. 2012;20: 376–81.
15. Shahriaree H. O'Connor's textbook of arthroscopic surgery. Philadelphia: Lippincott; 1992.
16. Li Y, Hua Y, Fang J, Wang C, Qiao L, Wan C, et al. Performance of different scan protocols of fetal echocardiography in the diagnosis of fetal congenital heart disease: a systematic review and meta-analysis. PLoS One. 2013;8:e65484.
17. Dexheimer Neto FL, Andrade JM, Raupp AC, Townsend Rda S, Beltrami FG, Brisson H, et al. Diagnostic accuracy of the bedside lung ultrasound in emergency protocol for the diagnosis of acute respiratory failure in spontaneously breathing patients. J Bras Pneumol. 2015;41:58–64.
18. Nazerian P, Tozzetti C, Vanni S, Bartolucci M, Gualtieri S, Trausi F, et al. Accuracy of abdominal ultrasound for the diagnosis of pneumoperitoneum in patients with acute abdominal pain: a pilot study. Crit Ultrasound J. 2015;7:15.
19. Brittberg M, Winalski CS. Evaluation of cartilage injuries and repair. J Bone Joint Surg Am. 2003;85-A(Suppl 2):58–69.
20. Aisen AM, McCune WJ, MacGuire A, Carson PL, Silver TM, Jafri SZ, et al. Sonographic evaluation of the cartilage of the knee. Radiology. 1984; 153:781–4.
21. Altman DG, Bland JM. Diagnostic tests 2: predictive values. BMJ. 1994; 309:102.
22. Kundel HL, Polansky M. Measurement of observer agreement. Radiology. 2003;228:303–8.
23. Jiang F, Xu B, Zhang XS, Wang L, Wen CJ. Feasibility of the femoral condylar cartilage ultrasound imaging. Acta Univ Med Anhui. 2003;38:144–6.
24. Outerbridge RE. The etiology of chondromalacia patellae. J Bone Joint Surg Br. 1961;43-B:752–7.
25. Goodfellow J, Hungerford DS, Zindel M. Patello-femoral joint mechanics and pathology. 1. Functional anatomy of the patello-femoral joint. J Bone Joint Surg Br. 1976;58:287–90.
26. Roemer FW, Crema MD, Trattnig S, Guermazi A. Advances in imaging of osteoarthritis and cartilage. Radiology. 2011;260:332–54.
27. Ostergaard M, Court-Payen M, Gideon P, Wieslander S, Cortsen M, Lorenzen I, et al. Ultrasonography in arthritis of the knee. A comparison with MR imaging. Acta Radiol. 1995;36:19–26.
28. Tarhan S, Unlu Z. Magnetic resonance imaging and ultrasonographic evaluation of the patients with knee osteoarthritis: a comparative study. Clin Rheumatol. 2003;22:181–8.
29. Cicuttini FM, Wluka AE, Stuckey SL. Tibial and femoral cartilage changes in knee osteoarthritis. Ann Rheum Dis. 2001;60:977–80.
30. Kim HK, Babyn PS, Harasiewicz KA, Gahunia HK, Pritzker KP, Foster FS. Imaging of immature articular cartilage using ultrasound backscatter microscopy at 50 MHz. J Orthop Res. 1995;13:963–70.
31. Roemer FW, van Holsbeeck M, Genant HK. Musculoskeletal ultrasound in rheumatology: a radiologic perspective. Arthritis Rheum. 2005;53:491–3.
32. Kijowski R, Blankenbaker DG, Davis KW, Shinki K, Kaplan LD, De Smet AA. Comparison of 1.5- and 3.0-T MR imaging for evaluating the articular cartilage of the knee joint. Radiology. 2009;250:839–48.
33. Kijowski R, Blankenbaker DG, Woods MA, Shinki K, De Smet AA, Reeder SB. 3.0-T evaluation of knee cartilage by using three-dimensional IDEAL GRASS imaging: comparison with fast spin-echo imaging. Radiology. 2010;255:117–27.
34. Duc SR, Pfirrmann CW, Schmid MR, Zanetti M, Koch PP, Kalberer F, et al. Articular cartilage defects detected with 3D water-excitation true FISP: prospective comparison with sequences commonly used for knee imaging. Radiology. 2007;245:216–23.
35. Disler DG, McCauley TR, Wirth CR, Fuchs MD. Detection of knee hyaline cartilage defects using fat-suppressed three-dimensional spoiled gradient-echo MR imaging: comparison with standard MR imaging and correlation with arthroscopy. AJR Am J Roentgenol. 1995;165:377–82.
36. Eckstein F, Hudelmaier M, Wirth W, Kiefer B, Jackson R, Yu J, et al. Double echo steady state magnetic resonance imaging of knee articular cartilage at 3 Tesla: a pilot study for the osteoarthritis initiative. Ann Rheum Dis. 2006; 65:433–41.

14

Transforaminal endoscopic discectomy versus conventional microdiscectomy for lumbar discherniation: a systematic review and meta-analysis

Bin Zhang[1†], Shen Liu[1†], Jun Liu[1,2†], Bingbing Yu[1], Wei Guo[1], Yongjin Li[1], Yang Liu[1], Wendong Ruan[1], Guangzhi Ning[1] and Shiqing Feng[1*]

Abstract

Background: The open microdiscectomy is the most common surgical procedure for the decompression of radiculopathy caused by lumbar disk herniation. To date, a variety of minimally invasive (MI) techniques have been developed. In the last decades, endoscopic techniques have been developed to perform discectomy. The transforaminal endoscopic discectomy (TED) with posterolateral access evolved out of the development of endoscopic techniques.

Methods: A systematic literature search was performed using the PubMed, EMBASE, and Cochrane Library databases for trials written in English. The randomized trials and observational studies that met our inclusion criteria were subsequently included. Two reviewers respectively extracted data and estimated the risk of bias. All statistical analyses were performed using Review Manager 5.3.

Results: Five prospective and four retrospective studies involving 1527 patients were included. The results of the meta-analysis indicated that there were significant differences between the two groups in length of hospital stay (MD = − 8.41, 95% CI − 10.26, − 6.56; p value < 0.00001). However, there were no significant differences in the leg visual analog scale (VAS) scores, the Oswestry Disability Index (ODI) scores, and the incidence of complications and recurrence.

Conclusions: The transforaminal endoscopic discectomy is superior to open microdiscectomy in the length of hospital stay. However, there were no differences in leg pain, functional recovery, and incidence of complications between TED and MD in treating LDH.

Keywords: Transforaminal endoscopic discectomy, Conventional microdiscectomy, Meta-analysis

Background

Lumbar disk herniation (LDH) is a common medical condition with a pathological process that leads to spinal surgery. The fibrous ring of an intervertebral disk is fractured and allows the soft central portion, the nucleus pulposus, to bulge out beyond the damaged fibrous rings. LDH is considered to be the most prevalent spinal disk herniation and always causes a series of signs and symptoms. One of the most challenging medical problems is sciatica symptoms. Sciatica affects millions of individuals worldwide [1]. The nerve root compression caused by the bulge of the nucleus pulposus and the secondary inflammatory reaction represent two crucial factors that result in lumbosacral radicular syndrome [2]. With the aggravation of LDH, incontinence may develop [3].

Currently, early conservative treatment is used when the symptoms are not serious. However, surgery is adopted

* Correspondence: sqfeng@tmu.edu.cn
†Bin Zhang, Shen Liu and Jun Liu contributed equally to this work.
[1]Department of Orthopedics, Tianjin Medical University General Hospital, No. 154 Anshan Road, Heping District, Tianjin 300052, People's Republic of China
Full list of author information is available at the end of the article

when conservative treatment fails, or complaints worsen over time [4, 5]. In 1934, lumbar disk herniation was the first condition treated surgically by performing an open laminectomy and discectomy [6]. With the introduction of the microscope, the open lumbar discectomy was refined into open microdiscectomy (MD) [7]. Currently, the open microdiscectomy is the most common surgical procedure for decompression of radiculopathy caused by lumbar disk herniation [8]. Since then, a variety of minimally invasive (MI) techniques have been developed. The minimally invasive techniques provide a similar view with a small incision and better cosmetic results [9, 10]. In the last decades, endoscopic techniques have been developed to perform discectomy under direct view and local anesthesia. The transforaminal endoscopic discectomy (TED) with posterolateral access evolved out of the development of endoscopic techniques [11–15]. The lateral access of transforaminal endoscopic discectomy to the spinal canal under continuous visualization has been developed since the late 1990s [16].

The indications for transforaminal endoscopic treatment are similar to classical open microdiscectomy procedures [17, 18]. However, a controversy remains over whether TED or MD should be utilized in clinical practice. It is therefore necessary to compare the clinical efficacies of different procedures to generate data that can be used to formulate clinical guidelines. Our goal was to systematically review, grade, and perform a meta-analysis of existing comparative studies. In this review, we compared the safety and efficacy of TED and MD for treating LDH patients.

Methods

Study design

The standards set by the Preferred Reporting Items for Systematic Reviews and Meta-Analyses (PRISMA) guidelines were used to construct this systematic review. The 27-item checklist and 4-phase flow diagram of PRISMA were both consulted.

Literature search

The PubMed, EMBASE, and Cochrane Library databases were searched up to January 2017 to identify studies comparing transforaminal endoscopic discectomy with microdiscectomy for the treatment of lumbar disk herniation. The search terms included "transforaminal endoscopic discectomy," "microdiscectomy," "endoscopic," "minimally invasive," and "lumbar disk herniation."

References from each article directly comparing the two kinds of surgeries, in addition to review articles discussing the safety and efficacy of the two procedures, were cross-referenced to identify additional relevant studies.

Inclusion and exclusion criteria

For inclusion in the systematic review, the articles were required to meet the following eligibility criteria: (1) patients suffering from lumbar disk herniation; (2) papers reporting the results of clinical studies evaluating transforaminal endoscopic discectomy and microdiscectomy; (3) patients followed for a minimum of 2 weeks; and (4) papers published in English prior to January 2017. Randomized controlled trials (RCTs) were identified as the primary studies for analysis. For inclusion in statistical analysis, the patients in a particular study must have been randomized to either TED or MD groups. Studies were excluded from the analysis if they included patients who had an infection, traumatic fracture, previous spinal surgery at the same disk level, and spinal stenosis among other conditions. The inclusion criteria for each study are listed in Table 1.

Table 1 Summary of study criteria—prospective studies and retrospective studies

Study	Study type	Sample size	Av. age	Mean duration of follow-up (months)	Gender (M/F)	Level
Hermantin et al. [20]	RCT	60	39 vs. 40	31(19–42) vs. 32(21–42)	22:8/17:13	L2-L3L3-L4L4-L5L5-S1
Mayer and Brock [21]	RCT	40	39.8 ± 10.4 vs. 42.7 ± 10	6.9	12:8/14:6	L2-L3L3-L4L4-L5
Ruetten et al. [10]	RCT	129	43	24	–	L1-L2L2-L3L3-L4L4-L5L5-S1
Gibson et al. [22]	RCT	140	42.0 ± 9 vs. 39 ± 9	24	30:40/40:30	L3-L4L4-L5L5-S1
Akçakaya et al. [27]	RCT	30	44.1	–	–	–
Kim et al. [23]	Retro	902	34.9 vs. 44.4	23.6	188:107/ 392:215	L1-L2L2-L3L3-L4L4-L5L5-S1
Lee et al. [24]	Retro	60	39.3 vs. 39.6	38.2(32–45) vs. 36.8(35–42)	22: 8/22: 8	L4-L5L5-S1
Ahn et al. [25]	Retro	66	22.41 ± 1.68 vs. 22.18 ± 1.51	13.69 + 1.26 vs. 13.41 + 1.02	32:0/34:0	L4-L5
Hsu et al. [26]	Retro	100	–	20.4	–	L1-L2L2-L3L3-L4L4-L5

Risk of bias

The risk of bias of the Cochrane Handbook for Systematic Reviews of Interventions was evaluated by using the risk of bias tool implemented in Review Manager 5.3. The included RCTs were evaluated for the risk of bias, which included assessments of adequate sequence generation, allocation of concealment, blinding, incomplete outcome data, and freedom from other biases. The judgment of each entry involved assessing the risk of bias as "low risk," "high risk," or "unclear risk," indicating either a lack of information or uncertainty over the potential for bias. Two reviewers independently assessed each RCT, and any disagreements were resolved by discussion and consensus.

Data extraction

Two authors independently extracted the following data. Any disagreements were resolved via discussion among the three reviewers. The data extracted from the studies included the following: study characteristics, types of interventions, follow-up duration, and outcome parameters.

Outcome measures

The "degree of pain relief" (visual or verbal analog pain scale (VAS) score) and the functional improvement (Oswestry Disability Index (ODI)) were the primary outcome measures of the effectiveness of the surgeries. The secondary outcome measures were average duration of surgery, complications, hospital stay, recurrence, and satisfactory outcome.

Statistical analysis

The data were collected and analyzed using Review Manager 5.3. Differences in pain, functional improvement, average duration of surgery, and hospital stay between the TED and MD groups were analyzed using the independent samples t test under a random-effects model. Risk ratios (RRs) and 95% confidence intervals (CIs) were used to evaluate the dichotomous outcomes, such as the incidence of complications. The differences are displayed using a forest plot. The I^2 statistic [19] (ranging from 0 to 100%) was applied to quantify between-study heterogeneity that was not attributed to chance ($I^2 = 0$–25%, no heterogeneity; $I^2 = 25$–50%, moderate heterogeneity; $I^2 = 50$–75%, large heterogeneity; and $I^2 = 75$–100%, extreme heterogeneity). A p value < 0.05 was considered statistically significant.

Results

Literature search

A total of 2397 records were identified through the PubMed, EMBASE, and the Cochrane Library database. Following the exclusion of 369 duplicate items, 2381 articles were screened for review, and 42 that met the inclusion criteria were selected. A total of 33 full-text articles were excluded due to either the absence of a comparison between transforaminal endoscopic discectomy and conventional microdiscectomy or the absence of an appropriate statistical analysis. Nine studies [10, 20–27] were ultimately included in the meta-analysis (Fig. 1).

Risk of bias in included studies

We used the risk of bias tool implemented in Review Manager 5.3 to evaluate the risk of bias of the Cochrane Handbook for Systematic Reviews of Interventions. The particular information of the risk of bias of the included articles is demonstrated in Fig. 2. Four [10, 20–22] of five studies comprehensively

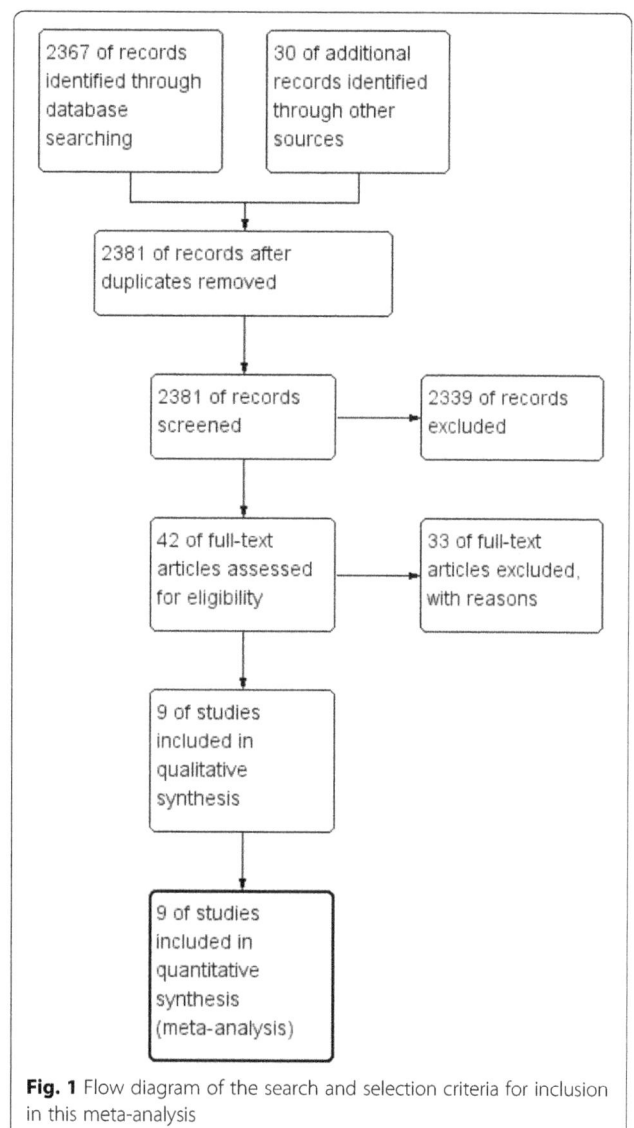

Fig. 1 Flow diagram of the search and selection criteria for inclusion in this meta-analysis

described the generation of a randomized sequence. The patients were not blinded to the treatment allocation in one study [10], which consisted of four indistinct studies [20–22, 27]. One article [27] displayed a high risk of bias for the incomplete outcomes. The rest of the included articles displayed a low risk of bias for the incomplete outcomes, selective outcome reporting, and other biases.

Demographics of the studies included in the review

Five [10, 20–22, 27] of the nine studies were prospective studies, and four [24–26, 28, 29] were retrospective studies. These studies included 1527 patients, 399 of whom were included in the prospective studies, and 1128 of whom were included in the retrospective studies. Statistical analysis was performed in the five prospective studies and four retrospective studies. Differences in age, gender, and level were noted; however, these differences were not statistically significant. Follow-up periods ranged from 6.9 to 24 months in duration (Table 1).

Outcome analyses: leg pain

VAS scores were available in two of the RCT studies. Mayer and Brock [21] show that the VAS scores were 8.23 ± 1.3 and 7.67 ± 1.9 in the TED and MD groups at 2 years postoperation, respectively. Both groups showed a significant difference between preoperative and postoperative scores. Gibson et al. [22] showed that the VAS scores were 1.9 ± 2.6 and 3.5 ± 3.1 in the TED and MD groups at 2 years postoperation, respectively. Meta-analyses were performed in these two studies. Although the heterogeneity was high (I^2 up to 89%), slightly better leg pain relief was observed in the TED group at 2 years and no differences were noted after 2 years of follow-up (Fig. 3a).

Two retrospective studies [25, 26] reported VAS scores (Fig. 3b). Meta-analyses were also performed in these two studies. Although the I^2 was low, the credibility was not high. Similar outcomes were reported in these two retrospective studies compared to the RCT studies. No significant differences were observed between the TED and MD groups (SMD = -0.13, 95% CI -0.58, 0.33; $p = 0.58$).

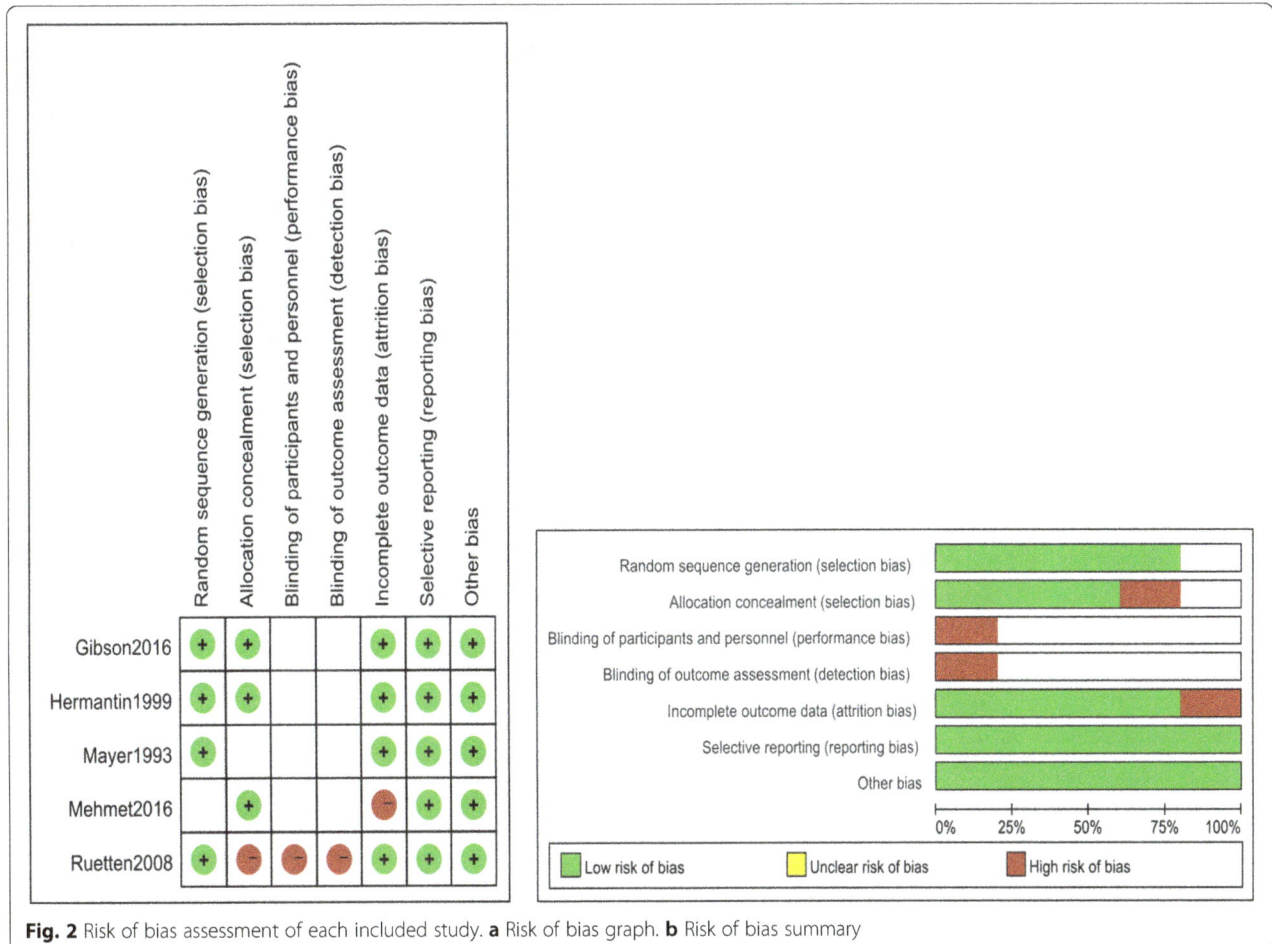

Fig. 2 Risk of bias assessment of each included study. **a** Risk of bias graph. **b** Risk of bias summary

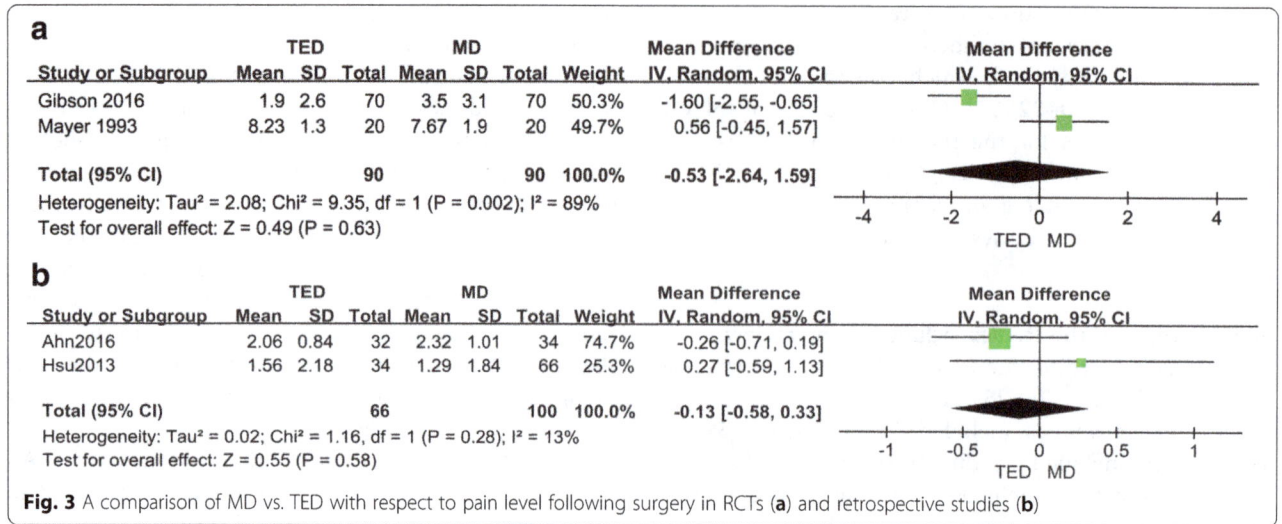

Fig. 3 A comparison of MD vs. TED with respect to pain level following surgery in RCTs (**a**) and retrospective studies (**b**)

Outcome analyses: functional recovery

Function was measured using an ODI. Only two retrospective studies [25, 26, 28] had reported the ODI scores. Ahn et al. [25] reported that the ODI scores were 9.63 ± 2.31 and 10.68 ± 2.67 in the TED and MD groups, respectively. Hsu et al. [26] reported that the ODI was 6.42 ± 9.82 and 3.29 ± 6.94 in the TED and MD groups, respectively. There were no significant differences between the TED and MD groups (Fig. 4).

Operative time

The average duration of surgery was available in two of the RCT studies. Mayer and Brock [21] showed that the operative time was 40.7 ± 11.3 and 58.2 ± 15.2 min in the TED and MD groups, respectively. Gibson et al. [22] showed that the VAS scores were 28 ± 11 and 29 ± 12 min in the TED and MD groups, respectively. Meta-analyses were performed in these two studies. Although a shorter operative time was observed in the TED group, there were no significant differences between the two groups (Fig. 5).

Stay in hospital

Only two retrospective studies [24, 25] reported hospital stay (Fig. 6). Meta-analyses were performed in these two

studies. Both studies reported a shorter hospital stay in the TED group vs. the MD group. The time was 19.5 ± 30.12 vs. 71.96 ± 60.05 and 7.5 ± 2.63 vs. 15.65 ± 4.8 h, respectively. The differences between the TED and MD groups was statistically significant (MD = -8.41, 95% CI $-10.26, -6.56$; $p < 0.00001$).

Complications

Both the RCT and retrospective studies recorded the postoperative complications (Fig. 7a). The conditions related to the complications were available in three of the RCT studies [10, 20, 22]. There were no complications reported in the articles of Hermantin et al. [20] and Gibson et al. [22]. No complications were reported in the TED group, but four complications and three complications were reported in the MD group [10, 22]. No significant differences were reported between the TED and MD groups (RR = 0.23, 95% CI 0.01, 4.13; $p = 0.32$).

Three retrospective studies [23, 25, 26] reported complications (Fig. 7b). Meta-analyses were also performed in these three studies. Similar outcomes were reported in these three retrospective studies compared to the RCT studies. However, the rate of complications was slightly higher in the MD group; differences between the TED and MD groups were not statistically significant.

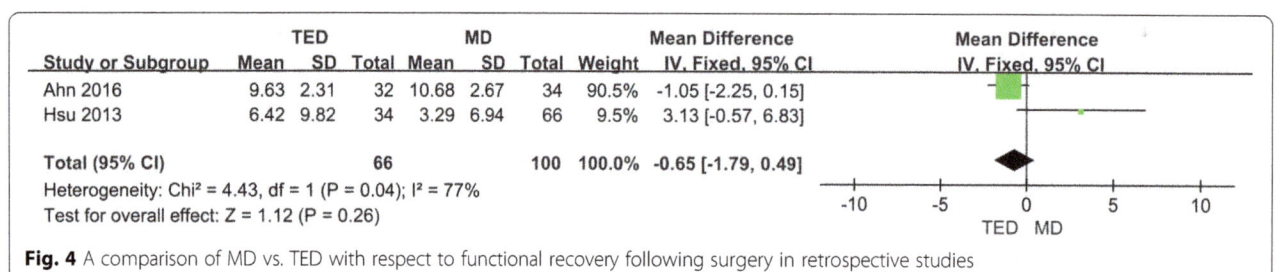

Fig. 4 A comparison of MD vs. TED with respect to functional recovery following surgery in retrospective studies

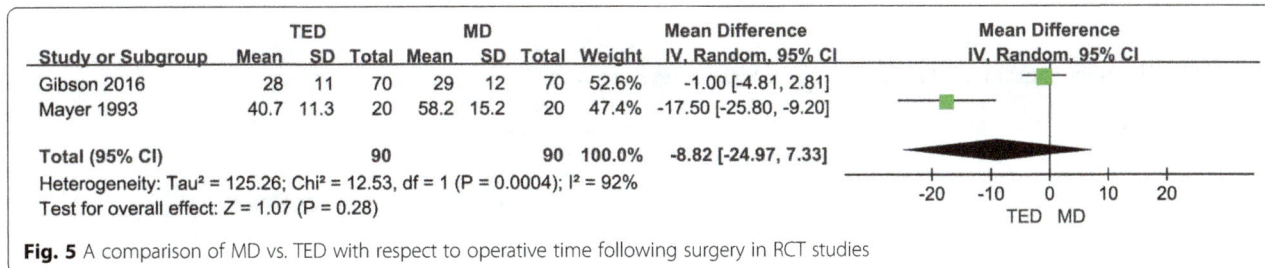

Fig. 5 A comparison of MD vs. TED with respect to operative time following surgery in RCT studies

Rate of recurrence

The recurrence was recorded in three of the RCT studies [10, 21, 22]. All the RCT studies reported a higher rate of recurrence in the TED group. No significant differences were observed between the TED and MD groups (RR = 1.77, 95% CI 0.66, 4.8; p = 0.26) (Fig. 8a).

Four retrospective studies [23–26] reported recurrence. Similar outcomes were observed in these four retrospective studies compared to the RCT studies. A higher rate of recurrence was observed in the TED group, and the difference between the TED and MD groups was statistically significant (RR = 1.65, 95% CI 1.08, 2.53; p = 0.02) (Fig. 8b).

Discussion

Lumbar open microdiscectomy is a popular procedure for the surgical treatment of lumbar disk herniation [28]. However, the open microdiscectomy surgery often requires a large incision to provide optimal vision. During the surgery, the paravertebral muscles are retracted, and the spinal lamina and facet joint are removed. This surgery can cause scarring and instability of the spine, which causes clinical symptoms in 10% or more of patients [29]. The transforaminal endoscopic discectomy was developed in the 1990s. Compared to the open microdiscectomy, it has several advantages. The TED can be performed under local anesthesia; thus, the rate of anesthesia-associated complications is low. The risk of scar formation and instability of the spine is also decreased [30–33]. A review [34] of the comparisons between TED and MD showed that TED was strongly favored. It is therefore necessary to compare the clinical efficacies of the different procedures to generate data that help surgeons make clinical decisions and develop optimal treatments.

We summarized the results of studies comparing transforaminal endoscopic discectomy and open microdiscectomy and performed a meta-analysis to compare the effectiveness and safety of these two surgeries for treating lumbar disk herniation. We analyzed the effectiveness of these two procedures by evaluating improvements in patients' pain, functional scores, average duration of surgery, and hospital stay. We also analyzed the safety of these two procedures by evaluating complications and recurrence of LDH. We included five prospective studies and four retrospective studies involving 1527 patients in our analysis (Table 2).

No significant difference in both leg pain and function recovery was observed between TED and MD. Both RCTs and retrospective studies support the evidence that the transmuscular approach to the transforaminal endoscopic discectomy is as effective as the conventional open microdiscectomy requiring paravertebral muscle retraction. It can be explained that the clinical symptoms were caused by the decompression of the nerve root due to the herniated disk [35]. Both surgical procedures can remove nerve compression. However, several studies [36] suggested that clinical outcomes were associated with paravertebral muscle injury. Additionally, some factors such as different sampling dates, different peri- and intraoperative procedures, and different surgeons may have influenced the clinical outcomes.

The results in operative times and length of hospital stay were difficult to interpret. Although the operative times of the TED group was slightly shorter than the MD group, no significant difference was observed between TED and MD groups. The differences in how operative time was defined are important. Whether the anesthesia time was considered into the operative time,

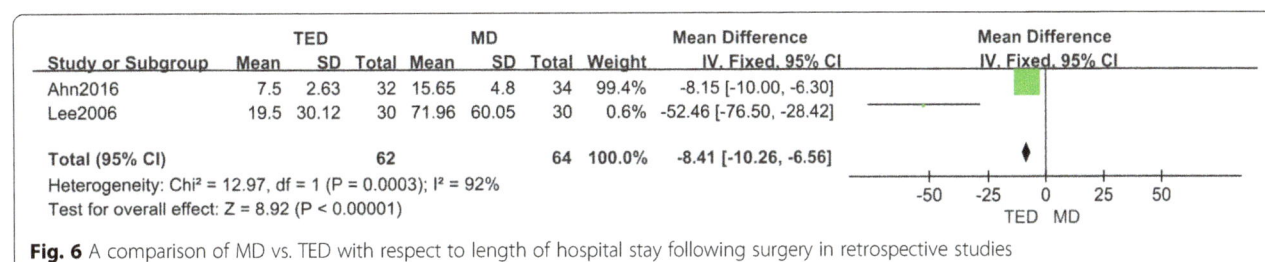

Fig. 6 A comparison of MD vs. TED with respect to length of hospital stay following surgery in retrospective studies

a

Study or Subgroup	TED Events	Total	MD Events	Total	Weight	Risk Ratio M-H, Random, 95% CI
Gibson2016	0	70	0	70		Not estimable
Hermantin1999	0	30	0	30		Not estimable
Ruetten2008	0	42	4	87	100.0%	0.23 [0.01, 4.13]
Total (95% CI)		**142**		**187**	**100.0%**	**0.23 [0.01, 4.13]**
Total events	0		4			

Heterogeneity: Not applicable
Test for overall effect: Z = 1.00 (P = 0.32)

b

Study or Subgroup	TED Events	Total	MD Events	Total	Weight	Risk Ratio M-H, Random, 95% CI
Ahn2016	4	32	4	34	72.0%	1.06 [0.29, 3.90]
Hsu2013	1	34	1	66	16.2%	1.94 [0.13, 30.09]
Kim 2007	0	295	1	607	11.9%	0.68 [0.03, 16.76]
Total (95% CI)		**361**		**707**	**100.0%**	**1.11 [0.37, 3.35]**
Total events	5		6			

Heterogeneity: Tau² = 0.00; Chi² = 0.25, df = 2 (P = 0.88); I² = 0%
Test for overall effect: Z = 0.19 (P = 0.85)

Fig. 7 A comparison of MD vs. TED with respect to complications following surgery in RCTs (**a**) and retrospective studies (**b**)

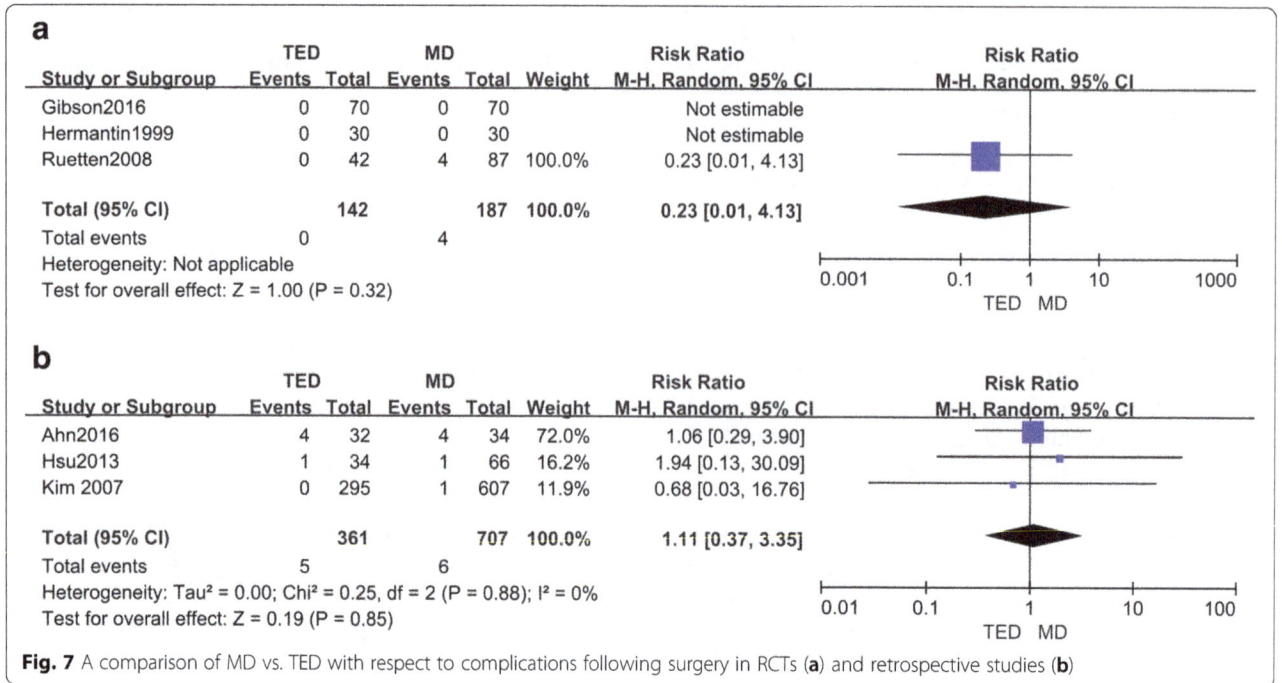

it had a large influence on operative time. Moreover, the variability in the techniques used was also a factor [37]. The length of hospital stay was much shorter in the TED group compared to that in the MD group. Transforaminal endoscopic discectomy may be associated with less muscle damage, among other outcomes [38], which allows the early recovery of patients. Additionally, economic factors should be considered.

In this meta-analysis, no significant difference in rates of total complications was observed between the two groups. Some studies [25, 26] suggested that the TED approach would be associated with a higher rate of complications. A limited surgical exposure leads to difficulty in surgery, and therefore, it is easier to cause nerve damage and other complications [39]. However, other research suggests the opposite because the small incision

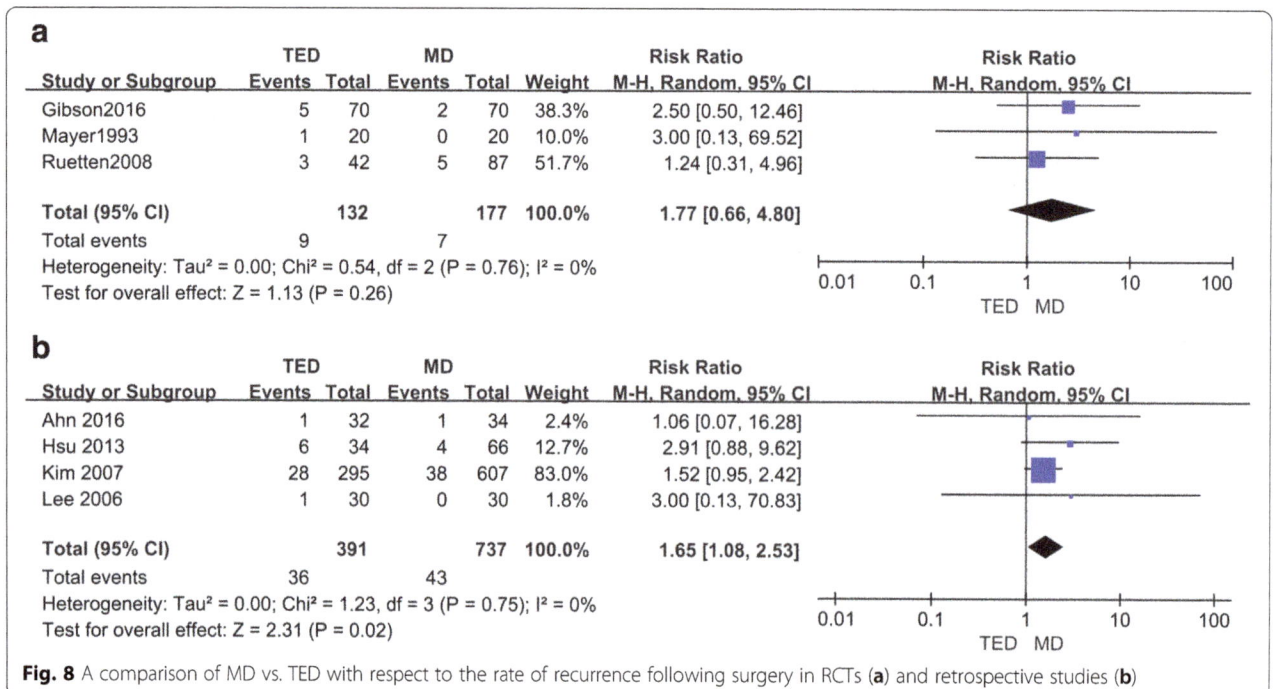

a

Study or Subgroup	TED Events	Total	MD Events	Total	Weight	Risk Ratio M-H, Random, 95% CI
Gibson2016	5	70	2	70	38.3%	2.50 [0.50, 12.46]
Mayer1993	1	20	0	20	10.0%	3.00 [0.13, 69.52]
Ruetten2008	3	42	5	87	51.7%	1.24 [0.31, 4.96]
Total (95% CI)		**132**		**177**	**100.0%**	**1.77 [0.66, 4.80]**
Total events	9		7			

Heterogeneity: Tau² = 0.00; Chi² = 0.54, df = 2 (P = 0.76); I² = 0%
Test for overall effect: Z = 1.13 (P = 0.26)

b

Study or Subgroup	TED Events	Total	MD Events	Total	Weight	Risk Ratio M-H, Random, 95% CI
Ahn 2016	1	32	1	34	2.4%	1.06 [0.07, 16.28]
Hsu 2013	6	34	4	66	12.7%	2.91 [0.88, 9.62]
Kim 2007	28	295	38	607	83.0%	1.52 [0.95, 2.42]
Lee 2006	1	30	0	30	1.8%	3.00 [0.13, 70.83]
Total (95% CI)		**391**		**737**	**100.0%**	**1.65 [1.08, 2.53]**
Total events	36		43			

Heterogeneity: Tau² = 0.00; Chi² = 1.23, df = 3 (P = 0.75); I² = 0%
Test for overall effect: Z = 2.31 (P = 0.02)

Fig. 8 A comparison of MD vs. TED with respect to the rate of recurrence following surgery in RCTs (**a**) and retrospective studies (**b**)

Table 2 Summary of information of the prospective studies and retrospective studies

Study	Low-back pain	Leg pain	ODI	Recurrence	Hospital stay	Complications	Average duration of surgery (min)
Hermantin et al. [20]	–	1.2 vs. 1.9	–	–	–	0 vs. 0	–
Mayer and Brock [21]	10/19 vs. 15/20	8.23 ± 1.3 vs. 7.67 ± 1.9	–	1/20 vs. 0/20	–	–	40.7 ± 11.3 vs. 58.2 ± 15.2
Ruetten et al. [10]	–	–	–	3 vs. 5	–	0 vs. 4	–
Gibson et al. [22]	2.50 ± 2.5 vs. 3.0 ± 2.8	1.9 ± 2.6 vs. 3.5 ± 3.1	18 ± 17 vs. 22 ± 20	5 vs. 2	0.7 ± 0.7 vs. 1.4 ± 1.3 days	0 vs. 0	28 ± 11 vs. 29 ± 12
Mehmet [27]	–	–	–	–	1.13 vs. 1.2 days	–	94 vs. 71
Kim et al. [23]	–	–	–	28/295 vs. 38/607	–	0 vs. 1	–
Lee et al. [24]	–	–	–	1 vs. 0	19.5 ± 30.12 vs. 71.9 ± 60.05 h	–	42.6 ± 14.21 vs. 65.1 ± 23.17
Ahn et al. [25]	2.50 ± 0.62 vs. 2.91 ± 0.67	2.06 ± 0.84 vs. 2.32 ± 1.01	9.63 ± 2.31 vs. 10.68 ± 2.67	1 vs. 1	7.50 ± 2.63 vs. 15.65 ± 4.80 h	4 vs. 4	48.66 ± 6.45 vs. 53.71 ± 8.49
Hsu et al. [26]		1.56 ± 2.18 vs. 1.29 ± 1.84	6.42 ± 9.82 vs. 3.29 ± 6.94	6 vs. 4		1 vs. 1	86.5 ± 45.9 vs. 48.1 ± 9.2

and minimal internal tissue damage make it possible for a shorter recovery period and minimization of scar tissue [40, 41]. No significant difference in rates of recurrence was observed between the two groups.

One limitation of this study was the small number of RCTs. Although five RCTs were included in this article, different outcomes could only be extracted from a few studies. It made assessing the effectiveness and safety of the interventions on the different surgical approaches difficult. Another limitation of this review was that clinical heterogeneity, which cannot be resolved completely, may be associated with inconsistency of outcomes.

Conclusions

Our study demonstrated that transforaminal endoscopic discectomy was superior to open microdiscectomy in the length of hospital stay. However, there was no difference in leg pain, functional recovery, and incidence of complications between TED and MD in treating LDH. Prior to selecting a surgical procedure for the management of LDH, the benefits and risks of the procedure discussed herein must be taken into consideration. Additional studies must be performed to guide the clinical decision-making process.

Abbreviations
LDH: Lumbar disk herniation; MD: Microdiscectomy; MI: Minimally invasive; PRISMA: Preferred Reporting Items for Systematic Reviews and Meta-Analyses; SMD: Standardized mean differences; TED: Transforaminal endoscopic discectomy

Acknowledgements
The authors are grateful to the participants and researchers of the primary studies identified for the present review. They would like to thank the editorial board of *Journal of Orthopaedic Surgery and Research* for the review and critique, which aided in improving the manuscript. The authors alone are responsible for the views expressed, which are not necessarily reflected by any institution.

Funding
This work was supported by the National Natural Science Foundation of China (81501899); the State Key Program of the National Natural Science Foundation of China (81330042); the Special Program for Sino-Russian Joint Research Sponsored by the Ministry of Science and Technology, China (2014DFR31210); the Key Program Sponsored by the Tianjin Science and Technology Committee, China (13RCGFSY19000, 14ZCZDSY00044); the Science Foundation of Tianjin Medical University for Young Scholar (2014KYQ01); and the Science Foundation of Tianjin Medical University General Hospital for Young Scholar (ZYYFY2014037).

Authors' contributions
BZ and SL conceived the study design. JL and BBY performed the study, collected the data, and contributed to the study design. BZ and LJ prepared the manuscript. SQF and SL edited the manuscript. All authors read and approved the final manuscript.

Competing interests
The authors declare that they have no competing interests.

Author details
[1]Department of Orthopedics, Tianjin Medical University General Hospital, No. 154 Anshan Road, Heping District, Tianjin 300052, People's Republic of China. [2]Department of Orthopedics, First Affiliated Hospital of Gannan Medical University General Hospital, No. 23 Qingnian Road, Zhanggong District, Ganzhou 341000, People's Republic of China.

References

1. Konstantinou K, Dunn KM. Sciatica: review of epidemiological studies and prevalence estimates. Spine. 2008;33:2464–72.

2. Boonstra AM, Preuper HRS, Reneman MF, Posthumus JB, Stewart RE. Reliability and validity of the visual analogue scale for disability in patients with chronic musculoskeletal pain. Int J Rehabil Res. 2008;31:165–9.

3. Ma D, Liang Y, Wang D, Liu Z, Zhang W, Ma T, et al. Trend of the incidence of lumbar disc herniation: decreasing with aging in the elderly. Clin Interv Aging. 2013;8:1047–50.

4. Lequin MB, Verbaan D, Jacobs WC, Brand R, Bouma GJ, Vandertop WP, et al. Surgery versus prolonged conservative treatment for sciatica: 5-year results of a randomised controlled trial. BMJ Open. 2013;3:13–7.

5. Awad JN, Moskovich R. Lumbar disc herniations: surgical versus nonsurgical treatment. Clin Orthop Relat Res. 2006;443:183–97.

6. Mixter W, Barr J. Rupture of the intervertebral disc with involvement of the spinal canal. N Engl J Med. 1934;211:210–5.

7. Caspar W. A new surgical procedure for lumbar disc herniation causing less tissue damage through a microsurgical approach. In: Wüllenweber R, Brock M, Hamer J, Klinger M, Spoerri O, editors. Lumbar disc adult hydrocephalus. Berlin, Heidelberg: Springer; 1977. p. 74–80.

8. Koebbe CJ, Maroon JC, Abla A, El-Kadi H, Bost J. Lumbar microdiscectomy: a historical perspective and current technical considerations. Neurosurg Focus. 2002;13:E3.

9. Ruetten S, Komp M, Merk H, Godolias G. Use of newly developed instruments and endoscopes: full-endoscopic resection of lumbar disc herniations via the interlaminar and lateral transforaminal approach. J Neurosurg Spine. 2007;6:521–30.

10. Ruetten S, Komp M, Merk H, Godolias G. Full-endoscopic interlaminar and transforaminal lumbar discectomy versus conventional microsurgical technique: a prospective, randomized, controlled study. Spine. 2008;33:931–9.

11. Deen HG. Posterolateral endoscopic excision for lumbar disc herniation: surgical technique, outcome, and complications in 307 consecutive cases. Spine. 2002;27:2081–2.

12. Tsou PM, Yeung AT. Transforaminal endoscopic decompression for radiculopathy secondary to intracanal noncontained lumbar disc herniations: outcome and technique. Spine J. 2002;2:41–8.

13. Mathews HH. Transforaminal endoscopic microdiscectomy. Neurosurg Clin N Am. 1996;7:59–63.

14. Lew SM, Mehalic TF, Fagone KL. Transforaminal percutaneous endoscopic discectomy in the treatment of far-lateral and foraminal lumbar disc herniations. J Neurosurg. 2001;94:216–20.

15. Kambin P, Casey K, O'Brien E, Zhou L. Transforaminal arthroscopic decompression of lateral recess stenosis. J Neurosurg. 1996;84:462–7.

16. Ruetten S, Komp M, Godolias G. An extreme lateral access for the surgery of lumbar disc herniations inside the spinal canal using the full-endoscopic uniportal transforaminal approach-technique and prospective results of 463 patients. Spine. 2005;30:2570–8.

17. Choi G, Lee SH, Bhanot A, Raiturker PP, Chae YS. Percutaneous endoscopic discectomy for extraforaminal lumbar disc herniations: extraforaminal targeted fragmentectomy technique using working channel endoscope. Spine. 2007;32:E93–9.

18. Kambin P, O'Brien E, Zhou L, Schaffer JL. Arthroscopic microdiscectomy and selective fragmentectomy. Clin Orthop Relat Res. 1998;347:150–67.

19. Higgins JP, Thompson SG. Quantifying heterogeneity in a meta-analysis. Stat Med. 2002;21:1539–58.

20. Hermantin FU, Peters T, Quartararo L, Kambin P. A prospective, randomized study comparing the results of open discectomy with those of video-assisted arthroscopic microdiscectomy. J Bone Joint Surg Am. 1999;81:958–65.

21. Mayer HM, Brock M. Percutaneous endoscopic discectomy: surgical technique and preliminary results compared to microsurgical discectomy. J Neurosurg. 1993;78:216–25.

22. Gibson JNA, Subramanian AS, Scott CEH. A randomised controlled trial of transforaminal endoscopic discectomy vs microdiscectomy. Eur Spine J. 2017;26:847–56.

23. Kim MJ, Lee SH, Jung ES, Son BG, Choi ES, Shin JH, et al. Targeted percutaneous transforaminal endoscopic diskectomy in 295 patients: comparison with results of microscopic diskectomy. Surg Neurol. 2007;68:623–31.

24. Lee SH, Chung SE, Ahn Y, Kim TH, Park JY, Shin SW. Comparative radiologic evaluation of percutaneous endoscopic lumbar discectomy and open microdiscectomy: a matched cohort analysis. Mt Sinai J Med. 2006;73:795–801.

25. Ahn SS, Kim SH, Kim DW, Lee BH. Comparison of outcomes of percutaneous endoscopic lumbar discectomy and open lumbar microdiscectomy for young adults: a retrospective matched cohort study. World Neurosurg. 2016;86:250–8.

26. Hsu HT, Chang SJ, Yang SS, Chai CL. Learning curve of full-endoscopic lumbar discectomy. Eur Spine J. 2013;22:727–33.

27. Akcakaya MO, Yorukoglu AG, Aydoseli A, Aras Y, Sabanci PA, Altunrende ME, et al. Serum creatine phosphokinase levels as an indicator of muscle injury following lumbar disc surgery: comparison of fully endoscopic discectomy and microdiscectomy. Clin Neurol Neurosurg. 2016;145:74–8.

28. Schizas C, Tsiridis E, Saksena J. Microendoscopic discectomy compared with standard microsurgical discectomy for treatment of uncontained or large contained disc herniations. Neurosurgery. 2005;57:357–60.

29. Fritsch EW, Heisel J, Rupp S. The failed back surgery syndrome: reasons, intraoperative findings, and long-term results: a report of 182 operative treatments. Spine. 1996;21:626–33.

30. Choi i, Ahn JO, So WS, Lee SJ, Choi IJ, Kim H. Exiting root injury in transforaminal endoscopic discectomy: preoperative image considerations for safety. Eur Spine J. 2013;22:2481–7.

31. Gempt J, Jonek M, Ringel F, Preuss A, Wolf P, Ryang Y. Long-term follow-up of standard microdiscectomy versus minimal access surgery for lumbar disc herniations. Acta Neurochir. 2013;155:2333–8.

32. Peng CW, Yeo W, Tan SB. Percutaneous endoscopic discectomy: clinical results and how it affects the quality of life. J Spinal Disord Tech. 2010;23:425–30.

33. Rahimi-Movaghar V, Rasouli M, Shokraneh F, Moradi-Lakeh M, Vakaro A, Sadeghi-Naini M. Minimally invasive discectomy versus microdiscectomy/discectomy for symptomatic lumbar disc herniation. J Inj Violence Res. 2012;4:61.

34. Gibson JN, Cowie JG, Iprenburg M. Transforaminal endoscopic spinal surgery: the future 'gold standard' for discectomy? A review. Surgeon. 2012;10:290–6.

35. Kamble PC, Sharma A, Singh V, Natraj B, Devani D, Khapane V. Outcome of single level disc prolapse treated with transforaminal steroid versus epidural steroid versus caudal steroids. Eur Spine J. 2016;25:217–21.

36. Kotil K, Tunckale T, Tatar Z, Koldas M, Kural A, Bilge T. Serum creatine phosphokinase activity and histological changes in the multifidus muscle: a prospective randomized controlled comparative study of discectomy with or without retraction. J Neurosurg Spine. 2007;6:121–5.

37. Lee DY, Lee SH. Learning curve for percutaneous endoscopic lumbar discectomy. Neurol Med Chir. 2008;48:383–8.

38. Songer MN, Ghosh L, Spencer DL. Effects of sodium hyaluronate on peridural fibrosis after lumbar laminotomy and discectomy. Spine. 1990;15:550–4.

39. Arts MP, Nieborg A, Brand R, Peul WC. Serum creatine phosphokinase as an indicator of muscle injury after various spinal and nonspinal surgical procedures. J Neurosurg Spine. 2007;7:282–6.

40. Knight MT, Ellison DR, Goswami A, Hillier VF. Review of safety in endoscopic laser foraminoplasty for the management of back pain. J Clin Laser Med Surg. 2001;19:147–57.

41. Knight MT, Goswami A, Patko JT, Buxton N. Endoscopic foraminoplasty: a prospective study on 250 consecutive patients with independent evaluation. J Clin Laser Med Surg. 2001;19:73–81.

15

Proximal third humeral shaft fractures fixed with long helical PHILOS plates in elderly patients: benefit of pre-contouring plates on a 3D-printed model—a retrospective study

Qiuke Wang[1†], Jian Hu[2†], Junjie Guan[1], Yunfeng Chen[1*] and Lei Wang[1*]

Abstract

Background: To explore the clinical efficacy of 3D printing fracture models to assist in creating pre-contoured plates to treat proximal third humeral shaft fractures.

Methods: We retrospectively identified proximal third humeral shaft fractures treated between February 2012 and February 2015. The patients were divided into two groups according to the treatment procedure: a Synbone group and a 3D-printed group. In the Synbone group, long proximal humeral internal locking system plates were pre-contoured into helical shape on Synbones before surgery, while in the 3D-printed group, they were contoured on 3D-printed bone models. The pre-contoured plates were sterilized before surgery and were then used for fracture fixation during surgery. Duration of surgeries, blood loss volumes, the incidence of complications, and the time to fracture union were recorded, and functional outcomes were assessed by the Constant-Murley shoulder score and the Mayo Elbow Performance Score (MEPS) at 1-year follow-up.

Results: The subjects comprised 46 patients; 25 patients were allocated to the Synbone group and the remaining 21 to the 3D-printed group. There was no significant difference between the baseline characteristics of the two groups. At the 1-year follow-up visit, all fractures were healed and showed a satisfactory outcome. There were no instances of iatrogenic radial nerve injury, and there was no significant difference between the two groups with regard to fracture union time, Constant-Murley score, or MEPS score. Surgery duration was significantly shorter in the 3D-printed group compared to the Synbone group (42.62 vs. 60.36 min, $P = 0.001$), and the 3D-printed group lost less blood during surgery (105.19 vs. 120.80 ml, $P = 0.001$). In addition, in the 3D-printed group, 9 surgeries were finished by senior attending doctors and 12 were finished by junior attending doctors; however, there was no significant difference between the 1-year outcomes of the two grades of surgeons.

Conclusions: Our results show that the 3D printing technique is helpful in shortening the duration of surgery, reducing blood loss volume, and in making this surgical procedure easier for less-experienced surgeons.

Keywords: Helical plate, Humeral fracture, 3D-printed, MIPO

* Correspondence: drchenyunfeng@sina.com; wanglei2264@126.com
†Qiuke Wang and Jian Hu contributed equally to this work.
[1]Department of Orthopedic Surgery, Shanghai Jiao Tong University Affiliated Sixth People's Hospital, 600 Yishan Road, Shanghai 200233, People's Republic of China
Full list of author information is available at the end of the article

Background

Humeral shaft fractures account for approximately 3% of all bone fractures [1–4], and for most of these, non-operative treatment with a functional brace is recommended. However, the non-union rate of fractures in the proximal third of the humerus is relatively higher than for those in other regions with conservative treatment, and shoulder stiffness problems tend to appear after long-term external fixation [2, 5–7]. Moreover, clinical studies have reported that approximately 49.3% of proximal third humeral shaft fractures extend into the humeral head, which is difficult to verify on X-ray and should be treated with stable fixation [6]. Thus, surgery should be considered as an alternative plan for proximal third humeral shaft fractures.

The helical plating technique was first reported to be used in cases of proximal third humeral shaft non-union in 1999 [8]. This technique was developed and successfully used to treat proximal humeral shaft fractures [9–14]. The helical-shaped design is mainly aimed at minimizing the risk of radial nerve injury, because the plate roughly parallels the nerve from the proximal to the distal humerus. The locking plate is twisted approximately 90° to lie on the lateral aspect of the greater tuberosity proximally and the anterior or anteromedial aspect of the humeral shaft distally, so theoretically, most of the deltoid muscle attachment can be preserved and the radial nerve should not be entrapped in the distal approach. With concerns about soft tissue compromise, the minimally invasive plate osteosynthesis (MIPO) technique is considered to be an essential component of this surgery. In order to fix the fractures in the proximal humerus and the proximal third of the shaft simultaneously, we recommend long helical proximal humeral internal locking system (PHILOS) plate (DePuy Synthes, Zuchwil, Switzerland) rather than normal metaphyseal locking plate, and its safety and efficacy have been proven in our previous study [11].

Although the outcomes of this novel technique are satisfactory, we found it difficult to pre-contour a PHILOS plate for personalized application. Even though we molded the plate on a Synbone (Synbone AG, Malans, Switzerland) before surgery, it was always necessary to adjust its shape during the operation, which wasted much time, especially in the case of elderly patients. Old patients, in whom fractures were likely to be combined with severe osteoporosis, in our country are more likely to have a much shorter humerus than the standard Synbone. Consequently, we considered that a personalized 3D-printed model would be helpful in producing a better matched long helical PHILOS plate before surgery.

The purpose of this study was to investigate the benefit of pre-contouring long helical PHILOS plates on 3D-printed models for the treatment of proximal third humeral shaft fractures in elderly patients. We hypothesized

that this individualized treatment plan would reduce the technical challenge, shorten the duration of surgery, and reduce blood loss volume.

Methods

Patients

We retrospectively identified patients, treated with long helical PHILOS plates between February 2012 and February 2015, from our trauma center's database. Inclusion criteria were (I) aged 65 years or above, (II) presence of proximal third humeral shaft fractures (unilateral), (III) treated by the MIPO technique with a long helical PHILOS plate, and (IV) more than 12 months follow-up after surgery with complete follow-up data. Exclusion criteria included pathological fractures, open fractures, multiple fractures, or the presence of other diseases affecting the same upper limb.

Ultimately, 46 patients were included, and data regarding their medical histories, functional evaluations, and regular radiographic examinations were collected. All fractures were classified according to the AO/ASIF classification system [15]. Medical history information included gender, age, and surgical information (plate pre-contoured on a Synbone or 3D-printed model, the name of the surgeon, duration of surgery, and blood loss volume during surgery).

3D-printed model and plate preparation

A bilateral humerus CT scan (1-mm layer interval) was taken from patients in the 3D-printed group, and CT data was extracted for constructing the 3D-printed model, using medical 3D processing software (Mimics 16.0, Materialise, Belgium). The scapula, clavicle, and relative soft tissue were separated. A mirror image of the intact side was used to simulate the other side, and the models were printed using a 3D-printing machine (Lite, RS6000, UnionTech, Shanghai, China) with ultraviolet rays (UV) curable resin material. Total preparation time of a 3D bone model was approximately 3 h as long as the CT data is available.

In the 3D-printed group, a long PHILOS plate was pre-contoured on an intact 3D-printed model, to ensure that it could be used on the fractured bone. In the Synbone group, the plate was pre-contoured on a standard Synbone model. The plate was twisted at approximately 60–90° (starting at the superior part of the humeral deltoid tuberosity), while the proximal part of the plate was located on the lateral side of the greater tubercle and the distal part on the anterior side of the distal humerus. Then, the contoured helical plate was sterilized on the day before the surgery. The 3D-printed models and the helical plate used in an elderly Asian female patient are shown in Fig. 1, and it is obvious that the true humerus is much shorter than the Synbone.

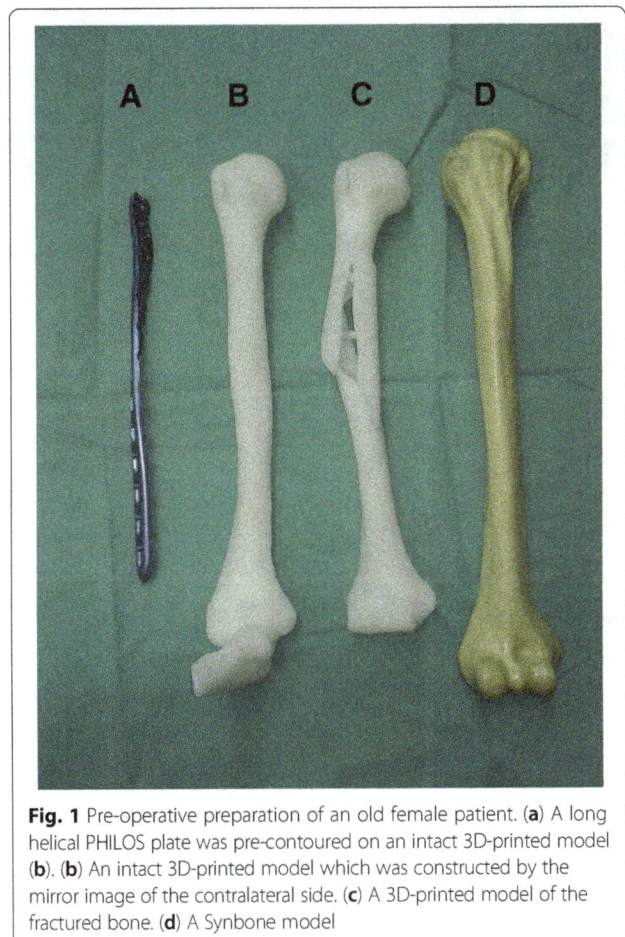

Fig. 1 Pre-operative preparation of an old female patient. (**a**) A long helical PHILOS plate was pre-contoured on an intact 3D-printed model (**b**). (**b**) An intact 3D-printed model which was constructed by the mirror image of the contralateral side. (**c**) A 3D-printed model of the fractured bone. (**d**) A Synbone model

Surgical procedure

The basic surgical steps were similar for the two groups and were as described in our previous study [11]. After general anesthesia or brachial plexus block anesthesia, the patient was placed in the beach-chair position, with the upper limb in full supination, and an anterolateral acromial approach (ALA) was performed with a 5-cm skin incision proximally, while the anterior approach was performed with a 5-cm skin incision distally by splitting the brachialis longitudinally just along the lateral side of the biceps brachii. The site of the distal approach was decided according to the length of the pre-contoured plate. During the distal anterior approach, care was taken not to injure the musculocutaneous nerve, which lies between the biceps and the brachialis; the dissection through the brachialis was performed bluntly but gently, without routine nerve exposure. An extraperiosteal tunnel was made to connect with both approaches, from the lateral part of the greater tubercle proximally to the anterior part of the humerus distally. The key point was that, in order to protect the deltoid attachment point, the tunnel did not pass through the humeral deltoid tuberosity but across it anteriorly. Using the MIPO technique, the pre-contoured

helical long PHILOS plate was then inserted from the proximal approach, passed through the tunnel distally, and fixed on the humerus with locking screws through the ALA approach proximally (five or more screws inserted). According to AO principles, at least two or three screw holes should be left open over the fracture to decrease stress concentration [15]. So, usually, three to four screws were inserted distally according to the different fracture types (Fig. 2). Finally, intraoperative fluoroscopy was used to ensure a correct fracture reduction and positioning of the plate. Some adjustments were required if the fluoroscopy results were unsatisfactory. The name of the surgeon, duration of surgery (from incision to skin closure), and blood loss volume were recorded.

Rehabilitation and follow-up

After surgery, all patients were recommended the same rehabilitation plan. They were allowed to perform passive range of motion exercises immediately, and active exercises were allowed after 2 weeks. Patients were recommended to attend follow-up visits at 4 weeks, 12 weeks, 6 months, and 12 months after surgery. At each follow-up visit, a regular X-ray examination was taken, and at the 12-month follow-up, functional evaluation was added.

Statistical analysis

Categorical variables in each group are presented as count (percentage), and continuous variables are presented as mean ± standard deviation. All categorical variables were compared directly to each other using the chi-square test or Fisher's exact tests. For continuous variables, Student's two-tailed t tests were conducted. Results were considered significant when $P < 0.05$. The analysis was performed using the statistical program SPSS version 21 (IBM Corp., Armonk, NY, USA).

Results

Among the 46 enrolled patients, 25 patients were treated with plates pre-contoured on standard Synbone before surgery, and the remaining 21 were contoured on 3D-printed models. Since we chose older patients to form our study population, the mean age of all patients was 71.45 years: 71.84 years in the Synbone group and 71.00 years in the 3D-printed group. The Synbone group consisted of 7 males and 18 females; 40% of these patients presented with a fracture that extended to the proximal humerus, and the mean follow-up time was 18.48 months. Twenty-one patients were allocated to the 3D-printed group, 7 were males and 14 were females; in 42.9% of cases, the proximal humerus was involved, and the mean follow-up time was 16.95 months. The two groups were considered homogeneous since there were no significant differences between these baseline characteristics (Table 1).

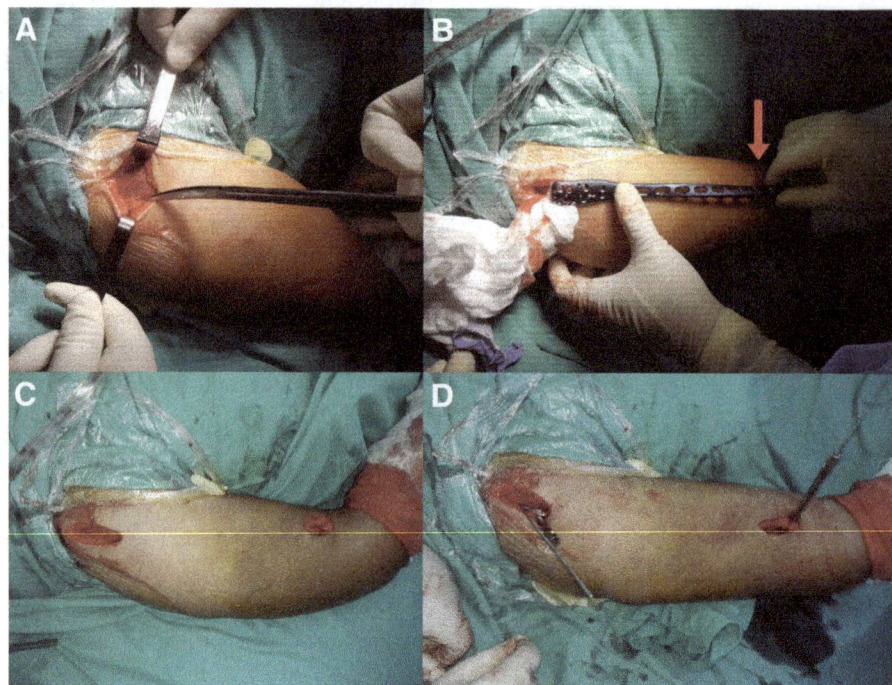

Fig. 2 Surgical procedure. **a** An anterolateral acromial approach (ALA) was performed with a 5-cm skin incision proximally. **b** The site of distal approach was decided according to the length of the pre-contoured plate (red arrow). **c** Two approaches were made. **d** An extraperiosteal tunnel was made to connect both approaches, and the plate was placed with MIPO technique

At the 1-year follow-up visit, all fractures were healed and showed a satisfactory outcome with respect to the radiographic examinations (Fig. 2). There were no significant differences between the two groups with regard to the fracture union time, Constant-Murley score or Mayo Elbow Performance Score (MEPS) (Table 2). One

patient in the Synbone group suffered shoulder impingement, and another one in the 3D-printed group presented with a superficial infection after surgery (Fig. 3). There were no instances of iatrogenic radial nerve injury or other major complications.

All surgeries in the Synbone group were finished by senior attending doctors, while in the 3D-printed group, 9 surgeries were finished by senior attending doctors and 12 were finished by junior attending doctors. The duration of surgery was significantly shorter in the 3D-printed group than in the Synbone group (42.62 vs. 60.36, $P = 0.001$). In addition, patients in the 3D-printed group lost significantly less blood during surgery (105.19

Table 1 Baseline characteristics of the Synbone group and 3D-printed group

	Synbone group	3D-printed group	P value
Age	71.84 ± 4.81	71.00 ± 5.81	0.594
Gender			0.695
Male	7 (28%)	7 (33.3%)	
Female	18 (72%)	14 (66.7%)	
Proximal humerus involved			0.845
Yes	10 (40%)	9 (42.9%)	
No	15 (60%)	12 (57.1%)	
Fracture type (AO/OTA)			0.782
A	4 (8.7%)	3 (6.5%)	
B	13 (28.3%)	13 (28.3%)	
C	8 (17.4%)	5 (10.9%)	
Follow-up months	18.48 ± 6.25	16.95 ± 5.12	0.367

Table 2 Outcomes of the Synbone group and 3D-printed group

	Synbone group	3D-printed group	P value
Time to fracture union (weeks)	16.16 ± 3.65	15.70 ± 2.96	0.976
Constant-Murley score	76.80 ± 6.67	76.95 ± 6.03	0.936
MEPS score	96.80 ± 3.79	94.32 ± 4.02	0.928
Duration of surgery (min)	60.36 ± 10.20	42.62 ± 7.61	0.001*
Blood loss volume (ml)	120.80 ± 10.61	105.19 ± 14.67	0.001*
Surgeon			
Senior attending doctor	25	9	
Junior attending doctor	0	12	

*Differences are statistically significant

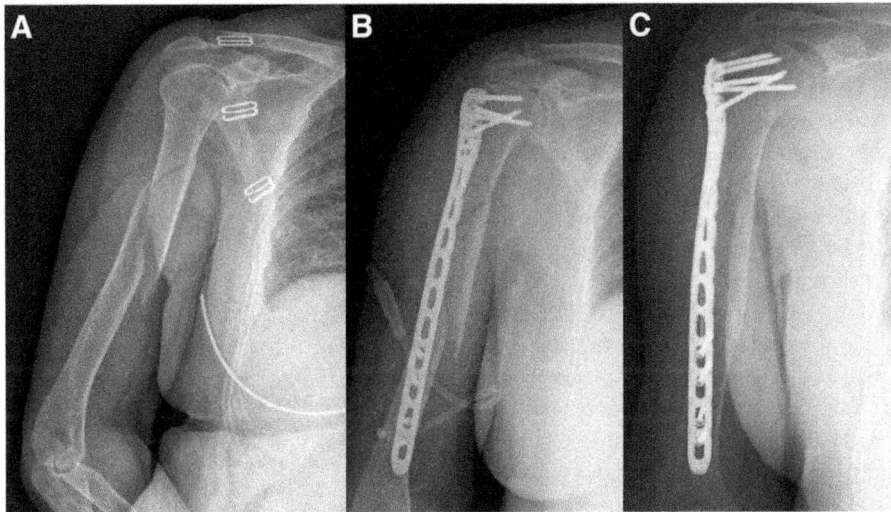

Fig. 3 A patient, suffered proximal third humeral shaft fracture from a simple fall, was allocated to the 3D-printed group. **a** Pre-operative X-ray examination. **b** The first day after surgery. **c** The completely healed fracture at 1-year follow-up

vs. 120.80 ml, $P = 0.001$) (Table 2). In the 3D-printed group, there were no significant differences between the baseline characteristics of the two grades of surgeons. However, we also found no significant difference between the outcomes (Table 3).

Discussion

The optimal treatment for humeral shaft fracture remains controversial. Although a large proportion of these fractures can be treated without surgery, a recent study, involving a randomized controlled trial, compared bridge plate with functional brace fixation for humeral shaft fractures and concluded that surgical plating has a statistically significant advantage with a better DASH score, lower non-union rate, and lower residual deformity rate [1]. As for proximal third humeral shaft fractures, they were

Table 3 Outcomes of the two grades of surgeons of the 3D-printed group

	Senior attending doctor	Junior attending doctor	P value
Age	70.56 ± 6.02	71.33 ± 5.88	0.770
Gender (male/female)	2/7	5/7	0.642
Fracture type (A/B/C)	2/4/3	1/9/2	0.355
Proximal humerus involved (yes/no)	5/4	7/5	0.899
Time to fracture union (weeks)	15.78 ± 2.11	16.50 ± 3.53	0.593
Constant-Murley score	77.33 ± 6.75	76.67 ± 5.74	0.809
MEPS score	97.22 ± 2.63	96.67 ± 4.92	0.763
Duration of surgery (min)	39.89 ± 8.07	44.67 ± 6.88	0.160
Blood loss volume (ml)	107.00 ± 18.01	103.83 ± 12.26	0.637

thought to be complicated with a higher non-union rate when treated conservatively compared with middle and distal fractures [2, 5, 16]. Since the helical plating technique was introduced for the treatment of humeral fractures, some studies have shown that this technique resulted in increased stiffness compared to fixation with a straight plate under torsional loading and produced satisfactory clinical outcomes [14, 17]. However, how to produce a suitable helical plate for each individual patient is a big question for surgeons. Previous studies have proven that the 3D printing technique is a good tool for designing surgical plans and pre-contouring plates used to treat other bone fractures [18–20]. Our results demonstrate the benefit of pre-contouring plates on a 3D-printed model for this special technique.

In this study, all kinds of fractures (from type A to type C) were treated by helical plating technique, and satisfactory outcomes were obtained. It was coincident with our previous cadaveric study results [11], so we thought this special technique was a good choice for these fractures. Previously, Stedtfeld and Biber reported that approximately 49.3% of the proximal third humeral shaft fractures extend into the humeral head and that this type of fracture cannot be characterized by conventional AO classification [6]. In our study, a total of 41.3% (19/46) of fractures involved the proximal humerus, a rate slightly lower compared with their report, but still a high rate of these fractures. Consequently, attention should be paid on the proximal third humeral shaft fractures since about half of them need adequate proximal fixation.

At the 1-year follow-up visit, all fractures were healed and none of the patients had suffered non-union, an outcome better than that reported for other treatment methods [1, 2, 5, 9, 21–23]. The mean union times of the

Synbone group and the 3D-printed groups were 16.16 and 15.57 weeks, respectively, which was similar to other studies even though our patients were older than in other studies [11, 17, 24]. Functional evaluations were satisfactory but were worse than those reported by others who conducted the same surgeries (Constant-Murley score 76.80, 76.95 vs. 88.6) [13, 17]. This may be attributed to the fact that our population was much older, so that humeral fracture might be combined with rotator cuff degeneration in our enrolled patients.

The primary outcomes of this study were that surgical duration and blood loss were reduced by the use of a 3D-printed model for pre-contouring the plates before surgery. This result was consistent with our hypothesis and can be explained by the fact that the humeri of older patients in our country are much shorter than the standard Synbone, requiring surgeons to adjust the plates during surgery. Since the 3D-printed model represented the actual size of the bone, the plates pre-contoured on these models were always suitable for fixing the fractures. Because of MIPO technique application, there was only 15 ml of blood loss difference between the two groups; maybe it was not clinically relevant, but on the whole, it reduced 12.5% of blood loss volume and presented a small part of the benefit of 3D-printed technique.

We compared the outcomes between the two grades of surgeons in the 3D-printed group. Although senior attending doctors are much more experienced than junior attending doctors, the results showed that there was no significant difference between them in terms of outcome. We believed that the 3D printing technique would make this novel technique much easier and make it available for use by less specialized surgeons. However, since all fractures in the Synbone group were finished by senior attending doctors, it was impossible to compare the results with a control group.

There are some limitations to this study: (I) the retrospective design limits the level of evidence and only represents one single center; (II) some patients who died within 1 year of surgery are excluded from this study, which may influence the final results; (III) all these surgeries were finished by surgeons in one trauma center, so personal differences cannot be avoided; and (IV) this study only included Asian population, and maybe the results could be challenged by other races because of different skeletal sizes.

Conclusions

Our results demonstrated that pre-contouring plates into a helical shape on a 3D-printed model was helpful in shortening the duration of surgery and reducing blood loss volume. In addition, the 3D printing technique could make this surgical procedure easier, enabling a widespread application for the treatment of proximal third humeral shaft fractures.

Abbreviations
3D print: Three-dimensional print; MIPO: Minimally invasive plate osteosynthesis; UV: Ultraviolet rays

Acknowledgements
We would like to thank Jianqing Li of The First Affiliated Hospital of Soochow University for the language modification.

Funding
This study is supported by a grant from Medical Engineering Cross Foundation of Shanghai Jiao Tong University (Grant YG2016MS18) and Three-year Project for Enhancing Clinical and Innovative Competence of Municipal Hospitals (Grant No. 16CR3042A).

Authors' contributions
QKW, JH, LW, and YFC designed the study. JJG collected the data. QKW performed the statistical analysis and was a major contributor in writing the manuscript. All authors read and approved the final manuscript.

Competing interests
The authors declare that they have no competing interests.

Author details
[1]Department of Orthopedic Surgery, Shanghai Jiao Tong University Affiliated Sixth People's Hospital, 600 Yishan Road, Shanghai 200233, People's Republic of China. [2]Department of Pathology, Shanghai Eighth People's Hospital, 8 Caobao Road, Shanghai 200233, People's Republic of China.

References

1. Matsunaga FT, Tamaoki MJ, Matsumoto MH, Netto NA, Faloppa F, Belloti JC. Minimally invasive osteosynthesis with a bridge plate versus a functional brace for humeral shaft fractures: a randomized controlled trial. J Bone Joint Surg Am. 2017;99:583–92.
2. Ali E, Griffiths D, Obi N, Tytherleigh-Strong G, Van Rensburg L. Nonoperative treatment of humeral shaft fractures revisited. J Shoulder Elb Surg. 2015;24:210–4.
3. Ekholm R, Tidermark J, Tornkvist H, Adami J, Ponzer S. Outcome after closed functional treatment of humeral shaft fractures. J Orthop Trauma. 2006;20:591–6.
4. Balfour GW, Mooney V, Ashby ME. Diaphyseal fractures of the humerus treated with a ready-made fracture brace. J Bone Joint Surg Am. 1982;64:11–3.
5. Court-Brown CM, McQueen MM. Nonunions of the proximal humerus: their prevalence and functional outcome. J Trauma. 2008;64:1517–21.
6. Stedtfeld HW, Biber R. Proximal third humeral shaft fractures -- a fracture entity not fully characterized by conventional AO classification. Injury. 2014; 45(Suppl 1):S54–9.
7. Papasoulis E, Drosos GI, Ververidis AN, Verettas DA. Functional bracing of humeral shaft fractures. A review of clinical studies. Injury. 2010;41:e21–7.
8. Gill DR, Torchia ME. The spiral compression plate for proximal humeral shaft nonunion: a case report and description of a new technique. J Orthop Trauma. 1999;13:141–4.
9. Moon JG, Kwon HN, Biraris S, Shon WY. Minimally invasive plate osteosynthesis using a helical plate for metadiaphyseal complex fractures of the proximal humerus. Orthopedics. 2014;37:e237–43.
10. Yang KH. Helical plate fixation for treatment of comminuted fractures of the proximal and middle one-third of the humerus. Injury. 2005;36:75–80.
11. Wang QK, Xu YF, Wang YC, Zhang S, Chen YF, Wang L. Tips and tricks of long helical PHILOS plating on proximal humeral diaphyseal and metaphyseal fractures using the MIPO technique in elderly patients: a cadaveric study and clinical experience. Int J Clin Exp Med. 2017;10:6489–95.

12. Perren SM, Regazzoni P, Fernandez AA. Biomechanical and biological aspects of defect treatment in fractures using helical plates. Acta Chir Orthop Traumatol Cechoslov. 2014;81:267–71.

13. Gardner MJ, Griffith MH, Lorich DG. Helical plating of the proximal humerus. Injury. 2005;36:1197–200.

14. Krishna KR, Sridhar I, Ghista DN. Analysis of the helical plate for bone fracture fixation. Injury. 2008;39:1421–36.

15. Marsh JL, Slongo TF, Agel J, Broderick JS, Creevey W, DeCoster TA, Prokuski L, Sirkin MS, Ziran B, Henley B, Audigé L. Fracture and dislocation classification compendium – 2007: orthopaedic trauma association classification, database and outcomes committee. J Orthop Trauma. 2007;21:S1–133.

16. Niall DM, O'Mahony J, McElwain JP. Plating of humeral shaft fractures—has the pendulum swung back? Injury. 2004;35:580–6.

17. Tan JC, Kagda FH, Murphy D, Thambiah JS, Khong KS. Minimally invasive helical plating for shaft of humerus fractures: technique and outcome. Open Orthop J. 2012;6:184–8.

18. You W, Liu LJ, Chen HX, Xiong JY, Wang DM, Huang JH, et al. Application of 3D printing technology on the treatment of complex proximal humeral fractures (Neer3-part and 4-part) in old people. Orthop Traumatol Surg Res. 2016;102:897–903.

19. Yang L, Grottkau B, He Z, Ye C. Three dimensional printing technology and materials for treatment of elbow fractures. Int Orthop. 2017;41:2381–7.

20. Omar M, Zeller AN, Gellrich NC, Rana M, Krettek C, Liodakis E. Application of a customized 3D printed reduction aid after external fixation of the femur and tibia: technical note. Int J Med Robot. 2017;13:e1803.

21. Ring D, Chin K, Taghinia AH, Jupiter JB. Nonunion after functional brace treatment of diaphyseal humerus fractures. J Trauma. 2007;62:1157–8.

22. McCormack RG, Brien D, Buckley RE, McKee MD, Powell J, Schemitsch EH. Fixation of fractures of the shaft of the humerus by dynamic compression plate or intramedullary nail. A prospective, randomised trial. J Bone Joint Surg Br. 2000;82:336–9.

23. Singh AK, Narsaria N, Seth RR, Garg S. Plate osteosynthesis of fractures of the shaft of the humerus: comparison of limited contact dynamic compression plates and locking compression plates. J Orthop Traumatol. 2014;15:117–22.

24. Aksu N, Karaca S, Kara AN, Isiklar ZU. Minimally invasive plate osteosynthesis (MIPO) in diaphyseal humerus and proximal humerus fractures. Acta Orthop Traumatol Turc. 2012;46:154–60.

16

Are three-dimensional patient-specific cutting guides for open wedge high tibial osteotomy accurate? An in vitro study

Mathias Donnez[1,2,3]* (iD), Matthieu Ollivier[1,2], Maxime Munier[2], Philippe Berton[3], Jean-Pierre Podgorski[3], Patrick Chabrand[1,2] and Sébastien Parratte[1,2]

Abstract

Background: The aim of this in vitro study was to assess the accuracy of three-dimensional patient-specific cutting guides for open wedge high tibial osteotomy (OWHTO) to provide the planned correction in both frontal and sagittal planes.

Methods: Ten cadaveric tibias underwent OWHTO performed using a patient-specific cutting guide based on 3D preoperative planning. An initial CT scan of the tibias was performed, and after segmentation, 3D geometrical models of the pre-OWHTO tibias were obtained. Reference planes were defined, and OWHTO virtually planned to then design patient-specific cutting guides. OWHTO were performed using the patient-specific cutting guides. The patient-specific cutting guide controls the cut and the correction of the OWHTO in both planes. 3D models of post-OWHTO tibias were created after a postoperative CT scan. Geometrical post-OWHTO 3D models were superimposed on pre-OWHTO 3D models. Mechanical medial proximal tibial angle (mMPTA) in the frontal plane and posterior tibial slope (PTS) in the sagittal plane were compared between planned-OWHTO and post-OWHTO 3D reconstructions relative to the pre-OWHTO reference planes and axis. Pearson's and Lin's correlation tests were performed to assess precision and accuracy of patient-specific cutting guides.

Results: The mean difference between post-OWHTO and planned-OWHTO was 0.2° (max 0.5°, SD 0.3°) in the frontal plane and − 0.1° (max 0.8°, SD 0.5°) in the sagittal plane. Statistically significant correlations were found between the planned-OWHTO and post-OWHTO configurations for the mMPTA ($p < 0.0001$) and PTS ($p < 0.0001$) measurements, and the bias correction factor was 0.99 in both planes.

Conclusions: 3D patient-specific cutting guides for OWHTO-based 3D virtual planning is a reliable and accurate method of achieving multiplanar correction in both frontal and sagittal planes.

Keywords: Knee surgery, Osteoarthrosis, Medial gonarthrosis, Osteotomy, Open wedge high tibial osteotomy, Patient-specific, Accuracy, Tibial slope correction

Background

Open wedge high tibial osteotomy (OWHTO) has been described as an efficient conservative surgical treatment preserving the bone stock for patients with moderate medial gonarthrosis and lower leg malalignment [1, 2].

The objective of the OWHTO is to correct lower leg malalignment in both the frontal and sagittal tibial planes to limit the overload of the medial compartment. Accurate correction is essential to its success as under correction leads to persistent pain and over correction to functional limitations [3, 4].

Different methods and instrumentations have been developed to help the surgeon to achieve the planned correction [3, 5–7].

Conventional methods use standard instrumentation to open the osteotomy [5, 6]. Frontal correction can then

---

* Correspondence: mathias.donnez@gmail.com
[1]Aix Marseille Univ, CNRS, ISM, Marseille, France
[2]Aix Marseille Univ, APHM, CNRS, ISM, Sainte-Marguerite Hospital, Institute for Locomotion, Department of Orthopaedics and Traumatology, Marseille, France
Full list of author information is available at the end of the article

be managed intraoperatively by measuring the opening angle or opening gap and comparing it to the preoperative plan [8–10], or by using a radiopaque cable under fluoroscopy to control lower limb alignment [9, 11–13]. The control of the correction for both the frontal and the sagittal planes at the same time with standard instrumentations remains challenging [14–16]. Computer-assisted surgery (CAS) for OWHTO was validated experimentally in vitro by Hankemeier et al. [7] and subsequently used in clinical studies [3, 17–21]. CAS allows real-time control of the correction. All these studies reported better accuracy and reliability for CAS than for conventional or cable methods, but with increased surgical time and a control of the global alignment of the limb but not of tibia only and not the posterior tibial slope (PTS).

While frontal plane correction is most often described for osteotomy management, PTS management in the sagittal plane is essential to preserve biomechanics [22–24]. Song et al. [19] reported that PTS is unchanged if the anterior opening is equal to 67% of the medial opening. However, this evaluation is complex to perform during surgery, and patient-specific instruments may help the surgeon to manage both the sagittal and the frontal plane correction during surgery [25, 26].

Using an experimental setup, three-dimensional patient-specific cutting guides were reported to be more accurate than free-hand technique to perform an osteotomy cut and drill in a synthetic bone [27]. The use of patient-specific cutting guides for OWHTO was also reported recently in three studies realized on small series of patients [25, 26, 28]. All three clinical studies reported good accuracy and reliability of the procedure. Planning procedures for OWHTO were carried out either on 2D long-leg radiographs [28] or from a 3D model [25, 26]. Pérez-Mañanes et al. used CT images to obtain the 3D tibial surface and to position two K-wires to lead the cut, and the correction was planned using two additional wedges.

To avoid the disappointing clinical results observed with patient-specific instrumentation for total knee arthroplasty, we wanted to evaluate in vitro this new technique. After developing a specific patient-specific guide to control both the cut and the correction adapted for a specific OWHTO plate, it was our aim to evaluate the accuracy of the system in an in vitro CT scan-controlled study. Our hypothesis was that the patient-specific cutting guide for OWHTO can provide an accurate correction in both the frontal and sagittal planes.

Methods

Study design

In this in vitro study, ten frozen cadaveric specimens' tibias (eight females and two males aged from 70 to 99, average age 88, 5 right sides) were obtained from our Department of Anatomy at the Aix-Marseille University School of Medicine (Table 1). The subjects were all preserved in Winckler liquid [29, 30]. All soft tissues were removed, except the patellar tendon insertion.

OWHTO preoperative planning

All specimens were scanned using a standardized CT scan protocol (Discovery 710, GE Medical System, CERIMED, Marseille, France). The following acquisition parameters were used both prior and after the HTO: 120 kV, 400 mA, and 0.625-mm-thick slices. DICOM images were imported into Mimics 17.0 software (Materialise®, Leuven, Belgium), and 3D geometrical models of the tibias were created (Pre-OWHTO configurations, Fig. 1).

Anatomical landmarks, anatomical reference planes, and the mechanical axis of the tibia were defined on the 3D models according to Lee et al. [31]. Preoperative mechanical medial proximal tibial angle (mMPTA) and medial PTS were measured (Fig. 2). mMPTA measures the varus deformation of the tibia. PTS measures the sagittal orientation of the proximal tibia. For each specimen, a correction for proximal tibial bony deformity, when present, was determined in both the frontal and the sagittal planes. For specimens with optimal tibial mechanical alignment, a random correction was applied. Each preoperative 3D tibia model was imported to a specially designed 3D planning tool for OWHTO. A cutting plane was positioned, and OWHTO was simulated with respect to the frontal and sagittal plane corrections previously determined (planned-OWHTO configurations, Fig. 1). The Activmotion-2 plate (Newclip Technics®, Haute-Goulaine, France) was positioned on the anteromedial surface of the tibia following the manufacturer's recommendations. The plate contains four locking screws above and four locking screws below the osteotomy cut. Then, a patient-specific cutting guide was designed for each tibia based on the OWHTO simulation. Patient-specific cutting

Table 1 Specimen description

Specimen	Gender	Age	Side	Pre-OWHTO mMPTA (°)	Pre-OWHTO PTS (°)
G068	F	99	R	89.6	7.9
G131	F	78	R	88.5	2.1
G059	F	95	L	84.2	5.3
G141	F	99	L	88.0	2.4
G115	M	88	R	86.9	4.7
G111	F	89	R	88.5	2.9
G119	M	90	R	88.1	4.5
G113	F	84	L	89.5	7.6
G136	F	90	L	90.3	4.2
G117	F	70	L	83.6	9.8

Demographic data, pre-OWHTO measurements

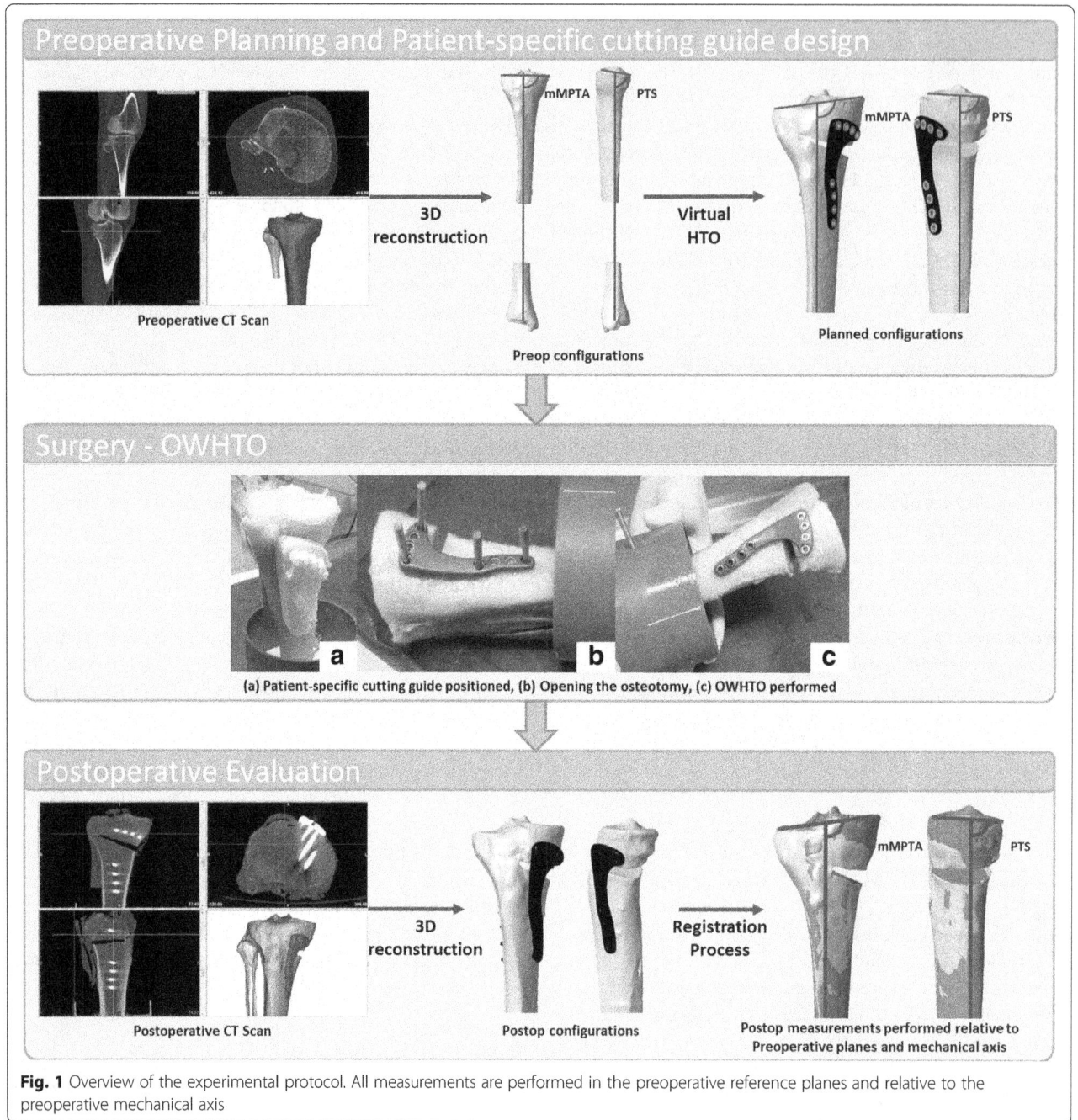

Fig. 1 Overview of the experimental protocol. All measurements are performed in the preoperative reference planes and relative to the preoperative mechanical axis

guides took into account the tibial anatomy, the position of the cutting plane, the amount of correction planned in all planes, and the plate location. All patient-specific cutting guides were 3D printed.

OWHTO
Specimens were thawed overnight. All OWHTO were performed by one surgeon (MM) using the patient-specific cutting guides [26]. Then, the same CT scan protocol was used to assess the tibias after OWHTO. Post-OWHTO 3D geometrical models were created

with Mimics 17.0 software (post-OWHTO configurations, Fig. 1).

Registration process
For each specimen, the distal part of the post-OWHTO tibia was superimposed on the distal part of the pre-OWHTO tibia using an iterative closest point (ICP) algorithm (Fig. 3). This registration process ensured that measurement references for all models of each tibia were the same. Then, mMPTA and PTS were measured on both the planned-OWHTO and the post-OWHTO

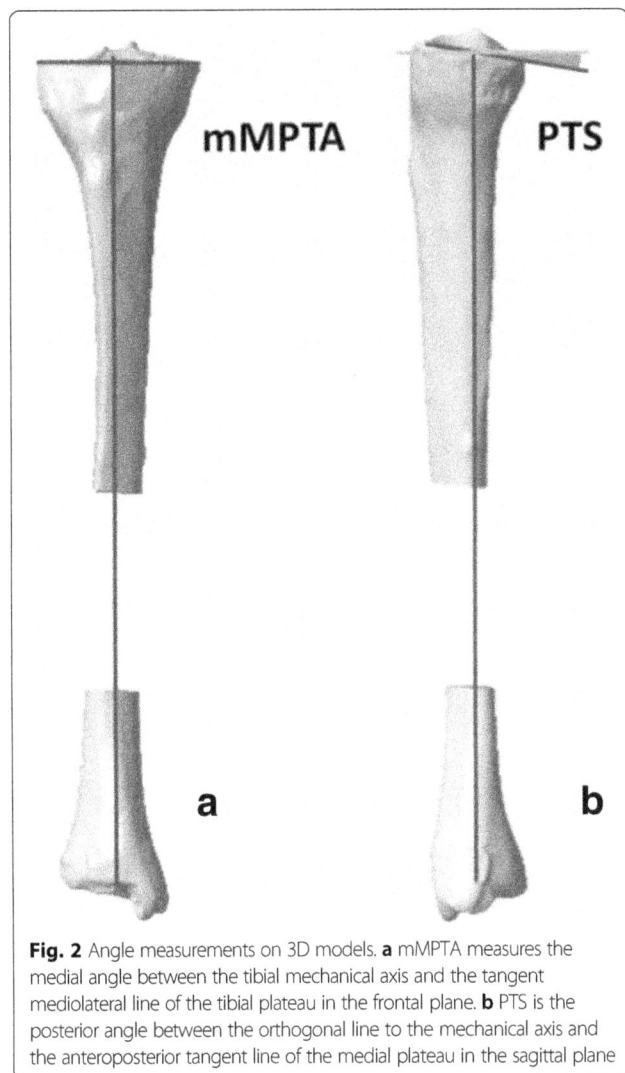

Fig. 2 Angle measurements on 3D models. **a** mMPTA measures the medial angle between the tibial mechanical axis and the tangent mediolateral line of the tibial plateau in the frontal plane. **b** PTS is the posterior angle between the orthogonal line to the mechanical axis and the anteroposterior tangent line of the medial plateau in the sagittal plane

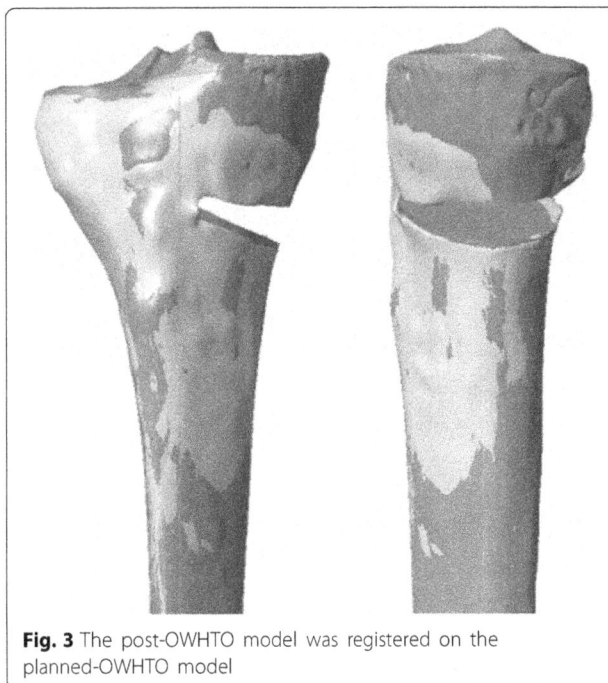

Fig. 3 The post-OWHTO model was registered on the planned-OWHTO model

configuration. For maximum reproducibility of measurements, both planned and postoperative angles were measured in the frontal and sagittal pre-OWHTO planes relative to the pre-OWHTO tibial mechanical axis.

Planned-OWHTO and post-OWHTO configurations were compared to assess the precision and the accuracy provided by the patient-specific cutting guides for OWHTO.

Statistical analysis

Statistical analysis was performed between the planned-OWHTO and the post-OWHTO mMPTA, and between the planned-OWHTO and the post-OWHTO PTS. Correlation analyses were performed using Pearson's correlation test to assess the precision reached by the patient-specific cutting guides. Accuracy was assessed by the calculation of the bias correction factor (C_b) given by Lin's correlation test [32].

Significance was considered at $p < 0.05$. The 95% confidence intervals (CI) were presented. Statistical analysis was performed on R software.

Results

The mean pre-OWHTO mMPTA was 87.7° (SD 2.2°), and the mean pre-OWHTO PTS was 5.1° (SD 2.6°). A mean 7.3° (SD 1.3°) correction in the frontal plane and a 3.3° (SD 2.7°) correction in the sagittal plane were thus planned. For all specimens, the positioning of the patient-specific cutting guides on the bone was possible in accordance with the planning. All patient-specific cutting guides fitted the tibial surface, so all OWHTO were performed as planned.

Differences between the post-OWHTO and planned-OWHTO configurations were calculated. The mean difference between the post-OWHTO and planned-OWHTO configurations was 0.2° (from − 0.3° to 0.5°, SD 0.3°) in the frontal plane, and − 0.1° (from − 0.7° to 0.8°, SD 0.5°) in the sagittal plane (Table 2).

According to Pearson's correlation tests, a statistically significant correlation was found between the planned-OWHTO and post-OWHTO configurations, for the mMPTA measurements with a correlation coefficient of 0.99 (95% CI, 94−99%, $p < 0.0001$), and for the PTS measurements with a correlation coefficient of 0.97 (95% CI, 86−99%, $p < 0.0001$) (Fig. 4).

Bias coefficient C_b was 0.99 in both the frontal and sagittal planes (Table 3).

Discussion

OWHTO success remains on accurate correction in order to avoid persistent pain or functional limitations [3, 4]. This in vitro study aimed to investigate the accuracy in both the frontal and sagittal planes provided by

Table 2 Angular measurements

Specimen	Pre-OWHTO		Corrections		Planned-OWHTO		Post-OWHTO		Planned-OWHTO vs post-OWHTO	
	mMPTA (°)	PTS (°)	mMPTA (°)	PTS (°)	mMPTA (°)	PTS (°)	mMPTA (°)	PTS (°)	mMPTA (°)	PTS (°)
G068	89.6	7.9	8	5	97.3	3.0	97.0	3.5	0.3	− 0.5
G131	88.5	2.1	6	0	94.5	2.1	94.7	2.3	− 0.2	− 0.2
G059	84.2	5.3	8	0	92.9	5.2	92.9	4.4	0.0	0.8
G141	88.0	2.4	9	3	97.0	− 0.7	96.6	− 0.6	0.4	− 0.1
G115	86.9	4.7	8	4	95.2	0.7	94.7	1.2	0.5	− 0.5
G111	88.5	2.9	7	3	95.1	− 0.1	95.2	0.3	− 0.1	− 0.4
G119	88.1	4.5	6	4	94.1	0.6	93.6	0.9	0.5	− 0.3
G113	89.5	7.6	5	6	94.1	1.7	93.7	1.1	0.4	0.6
G136	90.3	4.2	7	0	97.3	4.1	97.6	3.9	− 0.3	0.2
G117	83.6	9.8	9	8	92.2	1.9	91.8	2.6	0.4	− 0.7

Pre-OWHTO measurements, planned corrections, planned-OWHTO measurements, post-OWHTO measurements, and absolute difference between planned-OWHTO and post-OWHTO configurations

patient-specific cutting guides with respect to 3D planning of OWHTO. The hypothesis that patient-specific cutting guides can provide the planned correction in both the frontal and sagittal planes was confirmed in this CT scan-controlled in vitro study.

In this patient-specific procedure for OWHTO, bone deformation angles were measured with respect to the anatomical reference planes determined using the procedure of Lee et al. [31] in order to mimic clinical practice. Clinical studies report several methods of finding anatomical reference points and measuring deformation angles [25]. Seeking to achieve maximum reliability and to measure only the correction provided by the patient-specific cutting guide, all measurements were performed relative to the same axis and in the same planes for the pre-OWHTO, planned-OWHTO, and post-OWHTO configurations. Unlike Munier et al., who performed measurements separately on the preoperative and postoperative 3D configurations, and then compared how far the two configurations differed from the planned correction, we performed our measurements relative to the preoperative mechanical axis. This was made possible by the registration process we used to superimpose the post-OWHTO configuration on the

planned-OWHTO configuration. As our objective was to assess the amount of correction, it was vital to keep the reference definition the same for both planned-OWHTO and post-OWHTO configurations.

Intraoperative methods to control correction are varied, have limited accuracy, and mainly focus on the frontal plane correction. In their review of the literature, Van Den Bempt et al. reported ranges of accuracy in the frontal plane from several clinical studies [4]. For conventional methods, the mean amplitude of the range of accuracy was 5.6° (from 4° to 8°) [33–37], whereas using the CAS method, it was 5.5° (from 4° to 7°) [10, 17, 38–41]. Irrespective of the range of accuracy chosen by the authors, the literature reports a mean 32% of outlier patients when authors used conventional methods [9, 10, 17, 21, 34–37, 40, 42–45] and 22% when they used CAS [10, 17, 21, 38–42, 44, 46]. Some in vitro studies find CAS to be accurate for OWHTO. On a single synthetic bone and with a statistical model, Keppler et al. [47] evaluated a mean error of 0.7° in the frontal plane between the postoperative results and the target. Wang et al. [48] performed OWHTO with several amounts of correction in a synthetic bone using CAS and reported 0.4° accuracy in the frontal plane. Both authors validated their

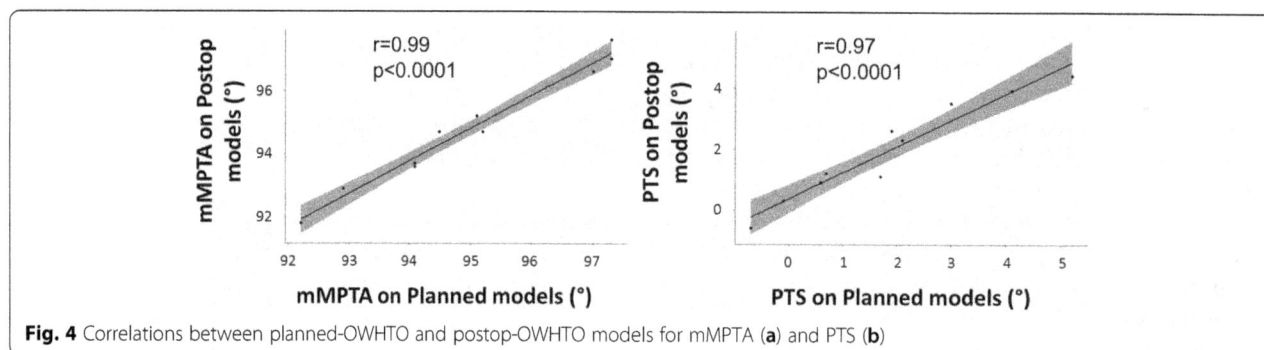

Fig. 4 Correlations between planned-OWHTO and postop-OWHTO models for mMPTA (**a**) and PTS (**b**)

Table 3 Statistical analysis results

	Pearson's correlation coefficient	C_b
mMPTA	0.99 (95% CI, 94–99%)	0.99
PTS	0.97 (95% CI, 86–99%)	0.99

Pearson's correlation coefficient and bias correction factor C_b between planned-OWHTO and post-OWHTO configurations

experimental work in a preliminary clinical study, on five and four patients. They both found a mean error of 1° in the frontal plane. On a single cadaveric specimen, Lützner et al. [49] evaluated the accuracy of CAS to measure lower limb alignment. They found a mean error of 0.6° in the frontal plane. Hankemeier et al. [7] performed OWHTO on 20 legs randomly assigned to CAS or a conventional method. They reported better accuracy and less variability than with a cable method. Among clinical studies using patient-specific cutting guides, Menetrey et al. [20] evaluated the frontal plane correction, based on 2D measurements for planning. Their patient-specific cutting guide only incorporates the cutting plane position, the correction being guided by two additional wedges. They found 0.5° accuracy (from 0° to 1.2°) in the frontal plane. Patient-specific cutting guides containing both the cutting plane planning and the correction were used in two other studies [19, 21]. In one, Munier et al. performed a postoperative 3D evaluation of their patients. Overall, they found similar accuracy for both 2D and 3D measurements by reproducing the measurement protocol on the postoperative model [26] around 0.0° (from – 1.7° to 1.8°, SD 1.1°) in the frontal plane. In the other study, Victor and Premanathan [25] reported a mean difference of 0.1° (from – 1° to 1°, SD – 0.1°) in the frontal plane.

Controlling the sagittal plane correction is essential to preserve knee biomechanics [23–25], but conventional methods have limited accuracy, remaining on gap measurements [15, 19]. Using CAS on synthetic bones, a mean error of 0.9° [47] and a 0.5° accuracy [48] were reported in the sagittal plane. Using patient-specific cutting guides, an accuracy around 0.3° (from – 2° to 3.2°, SD 1.4°) [26] and a mean difference of – 0.1° (from – 3° to 2°, SD 1.2°) [25] in the sagittal plane were reported.

In this study, the patient-specific OWHTO procedure includes 3D preoperative planning of the surgery and the design of a patient-specific cutting guide which takes into account the tibial anatomy, the position of the cutting plane, the amount of correction planned in all planes, and the plate location. The mean differences between the planned-OWHTO and post-OWHTO models are 0.2° (from – 0.3° to 0.5°, SD 0.3°) in the frontal plane and – 0.1° (from – 0.7° to 0.8°, SD 0.5°) in the sagittal plane. OWHTO outcomes are compared with the planning by superimposing the post-HTO 3D reconstruction on the planning 3D model. This enabled to assess the accuracy of

patient-specific cutting guides. Findings of the present study suggest that PTS is managed with accuracy, which is important for the management of cruciate ligament balance [23, 25].

One limitation of our study is the small number of specimens used. Moreover, not all specimens had a sufficient varus deformation in their proximal tibia to be considered as candidates for OWHTO. However, different degrees of correction consistent with clinical practice were planned in both the frontal and sagittal planes. We also departed from clinical practice in performing all the measurements on 3D models. This was possible thanks to the cadaveric nature of the specimens. This enabled us to assess precision and accuracy by comparing post-OWHTO and planned-OWHTO 3D models, thereby avoiding measurement errors related to 2D radiography. The preoperative CT scan required for this procedure could be another limitation for direct clinical application, not being necessary in conventional or CAS procedures. However, Menetrey et al. [20] reported that the patient-specific cutting guide reduced the use of intraoperative fluoroscopy from 55 images on average (range, 41–73) in conventional methods to 8 (range, 6–14), as well as requiring less surgical time.

Conclusion

OWHTO is demanding surgery, and accuracy of the correction in both frontal and sagittal planes is essential to its success. This study shows that combining 3D planning with patient-specific cutting guides for OWHTO is a reliable and accurate method of achieving multiplanar correction in both the frontal and the sagittal planes. Further randomized clinical studies should be carried out to validate these experimental results and evaluate the risk-benefit ratio of the preoperative CT scan, and the reduction in surgical time.

Acknowledgements
We would like to thank Pauline Brige (CERIMED, Aix-Marseille University, Marseille, France) for her help in the CT acquisitions. We also thank Marjorie Sweetko for re-reading the English of this manuscript.

Authors' contributions
MD participated in the conception and design of the study and in the acquisition and interpretation of the data and was a major contributor in writing the manuscript. MO participated in the conception of the study and in the acquisition of the data and was a major contributor in writing the manuscript. MM performed the OWHTO and participated in the acquisition and interpretation of the data. PB and JPP participated in the conception and design of the study. SP and PC were involved in the conception and design of the study and in the critical revision of the manuscript. All authors read and approved the final manuscript.

Competing interests
The authors declare that they have no competing interests.

Author details

[1]Aix Marseille Univ, CNRS, ISM, Marseille, France. [2]Aix Marseille Univ, APHM, CNRS, ISM, Sainte-Marguerite Hospital, Institute for Locomotion, Department of Orthopaedics and Traumatology, Marseille, France. [3]Newclip Technics, Haute-Goulaine, France.

References

1. Flecher X, Parratte S, Aubaniac J-M, J-NA A. A 12-28-year followup study of closing wedge high tibial osteotomy. Clin Orthop. 2006;452:91–6. https://doi.org/10.1097/01.blo.0000229362.12244.f6.

2. Amendola A, Bonasia DE. Results of high tibial osteotomy: review of the literature. Int Orthop. 2010;34:155–60. https://doi.org/10.1007/s00264-009-0889-8.

3. Saragaglia D, Chedal-Bornu B, Rouchy RC, Rubens-Duval B, Mader R, Pailhé R. Role of computer-assisted surgery in osteotomies around the knee. Knee Surg Sports Traumatol Arthrosc. 2016;24:3387–95. https://doi.org/10.1007/s00167-016-4302-z.

4. Van den Bempt M, Van Genechten W, Claes T, Claes S. How accurately does high tibial osteotomy correct the mechanical axis of an arthritic varus knee? A systematic review. Knee. 2016;23:925–35. https://doi.org/10.1016/j.knee.2016.10.001.

5. Lobenhoffer P, Agneskirchner JD. Improvements in surgical technique of valgus high tibial osteotomy. Knee Surg Sports Traumatol Arthrosc. 2003;11:132–8. https://doi.org/10.1007/s00167-002-0334-7.

6. Staubli AE, Jacob HAC. Evolution of open-wedge high-tibial osteotomy: experience with a special angular stable device for internal fixation without interposition material. Int Orthop. 2010;34:167–72. https://doi.org/10.1007/s00264-009-0902-2.

7. Hankemeier S, Hufner T, Wang G, Kendoff D, Zeichen J, Zheng G, et al. Navigated open-wedge high tibial osteotomy: advantages and disadvantages compared to the conventional technique in a cadaver study. Knee Surg Sports Traumatol Arthrosc. 2006;14:917–21. https://doi.org/10.1007/s00167-006-0035-8.

8. Elson DW, Petheram TG, Dawson MJ. High reliability in digital planning of medial opening wedge high tibial osteotomy, using Miniaci's method. Knee Surg Sports Traumatol Arthrosc. 2015;23:2041–8. https://doi.org/10.1007/s00167-014-2920-x.

9. Yoon S-D, Zhang G, Kim H-J, Lee B-J, Kyung H-S. Comparison of cable method and Miniaci method using picture archiving and communication system in preoperative planning for open wedge high tibial osteotomy. Knee Surg Relat Res. 2016;28:283–8. https://doi.org/10.5792/ksrr.16.052.

10. Schröter S, Ihle C, Elson DW, Döbele S, Stöckle U, Ateschrang A. Surgical accuracy in high tibial osteotomy: coronal equivalence of computer navigation and gap measurement. Knee Surg Sports Traumatol Arthrosc. 2016;24:3410–7. https://doi.org/10.1007/s00167-016-3983-7.

11. Fujisawa Y, Masuhara K, Shiomi S. The effect of high tibial osteotomy on osteoarthritis of the knee. An arthroscopic study of 54 knee joints. Orthop Clin North Am. 1979;10:585–608.

12. Dugdale TW, Noyes FR, Styer D. Preoperative planning for high tibial osteotomy. The effect of lateral tibiofemoral separation and tibiofemoral length. Clin Orthop. 1992;274:248–64.

13. Kim MS, Son JM, Koh IJ, Bahk JH, In Y. Intraoperative adjustment of alignment under valgus stress reduces outliers in patients undergoing medial opening-wedge high tibial osteotomy. Arch Orthop Trauma Surg. 2017:1–11. https://doi.org/10.1007/s00402-017-2729-4.

14. Hernigou P. Open wedge tibial osteotomy: combined coronal and sagittal correction. Knee. 2002;9:15–20. https://doi.org/10.1016/S0968-0160(01)00111-9.

15. Noyes FR, Goebel SX, West J. Opening wedge tibial osteotomy: the 3-triangle method to correct axial alignment and tibial slope. Am J Sports Med. 2005;33:378–87.

16. Hinterwimmer S, Beitzel K, Paul J, Kirchhoff C, Sauerschnig M, von Eisenhart-Rothe R, et al. Control of posterior tibial slope and patellar height in open-wedge valgus high tibial osteotomy. Am J Sports Med. 2011;39:851–6. https://doi.org/10.1177/0363546510388929.

17. Saragaglia D, Roberts J. Navigated osteotomies around the knee in 170 patients with osteoarthritis secondary to genu varum. Orthopedics. 2005;28:s1269–74.

18. Maurer F, Wassmer G. High tibial osteotomy: does navigation improve results? Orthopedics. 2006;29:S130–2.

19. Song E-K, Seon J-K, Park S-J. How to avoid unintended increase of posterior slope in navigation-assisted open-wedge high tibial osteotomy. Orthopedics. 2007;30:S127–31.

20. Menetrey J, Duthon V, Fritschy D. Computer-assisted open-wedge high tibial osteotomy. Oper Tech Orthop. 2008;18:210–4. https://doi.org/10.1053/j.oto.2008.12.003.

21. Chang J, Scallon G, Beckert M, Zavala J, Bollier M, Wolf B, et al. Comparing the accuracy of high tibial osteotomies between computer navigation and conventional methods. Comput Assist Surg Abingdon Engl. 2017;22(1):–8. https://doi.org/10.1080/24699322.2016.1271909.

22. Rodner CM, Adams DJ, Diaz-Doran V, Tate JP, Santangelo SA, Mazzocca AD, et al. Medial opening wedge osteotomy and the sagittal plane. Am J Sports Med. 2006;34:1431–41. https://doi.org/10.1177/0363546506287297.

23. Martineau PA, Fening SD, Miniaci A. Anterior opening wedge high tibial osteotomy: the effect of increasing posterior tibial slope on ligament strain. Can J Surg. 2010;53:261–7.

24. Akamatsu Y, Sotozawa M, Kobayashi H, Kusayama Y, Kumagai K, Saito T. Usefulness of long tibial axis to measure medial tibial slope for opening wedge high tibial osteotomy. Knee Surg Sports Traumatol Arthrosc. 2014:1–7. https://doi.org/10.1007/s00167-014-3403-9.

25. Victor J, Premanathan A. Virtual 3D planning and patient specific surgical guides for osteotomies around the knee. Bone Jt J. 2013;95-B:153–8. https://doi.org/10.1302/0301-620X.95B11.32950.

26. Munier M, Donnez M, Ollivier M, Flecher X, Chabrand P, Argenson J-N, et al. Can three-dimensional patient-specific cutting guides be used to achieve optimal correction for high tibial osteotomy? Pilot study. Orthop Traumatol Surg Res n.d. doi:https://doi.org/10.1016/j.otsr.2016.11.020.

27. Sys G, Eykens H, Lenaerts G, Shumelinsky F, Robbrecht C, Poffyn B. Accuracy assessment of surgical planning and three-dimensional-printed patient-specific guides for orthopaedic osteotomies. Proc Inst Mech Eng [H]. 2017;231:499–508. https://doi.org/10.1177/0954411917702177.

28. Pérez-Mañanes R, Burró J, Manaute J, Rodriguez F, Martín J. 3D surgical printing cutting guides for open-wedge high Tibial osteotomy: do it yourself n.d. doi:https://doi.org/10.1055/s-0036-1572412.

29. Winckler G. Manuel d'anatomie topographique et fonctionnelle. Masson et Cie Niort, impr. Soulisse et Cassegrain. 1964.

30. Crandall J. The preservation of human surrogates for biomechanical studies: University of Virginia; 1994.

31. Lee YS, Park SJ, Shin VI, Lee JH, Kim YH, Song EK. Achievement of targeted posterior slope in the medial opening wedge high tibial osteotomy: a mathematical approach. Ann Biomed Eng. 2009;38:583–93. https://doi.org/10.1007/s10439-009-9860-5.

32. Lin LI-K. A concordance correlation coefficient to evaluate reproducibility. Biometrics. 1989;45:255–68. https://doi.org/10.2307/2532051.

33. Magyar G, Ahl TL, Vibe P, Toksvig-Larsen S, Lindstrand A. Open-wedge osteotomy by hemicallotasis or the closed-wedge technique for osteoarthritis of the knee. J Bone Jt Surg Br. 1999;81-B:444–8.

34. Brouwer RW, Bierma-Zeinstra SMA, van Raaij TM, Verhaar J a N. Osteotomy for medial compartment arthritis of the knee using a closing wedge or an opening wedge controlled by a Puddu plate. Bone Jt J. 2006;88-B:1454–9. https://doi.org/10.1302/0301-620X.88B11.17743.

35. Hankemeier S, Mommsen P, Krettek C, Jagodzinski M, Brand J, Meyer C, et al. Accuracy of high tibial osteotomy: comparison between open- and closed-wedge technique. Knee Surg Sports Traumatol Arthrosc. 2009;18:1328–33. https://doi.org/10.1007/s00167-009-1020-9.

36. Brosset T, Pasquier G, Migaud H, Gougeon F. Opening wedge high tibial osteotomy performed without filling the defect but with locking plate fixation (TomoFix™) and early weight-bearing: prospective evaluation of bone union, precision and maintenance of correction in 51 cases. Orthop Traumatol Surg Res OTSR. 2011;97:705–11. https://doi.org/10.1016/j.otsr.2011.06.011.

37. Duivenvoorden T, Brouwer RW, Baan A, Bos PK, Reijman M, Bierma-Zeinstra SMA, et al. Comparison of closing-wedge and opening-wedge high tibial osteotomy for medial compartment osteoarthritis of the knee: a randomized controlled trial with a six-year follow-up. J Bone Joint Surg Am. 2014;96:1425–32. https://doi.org/10.2106/JBJS.M.00786.

38. Bae DK, Song SJ, Yoon KH. Closed-wedge high tibial osteotomy using computer-assisted surgery compared to the conventional technique. Bone Jt J. 2009;91-B:1164–71. https://doi.org/10.1302/0301-620X.91B9.22058.

39. Gebhard F, Krettek C, Hüfner T, Grützner PA, Stöckle U, Imhoff AB, et al. Reliability of computer-assisted surgery as an intraoperative ruler in

navigated high tibial osteotomy. Arch Orthop Trauma Surg. 2011;131:297–302. https://doi.org/10.1007/s00402-010-1145-9.

40. Iorio R, Pagnottelli M, Vadalà A, Giannetti S, Sette PD, Papandrea P, et al. Open-wedge high tibial osteotomy: comparison between manual and computer-assisted techniques. Knee Surg Sports Traumatol Arthrosc. 2011; 21:113–9. https://doi.org/10.1007/s00167-011-1785-5.

41. Lee D-H, Nha K-W, Park S-J, Han S-B. Preoperative and postoperative comparisons of navigation and radiologic limb alignment measurements after high tibial osteotomy. Arthrosc J Arthrosc Relat Surg. 2012;28:1842–50. https://doi.org/10.1016/j.arthro.2012.05.881.

42. Stanley JC, Robinson KG, Devitt BM, Richmond AK, Webster KE, Whitehead TS, et al. Computer assisted alignment of opening wedge high tibial osteotomy provides limited improvement of radiographic outcomes compared to flouroscopic alignment. Knee. 2016;23:289–94. https://doi.org/10.1016/j.knee.2015.12.006.

43. Marti CB, Gautier E, Wachtl SW, Jakob RP. Accuracy of frontal and sagittal plane correction in open-wedge high tibial osteotomy. Arthrosc J Arthrosc Relat Surg. 2004;20:366–72. https://doi.org/10.1016/j.arthro.2004.01.024.

44. Lee D-H, Han S-B, Oh K-J, Lee JS, Kwon J-H, Kim J-I, et al. The weight-bearing scanogram technique provides better coronal limb alignment than the navigation technique in open high tibial osteotomy. Knee. 2014;21:451–5. https://doi.org/10.1016/j.knee.2012.09.003.

45. El-Azab HM, Morgenstern M, Ahrens P, Schuster T, Imhoff AB, Lorenz SGF. Limb alignment after open-wedge high tibial osteotomy and its effect on the clinical outcome. Orthopedics. 2011;34:e622–8. https://doi.org/10.3928/01477447-20110826-02.

46. Lee D-H, Park S-C, Park H-J, Han S-B. Effect of soft tissue laxity of the knee joint on limb alignment correction in open-wedge high tibial osteotomy. Knee Surg Sports Traumatol Arthrosc. 2016;24:3704–12. https://doi.org/10.1007/s00167-015-3682-9.

47. Keppler P, Gebhard F, Grützner PA, Wang G, Zheng G, Hüfner T, et al. Computer aided high tibial open wedge osteotomy. Injury. 2004;35:68–78. https://doi.org/10.1016/j.injury.2004.05.013.

48. Wang G, Zheng G, Keppler P, Gebhard F, Staubli A, Mueller U, et al. Implementation, accuracy evaluation, and preliminary clinical trial of a CT-free navigation system for high tibial opening wedge osteotomy. Comput Aided Surg Off J Int Soc Comput Aided Surg. 2005;10:73–85. https://doi.org/10.3109/10929080500228837.

49. Lützner J, Groß A, Günther K, Kirschner S. Reliability of limb alignment measurement for high tibial osteotomy with a navigation system. Eur J Med Res. 2009;14:447–50. https://doi.org/10.1186/2047-783X-14-10-447.

17

The distal femur is a reliable guide for tibial plateau fracture reduction: a study of measurements on 3D CT scans in 84 healthy knees

Sorawut Thamyongkit[1,2], Laura M. Fayad[3], Lynne C. Jones[1], Erik A. Hasenboehler[1], Norachart Sirisreetreerux[1] and Babar Shafiq[1,4*]

Abstract

Background: Limited data have been published regarding the typical coronal dimensions of the femur and tibia and how they relate to each other. This can be used to aid in judging optimal operative reduction of tibial plateau fractures. The purpose of the present study was to quantify the width of tibial plateau in relation to the distal femur.

Methods: We reviewed 3D computed tomography (CT) scans taken between 2013 and 2016 of 42 patients (84 knees). We measured positions of the lateral tibial condyle with respect to the lateral femoral condyle (dLC) and the medial tibial condyle with respect to the medial femoral condyle (dMC) in the coronal plane. Positions of the articular edges of the lateral and medial tibia were also measured with respect to the femur (dLA and dMA).

Results: The mean (± standard deviation) measurements were as follows: dLC, − 0.1 ± 1.9 mm; dMC, − 4.7 ± 4.1 mm; dLA, 0.9 ± 1.0 mm; and dMA, 0.1 ± 1.5 mm. The mean (± standard deviation) ratio of tibial to femoral condylar width was 0.91 ± 0.03, and the ratio of tibial to femoral articular width was 1.01 ± 0.04.

Conclusions: The articular width of the tibia laterally and medially was slightly wider than the femoral articular width. These small differences and deviations indicate that the femur might be used as a reference to judge tibial plateau width reduction.

Keywords: Femoral condyle articular width, Knee, Reduction, Tibial articular width, Tibial plateau fracture

Background

Surgical outcomes after tibial plateau fracture are associated strongly with functional alignment, knee range of motion, and stability [1, 2]. The primary goals of tibial plateau fracture treatment are to restore the articular surface, sagittal and coronal alignment, and condylar width. Splitting of the lateral plateau causes a loss of lateral support for the lateral femoral condyle, leading to coronal instability and osteoarthritis [3]. Honkonen [4] found that condylar width is a predictor of clinical outcome. Residual increase in tibial condylar width after

treatment tends to affect outcomes adversely [4, 5]. Currently, the most common reference for intraoperative tibial condylar width reduction is the ipsilateral femur. Surgeons typically will drop a plumb line from the lateral femoral condyle and aim for reduction of the tibial plateau to within this line. Another goal is to align the lateral tibial articular edge with the femoral articular edge. Limited data have been published regarding the typical coronal dimensions of the femur and tibia and how they relate to each other with respect to condylar and articular width [6–8].

The purpose of this study was to quantify the relationship between measures of the distal femur and those of the proximal tibia such that they can be used to aid in judging optimal operative reduction of tibial plateau fractures. The reliability of three different means of

* Correspondence: bshafiq2@jhmi.edu
[1]Department of Orthopaedic Surgery, The Johns Hopkins University, 4940 Eastern Avenue, Baltimore, MD 21224, USA
[4]Department of Orthopaedic Surgery, The Johns Hopkins University, 601 N. Caroline St., Fl. 5, Baltimore, MD 21205, USA
Full list of author information is available at the end of the article

determining anterior-posterior (AP) view was also assessed. Our hypotheses were that (1) radiographic measurements of the distal femur would correspond reliably to those of the proximal tibia and could be used during surgery to judge fracture reduction and (2) that the posterior condylar tangent line view would provide the most reproducible AP view.

Methods
Patients

This is a retrospective review study (level of evidence: III). After obtaining institutional review board approval (IRB00105744), we reviewed computed tomography (CT) studies of patients who underwent knee CT. A total of 1465 CT studies, taken between June 2013 and May 2016, were available. We included patients aged 18–65 years who had CT scans of both knees for non-traumatic reasons, resulting in 138 patients. We excluded 96 patients who had femoral condyle hypoplasia or periarticular abnormalities such as tumors, rheumatoid arthritis, a history of fracture around the knee, a history of proximal tibia or distal femur surgery, or radiographic evidence of knee osteoarthritis of grade 2 or higher (according to the Kellgren and Lawrence classification [9]). CT images of 84 healthy knees in 42 patients (23 women) with a mean (± standard deviation) age of 48 ± 15 years were analyzed (Fig. 1).

CT technique

CT scans were performed using the Flash or Somatom Sensation 64 (Siemens Medical Systems, Malvern, PA). Images were exported to a picture archiving and communication system with three-dimensional (3D) postprocessing software (Carestream Vue PACS, Carestream Health, Rochester, NY). 3D models of the knee were created from thin-section, 0.75-mm axial cuts. All measurements were made on the resultant models.

3D CT imaging was used instead of plain radiographs, because all images could be rotated reproducibly to anterior-posterior (AP) views commonly used intraoperatively. Image rendering and image transparency were then adjusted such that two-dimensional images similar to those seen fluoroscopically were used for measurements.

Measurements

All measurements were taken in the coronal view to simulate an AP view by fluoroscopy. The following reference methods were used to define coronal views: (1) patella-in-center (PIC-AP) view, which was a coronal view of the knee with the patella centered between the distal femoral condyles; (2) fibular coverage (FC-AP) view, which was a coronal view of the knee with 50% overlap of the fibular head; and (3) posterior condylar tangent line (PCT-AP) view, which was 90° to the true lateral view of the distal femur (true lateral view of the distal femur was defined as

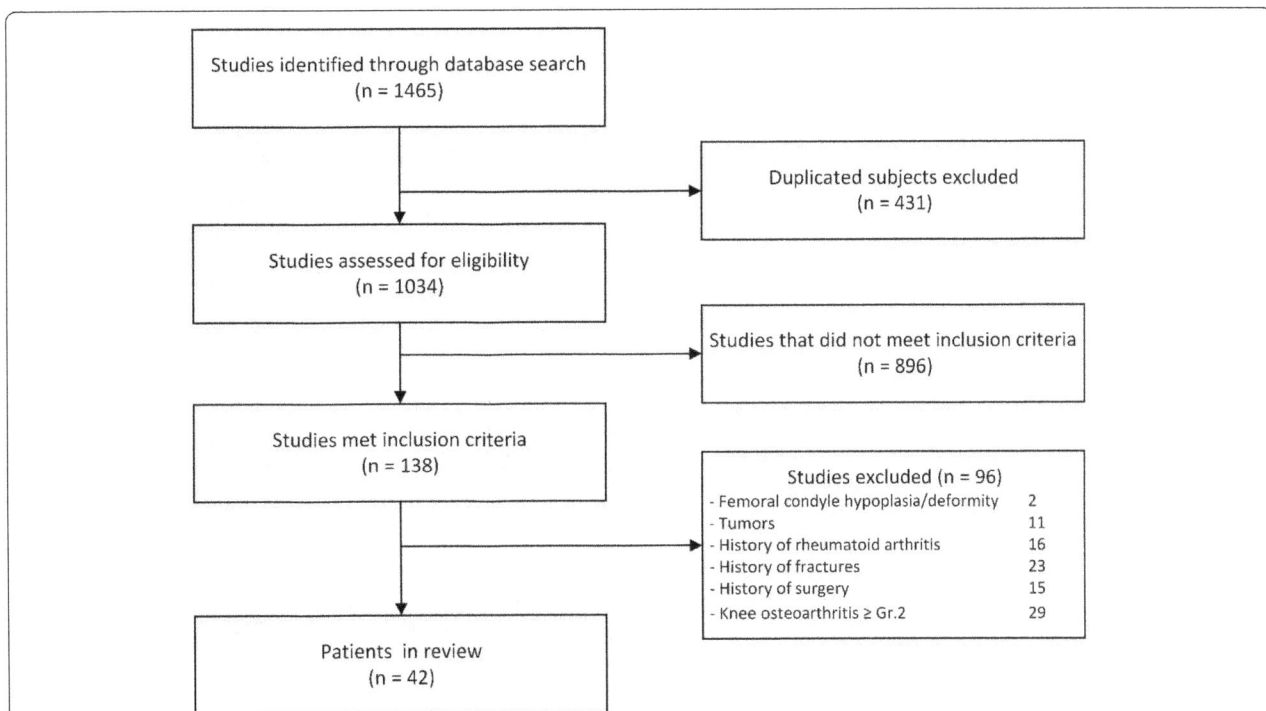

Fig. 1 Flow diagram showing selection of 42 patients who underwent knee CT scans for nontraumatic reasons between June 2013 and May 2016

the view that shows complete superimposition of the posterior aspects of the femoral condyles) (Fig. 2).

The following six comparisons were made and recorded in millimeters (Figs. 3 and 4): dLA, horizontal distance from the lateral femoral articular edge to the lateral tibial articular edge; dLC, horizontal distance from the lateral femoral condyle to the lateral tibial condyle; dMA, horizontal distance from the medial femoral articular edge to the medial tibial articular edge; dMC, horizontal distance from the medial femoral condyle to the medial tibial condyle; percent of fibular coverage by tibia on PIC-AP and PCT-AP; and tibial to femoral articular width ratio.

The first 20 patients' images were evaluated independently twice, at 2-week intervals, by the senior author, the

first author, and one additional author to determine inter- and intraobserver reliability. The measurement methods are detailed in Table 1.

Statistical analysis

According to the results of a study by Mensch and Amstutz [10], the required sample size was determined to be 35 subjects. This sample size allowed detection of a difference of 3 mm with 80% power and a two-sided α value of 0.05. Inter- and intraobserver correlation was evaluated to determine reliability using intraclass correlation coefficients (ICCs) (values greater than 0.8 are considered excellent agreement). Categorical data were analyzed using the Fisher exact test. Continuous data

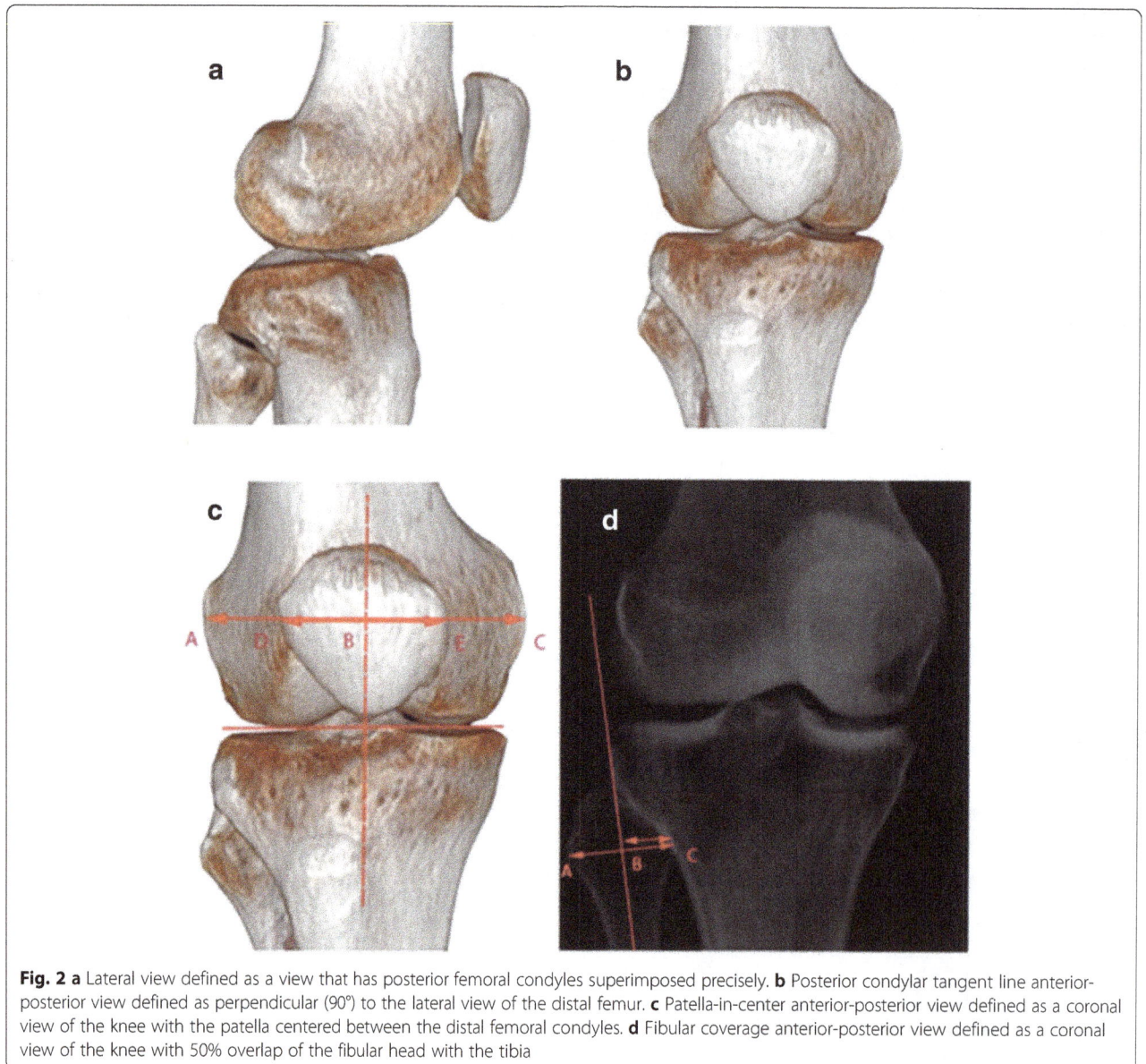

Fig. 2 a Lateral view defined as a view that has posterior femoral condyles superimposed precisely. **b** Posterior condylar tangent line anterior-posterior view defined as perpendicular (90°) to the lateral view of the distal femur. **c** Patella-in-center anterior-posterior view defined as a coronal view of the knee with the patella centered between the distal femoral condyles. **d** Fibular coverage anterior-posterior view defined as a coronal view of the knee with 50% overlap of the fibular head with the tibia

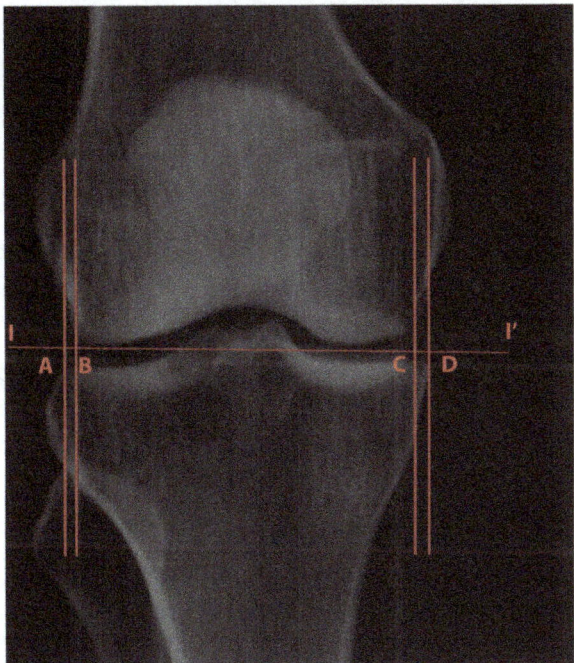

Fig. 3 Knee measurements. A–B, horizontal distance between lateral femoral articular edge and lateral tibial articular edge (dLA); C–D, horizontal distance between medial femoral articular edge to medial tibial articular edge (dMA); I–I', distal femoral joint line

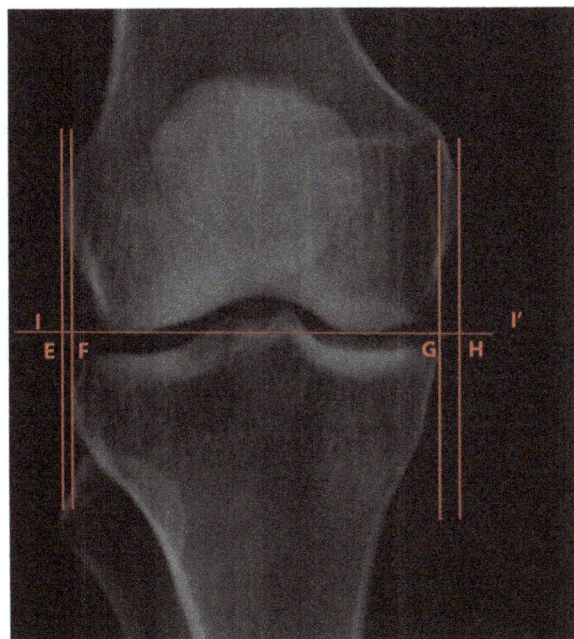

Fig. 4 Knee measurements. E–F, horizontal distance between lateral femoral condyle edge and lateral tibial condyle edge (dLC); G–H, horizontal distance between medial femoral condyle edge to medial tibial condyle edge (dMC); I–I', distal femoral joint line

were summarized as means and standard deviations and analyzed using Student t tests or analysis of variance.

Results

The inter- and intraobserver reliability of measurements on the three coronal views were evaluated. The PCT-AP view had more good-to-excellent interobserver ICC values (> 0.6) than the PIC-AP and FC-AP views ($p = 0.012$) (Table 2). Although intraobserver ICC values were not significantly different between views, most intraobserver ICC values were good-to-excellent in PCT-AP views. Therefore, we chose to analyze measurements performed using the PCT-AP view.

Using the PCT-AP view, the mean ratio of tibial to femoral condylar width was 0.91 ± 0.03, and the ratio of tibial to femoral articular width was 1.01 ± 0.04. This demonstrates that the overall femoral condyle width is slightly greater than the tibia, whereas the overall tibial articular width is slightly greater than the femur.

The mean dLC was − 0.1 ± 1.9 mm, and the mean dLA was 0.9 ± 1.0 mm. This demonstrates that when looking at the lateral side only, the lateral tibial condyle is slightly smaller than the femur, whereas the lateral tibial articular edges are wider than the femur.

The percentages of the fibula covered by the tibia in both PIC-AP and PCT-AP views were more than 50% (56% ± 11% and 67% ± 12%, respectively) (Table 3). This suggests that the 50% fibula coverage view does not correspond reliably to the most reproducible AP view, namely the PCT-AP view, and should therefore not be used as a method of judging a good AP view.

Discussion

The most reproducible AP view for making anatomic measurements was the PCT-AP view, which had higher inter- and intraobserver reliability than measurements taken in the PIC-AP and FC-AP views. Thus, we decided to analyze and report all measurements on the PCT-AP view. The results show that the contralateral tibial plateau and the ipsilateral distal femur might conceivably be used as references for tibial plateau fracture reduction. We found that the lateral articular edge of the tibia was slightly lateral to the lateral articular edge of the femur (mean dLA, 0.9 ± 1 mm). This suggests that attempting to reduce the lateral tibial condylar or articular edges to within the margins of the corresponding femoral edges will result in over-reduction. Thus, in fracture reduction, the lateral tibial plateau articular edge should be slightly more lateral and not medial to the lateral articular edge of the distal femur. Similarly, the medial articular edge of the tibia should be slightly more medial and not lateral to the medial articular edge of the femur (mean dMA, 0.1 ± 1.5 mm). Although the size of the distal femur and proximal tibia may differ between men and

Table 1 Description of distal femur and proximal tibia measurements

Measure	Description
Distance	
Lateral femoral articular edge to lateral tibial articular edge (dLA)	Horizontal distance between the most lateral femoral articular edge to the most lateral tibial articular edge, parallel to the joint line, on coronal view.[1]
Lateral femoral condyle to lateral tibial condyle (dLC)	Horizontal distance between the most lateral femoral condyle to the lateral tibial condyle, parallel to the joint line, on coronal view.[2]
Medial femoral articular edge to medial tibial articular edge (dMA)	Horizontal distance between the most medial femoral articular edge to the most medial tibial articular edge, parallel to the joint line, on coronal view.[3]
Medial femoral condyle to medial tibial condyle (dMC)	Horizontal distance between the most medial femoral condyle to the medial tibial condyle, parallel to the joint line, on coronal view.[4]
Articular width ratio	Tibial articular width (distance between the most medial to the most lateral of tibial articular edge, parallel to the joint line, on coronal view) divided by femoral articular width (distance between the most medial to the most lateral of femoral articular edge, parallel to the joint line, on coronal view)
Percentage	
Fibular coverage in PIC-AP view	Percentage of fibular coverage by tibia on coronal view. The widest aspect of the fibular head was measured perpendicular to the fibular axis. A vertical line was made at the most lateral edge of the tibia and parallel to the fibular axis. Fibular coverage was defined as percentage of fibular head width transected to the vertical line from the tibial edge. Coronal view was defined as patella-in-center between the medial and lateral epicondyle of distal femur.
Fibular coverage in PCT-AP view	Percentage of fibular coverage by tibia on coronal view. Widest aspect of fibular head was measured perpendicular to the fibular axis. A vertical line was made at the most lateral edge of the tibia and parallel to the fibular axis. Fibular coverage was defined as percentage of fibular head width transected to the vertical line from the tibial edge. Coronal view was defined as 90° to the lateral view of the distal femur (posterior aspects of the femoral condyles are superimposed).

AP anterior-posterior, *PCT* posterior condylar tangent, *PIC* patella-in-center

[1] A positive value means the lateral tibial articular edge is more lateral compared with the femur; a negative value means the femoral articular edge is more lateral compared with the tibia

[2] A positive value means the lateral tibial condyle is more lateral compared with the femur; a negative value means the lateral femoral condyle is more lateral compared with the tibia

[3] A positive value means the medial tibial articular edge is more medial compared with the femur; a negative value means the medial femoral articular edge is more medial compared with the tibia

[4] A positive value means the medial tibial condyle is more medial compared with the femur; a negative value means the femoral condyle is more medial compared with the tibia

women, there were no significant differences in dMC, dLC, dMA, and articular width ratio between men and women. Understanding these anatomic relationships may help orthopedic surgeons improve the accuracy of tibial plateau fracture reduction during surgery.

Previous studies found that an increase in the original width of the tibial plateau by more than 5 mm, or 105% compared with the femoral condylar width, is related to long-term development of degenerative lesions of the meniscus and poor outcomes [4, 5]. During tibial plateau fracture surgery, many surgeons use the ipsilateral femoral condyle or contralateral tibial plateau width as the reference width [11–17]. The contralateral tibial plateau may be more suitable as a template for repair of tibial plateau fractures because surgeons typically assume the two sides are identical. However, unequal size of the distal femoral width for each specimen in a cadaveric study has been reported [18] and may indicate a possibility of unequal size of the tibial plateaus in each individual. The drawbacks of using the contralateral knee radiograph to assess reduction are the additional radiation exposure to patients and the need for additional measurements for comparison.

Table 2 Intraclass correlation coefficients for interobserver and intraobserver reliability in three AP views

Measure	Interobserver reliability			*p*	Intraobserver reliability			*p*
	PCT-AP	PIC-AP	FC-AP		PCT-AP	PIC-AP	FC-AP	
dMC	0.71	0.61	0.50	0.012	0.67	0.57	0.63	0.253
dLC	0.84	0.44	0.44		0.70	0.81	0.76	
dMA	0.75	0.59	0.46		0.72	0.30	0.60	
dLA	0.75	0.51	0.20		0.47	0.13	0.25	

Values greater than 0.6 are considered good-to-excellent agreement

AP anterior-posterior, *dLA* distance from lateral femoral articular edge to lateral tibial articular edge, *dLC* distance from lateral femoral condyle to lateral tibial condyle, *dMA* distance from medial femoral articular edge to medial tibial articular edge, *dMC* distance from medial femoral condyle to medial tibial condyle, *FC* fibular coverage

Table 3 Morphologic measurements of 84 knees in 42 patients

Measure	Total	Side		p value	Sex		p value
		Left	Right		Male	Female	
Distance, mm							
dMC	− 4.7[a] (4.1)	− 4.5 (3.0)	− 5.0 (5.2)	0.583	− 0.6 (0.6)	− 0.4 (0.2)	0.082
dLC	− 0.1[b] (1.9)	− 0.9 (1.7)	− 0.9 (2.1)	0.958	0.0 (0.2)	− 0.1 (0.2)	0.317
dMA	0.1 (1.5)	0.0 (1.3)	0.2 (1.4)	0.443	0.0 (0.2)	0.0 (0.1)	0.076
dLA	0.9 (1.0)	1.0 (1.0)	0.8 (1.1)	0.408	0.1 (0.1)	0.1 (9.8)	0.836
Fibular coverage, %							
PIC-AP	56 (11)	56 (10)	57 (12)	0.860	59 (12)	54 (10)	0.295
PCT-AP	67 (12)	67 (12)	67 (12)	0.887	69 (13)	65 (2.4)	0.073
Articular width ratio	1.01 (0.04)	1.01 (0.04)	1.02 (0.05)	0.231	1.01 (0.05)	1.02 (0.04)	0.079

The negative values for the tibia indicate that the tibia was narrower than the femur in the coronal plane. Data are the mean, and data in parenthesis are standard deviation

AP anterior-posterior, dLA distance from lateral femoral articular edge to lateral tibial articular edge, dLC distance from lateral femoral condyle to lateral tibial condyle, dMA distance from medial femoral articular edge to medial tibial articular edge, dMC distance from medial femoral condyle to medial tibial condyle
[a]The medial femoral condyle was medial to the medial tibial condyle
[b]The lateral femoral condyle was lateral to the lateral tibial condyle

Conversely, using the distal femur as a reference does not require a second radiograph and could be a simple landmark for reduction of the proximal tibial plateau fracture.

One explanation for the discrepancy in reliability is that the PIC-AP view depends on subjective assessment of the position of the patella in the trochlea. In the FC-AP view, the percentage of fibular coverage was higher when the knee had more external rotation and lower when the knee had more internal rotation. Thus, the FC-AP view had different rotation depending on each subject's anatomy and may not have been 90° to the lateral view. In our study, PIC-AP and FC-AP views had more internal rotation compared with PCT-AP. These results support the recommendation that surgeons use the PCT-AP view because measurements taken in this view are more reliable and reproducible than those taken in the PIC-AP and FC-AP views.

There are several limitations to this study. First, we included a small number of patients (84 knees in 42 subjects) because we included only patients who had bilateral CT scans of healthy knees. Significant differences may be found in a larger study population. However, the magnitude of the difference in these measurements is likely to be small. Second, these measurements may be difficult to apply in patients who have deformity or osteoarthritic changes of the knee. Third, we used 3D CT imaging to represent AP views of two-dimensional images. A prospective study of measurements using intraoperative fluoroscopic images is needed to validate these results.

Conclusions

For intraoperative tibial plateau width reduction, the ipsilateral femoral condyle articular width is one of the reliable references. Importantly, both articular edges of the femur and tibia were almost overlapping or coincident on the AP view. The mean lateral tibial articular edge is slightly more lateral than the lateral femoral articular edge. These results support the recommendation that surgeons use the ipsilateral distal femur as one reference to guide proximal tibial fracture reduction.

Abbreviations
2D: Two-dimensional; 3D: Three-dimensional; AP: Anterior-posterior; CT: Computed tomography; dLA: Distance from lateral femoral articular edge to lateral tibial articular edge; dLC: Distance from lateral femoral condyle to lateral tibial condyle; dMA: Distance from medial femoral articular edge to medial tibial articular edge; dMC: Distance from medial femoral condyle to medial tibial condyle; FC: Fibular coverage; PCT: Posterior condylar tangent; PIC: Patella-in-center

Authors' contributions
ST contributed to the research design, acquisition and analysis of data, and wrote the manuscript. LF contributed to the acquisition of data and research design. LJ contributed to the analysis of data. EH contributed to the acquisition of data and critical revising of the manuscript. NS contributed to the acquisition of data. BS contributed to the research design, acquisition of data, and critical revising of the manuscript. All authors were fully involved in the study and approved the final version of this manuscript.

Competing interests
The authors declare that they have no competing interests.

Author details
[1]Department of Orthopaedic Surgery, The Johns Hopkins University, 4940 Eastern Avenue, Baltimore, MD 21224, USA. [2]Chakri Naruebodindra Medical Institute, Faculty of Medicine Ramathibodi Hospital, Mahidol University, 270 Rama VI Road, Ratchatewi, Bangkok 10400, Thailand. [3]Russell H. Morgan Department of Radiology and Radiological Science, The Johns Hopkins University, 601 North Caroline Street, Baltimore, MD 21224, USA. [4]Department of Orthopaedic Surgery, The Johns Hopkins University, 601 N. Caroline St., Fl. 5, Baltimore, MD 21205, USA.

References

1. Barei DP, Nork SE, Mills WJ, et al. Functional outcomes of severe bicondylar tibial plateau fractures treated with dual incisions and medial and lateral plates. J Bone Joint Surg Am. 2006;88:1713–21.
2. Malakasi A, Lallos SN, Chronopoulos E, et al. Comparative study of internal and hybrid external fixation in tibial condylar fractures. Eur J Orthop Surg Traumatol. 2013;23:97–103.
3. Rasmussen PS. Tibial condylar fractures. Impairment of knee joint stability as an indication for surgical treatment. J Bone Joint Surg Am. 1973;55:1331–50.
4. Honkonen SE. Indications for surgical treatment of tibial condyle fractures. Clin Orthop Relat Res. 1994;302:199–205.
5. Mattiassich G, Foltin E, Pietsch M, et al. Magnetic resonance evaluation in long term follow up of operated lateral tibial plateau fractures. BMC Musculoskelet Disord. 2015;16:168.
6. OF E, Kucukdurmaz F, Sayar S, et al. Anthropometric measurements of tibial plateau and correlation with the current tibial implants. Knee Surg Sports Traumatol Arthrosc. 2016;24:2990–7.
7. Shah DS, Ghyar R, Ravi B, Shetty V. 3D morphological study of the Indian arthritic knee: comparison with other ethnic groups and conformity of current TKA implant. OJRA. 2013;3:263–9.
8. Yue B, Varadarajan KM, Ai S, et al. Differences of knee anthropometry between Chinese and white men and women. J Arthroplast. 2011;26:124–30.
9. Kellgren JH, Lawrence JS. Radiological assessment of osteo-arthrosis. Ann Rheum Dis. 1957;16:494–502.
10. Mensch JS, Amstutz HC. Knee morphology as a guide to knee replacement. Clin Orthop Relat Res. 1975;112:231–41.
11. Ballmer FT, Hertel R, Notzli HP. Treatment of tibial plateau fractures with small fragment internal fixation: a preliminary report. J Orthop Trauma. 2000;14:467–74.
12. Dall'oca C, Maluta T, Lavini F, et al. Tibial plateau fractures: compared outcomes between ARIF and ORIF. Strategies Trauma Limb Reconstr. 2012;7:163–75.
13. El Barbary H, Abdel Ghani H, Misbah H, Salem K. Complex tibial plateau fractures treated with Ilizarov external fixator with or without minimal internal fixation. Int Orthop. 2005;29:182–5.
14. Hsu CJ, Chang WN, Wong CY. Surgical treatment of tibial plateau fracture in elderly patients. Arch Orthop Trauma Surg. 2001;121:67–70.
15. Kayali C, Ozturk H, Altay T, et al. Arthroscopically assisted percutaneous osteosynthesis of lateral tibial plateau fractures. Can J Surg. 2008;51:378–82.
16. Ramos T, Ekholm C, Eriksson BI, et al. The Ilizarov external fixator--a useful alternative for the treatment of proximal tibial fractures. A prospective observational study of 30 consecutive patients. BMC Musculoskelet Disord. 2013;14:11.
17. Zhai Q, Hu C, Luo C. Multi-plate reconstruction for severe bicondylar tibial plateau fractures of young adults. Int Orthop. 2014;38:1031–5.
18. Yoshioka Y, Siu D, TDV C. The anatomy and functional axes of the femur. J Bone Joint Surg Am. 1987;69:873–80.

Rationale and pre-clinical evidences for the use of autologous cartilage micrografts in cartilage repair

Marco Viganò[1†], Irene Tessaro[1†], Letizia Trovato[2*], Alessandra Colombini[1], Marco Scala[3], Alberto Magi[4], Andrea Toto[4], Giuseppe Peretti[1,5] and Laura de Girolamo[1]

Abstract

Background: The management of cartilage lesions is an open issue in clinical practice, and regenerative medicine represents a promising approach, including the use of autologous micrografts whose efficacy was already tested in different clinical settings. The aim of this study was to characterize in vitro the effect of autologous cartilage micrografts on chondrocyte viability and differentiation and perform an evaluation of their application in racehorses affected by joint diseases.

Materials and methods: Matched human chondrocytes and micrografts were obtained from articular cartilage using Rigenera® procedure. Chondrocytes were cultured in the presence or absence of micrografts and chondrogenic medium to assess cell viability and cell differentiation. For the pre-clinical evaluation, three racehorses affected by joint diseases were treated with a suspension of autologous micrografts and PRP in arthroscopy interventions. Clinical and radiographic follow-ups were performed up to 4 months after the procedure.

Results: Autologous micrografts support the formation of chondrogenic micromasses thanks to their content of matrix and growth factors, such as transforming growth factor β (TGFβ) and insulin-like growth factor 1 (IGF-1). On the other hand, no significant differences were observed on the gene expression of type II collagen, aggrecan, and SOX9. Preliminary data in the treatment of racehorses are suggestive of a potential in vivo use of micrografts to treat cartilage lesions.

Conclusion: The results reported in this study showed the role of articular micrografts in the promoting chondrocyte differentiation suggesting their potential use in the clinical practice to treat articular lesions.

Keywords: Micrografts, Cartilage repair, Regenerative medicine, Cartilage defects, Rigenera

Background

The management of cartilage lesions still represents a challenge for surgeons, due to the limited regenerative ability of cartilage, given its avascularity and hypocellularity. Additionally, cartilage defects can lead to the pathogenesis of osteoarthritis, resulting in pain and disability with a high economic and social impact in many developed countries [1]. Depending on the type of cartilage defect, different methodologies for cartilage repair and regeneration can be applied today, such as arthroscopic debridement [2], bone marrow stimulations [3], osteochondral autografts, or allograft [4]. Beyond these methodologies, autologous chondrocyte implantation (ACI) or matrix-induced autologous chondrocyte implantation (MACI) can represent valid approaches in the treatment of cartilage defects, to promote the formation of hyaline or hyaline-like cartilage and improve the pain and functional outcomes in most of treated patients. However, nowadays, the use of autologous chondrocytes is limited by the need to perform two-stage procedures and by the long recovery time required after surgery [5].

Recently, regenerative medicine approaches, based on cell therapy or tissue engineering, gather increasing interest, representing possible therapeutic alternatives.

* Correspondence: info@hbwsrl.com
†Marco Viganò and Irene Tessaro contributed equally to this work.
²Human Brain Wave, corso Galileo Ferraris 63, 10128 Turin, Italy
Full list of author information is available at the end of the article

Indeed, the use of live cells with appropriate scaffold and growth factors could allow for restoration of physiological tissue within small or large defects. Nevertheless, recent studies demonstrated that progenitors cells from cartilage are the preferred cell type for this kind of approach, since other cell types, such as bone marrow-derived mesenchymal stem cells, are not able to generate hyaline cartilage [6].

The Rigenera® procedure is an innovative clinical protocol to obtain autologous articular micrografts, containing both live cells and fragments of hyaline cartilage matrix, ready to use alone or in combination with the most common scaffolds. Previous studies have been reported that autologous micrografts are enriched of progenitor cells and maintain regenerative properties [7, 8]. The autologous micrografts are already used in dentistry [9, 10]and wound healing [11–15], reporting satisfactory results in terms of bone and dermal regeneration. Furthermore, some recent papers showed the effectiveness of micrografts also in the cartilage and cardiac regeneration [16, 17].

In this study, we provide an in vitro characterization of cartilage autologous micrografts properties on chondrocytes viability and differentiation, together with an evaluation of their pre-clinical application in racehorses affected by joint diseases, where autologous micrografts were used in combination with autologous platelet-rich plasma (PRP) to better vehicle the micrografts in the injured site and obtain a biocomplex ready to be used.

Joint diseases represent the main cause of reduced athletic function for racehorses and are characterized by a degenerative process involving several components of the joints including cartilage, subchondral bone, and articular capsule [18]. Anti-inflammatory and analgesic drugs represent the standard treatment for mild defects, while articular cartilage curettage, osteophyte removal or surgical arthroscopy, and arthrodesis can be indicated for severe cartilage and bone degeneration [19]. Nevertheless, while all these therapies effectively reduce symptoms, they are not able to restore the physiological conditions in cartilage tissue. Regenerative therapy for racehorses is assuming a growing interest for the significant economic impact on the horse industry, and racehorses can be a valuable large animal model for the evaluation of new therapies due to the interspecies similarities with humans in the thickness of the non-calcified cartilage of the stifle joint [20].

Materials and methods
Isolation of human primary chondrocytes and culture with micrografts
Human primary chondrocytes were isolated from eight samples of articular cartilage of femoral head of donor patients undergoing total hip arthroplasty. All individuals provided informed consent as per the Institutional Review Board approved procedure (M-SPER-014.ver7). Primary chondrocytes were isolated from articular cartilage (0.6–1.2 mg) using overnight incubation at 37 °C with 0.15% w/v type II collagenase (Worthington, NJ, USA) solution in DMEM (Sigma Aldrich, MO, USA) + 5% fetal bovine serum (FBS, Hyclone, Thermo-Fisher Scientific, MA, USA). Cells were then seeded at 5.000 cell/cm^2 for expansion. The autologous micrografts were obtained by Rigenera protocol after mechanical disaggregation using a medical disposable Rigeneracons (Human Brain Wave srl, Turin, Italy) [9]. Briefly, 200 mg of each sample was inserted in the Rigeneracons and minced for 5 min in a total of 5 ml of DMEM. The primary chondrocytes isolated by collagenase were cultured in four different conditions: DMEM supplemented with 10% FBS (control medium), control medium plus 10% v/v autologous micrografts, DMEM supplemented with 1% FBS and chondrogenic factors (chondrogenic medium), and chondrogenic medium plus 10% v/v autologous micrografts. For cell viability assay, only control medium and control medium with 10% v/v autologous micrografts were tested. Particles obtained after disaggregation with Rigenera ranged from 50 to 70 µm.

Cell viability
Cell viability was assessed at 1, 4, 7, and 14 days of incubation with the different media by MTT [3-(4,5-dimethylthiazol-2-yl)-2,5-diphenyltetrazolium bromide, Sigma-Aldrich] assay. Cells at passage 3 were cultured in 96-well plates at the density of 3.0×10^3 cells/cm^2; to perform the assay, a final concentration of 0.5 mg/mL MTT was added to the culture medium and incubated for 4 h at 37 °C; the medium was removed and 100% DMSO was added to each well to solubilize the precipitate. Absorbance was read at 570 nm.

Chondrogenetic differentiation assay
For chondrogenic differentiation, 5.0×10^5 cells were centrifuged at 250g for 5 min to obtain pellets. The pellets were cultured in four different media: control medium, DMEM supplemented with 100 U/ml penicillin, 100 µg/ml streptomycin, 0.29 mg/ml L-glutamine, 1 mM sodium pyruvate, 1.25 mg/ml human serum albumin (HAS; Sigma-Aldrich), and 10% FBS; chondrogenic medium, consisting of DMEM supplemented with 100 U/ml penicillin, 100 µg/ml streptomycin, 0.29 mg/ml L-glutamine, 1 mM sodium pyruvate, 1.25 mg/ml human serum albumin (HAS; Sigma-Aldrich), 1% ITS+1 containing 1.0 mg/ml insulin from bovine pancreas, 0.55 mg/ml human transferrin, 0.5 µg/ml sodium selenite, 50 mg/ml bovine serum albumin and 470 µg/ml linoleic acid (Sigma-Aldrich), 0.1 µM dexamethasone, 0.1 mM L-ascorbic acid-2-phosphate, and 10 ng/ml

TGF-β1 (PeproTech, Rocky Hill, NJ, USA) (Lopa S); control medium plus 10% *v/v* autologous micrografts; chondrogenic medium plus 10% *v/v* autologous micrografts. The medium was replaced every 3 days and cells cultured at 37 °C under a 5% CO_2 atmosphere for 4 weeks before the following evaluations.

Histology and immunohistochemistry

For the histological analysis, representative pellets from each sample and treatment ($n = 32$) were fixed in 10% neutral buffered formalin (Bio-Optica Milano SpA, Milan, Italy), embedded in paraffin blocks, and cut into 4-μm-thick sections. To detect sulfated glycosaminoglycans (GAGs), sections were stained with standard Alcian blue protocol (Bio-Optica). Briefly, slides were deparaffinized and rehydrated then stained with Alcian blue (pH 2.5; according to Mowry) for 30 min. The sections were then immersed in a sodium tetraborate solution for 10 min and counterstained with Mayer's hematoxylin, dehydrated, and mounted.

For immunohistochemical localization of collagen type I (COLL I) and collagen type II (COLL II), the sections were dewaxed and rehydrated, and a heat-induced antigen retrieval was applied using a microwave treatment for 5 min at 400 W in citrate buffer pH 6.0 (Thermo Fisher Scientific, Waltham, MA, USA). Then, the slides were treated with 3% H_2O_2 in absolute methanol for 10 min to quench endogenous peroxidases and successively with 3% *w/v* bovine serum albumin (BSA) in PBS for 30 min to inhibit non-specific reactivity. Biotinylated anti-COLL I (10 μg/ml; #7026, Chondrex Inc., Redmond, WA, USA) and biotinylated anti-COLL II (10 μg/ml; #7049, Chondrex Inc.) antibodies were applied overnight at 4 °C in a humid chamber upon sections. The primary antibodies were diluted in PBS with 1% *w/v* BSA and 0.3% *v/v* Tween 20 (Thermo Fisher Scientific). At the end of incubation, biotinylated antibodies were detected with streptavidin conjugated to horseradish peroxidase (Abcam, Cambridge, UK) and then with HIGHDEF® yellow IHC chromogen (Enzo Life Sciences Inc., Farmingdale, NY, USA). All sections were finally weakly counterstained with Mayer's hematoxylin, dehydrated, and mounted. For negative control, the primary antibody was omitted. Photomicrographs were taken with an Olympus IX71 light microscope and an Olympus XC10 camera (Japan).

GAGs deposition

Glycosaminoglycans (GAG) content was evaluated by dimethylmethylene blue (DMMB) assay. Briefly, the pellets were digested at 60 °C for 16 h in PBE buffer (100 mM Na2HPO4, 10 mM Na EDTA, pH 6.8) containing 1.75 mg/ml L-cysteine (Sigma-Aldrich) and 14.2 U/ml papain (Worthington, Lakewood, NJ, USA). The obtained extracts were incubated with 16 mg/l dimethylmethylene blue (Sigma-Aldrich), and absorbance was read at 500 nm (Perkin Elmer Victor X3 microplate reader). For normalization purposes, DNA content evaluation was performed on each sample by CyQUANT Kit (Life Technologies), following manufacturer's instructions. Data are presented as microgram of GAGs per microgram of DNA.

Quantitative real time-PCR

Total RNA was isolated from cells using TriReagent (Life Technologies) and cDNA was synthesized from 1 μg of total RNA by reverse transcription (RT) reaction. The expression of type II collagen (*COL2A1*), *SOX9*, and aggrecan (*ACAN*) mRNAs was measured by real-time RT-PCR, using TaqMan reagents (Life Technologies). The calculations of the results were carried out according to the $2^{\Delta Ct}$ methods. GAPDH was used as an internal control for data normalization [21].

Growth factors measurement

Immediately after micrograft production with the Rigenera protocol, an aliquot of the micrograft suspension was frozen at − 20 °C. Transforming growth factor β (TGFβ) and insulin-like growth factor 1 (IGF-1) concentrations in the micrograft suspensions were measured by commercially available ELISA kit, according to the manufacturer's instructions (Peprotech, UK).

Horses

Three horses (1 gelding and 2 thoroughbreds) aged from 3 to 5 years (4.4 ± 1.5) with intra-articular lesions were treated. Their characteristics, before and after treatment, are provided in Table 1.

Preparation of equine platelet-rich plasma (PRP)

Autologous PRP was prepared as previously described [22]. Briefly, two units of 450 ml of blood are collected from the horses through a standard triple-bag system, a method that allows easily the removal of 450–900 ml of blood. Sampling was done from the jugular vein after trichotomy and disinfection of the area. Blood was centrifuged at 1450 rpm for 10 min at 20 °C, in order to obtain the separation of red blood cells from plasma containing platelets and the factors that lead to the formation of a clot. Plasma is then centrifuged at 3000 rpm for 20 min at 20 °C, thus obtaining the separation of a platelet pellet and platelet-poor plasma (PPP). The platelets are then re-suspended in 30–35 ml of PPP in order to have a PRP with a platelet concentration of about 1×106 platelets/μl. The bag containing the PRP is placed on a platelet agitator under constant agitation at room temperature and after about 2 h transferred under a sterile hood to dispense the platelet concentrate into

Table 1 Baseline characteristics of horses before and after treatment

Horses	Sex and breed	Diagnosis	AAEP lameness scale (before treatment)	AAEP lameness scale (after treatment)
1	Gelding, quarter horse	Middle-carpal joint arthrosis, severe cartilage erosions, and detachment on radial and third carpal bone, radial bone fragments	3	0
2	Male, thoroughbred	Severe cartilage damage to the metacarpal-phalangeal joint, joint space reduction, early signs of bone proliferation associated with degenerative osteoarthritis at early stage	3	0
3	Female, thoroughbred	Cartilage ulcer of the dorsomedial eminence of the first phalanx. Linear erosions of metacarpal condyles. Cartilage thinning	2	1

AAEP American Association of Equine Practitioners

sterile tubes (Monovette, Sarstedt). The PRP product is stored at − 20 °C until use.

Use of equine autologous micrografts and PRP in arthroscopy interventions

Equine autologous micrografts were prepared as previously described using Rigenera protocol. Briefly, a small piece of intra-articular cartilage (weight 0.0230 g) was collected by endoscopic procedure and disaggregated by Rigeneracons medical device for 5 min for three times adding 1.5 ml of sterile physiological solution (Fig. 1a–d). The chondrocyte-derived micrografts were then mixed to 10 ml of PRP (Fig. 1d) and after an arthroscopic curettage injected in the articular lesions of horses (Fig. 1e). After the procedure, the skin is disinfected with iodine product and dressed with cotton gauze and a Vetrap-type bandage

strip. The dressing remains in situ for 48 h. A clinical follow-up was performed every week, while the radiographic follow-up was performed between 4 and 6 months after arthroscopy.

Statistical analysis

All data are reported as means ± SD. Statistical difference between two groups was determined by one-way ANOVA or t test, when appropriate. The significance was established for a p value ≤ 0.05.

Results

Effect of autologous micrografts on chondrocyte differentiation and viability

The effect of micrografts on cell viability was evaluated after 10 days of culture, and no significant interference

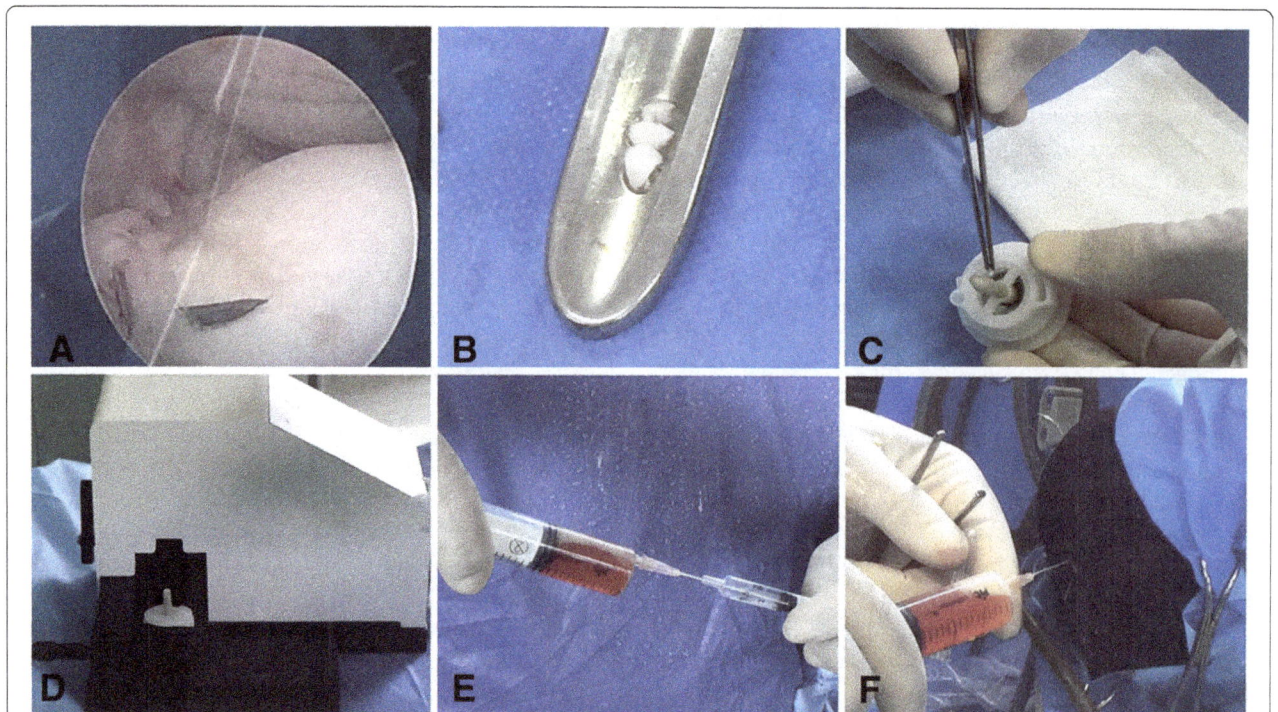

Fig. 1 Collection of equine autologous micrografts. **a, b** During the arthroscopy intervention, a small piece of intra-articular cartilage was collected by endoscopic procedure. **c, d** The intra-articular cartilage was inserted in Rigeneracons disposable and disaggregated for 2 min by a rotation process triggered by Rigenera machine. **e, f** The micrografts obtained were mixed to autologous PRP and directly injected on the lesion

was observed comparing cells cultured in the presence and absence of cartilage micrografts (Fig. 2a). The chondrocyte differentiation was evaluated by histology and immunohistochemistry on human primary chondrocyte pellets cultured in the presence or absence of autologous micrografts. The micromasses cultured in the presence of micrografts showed higher dimension and positivity to Alcian blue staining with respect to control samples. When cultured in a chondrogenic medium, these differences were less obvious, but the action of micrografts in favoring cell harboring was confirmed (Fig. 2b). In addition, a DMMB assay revealed that GAGs content was significantly increased in the cells cultured with micrografts in standard culture conditions ($p < 0.01$)

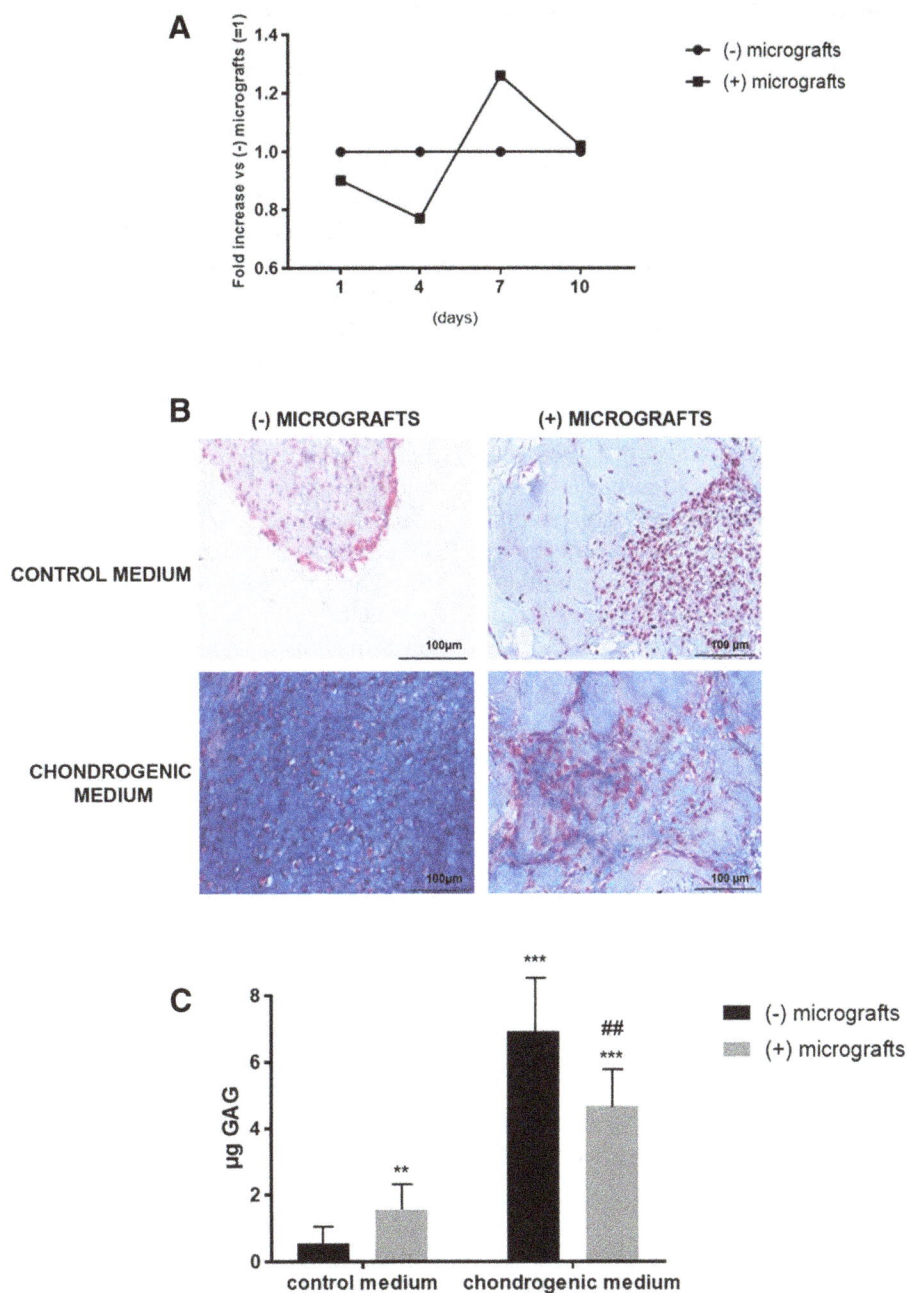

Fig. 2 Chondrogenic differentiation. a Cell viability evaluated after 10 days of culture in the presence or absence of autologous micrografts. The results are expressed as fold increase with respect to chondrocytes cultured without micrografts (= 1). b Alcian blue staining to evaluate the chondrogenic differentiation of cells cultured in the control or chondrogenic medium with or without autologous micrografts (magnification × 20). c GAGs deposition in cells cultured in the control or chondrogenic medium with or without autologous micrografts (**$p < 0.01$, ***$p < 0.001$ vs cells in the control medium without micrografts; ## $p < 0.01$ vs cells in the chondrogenic medium without micrografts)

(Fig. 2c). Nevertheless, a decrease was observed in chondrogenic medium plus micrografts cultured pellets with respect to samples maintained in chondrogenic medium alone. Despite this difference resulted statistically significant ($p < 0.01$), the differentiation ability was not prevented as demonstrated by the great increase in GAGs content observed in these pellets when compared to control cells ($p < 0.001$) (Fig. 2c).

Finally, immunohistochemistry analysis revealed a strong presence of type II collagen in the chondrocytes plus micrografts with respect to those without micrografts, both in the control or chondrogenic medium (Fig. 3). As expected, the cells are negative for type I collagen (Fig. 4), confirming the lack of trans-differentiation events.

Evaluation of the cartilage-specific gene expression

Type II collagen and aggrecan are critical components for cartilage structure. We evaluated their expression in human primary chondrocytes showing that in the chondrogenic medium, the expression of these markers increases with respect to samples cultured in control medium, in the presence or absence of autologous micrografts. The expression of the cartilage-specific transcription factor SOX9 resulted more expressed in samples treated with chondrogenic medium and micrografts, with respect to all the other culture conditions. Nevertheless, due to the high inter-donor variability, no statistically significant differences were found in the gene expression of these markers (Fig. 5a–c).

Autologous micrografts suspension contains cartilage trophic factors

The suspension of the autologous micrografts was assayed for cartilage trophic factors TGFβ and IGF-1. The mean content of TGFβ in all micrografts samples was 81.4 ± 88.2 pg/ml, while IGF-1 was 676.3 ± 212.7 pg/ml. All samples showed the presence of IGF-1, while only six out of eight samples showed the presence of TGFβ (Fig. 5d).

Use of autologous micrografts plus PRP for arthroscopic intervention in the sport racehorses

Autologous micrografts and PRP were used for arthroscopic intervention in sports racehorses affected by joint disease causing lameness. In the first horse, a severe cartilage erosion was observed (Fig. 6a) and the RX pre-intervention showed the presence of both middle-carpal arthrosis and an osteophyte on the dorsomedial edge of the radial bone with an articular fragment close to the third carpal bone (Fig. 6b). After 4 months from intervention, an improvement of articular, dorsomedial, and inter-carpal edge can be observed (Fig. 6c). In the second horse, a severe cartilaginous damage was observed (Fig. 6d) and the RX pre-intervention showed a reduced articular space and an early stage of degenerative arthrosis (Fig. 6e). After 4 months from micrografts plus PRP injection, an increase of articular and peri-articular proliferation was observed (Fig. 6f). For the third horse, the diagnosis of cartilagenous damage on the fetlock was confirmed by clinical evidences but not at a radiographic level showing no difference before and after the treatment (data not shown). In two cases, a complete resolution of lameness which allowed the recovery of sports race activity was observed (Additional files 1 and 2).

Discussion

The possibility to use biological strategies to enhance the cartilage regeneration ability in a one-step surgery would represent an important advance in the treatment of cartilage defects. Indeed, while the most used techniques are nowadays limited to microfractures for bone marrow stimulation or two-step surgeries for articular chondrocyte transplantation, the use of Rigenera® procedure would improve the feasibility of biological treatments in the field. The in vitro results reported in this study demonstrate that autologous micrografts do not affect chondrocyte viability and influence chondrocyte differentiation, as shown by both increased GAGs deposition and the presence of collagen II in primary human cells cultured in the presence of micrografts supporting the formation of chondrogenic micromasses and acting like a scaffold for chondrocyte harboring. From our experiments, the presence of IGF-1 and TGFβ in the product obtained by cartilage processing with Rigenera protocol also emerged; both factors were able to enhance cartilage repair in vivo by increasing proteoglycan synthesis and stimulating mesenchymal stem cell differentiation into chondrocytes, stimulate matrix synthesis, and reverse the catabolic effects of pro-inflammatory cytokines [23, 24].

Previous in vitro studies reported that micrografts maintained a high cell viability after mechanical disaggregation of different types of human tissues such as dental pulp, periosteum, and cardiac atrial appendage [7] and that they are able to differentiate in osteocytes, adipocytes, and chondrocytes [8].

In addition to in vitro data, the study provides positive preliminary results in the treatment of racehorses affected by joint diseases, suggesting an in vivo application of cartilage micrografts associated with PRP. The efficacy of micrografts in the cartilage repair was reported in previous human studies where the authors described the combined the use of autologous chondrocyte-derived micrografts and PRP to reconstruct not hyaline alar nasal cartilage and to promote cartilage regeneration in patients affected by external nasal valve collapse. In fact,

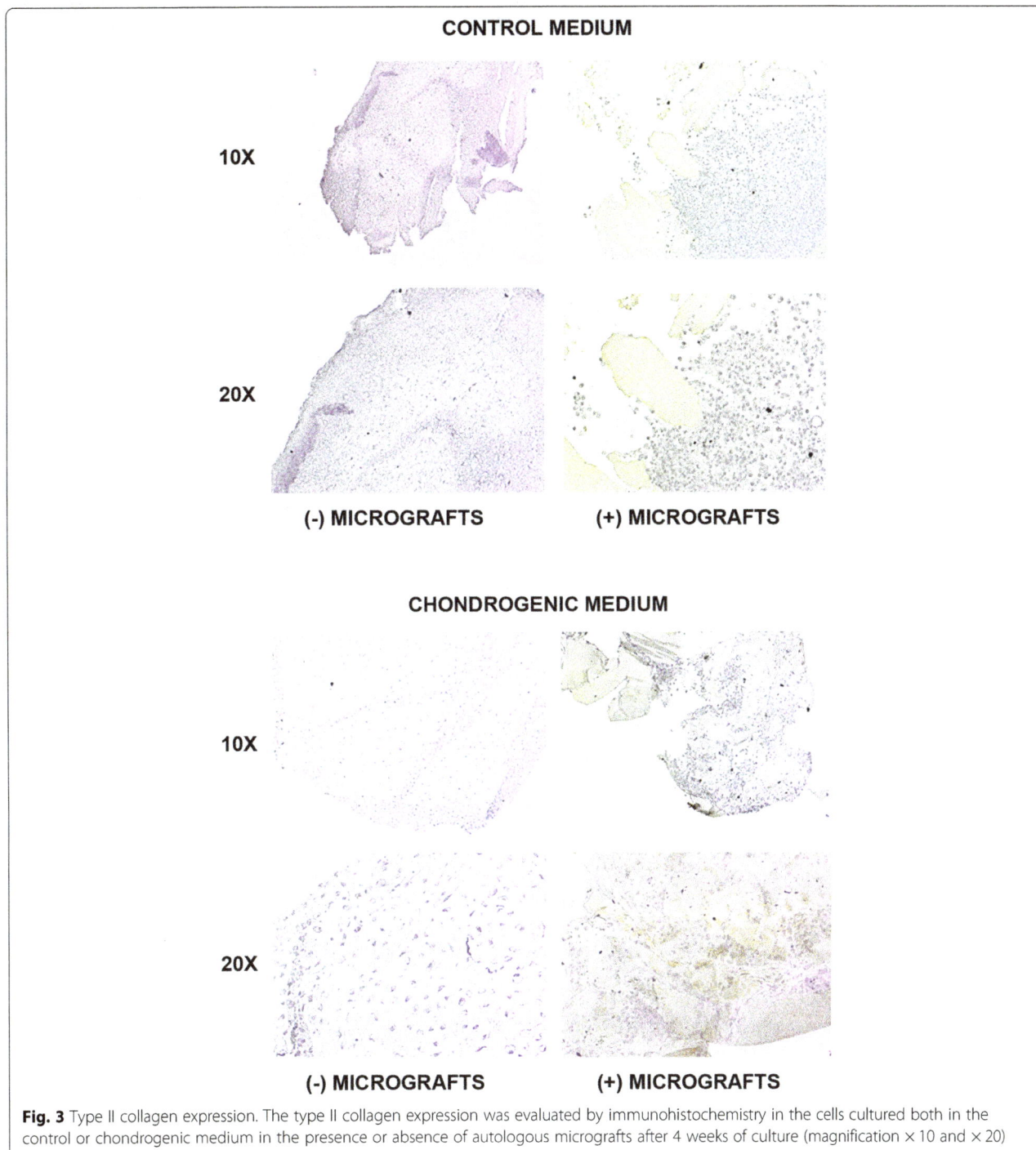

Fig. 3 Type II collagen expression. The type II collagen expression was evaluated by immunohistochemistry in the cells cultured both in the control or chondrogenic medium in the presence or absence of autologous micrografts after 4 weeks of culture (magnification × 10 and × 20)

the constructs of chondrocyte micrografts-PRP resulted in a persistent cartilage tissue with appropriate morphology, adequate central nutritional perfusion without central necrosis or ossification, and further augmented nasal dorsum without obvious contraction and deformation [16, 25].

To confirm the clinical efficacy of micrografts in the tissue repair/regeneration, several case series studies were performed in different clinical areas such as dentistry, dermatology, and wound care. To this regard, it has been reported that human dental pulp or periosteum-derived micrografts were able to promote the bone regeneration in the atrophic maxilla [9], to preserve the alveolar socket after tooth extraction by both reducing bone resorption and increasing new bone formation [10] and to promote sinus lift augmentation [26]. Autologous micrografts also improve the wound healing of complex post-operative and post-traumatic wounds [27] of post-surgical dehiscences

CONTROL MEDIUM

10X

20X

(-) MICROGRAFTS   (+) MICROGRAFTS

CHONDROGENIC MEDIUM

10X

20X

(-) MICROGRAFTS   (+) MICROGRAFTS

Fig. 4 Type I collagen expression. The type I collagen expression was evaluated by immunohistochemistry in the cells cultured both in the control or chondrogenic medium in the presence or absence of autologous micrografts after 4 weeks of culture (magnification × 10 and × 20)

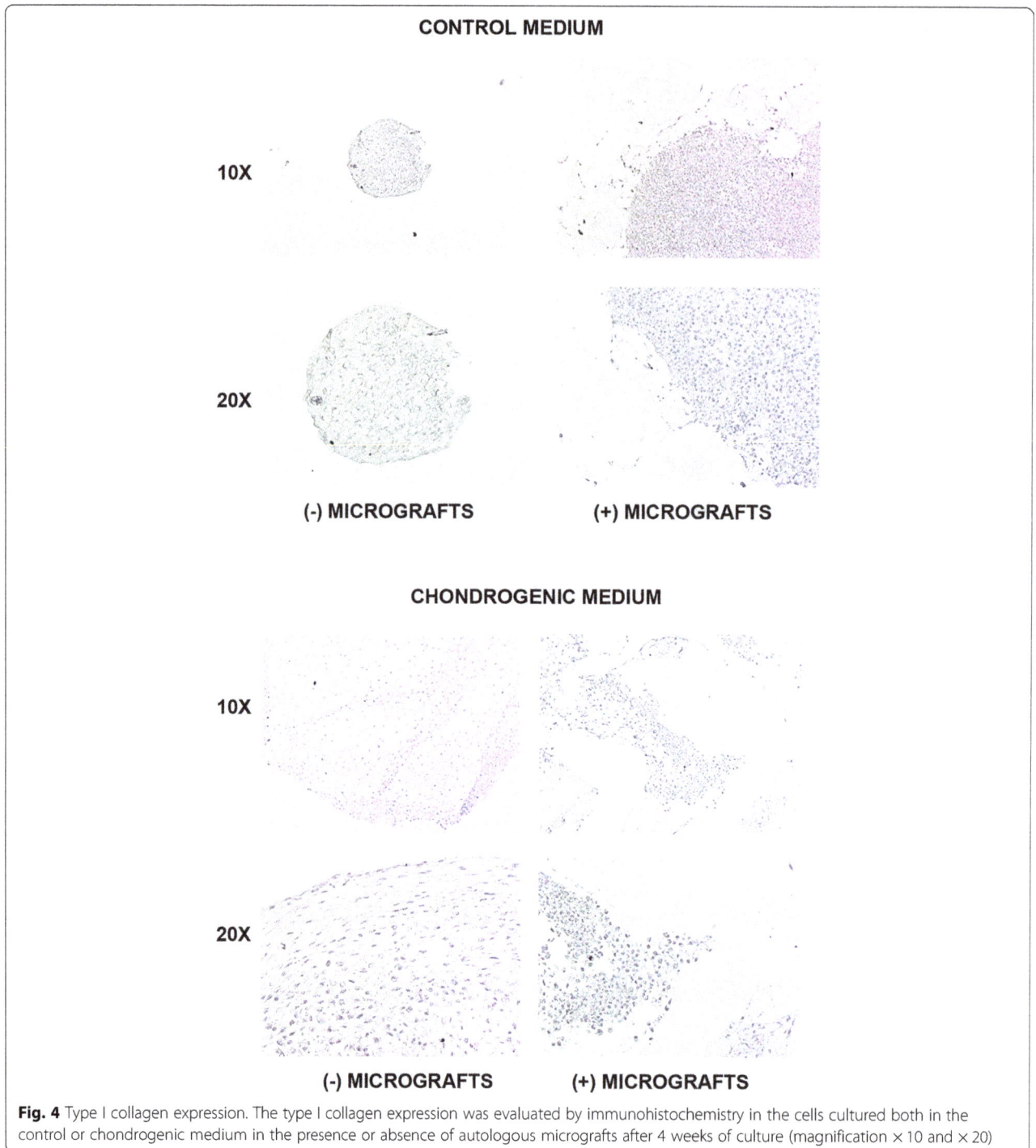

[11, 12] and chronic ulcers [13, 14]. Furthermore, micrografts were also used in the treatment of pathological and hypertrophic scars restoring the structural layers immediately below the epidermis and promoting the horizontal realignment of collagen fibers in the papillary dermis [15]. Finally, a very recent paper showed the ability of autologous micrografts to induce cardiac regeneration [17].

Joint healing can be improved by supplying stem cells, growth factors, and growth substrates at the site of injury. For example, several studies demonstrate that mesenchymal stem cells were effective in the bone and cartilage regeneration due their capacity to differentiate into osteocytes and chondrocytes and stimulate the synthesis of the chondrocyte extracellular matrix [28]. In previous studies, we showed that cells contained in the

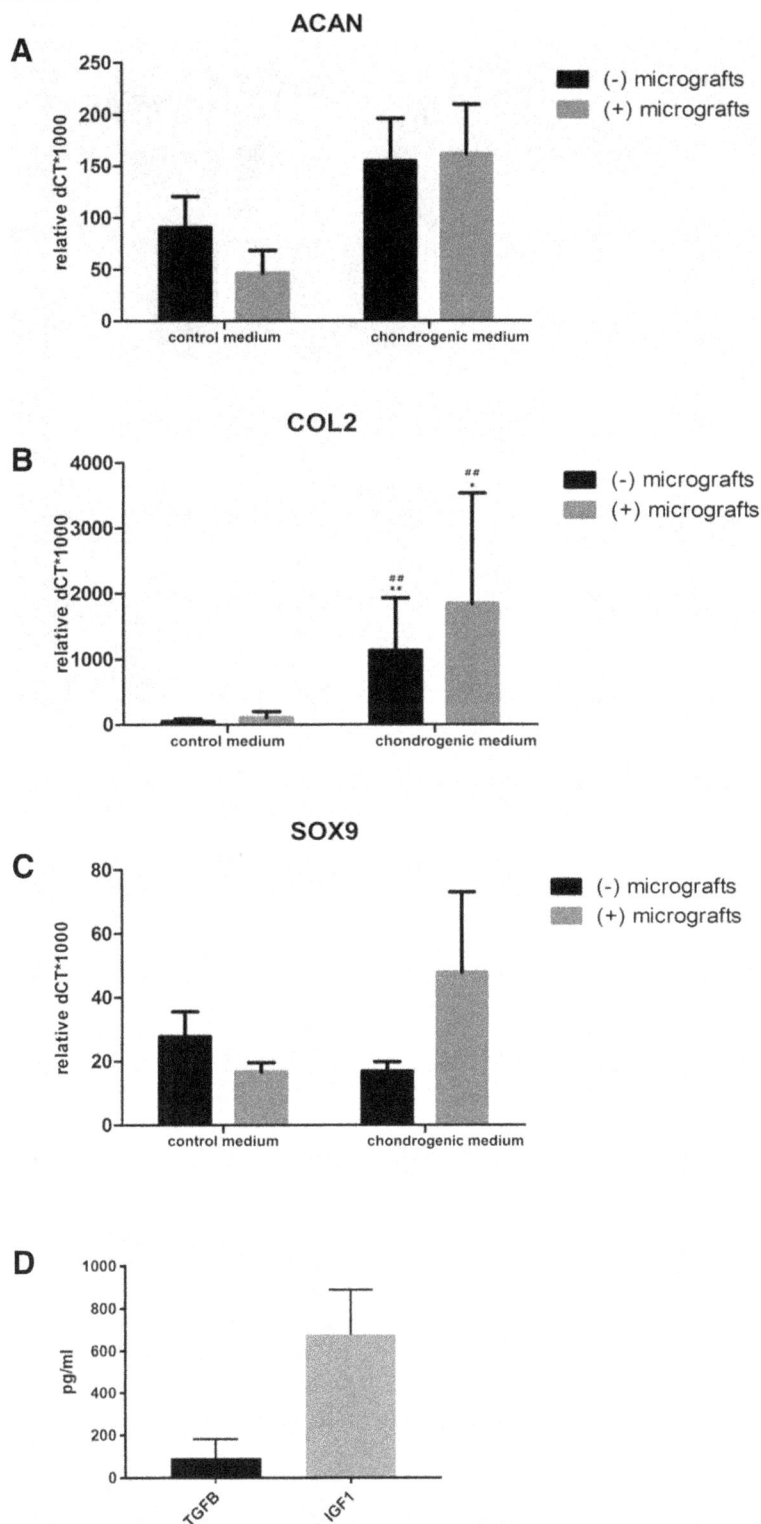

Fig. 5 Gene expression of ACAN, COL2, and SOX9 and measurement of cartilage trophic factors TGFβ and IGF-1. **a–c** mRNA expression of ACAN (aggrecan), COL2 (type II collagen), and SOX9 was evaluated in the cells cultured both in the control or chondrogenic medium in the presence or absence of autologous micrografts after 4 weeks of culture. The results are expressed as dCt vs. GAPDH. **d** The levels of cartilage trophic factors TGFβ and IGF-1 were measured by ELISA in the autologous micrografts suspension. $*p < 0.05$, $**p < 0.01$ vs control medium (–) micrografts; $^{##}p < 0.01$ vs control medium (+) micrografts

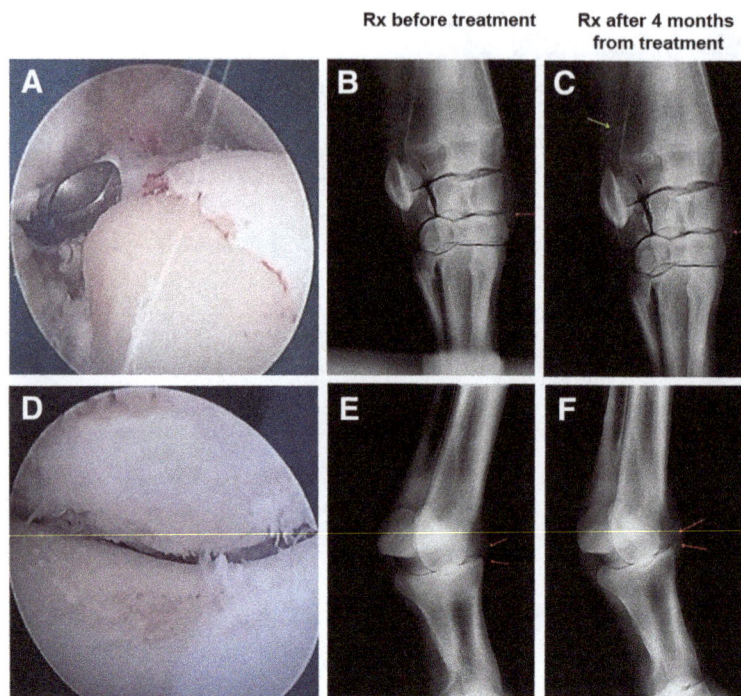

Fig. 6 Application of equine autologous micrografts in arthroscopy intervention. **a** Endoscopic image of left intercarpal joint showing the surface of the radial bone of the carpus after curettage and removal of the large portion of damaged cartilage. **b, c** Right front carpus, dorsolateral palmaro-medial X-ray pre- and post-intervention which evidences the radio-carpal joint, the middle carpal joint, and the proximal extremities of the metacarpal bones. Osteophyte on the dorsomedial edge of radial bone (yellow arrow) and articular fragment close to the third carpal bone (red arrows). **d** Endoscopic image of right metacarpal-phalangeal joint showing a severe damage to the articular cartilage. At the bottom, at the level of the lateral condyle of third metacarpal bone, and at the top, on the lateral portion of the proximal side eminence of the phalanx. **e, f** Right fetlock, dorsolateral palmaro-medial X-ray pre- and post-intervention which reports the metacarpal-phalangeal joint. Articular space and signs of bone proliferation before and after treatment (red arrows)

micrografts derived from different tissues express mesenchymal stem cells (MSCs) markers, such as CD90, CD73 and CD105, CD117, and CD44 [7, 8, 25], suggesting the presence of MSCs or tissue-specific progenitors within micrografts, as a possible explanation of their regenerative potential. Behind the stem cells, also the PRP containing both PDGF and TGF-β1 was shown to be effective in cartilage regeneration by promoting chondrocyte proliferation and synthesis of proteoglycan and type II collagen [29]. We reported in this study the pre-clinical application of autologous micrografts combined with PRP in the cartilage repair in racehorses, suggesting that a combined action of both these factors would be able to promote the osteochondral regeneration. In fact, PRP alone resulted effectively in the treatment of cartilage lesions only at short-term [30, 31], and it has been suggested that the combination with other approaches would allow for the stabilization of its beneficial effects [29]. Even if the known short-term effect of PRP may have masked the benefits of autologous cartilage micrografts, our in vivo data provide the first proof of concept for the use of the combination of these techniques in cartilage defects. Moreover, the use

of osteochondral autografts and allograft is already a well-established practice in the management of horse injuries, allowing the treatment of large defects, thanks to the immediate reconstruction of the articular surface by transfer of mature intact hyaline cartilage and the underlying subchondral bone. The success of this technique depends on the viability of chondrocytes in the graft and on the mechanical stability of the host–graft interface [32]. Furthermore, the use of osteochondral grafts transfer is limited by donor site availability in the autologous approach or joint congruency and host response in the case of allogeneic tissue [19]. The use of autologous micrografts overcomes some of these limitations, given that their collection is scarcely invasive, reducing donor site morbidity without influencing the grafts viability and overcoming the possible rejection issue related to allogeneic grafts.

Conclusion

Taken together, these results showed that autologous cartilage micrografts may promote cartilage repair, favoring chondrocytes harboring and growth, and they suggest their potential in the treatment of articular lesions in combination with PRP. However, further studies are needed to confirm the effectiveness of micrografts on cartilage repair/regeneration both alone or in combination with different approaches.

Abbreviations

ACAN: Aggrecan; ACI: Autologous chondrocyte implantation; BSA: Bovine serum albumin; COL2A1: Type II collagen; COLL I: Collagen type I; COLL II: Collagen type II; DMMB: Dimethylmethylene blue; DMSO: Dimethyl sulfoxide; FBS: Fetal bovine serum; GAGs: Glycosaminoglycans; HAS: Human serum albumin; IGF-1: Insulin-like growth factor 1; MACI: Matrix-induced autologous chondrocyte implantation; MTT: 3-(4,5-Dimethylthiazol-2-yl)-2,5-diphenyltetrazolium bromide; PPP: Platelet-poor plasma; PRP: Platelet-rich plasma; TGFβ: Transforming growth factor β

Acknowledgements
The authors thank Antonio Graziano for the coordination of in vitro and in vivo studies.

Funding
In vitro experiments were supported by the Human Brain Wave srl supplying Rigeneracons medical devices.

Authors' contributions
MV, IT, and AC participated in developing the experimental design, data interpretation, and analysis. LT drafted the manuscript. MS, AM, and AT performed in vivo experiments on horses. LdG and GP contributed to the developing of experimental design and editing of the manuscript. All authors read and approved the final submitted manuscript.

Competing interests
The author Letizia Trovato is a consultant of the Scientific Division of Human Brain Wave, the company owner of Rigenera™ technology. The other authors declare that they have no competing interests.

Author details
[1]IRCCS Istituto Ortopedico Galeazzi, via Riccardo Galeazzi 4, 20161 Milan, Italy. [2]Human Brain Wave, corso Galileo Ferraris 63, 10128 Turin, Italy. [3]Primus Gel srl, Via Casaregis, 30, 16129 Genoa, Italy. [4]Clinica Veterinaria San Rossore, via delle cascine 149, 56100 Pisa, Italy. [5]Department of Biomedical Sciences for Health, Università degli Studi di Milano, via Mangiagalli 31, 20133 Milan, Italy.

References

1. Ambra LF, de Girolamo L, Mosier B, Gomoll AH. Interventions for cartilage disease – current state of the art and emerging technologies. Arthritis Rheumatol. 2016. https://doi.org/10.1002/art.40094.
2. Badri A, Burkhardt J. Arthroscopic debridement of unicompartmental arthritis: fact or fiction? Clin Sports Med. 2014;33(1):23–41. https://doi.org/10.1016/j.csm.2013.08.008.
3. Steinwachs MR, Guggi T, Kreuz PC. Marrow stimulation techniques. Injury. 2008;39(Suppl 1):S26–31. https://doi.org/10.1016/j.injury.2008.01.042.
4. Brittberg M. Cell carriers as the next generation of cell therapy for cartilage repair: a review of the matrix-induced autologous chondrocyte implantation procedure. Am J Sports Med. 2010;38(6):1259–71. https://doi.org/10.1177/0363546509346395.
5. Devitt BM, Bell SW, Webster KE, Feller JA, Whitehead TS. Surgical treatments of cartilage defects of the knee: systematic review of randomised controlled trials. Knee. 2017;24(3):508–17. https://doi.org/10.1016/j.knee.2016.12.002.
6. Correa D, Lietman SA. Articular cartilage repair: current needs, methods and research directions. Semin Cell Dev Biol. 2017;62:67–77. https://doi.org/10.1016/j.semcdb.2016.07.013.
7. Trovato L, Monti M, Del Fante C, Cervio M, Lampinen M, Ambrosio L, Redi CA, Perotti C, Kankuri E, Ambrosio G, Rodriguez Y Baena R, Pirozzi G, Graziano A. A new medical device rigeneracons allows to obtain viable micro-grafts from mechanical disaggregation of human tissues. J Cell Physiol. 2015;230:2299–303.
8. Monti M, Graziano A, Rizzo S, Perotti C, Del Fante C, d'Aquino R, Redi C, Rodriguez Y, Baena R. In vitro and in vivo differentiation of progenitor stem cells obtained after mechanical digestion of human dental pulp. J Cell Physiol. 2017;232:548–55. https://doi.org/10.1002/jcp.25452.
9. Brunelli G, Motroni A, Graziano A, D'Aquino R, Zollino I, Carinci F. Sinus lift tissue engineering using autologous pulp micro-grafts: a case report of bone density evaluation. J Indian Soc Periodontol. 2013;17(5):644–7. https://doi.org/10.4103/0972-124X.119284.
10. D'Aquino R, Trovato L, Graziano A, Ceccarelli G, Cusella de Angelis G, Marangini A, Nisio A, Galli M, Pasi M, Finotti M, Lupi SM, Rizzo S, Rodriguez Y, Baena R. Periosteum-derived micro-grafts for tissue regeneration of human maxillary bone. J Transl Sci. 2016;2(2):125–9. https://doi.org/10.15761/JTS.1000128.
11. Baglioni E, Trovato L, Marcarelli M, Frenello A, Bocchiotti MA. Treatment of oncological post-surgical wound dehiscence with autologous skin micrografts. Anticancer Res. 2016;36(3):975–80.
12. Marcarelli M, Trovato L, Novarese E, Riccio M, Graziano A. Rigenera protocol in the treatment of surgical wound dehiscence. Int Wound J. 2017;14(1):277–81. https://doi.org/10.1111/iwj.12601.
13. Trovato L, Failla G, Serantoni S, Palumbo FP. Regenerative surgery in the management of the leg ulcers. J Cell Sci Ther. 2016;7:238. https://doi.org/10.4172/2157-7013.1000238.
14. De Francesco F, Graziano A, Trovato L, Ceccarelli G, Romano M, Marcarelli M, Cusella De Angelis GM, Cillo U, Riccio M, Ferraro GA. A regenerative approach with dermal micrografts in the treatment of chronic ulcers. Stem Cell Rev. 2017;13(1):149. https://doi.org/10.1007/s12015-016-9698-9.
15. Svolacchia F, De Francesco F, Trovato L, Graziano A, Ferraro GA. An innovative regenerative treatment of scars with dermal micrografts. J Cosmet Dermatol. 2016;15(3):245–53. https://doi.org/10.1111/jocd.12212.
16. Gentile P, Scioli MG, Bielli A, Orlandi A, Cervelli V. Reconstruction of alar nasal cartilage defects using a tissue engineering technique based on a combined use of autologous chondrocyte micrografts and platelet-rich plasma: preliminary clinical and instrumental evaluation. Plast Reconstr Surg Glob Open. 2016;4(10):e1027.
17. Lampinen M, Nummi A, Nieminen T, Harjula A, Kankuri E. Intraoperative processing and epicardial transplantation of autologous atrial tissue for cardiac repair. J Heart Lung Transplant. 2017;36(9):1020–2. https://doi.org/10.1016/j.healun.2017.06.002.
18. Branly T, Bertoni L, Contentin R, Rakic R, Gomez-Leduc T, Desancé M, Hervieu M, Legendre F, Jacquet S, Audigié F, Denoix JM, Demoor M, Galéra P. Characterization and use of equine bone marrow mesenchymal stem cells in equine cartilage engineering. Study of their hyaline cartilage forming potential when cultured under hypoxia within a biomaterial in the presence of BMP-2 and TGF-ß1. Stem Cell Rev. 2017. https://doi.org/10.1007/s12015-017-9748-y.
19. Cokelaere S, Malda J, van Weeren R. Cartilage defect repair in horses: current strategies and recent developments in regenerative medicine of the

equine joint with emphasis on the surgical approach. Vet J. 2016;214:61–71. https://doi.org/10.1016/j.tvjl.2016.02.005.

20. Barrett JG. A set of grand challenges for veterinary regenerative medicine. Front Vet Sci. 2016;3:20. https://doi.org/10.3389/fvets.2016.00020.

21. Lopa S, Ceriani C, Cecchinato R, Zagra L, Moretti M, Colombini A. Stability of housekeeping genes in human intervertebral disc, endplate and articular cartilage cells in multiple conditions for reliable transcriptional analysis. Eur Cell Mater. 2016;31:395–406.

22. Scala M, Lenarduzzi S, Spagnolo F, Trapasso M, Ottonello C, Muraglia A, Barla A, Squillario M, Strada P. Regenerative medicine for the treatment of Teno-desmic injuries of the equine. A series of 150 horses treated with platelet-derived growth factors. In Vivo. 2014;28(6):1119–23.

23. Freyria AM, Mallein-Gerin F. Chondrocytes or adult stem cells for cartilage repair: the indisputable role of growth factors. Injury. 2012;43(3):259–65. https://doi.org/10.1016/j.injury.2011.05.035.

24. Bernhard JC, Vunjak-Novakovic G. Should we use cells, biomaterials, or tissue engineering for cartilage regeneration? Stem Cell Res Ther. 2016;7(1): 56. https://doi.org/10.1186/s13287-016-0314-3.

25. Ceccarelli G, Gentile P, Marcarelli M, Balli M, Ronzoni FL, Benedetti L, Cusella De Angelis MG. In vitro and in vivo studies of alar-nasal cartilage using autologous micro-grafts: the use of the Rigenera® protocol in the treatment of an osteochondral lesion of the nose. Pharmaceuticals (Basel). 2017;10(2). https://doi.org/10.3390/ph10020053.

26. Rodriguez Y, Baena R, D'Aquino R, Graziano A, Trovato L, Aloise AC, Ceccarelli G, Cusella G, Pelegrine AA, Lupi SM. Autologous periosteum-derived micrografts and PLGA/HA enhance the bone formation in sinus lift augmentation. Front Cell Dev Biol. 2017;5:87. https://doi.org/10.3389/fcell.2017.00087.

27. Purpura V, Bondioli E, Graziano A, Trovato L, Melandri D, Ghetti M, Marchesini A, Cusella de Angelis MG, Benedetti L, Ceccarelli G, Riccio M. Tissue characterization after a new disaggregation method for skin micro-grafts generation. J Vis Exp. 2016;(109):e53579. https://doi.org/10.3791/53579.

28. Goldberg A, Mitchell K, Soans J, Kim L, Zaidi R. The use of mesenchymal stem cells for cartilage repair and regeneration: a systematic review. J Orthop Surg Res. 2017;12:39. https://doi.org/10.1186/s13018-017-0534-y.

29. Sermer C, Devitt B, Chahal J, Kandel R, Theodoropoulos J. The addition of platelet-rich plasma to scaffolds used for cartilage repair: a review of human and animal studies. Arthroscopy. 2015;31(8):1607–25. https://doi.org/10.1016/j.arthro.2015.01.027.

30. Serra CI, Soler C, Carrillo JM, Sopena JJ, Redondo JI, Cugat R. Effect of autologous platelet-rich plasma on the repair of full-thickness articular defects in rabbits. Knee Surg Sports Traumatol Arthrosc. 2013;21(8): 1730–6. https://doi.org/10.1007/s00167-012-2141-0 Erratum in: Knee Surg Sports Traumatol Arthrosc. 2014 Jul;22(7):1710. Carillo, Jose M [corrected to Carrillo, Jose M].

31. Filardo G, Kon E, Buda R, Timoncini A, Di Martino A, Cenacchi A, Fornasari PM, Giannini S, Marcacci M. Platelet-rich plasma intra-articular knee injections for the treatment of degenerative cartilage lesions and osteoarthritis. Knee Surg Sports Traumatol Arthrosc. 2011;19(4):528–35. https://doi.org/10.1007/s00167-010-1238-6.

32. Pallante AL, Chen AC, Ball ST, Amiel D, Masuda K, Sah RL, Bugbee WD. The in vivo performance of osteochondral allografts in the goat is diminished with extended storage and decreased cartilage cellularity. Am J Sports Med. 2012;40:1814–23.

19

Accurate determination of post-operative 3D component positioning in total knee arthroplasty: the AURORA protocol

Edgar A Wakelin[1*], Linda Tran[1], Joshua G Twiggs[1,2], Willy Theodore[1], Justin P Roe[3], Michael I Solomon[4], Brett A Fritsch[5] and Brad P Miles[1]

Abstract

Background: Successful component alignment is a major metric of success in total knee arthroplasty. Component translational placement, however, is less well reported despite being shown to affect patient outcomes. CT scans and planar X-rays are routinely used to report alignment but do not report measurements as precisely or accurately as modern navigation systems can deliver, or with reference to the pre-operative anatomy.

Methods: A method is presented here that utilises a CT scan obtained for pre-operative planning and a post-operative CT scan for analysis to recreate a computation model of the knee with patient-specific axes. This model is then used to determine the post-operative component position in 3D space.

Results: Two subjects were investigated for reproducibility producing 12 sets of results. The maximum error using this technique was $0.9° \pm 0.6°$ in rotation and 0.5 mm ± 0.3 mm in translation. Eleven subjects were investigated for reliability producing 22 sets of results. The intra-class correlation coefficient for each of the three axes of rotation and three primary resection planes was > 0.93 indicating excellent reliability.

Conclusions: Routine use of this analysis will allow surgeons and engineers to better understand the effect of component alignment as well as the placement on outcome.

Keywords: Registration, CT scan, Total knee arthroplasty, Alignment, Reliability, Reproducibility

Background

Dissatisfaction amongst total knee arthroplasty (TKA) is the result of a complex relationship between the patient anatomy, prosthesis design and position, and other patient-specific factors. Prosthesis malalignment has been linked to poor patient outcomes in which coronal and axial malalignment has been most closely studied [1, 2]. To have confidence in the correlation between component alignment and outcome, the method used to determine component placement must be accurate and reliable.

Component alignment refers to the angular difference between the prosthetic components and patient-derived antero-posterior (AP), medio-lateral (ML), and superior-inferior (SI) anatomic axes. This measurement has traditionally been the focus of post-operative analysis in

TKA due to the ease of measurement [3–5]. Component placement refers to the translational movement of the prosthetic components along these patient-specific axes. Due to difficulty in identifying the origin of these axes and accurately determining translation in space, component placement has been less well investigated. To understand the holistic effect of the TKA components on knee kinematics, both the alignment and placement must be taken into account. Here, we term the combination of component alignment and placement as 'component position'.

The pre-operative state of the patient is a critical source of missing data from most analyses which prevents accurate reporting of component position. Bony resections cannot be accurately determined from a post-op analysis alone, and as a result, there is very little data available on the outcome of TKA as a result of the modification of the anatomy [6, 7], highlighting the need

---

* Correspondence: edgar@kneesystems.com
[1]360 Knee Systems, Suite 3, Building 1, Sydney, NSW 2073, Australia
Full list of author information is available at the end of the article

for improved post-operative analysis techniques. Nevertheless, studies have investigated a range of movement and maximum flexion as a function of the posterior condylar offset (PCO) [8–10]. In these publications, a greater PCO resulted in higher maximum flexion due to reduced steric hindrance. Pre- and post-operative measurements however were limited by the use of ML X-rays, indicating that the relationship must be strong to overcome such errors.

Alteration of the joint line and flexion/extension gaps is associated with a change in joint kinematics [11] and patient outcome [12]. In these studies, patients with less change to the coronal joint line reported improved WOMAC and Knee Society Clinical Rating Scores. Identification of such changes however can be difficult, as the joint line and joint gaps can be modified without affecting the appearance of the component alignment [5]. To better understand the effect of bone resections and joint line and gap modification, accurate pre-operative geometry data is required. Similarly, Bengs and Scott [13] found that increasing the patella button thickness without increasing the patella resection decreased the maximum passive flexion. Identification of appropriate patella resection for a given button thickness would not be possible with traditional post-operative analysis techniques.

Traditional methods of assessing TKA component alignment, including short leg X-rays [14–16], long leg X-rays [17], and post-operative 3D imaging only [18–22], have been shown to suffer inaccuracies from anatomic variability and projection errors and difficulty in identifying patient-specific landmarks from the post-operative imaging. To improve landmarking and component placement accuracy, a pre-operative CT is required. Fortunately, CT imaging is rapidly becoming a standard of care in pre-operative planning for TKA [23] and is available for a wide range of patients. Pre-operative CT imaging allows a volumetric registration of the pre-operative and post-operative bones and component geometries in 3D space eliminating any anatomic assumptions and projection errors. The models can then be used to determine bony resections and component placement. A method to compare the pre-operative state of the knee to the post-operative component position and bone resections, in which accuracy has not been affected by component flare, has not yet been achieved.

Here, we introduce a method of 3D reconstruction which utilises both a pre-operative and post-operative CT scan to determine the post-operative component position in TKA. The method may be extended to any joint replacement and is termed here the Australian Universal Resection, Orientation, and Rotation Analysis (AURORA) protocol. Landmarks and bone models unaffected by component flare obtained from the pre-operative scan are transformed into the post-operative frame of reference. Component position as defined by the landmarked patient-specific axes and bony resections are reported. The reproducibility and reliability of this method are presented and compared to other post-operative analysis techniques.

Methods

CT protocol

A series of patients received long leg pre-operative CT scans for the routine pre-operative planning of TKA surgery [24] and to design patient-specific instrumentation. Ethics approval for all data collection and accessing information from a joint registry for this study was approved by Bellberry Ethics (Sydney, Australia) (approval 2012-03-710). The same protocol is followed for post-operative CT imaging. This protocol requires the patient to be in supine at the isocentre of the gantry, with both legs fully extended and parallel to the horizontal plane. The legs are straightened and maintained in a relaxed position. Image acquisition involves a full leg pass CT scan taken through both limbs with all images taken in the same field of view, see Fig. 1. This allows detection of any patient movement during the scanning process. Transverse slice thicknesses of 1.25 mm are taken, with less than 1 mm slices taken within the sagittal and coronal axis.

All patients investigated here had a TKA using OMNI APEX implants (Raynham, MA), from four different surgeons using four different techniques. Patients were randomly selected from a database of over 2000 TKA surgeries.

The CT dose is calculated by multiplying the dose-length-product (mGy.cm) provided as supporting information with the CT scan, by the length of the CT scan in which the patient is imaged. The dose value is then converted to an effective dose based on anatomic conversion coefficients presented by Saltybaeva et al. [25] to allow comparison between different CT protocols. Movement in the scan can affect both individual bone and long leg measurements. Movement is detected by an engineer assessing the scan before processing. All patients were randomly selected from a database of patients scanned over a 3-month period previously confirmed to have not moved.

Image processing and volumetric registration

3D reconstructed patient femur and tibia bones are generated within the pre-operative planning process through semi-automated segmentation, used to landmark and identify points of interest by biomedical engineers using the 3D imaging software, ScanIP (Simpleware, Exeter, UK). The patient bones are converted to stereolithography (STL) files and landmarked twice by different engineers. If any landmarks differ by a threshold value (in this case 4 mm), the landmark was reviewed by another trained engineer. Landmark references were used to define patient-specific bone axes and soft tissue attachment sites, see Fig. 2a. The

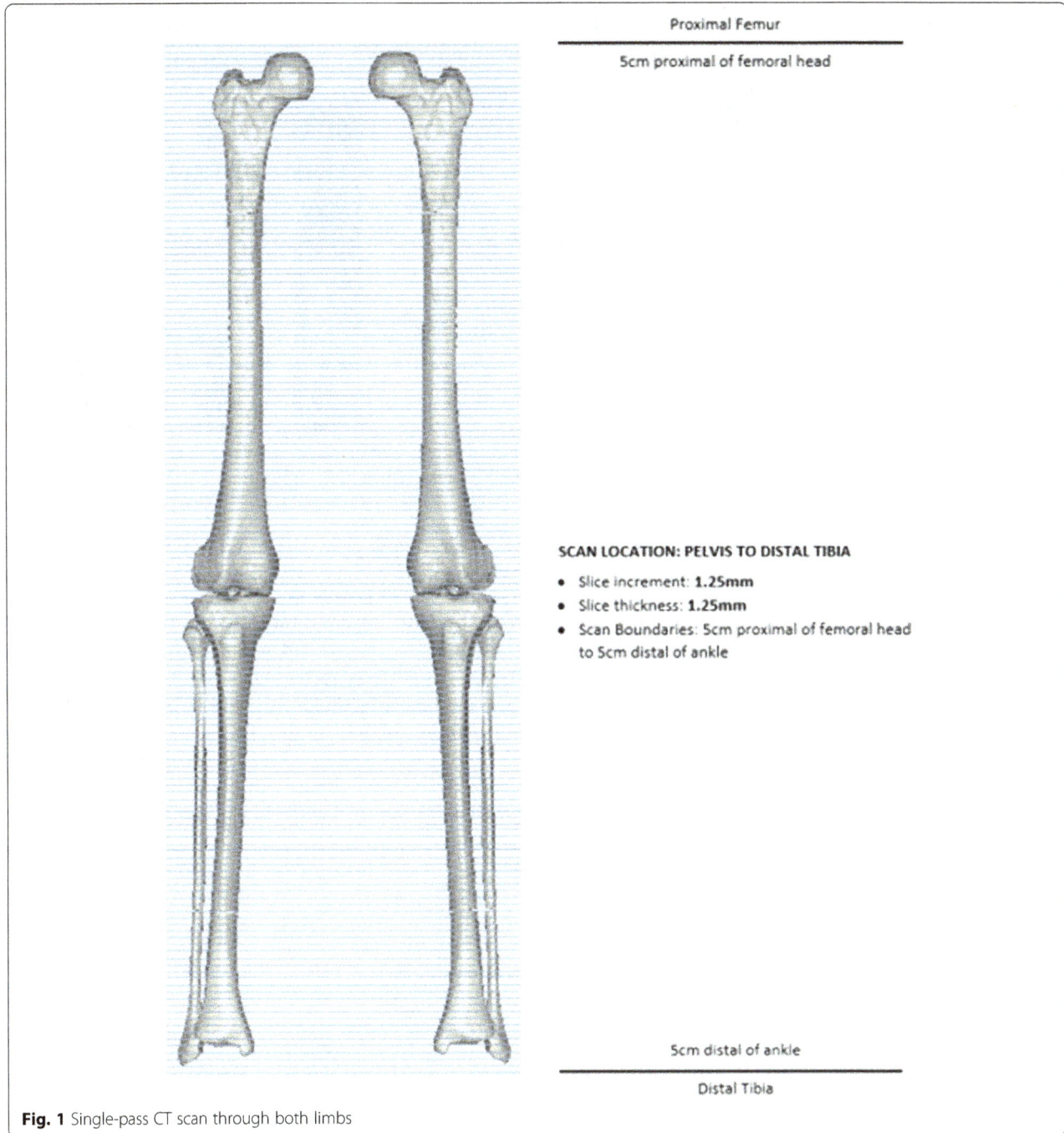

Proximal Femur

5cm proximal of femoral head

SCAN LOCATION: PELVIS TO DISTAL TIBIA

- Slice increment: **1.25mm**
- Slice thickness: **1.25mm**
- Scan Boundaries: 5cm proximal of femoral head to 5cm distal of ankle

5cm distal of ankle

Distal Tibia

Fig. 1 Single-pass CT scan through both limbs

femoral and hip centres are landmarked to define the mechanical axis of the femur. The tibial mechanical axis is defined from the midpoint of the lateral and medial malleoli to the midpoint of the medial 1/3 of the tubercle and posterior cruciate ligament (PCL) insertion. The tibial AP axis is defined along the medial 1/3 of the tubercle and PCL insertion, while the transepicondylar axis (TEA) is defined along the medial sulcus to the lateral epicondyle on the femur. These axes are used to define a frame of reference from which implant position may be calculated.

Using the post-operative full leg CT scan, the 3D post-operative femur and tibia bone sections unaffected by the component flare are segmented, see Fig. 2b. 3D registration is then performed, by registering the pre-operative femur and tibia models into the post-operative CT with reference to both the imaging and newly generated post-operative bone models, see Fig. 2c. Point-to-point registration is performed on CAD models of the implanted prosthesis and segmented prosthesis models from the CT, see Fig. 2c. All registration is refined using model outlines viewed

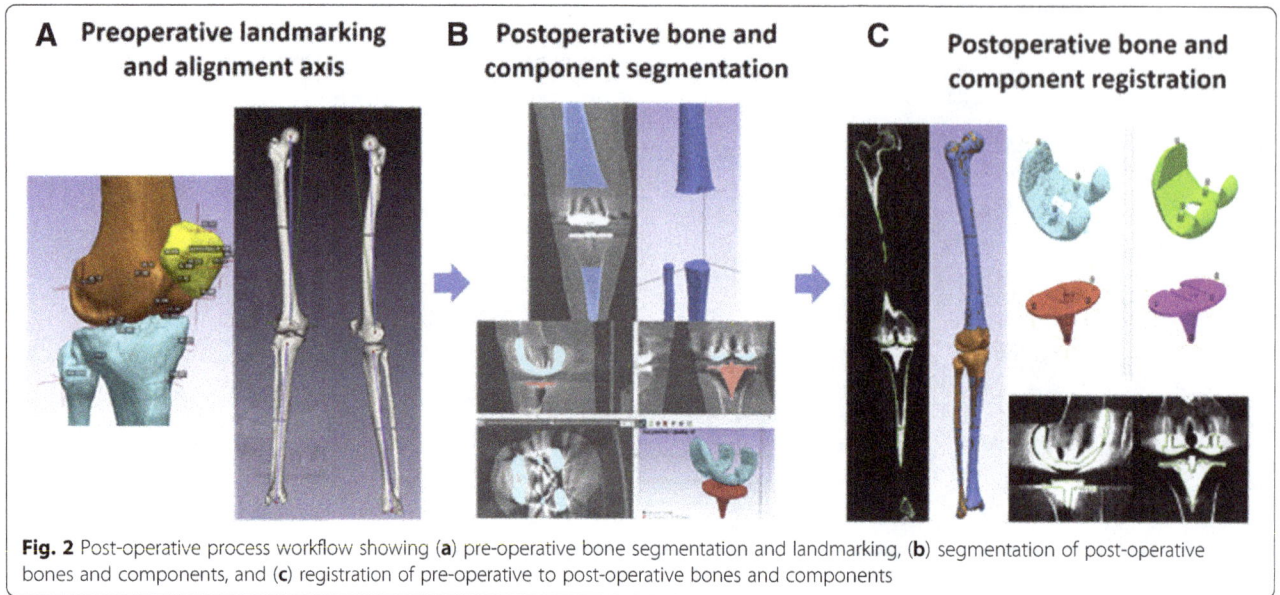

Fig. 2 Post-operative process workflow showing (**a**) pre-operative bone segmentation and landmarking, (**b**) segmentation of post-operative bones and components, and (**c**) registration of pre-operative to post-operative bones and components

in the full leg CT scan. A second engineer reviews both the registered femur and tibia bones and the femoral and tibial implant components to further refine both bone and implant positions within the CT scan.

Euler transform matrices are obtained from the resulting registered pre-operative bones and used to transform the pre-operative bone landmarks into the post-operative CT reference frame. Using the transformed landmark references, component alignment and placement are determined within the local reference frames from the defined axes of landmarks identified pre-operatively.

Accuracy testing
Reproducibility
Two primary TKR patients were processed post-operatively twice by three engineers in a 2-week period. Patient CT scans were segmented and registered by an engineer and then reviewed by a second engineer. The same case was processed again by the initial engineer on another day at a different time of day and then reviewed by a third engineer. This process was repeated across the three engineers for the two cases with alternating reviewers, and a total of 12 registrations was then analysed (see Fig. 3).

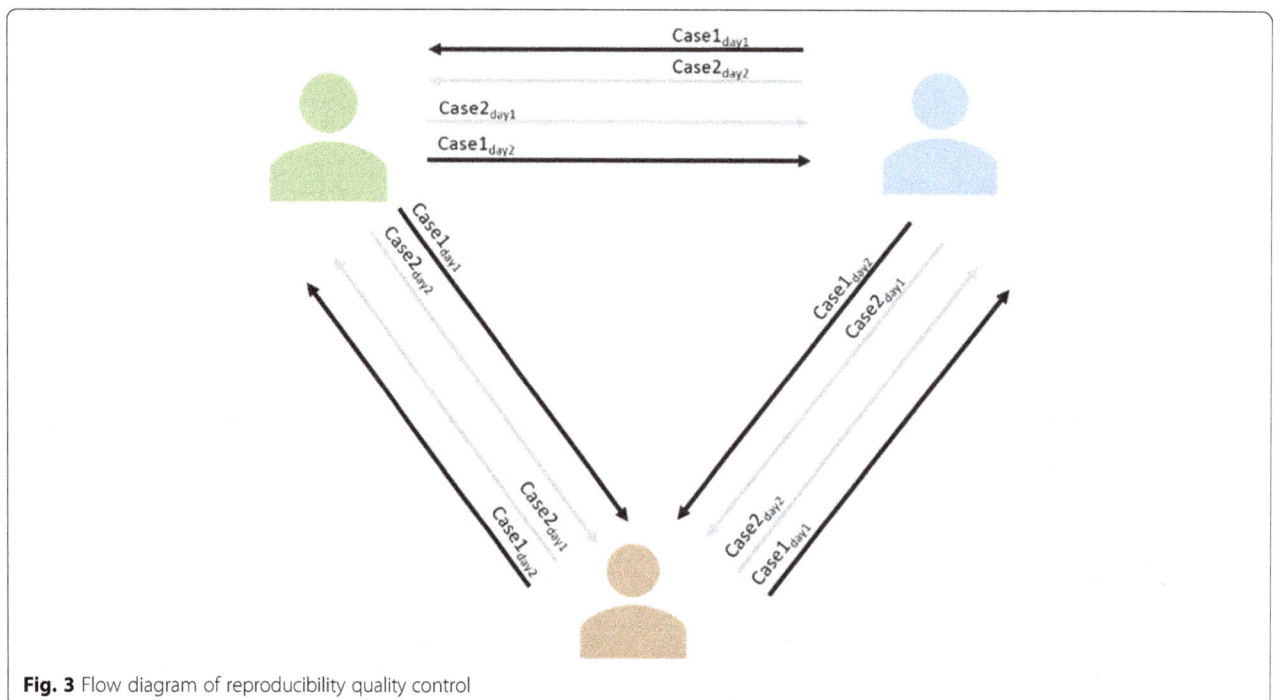

Fig. 3 Flow diagram of reproducibility quality control

Comparison of component alignment angles in flexion/extension (FE), varus/valgus (VV), and internal/external (IE) rotation, and component placement values by measuring the femoral medial and lateral, distal and posterior condyles, and the medial and lateral tibial plateau was recorded. Reproducibility was assessed from these angular and resection measurements by determining the maximum difference and standard deviation from the mean calculated for each patient, with the 95% confidence interval defined across both cases.

Reliability

To describe the interobserver reliability, 11 TKR patients were processed post-operatively between two engineers. Each case was reviewed by a third and fourth engineer, with refinement of the bone and component registration made by the reviewing engineer if necessary. A set of 22 results was produced for the comparison of the three rotation axes across two components and six resection measurements. The intra-class correlation coefficient (ICC) was calculated for each of the measurements. An ICC value of 1 shows perfect reliability, values greater than 0.9 indicates an excellent result, 0.81 to 0.9 is very good, 0.76 to 0.80 is good, 0.5 to 0.75 is moderate, and < 0.50 is considered to show poor reliability [26, 27].

Results

Radiation dose

The average effective radiation dose received per CT scan using this protocol is 1.24 ± 0.96 mSv. This dose is compared to other CT and radiography protocols in Fig. 4. The average received dose is lower than all protocols shown in the figure with the exception of the most recent Imperial Protocol [6] and a standard AP radiograph. The spread of values shown for the AURORA CT

protocol used here reflects the large range of patient sizes scanned. Smaller patients receive a correspondingly lower dose of radiation and vice versa for larger patients.

Using the AURORA protocol, patient movement in the CT scan may be detected at any point along the length of the bone. In previous methods, such as the Perth CT and Imperial protocols, movement in the mid-femur and mid-tibia will not be detected, leaving any measurements to propagate through the protocol as an error. In a database of CT scans obtained for the routine pre-operative planning of TKA, the rate of scans identified with movement over a 3-month period is 6.78% (total number of scans, 118). Of this fraction, all movement in the scans were detected in the mid-femur and mid-tibia regions.

Reproducibility

The alignment reproducibility results generated from three engineers processing two cases at two different time points which were then QC checked are shown in Table 1. The maximum difference from the mean angle is shown for each case. In both cases, the maximum difference is reported for tibial component axial rotation, of 0.9° for case 1 and 0.7° for case 2. In all other angles, the maximum difference in rotation is ≤ 0.5°. The confidence intervals in all cases are less than 0.3° with the exception of tibial tray IE rotation, which is 0.6° for case 1 and 0.4° for case 2.

The bony resection thicknesses are a proxy measure for the accuracy of measuring component placement and are shown in Table 2 for the distal medial and lateral condyles, posterior medial and lateral condyles, and tibial medial and lateral plateaus. The maximum difference from the mean resection is shown for each case. In both cases, the maximum difference is reported for the medial tibial plateau, of 0.5 mm for case 1 and 0.3 mm

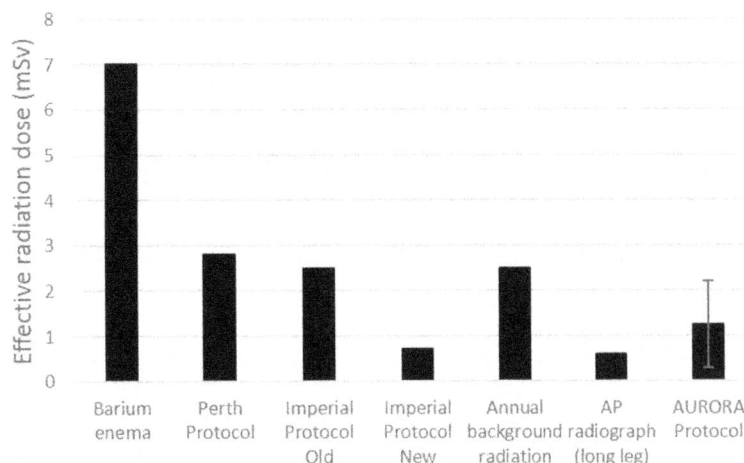

Fig. 4 Comparison of the AURORA CT protocol with a barium enema and other relevant protocols for determining prosthesis positioning. AURORA protocol dose is calculated from CT reports, and all other data taken from Henckel et al. [6]

Table 1 Reproducibility results showing the difference in calculated component angular alignment across two cases performed by three engineers at two different time points. The maximum average difference for each case and a 95% confidence interval are shown for all three axes of rotation for the femoral and tibial components

Case	Operator	Run	Femoral component alignment			Tibial component alignment		
			F/E	V/V	IE	F/E	V/V	IE
Case 1	Sim Eng A	Run 1	1.1	− 0.6	− 0.8	7.1	0.6	5.9
Case 1	Sim Eng A	Run 2	1.0	− 0.5	− 1.2	7.0	0.4	6.2
Case 1	Sim Eng B	Run 1	1.0	− 0.8	− 1.5	7.0	0.5	4.5
Case 1	Sim Eng B	Run 2	0.8	− 0.7	− 0.8	7.4	0.4	4.7
Case 1	Sim Eng C	Run 1	1.1	− 0.6	− 1.8	6.9	0.8	5.5
Case 1	Sim Eng C	Run 2	1.1	− 0.4	− 1.0	7.2	0.6	5.9
Maximum difference from average (°) ± 95% CI			**0.2 ± 0.1**	**0.2 ± 0.1**	**0.5 ± 0.3**	**0.3 ± 0.1**	**0.2 ± 0.1**	**0.9 ± 0.6**
Case 2	Sim Eng A	Run 1	1.9	− 0.9	0.1	8.2	1.5	3.0
Case 2	Sim Eng A	Run 2	2.3	− 0.8	− 0.1	7.7	1.8	2.7
Case 2	Sim Eng B	Run 1	2.3	− 0.7	− 0.2	7.9	1.7	1.7
Case 2	Sim Eng B	Run 2	2.1	− 0.8	0.4	8.4	1.4	2.8
Case 2	Sim Eng C	Run 1	2.0	− 0.7	− 0.2	7.9	1.0	2.3
Case 2	Sim Eng C	Run 2	1.8	− 0.8	0.0	8.4	1.5	2.8
Maximum difference from average (°) ± 95% CI			**0.3 ± 0.2**	**0.1 ± 0.1**	**0.3 ± 0.2**	**0.3 ± 0.2**	**0.4 ± 0.2**	**0.7 ± 0.4**

for case 2. In all other resections, the maximum difference in resection is ≤ 0.3 mm. The confidence intervals in all cases are less than 0.3 mm.

Reliability

The rotational alignments and bony resections for the femur and tibial components reported for 11 cases performed twice (each time by a team of two different engineers) are shown in Figs. 5 and 6. The ICC value is given for each alignment and resection variable. The lowest reported ICC variable is for femoral axial rotation, with an ICC of 0.93. These values are all above 0.9, indicating that across all rotations and resections in both the femur and tibia, the protocol reports excellent reliability.

Table 2 Reproducibility results showing the difference in calculated bony resection thicknesses (giving a measure of the accuracy of component placement) for the distal medial and lateral condyles, posterior medial and lateral condyles, and tibial medial and lateral plateaus across two cases performed by three engineers at two different time points. The maximum average difference for each case and a 95% confidence interval are shown for all resections

Case	Operator	Run	Femoral resections				Tibial resections	
			Lat. condyle	Med. condyle	Post. lat. condyle	Post. med. condyle	Lat. plateau	Med. plateau
Case 1	Sim Eng A	Run 1	6.5	6.0	10.0	10.3	11.2	10.0
Case 1	Sim Eng A	Run 2	6.2	5.7	10.0	10.7	10.3	9.0
Case 1	Sim Eng B	Run 1	6.1	5.4	10.2	11.1	10.5	9.3
Case 1	Sim Eng B	Run 2	6.8	6.1	10.2	10.6	11.1	9.8
Case 1	Sim Eng C	Run 1	6.2	5.7	9.5	10.7	10.7	9.6
Case 1	Sim Eng C	Run 2	6.4	6.0	9.9	10.3	11.1	9.9
Maximum difference from average (mm) ± 95% CI			**0.3 ± 0.2**	**0.4 ± 0.2**	**0.4 ± 0.2**	**0.4 ± 0.2**	**0.4 ± 0.2**	**0.5 ± 0.3**
Case 2	Sim Eng A	Run 1	6.0	7.4	10.9	10.3	11.0	6.7
Case 2	Sim Eng A	Run 2	6.2	7.8	10.8	10.3	11.1	7.0
Case 2	Sim Eng B	Run 1	6.1	7.7	10.6	10.2	10.9	6.7
Case 2	Sim Eng B	Run 2	6.1	7.6	10.8	9.9	11.2	6.9
Case 2	Sim Eng C	Run 1	5.9	7.5	11.0	10.6	11.0	6.3
Case 2	Sim Eng C	Run 2	6.0	7.4	10.9	10.4	10.9	6.6
Maximum difference from average (mm) ± 95% CI			**0.2 ± 0.1**	**0.2 ± 0.1**	**0.2 ± 0.1**	**0.2 ± 0.1**	**0.2 ± 0.1**	**0.3 ± 0.2**

Accurate determination of post-operative 3D component positioning in total knee...

163

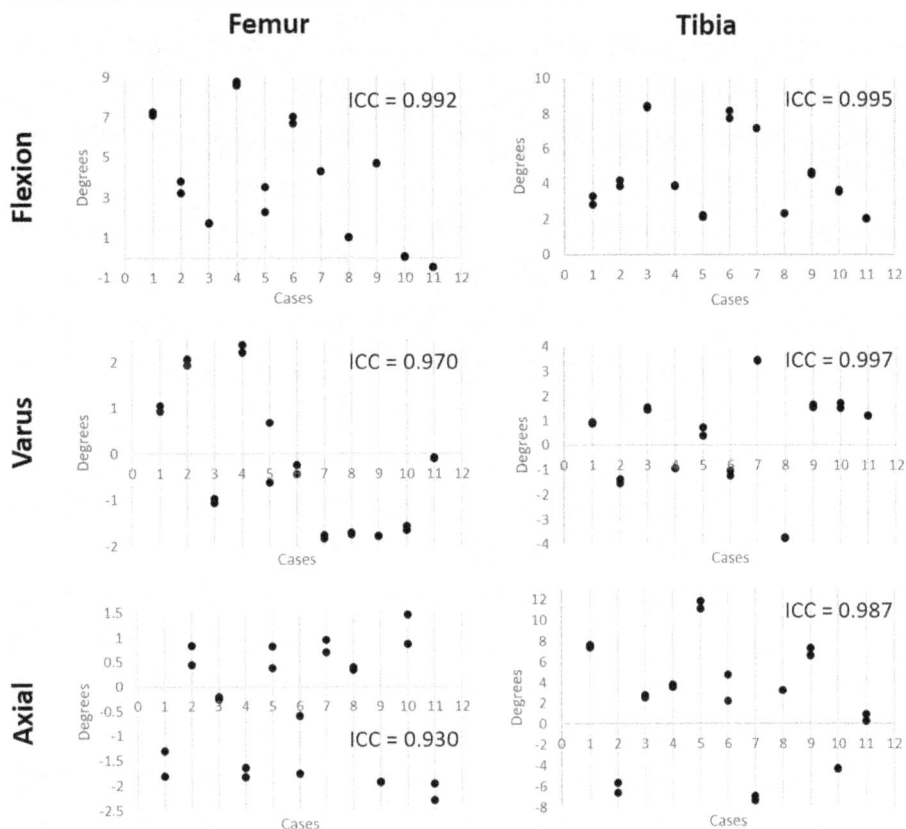

Fig. 5 Reliability testing for femur and tibia placement showing the coronal, axial, and sagittal rotation reported by the method across 11 cases performed by two engineers, followed by two additional engineers reviewing the placement. The ICC for each rotation in each component is reported. All values are greater than 0.9 indicating excellent reliability

Discussion

The maximum component alignment differences from the mean within this study are low compared to previous literature and provide a confidence interval up to tenfold narrower when compared to protocols in which individual CT slices were investigated [18, 19, 22, 28], or only post-operative CT scans were available [29, 30]. The maximum error of < 1° is similar to the protocols using more advanced techniques, such a computational edge detection; however, these studies did not include ICC coefficients, so an assessment of the repeatability was not possible [31]. The highest deviation from the mean was the tibial IE rotation at 0.9° and 0.7° for the two cases, with a confidence interval of 0.6° and 0.4°, respectively. These values represent an eightfold improvement in accuracy compared to previous attempts to measure tibial rotation [32]. Previous attempts have reported difficulty in measuring tibial IE rotation due to the variability in the landmarks required to define a useful axis [33]. By combining the pre-op and post-op CT, the landmarks that define the AP axis can be identified more easily than using post-op CTs alone. Although there may still be some debate over which landmarks

are the most appropriate, this method allows points to be defined that accurately reproduce an anatomic axis across multiple subjects. The origin of all axes may be redefined based on future literature if needed.

The resulting resection level measures of the femur and tibia also show high reproducibility, with the highest deviation seen for the medial tibial plateau resection at 0.5 mm and 0.3 mm between the two cases and confidence intervals of 0.6° and 0.4°, respectively. The magnitude of the error here, however, is only slightly above the other resections, indicating that there may not be a systematic reason for reduced accuracy when placing this component. Previous attempts have been made to investigate the effect on TKA outcome arising from resection levels. These studies have mainly focussed on the femur, particularly the posterior condylar offset [8, 34, 35]. These techniques however have primarily relied upon fluoroscopic images and planar X-rays which were discussed previously to be inaccurate, limiting the reliability of such studies.

Across both femoral and tibial component alignments and bony resections, this 3D pre-operative registration process shows excelled reliability, in which all ICC

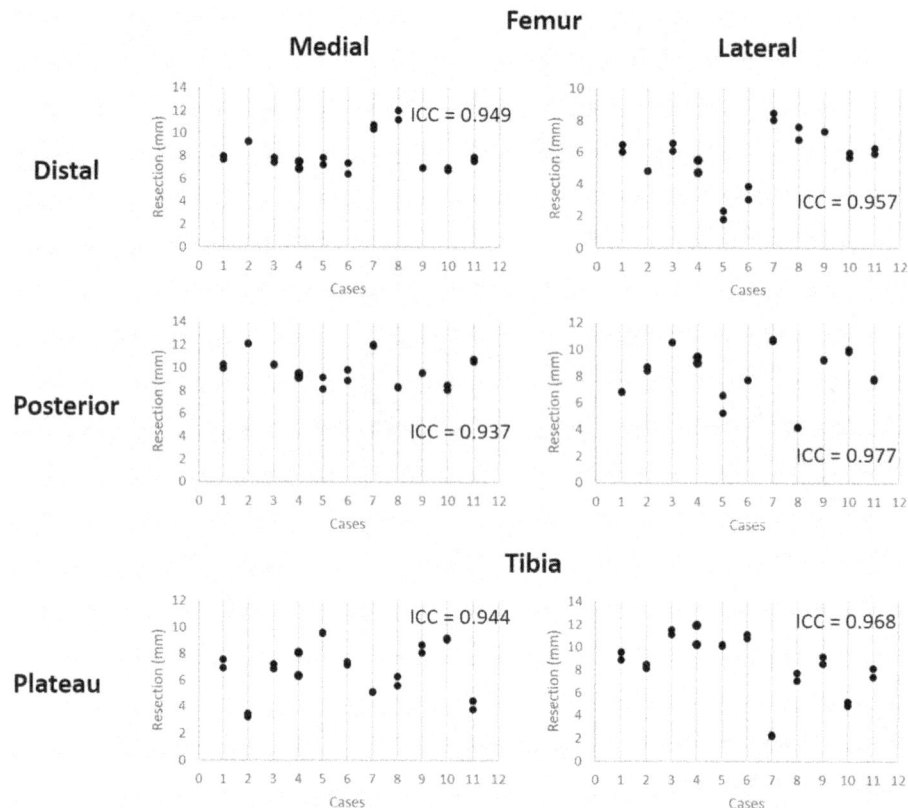

Fig. 6 Reliability testing for femur and tibia bony resections reported by the method across 11 cases performed by two engineers, followed by two additional engineers reviewing the placement. The ICC for each rotation in each component is reported. All values are greater than 0.9 indicating excellent reliability

values report greater than 0.93. The lowest reported ICC value of 0.93, resulting from the femoral axial IE rotation measure, is primarily due to the difficulty of post-operative registration of the femur component. The posterior condyles, which dominate the axial rotation positioning, of the APEX implant used in this study are thicker than the distal condyles (11 mm vs 9 mm) and tibial tray (~ 3 mm). As such, the CT flare is greater in these regions, reducing the accuracy of the registration. The ICC values reported here are consistently similar to or higher than other post-operative analysis techniques [7, 22, 36] indicating this method is not only accurate but suitable for routine post-processing by multiple users.

The high reproducibility and reliability of calculating both component alignment and bony resections performed by surgeons can lead to a better understanding of the influences of component alignment and component placement. The current literature has thoroughly reviewed the influence of component malalignment and poor patient outcomes [37–39]. Missing from all of these analyses, however, is an understanding of the patient's pre-operative anatomy, leading Hadi et al. [37] to conclude that there is a dubious link between component malalignment and patient outcomes. From this

post-operative analysis, we can begin to determine how the bony resections and the combination of component placement and alignment influence the outcome on a patient-specific level in greater detail. For example, the use of reliable bone resection measures from pre-operative bones may provide insight into the change of a patient's soft tissue profile post-surgery. From the pre-operative CT scans, comparative ligament lengths and change in length resulting from component alignment and placement can be investigated from landmarked attachment sites. CT scans in this analysis, however, are performed in a non-functional supine position, such that the distance between ligament attachment sites may not be representative of the functional length of the ligament. Functional imaging may be introduced to this workflow in the future to this issue without a change in post-processing techniques.

The proposed 3D registration process for post-operative analysis involves additional pre-operative CT imaging compared to other processes [6, 18]. Though this increases X-ray exposure to the patient, pre-operative planning, generally requiring a CT scan, is becoming the standard of care for TKA [23], such that the pre-operative scans are not for post-operative analysis alone. The protocol used here is a low-dose CT, with radiation exposure less than the typical yearly background radiation and similar to protocols currently in use [6]. All patient movement identified in pre-operative scans occurred in the mid-femur and mid-tibia regions, indicating that protocols which did not include the mid-femur and tibia sections would report inaccurate component placement. The resulting error in component position if these scans were used is the subject of further study.

Manual translation and rotation of the pre-operative bones and component geometries into the post-operative CT scan is reasonably labour intensive, requiring on average 60 min to complete, before the registration is quality control checked by a second engineer with additional experience. Further refinement of the proposed post-operative analysis process could include the use of an automated registration method. A preliminary automated registration process using the iterative closest point (ICP) method [30] was performed on these cases. The registration time was observed to reduce to approximately 2 min, from which the results were then fine-tuned by one engineer and quality control checked by a second engineer, representing a 30-fold decrease in time. Further development of the ICP method to optimise parameters around fitting regions of interest, reliability, and time for analysis may allow accurate post-operative analysis to be part of routine care and is the subject of future studies.

Joint infection and component loosening are a cause of dissatisfaction and revision surgery. Joint infection can be identified by swelling of the joint and pathology reports; however, these are not always conclusive. Combining component position as determined using the AURORA protocol with SPECT imaging could identify bone metabolism associated with infection or component movement [40]. Although current methods integrating SPECT imaging with CT do not improve the accuracy of determining component placement, such methods may be used to augment a pre-operative and post-operative CT 3D reconstruction to add metabolic activity.

The proposed post-operative 3D registration method described here has some limitations. The current time taken for this analysis as mentioned is approximately 60 min; this represents a high engineering burden and must be reduced to improve use in routine analysis. Commercially, TKA component geometry varies between medical device manufacturers, forming a significant part of their IP portfolio, as such, the component geometries must be obtained from the implant companies, which may be difficult—limiting the generalisability of this technique to engineering firms with a close relationship with implant companies. The reproducibility analysis performed here utilises two cases processed at multiple time points by multiple engineers of equal training. To better understand the reproducibility, particularly when processing outlier or severely pathological anatomy, a greater number of cases should be analysed.

Other methods to assess component position such as bi-planar X-rays followed by 2D to 3D registration offer a number of advantages over a CT, such as providing long leg assessments in a functional state [41]. Such techniques, however, may require fluoroscopic agents [42] and may only capture the region around the knee and are performed on apparatus less widely available than a traditional X-ray or CT machines, limiting its use [31].

Conclusion

Component alignment has been of great interest in total knee arthroplasty; however, the focus has previously been on achieved component alignment and identification of malalignment without regard for the component placement or pre-operative anatomy. The method presented here uses a low-dose CT scan to analyse the position and rotation of all components in 3D space, with a comparison to the pre-operative anatomy, allowing surgical changes to the joint to be determined. The method shows excellent reliability and reproducibility by removing the sources of error that are typically associated with post-operative total knee arthroplasty analysis. Routine use of this analysis in TKA as well as other joint replacement procedures will allow surgeons and engineers to better understand the effect of component alignment as well as the placement on outcome.

Abbreviations
3D: 3-Dimesional; AP: Antero-posterior; AURORA: Australian Universal Resection Orientation and Rotation Analysis; CT: Computed tomography; FE: Flexion-extension; ICC: Intra-class correlation coefficient; IE: Internal-external; ML: Medio-lateral; PCO: Posterior condylar offset; SI: Superior-inferior; STL: Stereolithographic language; TEA: Transepicondylar axis; TKA: Total knee arthroplasty; VV: Varus/valgus

Authors' contributions
EW and LT performed the statistical analysis and wrote the paper. JT and WT provided advice on the statistical methods and structured the protocol. JR, MS, and BF performed the TKA surgeries and provided clinical feedback on the utility of analysis. BM conceived the initial computational analysis and provided advice at all stages of the study. All authors read and approved the final manuscript.

Competing interests
All authors are employees or consultants of 360 Knee Systems.

Author details
[1]360 Knee Systems, Suite 3, Building 1, Sydney, NSW 2073, Australia. [2]Department of Biomedical Engineering, University of Sydney, Sydney, NSW 2006, Australia. [3]North Sydney Orthopaedic and Sports Medicine Centre, The Mater Hospital, North Sydney, NSW 2065, Australia. [4]Prince of Wales Private Hospital, Barker Street, Kensington, NSW 2030, Australia. [5]Sydney Orthopaedic Research Institute, 445 Victoria Ave, Sydney, NSW 2067, Australia.

References

1. Takahashi T, Ansari J, Pandit HG. Kinematically aligned total knee arthroplasty or mechanically aligned total knee arthroplasty. J Knee Surg. 2018. https://doi.org/10.1055/s-0038-1632378.
2. Abdel M, et al. Coronal alignment in total knee replacement: historical review, contemporary analysis, and future direction. Bone Joint J. 2014;96(7):857–62.
3. Panni AS, et al. Tibial internal rotation negatively affects clinical outcomes in total knee arthroplasty: a systematic review. Knee Surg Sports Traumatol Arthrosc. 2018;26(6):1636–44.
4. Kim Y-H, et al. The relationship between the survival of total knee arthroplasty and postoperative coronal, sagittal and rotational alignment of knee prosthesis. Int Orthop. 2014;38(2):379–85.
5. Carroll K, et al. Does restoration of joint line obliquity, tibial varus, and coronal alignment improve early clinical outcomes in TKA? Bone Joint J. 2016;98(SUPP 9):27.
6. Henckel J, et al. Very low-dose computed tomography for planning and outcome measurement in knee replacement. Bone Joint J. 2006;88(11):1513–8.
7. Hirschmann M, et al. The position and orientation of total knee replacement components: a comparison of conventional radiographs, transverse 2D-CT slices and 3D-CT reconstruction. J Bone Joint Surg Br. 2011;93(5):629–33.
8. Bellemans J, et al. Fluoroscopic analysis of the kinematics of deep flexion in total knee arthroplasty: influence of posterior condylar offset. J Bone Joint Surg Br. 2002;84(1):50–3.
9. Malviya A, et al. Predicting range of movement after knee replacement: the importance of posterior condylar offset and tibial slope. Knee Surg Sports Traumatol Arthrosc. 2009;17(5):491–8.
10. Clement N, et al. Posterior condylar offset is an independent predictor of functional outcome after revision total knee arthroplasty. Bone Joint Res. 2017;6(3):172–8.
11. Martin JW, Whiteside LA. The influence of joint line position on knee stability after condylar knee arthroplasty. Clin Orthop Relat Res. 1990;259:146–56.
12. Partington PF, et al. Joint line restoration after revision total knee arthroplasty. Clin Orthop Relat Res. 1999;367:165–71.
13. Bengs BC, Scott RD. The effect of patellar thickness on intraoperative knee flexion and patellar tracking in total knee arthroplasty. J Arthroplast. 2006;21(5):650–5.
14. Petersen TL, Engh GA. Radiographic assessment of knee alignment after total knee arthroplasty. J Arthroplast. 1988;3(1):67–72.
15. Petterwood J, et al. The immediate post-operative radiograph is an unreliable measure of coronal plane alignment in total knee replacement. Front Surg. 2014;1:1–6.
16. Park A, et al. The inadequacy of short knee radiographs in evaluating coronal alignment after total knee arthroplasty. J Arthroplast. 2016;31(4):878–82.
17. Holme T, et al. Quantification of the difference between 3D CT and plain radiograph for measurement of the position of medial unicompartmental knee replacements. Knee. 2011;18(5):300–5.
18. Chauhan S, et al. Computer-assisted total knee replacement a controlled cadaver study using a multi-parameter quantitative CT assessment of alignment (the Perth CT Protocol). J Bone Joint Surg Br. 2004;86(6):818–23.
19. Jazrawi LM, et al. The accuracy of computed tomography for determining femoral and tibial total knee arthroplasty component rotation. J Arthroplast. 2000;15(6):761–6.
20. Matziolis G, et al. A prospective, randomized study of computer-assisted and conventional total knee arthroplasty: three-dimensional evaluation of implant alignment and rotation. JBJS. 2007;89(2):236–43.
21. Mizu-Uchi H, et al. The evaluation of post-operative alignment in total knee replacement using a CT-based navigation system. Bone Joint J. 2008;90(8):1025–31.

22. Konigsberg B, et al. Inter- and intraobserver reliability of two-dimensional CT scan for total knee arthroplasty component malrotation. Clin Orthop Relat Res. 2014;472(1):212–7.
23. Victor J, et al. How precise can bony landmarks be determined on a CT scan of the knee? Knee. 2009;16(5):358–65.
24. Twiggs JG, et al. Patient variation limits use of fixed references for femoral rotation component alignment in total knee arthroplasty. J Arthroplast. 2018;33(1):67–74.
25. Saltybaeva N, et al. Estimates of effective dose for CT scans of the lower extremities. Radiology. 2014;273(1):153–9.
26. Walter S, Eliasziw M, Donner A. Sample size and optimal designs for reliability studies. Stat Med. 1998;17(1):101–10.
27. Koo TK, Li MY. A guideline of selecting and reporting intraclass correlation coefficients for reliability research. J Chiroprac Med. 2016;15(2):155–63.
28. Abu-Rajab RB, et al. Hip–knee–ankle radiographs are more appropriate for assessment of post-operative mechanical alignment of total knee arthroplasties than standard AP knee radiographs. J Arthroplast. 2015;30(4):695–700.
29. Hirschmann MT, et al. A novel standardized algorithm for evaluating patients with painful total knee arthroplasty using combined single photon emission tomography and conventional computerized tomography. Knee Surg Sports Traumatol Arthrosc. 2010;18(7):939–44.
30. Hu L, et al. 3D registration method based on scattered point cloud from B-model ultrasound image. In: International Conference on Innovative Optical Health Science: International Society for Optics and Photonics; 2017. https://doi.org/10.1117/12.2265976.
31. Kim Y, et al. Novel methods for 3D postoperative analysis of total knee arthroplasty using 2D–3D image registration. Clin Biomech. 2011;26(4):384–91.
32. Heyse TJ, Stiehl JB, Tibesku CO. Measuring tibial component rotation of TKA in MRI: what is reproducible? Knee. 2015;22(6):604–8.
33. Siston RA, et al. The high variability of tibial rotational alignment in total knee arthroplasty. Clin Orthop Relat Res. 2006;452:65–9.
34. Wang W, et al. Posterior condyle offset and maximum knee flexion following a cruciate retaining total knee arthroplasty. J Knee Surg. 2018. https://doi.org/10.1055/s-0038-1636912.
35. Degen RM, et al. Does posterior condylar offset affect clinical results following total knee arthroplasty? J Knee Surg. 2017;31(8):754–60.
36. van Houten A, et al. Measurement techniques to determine tibial rotation after total knee arthroplasty are less accurate than we think. Knee. 2018;25(4):663–8.
37. Hadi M, et al. Does malalignment affect patient reported outcomes following total knee arthroplasty: a systematic review of the literature. Springerplus. 2016;5(1):1201.
38. Valkering KP, et al. Effect of rotational alignment on outcome of total knee arthroplasty: a systematic review of the literature and correlation analysis. Acta Orthop. 2015;86(4):432–9.
39. Vandekerckhove PJ, et al. The current role of coronal plane alignment in total knee arthroplasty in a preoperative varus aligned population: an evidence based review. Acta Orthop Belg. 2016;82(1):129–42.
40. Rasch H, et al. 4D-SPECT/CT in orthopaedics: a new method of combined quantitative volumetric 3D analysis of SPECT/CT tracer uptake and component position measurements in patients after total knee arthroplasty. Skelet Radiol. 2013;42(9):1215–23.
41. Zeighami A, et al. Tibio-femoral joint contact in healthy and osteoarthritic knees during quasi-static squat: a bi-planar X-ray analysis. J Biomech. 2017;53:178–84.
42. Scarvell JM, Pickering MR, Smith PN. New registration algorithm for determining 3D knee kinematics using CT and single-plane fluoroscopy with improved out-of-plane translation accuracy. J Orthop Res. 2010;28(3):334–40.

20

The potent anti-inflammatory effect of Guilu Erxian Glue extracts remedy joint pain and ameliorate the progression of osteoarthritis in mice

Yen-Jung Chou[1,2,3], Jiunn-Jye Chuu[4], Yi-Jen Peng[5], Yu-Hsuan Cheng[4], Chin-Hsien Chang[6,7], Chieh-Min Chang[7] and Hsia-Wei Liu[2,3*]

Abstract

Background: Osteoarthritis (OA) is a slow progressing, degenerative disorder of the synovial joints. Guilu Erxian Glue (GEG) is a multi-component Chinese herbal remedy with long-lasting favorable effects on several conditions, including articular pain and muscle strength in elderly men with knee osteoarthritis. The present study aimed to identify the effects of Guilu Erxian Paste (GE-P) and Liquid (GE-L) extracted from Guilu Erxian Glue in anterior cruciate ligament transection (ACLT)-induced osteoarthritis mice, and to compare the effectiveness of different preparations on knee cartilage degeneration during the progression of osteoarthritis.

Methods: Male C57BL/6J mice underwent anterior cruciate ligament transection to induce mechanically destabilized osteoarthritis in the right knee. 4 weeks later, the mice were orally treated with PBS, celecoxib (10 mg/kg/day), Guilu Erxian Paste (100 or 300 mg/kg/day), and Guilu Erxian Liquid (100 or 300 mg/kg/day) for 28 consecutive days. Von Frey and open-field tests (OFT) were used to evaluate pain behaviors (mechanical hypersensitivity and locomotor performance). Narrowing of the joint space and osteophyte formation were examined radiographically. Inflammatory cytokine (IL-1β, IL-6, and TNF-α) levels in the articular cartilage were determined by quantitative real-time PCR. Histopathological examinations were conducted to evaluate the severity and extent of the cartilage lesions.

Results: Guilu Erxian Paste and Guilu Erxian Liquid (300 mg/kg/day) were significantly more effective ($p < 0.01$) than celecoxib (10 mg/kg/day) in decreasing secondary allodynia when compared to the saline-treated group ([#]$p < 0.05$). Open-field tests revealed no significant motor dysfunction between the Guilu Erxian Paste- and Guilu Erxian Liquid-treated mice compared to the saline-treated mice. Radiographic findings also confirmed that the administration of Guilu Erxian Paste and Guilu Erxian Liquid (100 and 300 mg/kg/day) significantly and dose-dependently reduced osteolytic lesions and bone spur formation in the anterior cruciate ligament transection-induced osteoarthritis mice when compared to the saline-treated group. Notably, Guilu Erxian Liquid (100 mg/kg/day) treatment significantly reduced the mRNA levels of IL-1β, IL-6, and TNF-α as well as relative the protein expression of IL-1β and TNF-α to the effect of celecoxib. Guilu Erxian Paste and Guilu Erxian Liquid (300 mg/kg/day) markedly attenuated cartilage destruction, surface unevenness, proteoglycan loss, chondrocyte degeneration, and cartilage erosion in the superficial layers ([##]$p < 0.01$ and [###]$p < 0.001$ respectively).

(Continued on next page)

---

* Correspondence: 079336@gmail.com
[2]Department of Life Science, Fu Jen Catholic University, New Taipei City, Taiwan
[3]Graduate Institute of Applied Science and Engineering, Fu Jen Catholic University, No. 510, Zhongzheng Rd., Xinzhuang Dist., New Taipei City 24205, Taiwan
Full list of author information is available at the end of the article

(Continued from previous page)

Conclusions: As expected, our findings suggest that the anti-inflammatory effects of Guilu Erxian Liquid (GE-L), following marked decrease on both IL-1β and TNF-α during the early course of post-traumatic osteoarthrosis (OA), may be of potential value in the treatment of osteoarthritis.

Keywords: Osteoarthritis, Anterior cruciate ligament, Guilu Erxian Glue, Knee, Articular cartilage, Mice

Background

Osteoarthritis (OA), the most frequent chronic musculo-skeletal disorder, is a slowly progressing disease characterized by articular cartilage degeneration, subchondral bone changes, osteophyte formation, low-grade synovial inflammation, and hypertrophic bone changes, leading to pain and functional deterioration [1, 2] . It is the most prevalent form of disease that involves cartilage degradation and periarticular bone responses, especially in the knee [3]. OA can affect every joint in the body; approximately 10–12% of the adult population is affected by this disease [4]. Individuals above 60 years of age present with the pathological features of OA in at least one joint, thus influencing the quality of life and resulting in enormous costs to the healthcare system [5]. Although OA is one of the most common disorders of the joints with a rising prevalence, it is difficult to treat the disease using current therapies [6, 7]. Given the complexity of this pathology, there are no pharmaceutical treatments that can slow the disease progression due to the limited knowledge about the pathogenesis of this condition [8, 9].

In the joint, the tissues containing nociceptors include primarily the joint capsule, ligaments, synovium, bone, and the outer edge of the menisci (in the knee) [10–12]. Inflammation lowers the threshold for nociception; while cytokines are being assessed as possible candidates for biochemical markers, inflammation is increasingly being considered as an important part of the pathophysiology of OA [13–15]. According to the American College of Rheumatology 2000 guidelines, patients with OA of the knee, a condition characterized by cartilage degradation, are often treated with steroids, non-steroidal anti-inflammatory drugs (NSAIDs), and cyclooxygenase-2 selective NSAIDs (e.g., celecoxib), which relieve pain and inflammation but are not capable of restoring tissues once OA has initiated [16, 17].

OA is a chronic progressive disease with complicated mechanisms that include inflammation, periarticular bone response, and cartilage degradation [18–20]. To date, the available pain treatments are limited in their efficacy and known to possess associated toxicities, none of which halts disease progression or regenerates damaged cartilage or bone [21]. Thus, current therapeutic strategies seek to ameliorate pain, offer chondroprotective or regenerative capability, and increase mobility, thereby representing the critically unmet needs. Notably, the anti-inflammation, anti-apoptosis, and anti-catabolism activities of several traditional Chinese medicines (TCM) provide a proposed medical option by modifying the disease and its symptoms in OA [22] .

Guilu Erxian Glue (GEG), which comprises four major components, *Testudinis Plastrum*, *Cornu Cervi*, *Lycii Fructus*, and *Ginseng Radix*, is a Chinese herbal remedy that has long-lasting favorable effects on aging, perimenopausal syndrome, and degenerative joint diseases in Asia [23–25]. Recent studies have also mentioned that GEG can stimulate the secretion of IGF-1 in osteoblasts and attenuate the bone resorption activity of osteoclasts in vitro [26], inhibit the formation of osteoclasts and bone pits in rats [27], and decrease articular pain and increase muscle strength in elderly men with knee OA [28]. However, knowledge about the mechanisms responsible for the beneficial effects of GEG in OA is limited.

Post-traumatic arthritis by bilateral transection of the anterior cruciate ligament (ACLT) is one of the most frequent causes of disability following joint trauma [29, 30]. Hence, in the present study, we developed a post-traumatic OA mouse model to investigate the pathophysiology of knee OA and the molecular characteristics of knee joint cartilage. During the course of the experiments, tests for mechanical hypersensitivity (von Frey test) and locomotor performance (open-field test) were used to evaluate pain behaviors associated with ACLT-induced OA mice. The present study aimed to identify the anti-nociceptive and anti-inflammatory effects of Guilu Erxian Paste (GE-P) and Guilu Erxian Liquid (GE-L) extracted from different preparations of GEG in ACLT-induced OA mice.

Methods
Chemicals and reagents

Celecoxib was produced by Pfizer Inc. (Manhattan, NY, USA), and Ketoprofen was produced by Swiss Co., Ltd. (Xinshi, TNN, Taiwan). Zoletil was purchased from Virbac (Grasse, Carros, France). Hematoxylin and eosin (HE), xylene, and paraffin were purchased from Thermo Fisher Scientific Inc. (Waltham, MA, USA). Safranin-O/fast green histochemical stain was obtained from ScienCell Research Laboratories. (Carlsbad, CA, USA). Designed Real-Time RT-PCR Primers (GAPDH, IL-6, IL-1β, and TNF-α) were ordered from Integrated DNA Technologies (Coralville, IA, USA). Phenol-Free Total RNA Purification Kit was purchased from AMRESCO (Solon, IA, USA). SYBR Green was ordered from Protech Technology Enterprise Co., Ltd. (Nangang,

TPE, Taiwan). The rabbit polyclonal antibodies-IL-1β and TNF-α, HRP-anti-rabbit IgG, and HRP anti-mouse IgG were from Santa Cruz Biotechnology, Inc. (Delaware, California, USA). Guilu Erxian Paste (GE-P) and Guilu Erxian Liquid (GE-L) were prepared (100 and 300 mg/kg/day, respectively) for treating the ACLT-induced OA mice.

Animals

Male C57BL/6J mice, 9 weeks of age (10 weeks at time of injury), were purchased from the National Laboratory Animal Center, Taiwan. All animals were maintained in laminar flow cabinets with free access to food and water under specific pathogen-free conditions in facilities approved by the Accreditation of Laboratory Animal Care and in accordance with the Institutional Animal Care and Use Committee of the Animal Research Committee of the Southern Taiwan University of Science and Technology, Tainan, Taiwan. Five mice per cage were fed with mouse chow and water ad libitum. The mice were acclimatized to the 12/12-h light–dark cycle conditions in the cages and were kept in the housing facility for a 1-week acclimation period before surgical injury.

Preparation of Guilu Erxian Glue extracts

The herbs and extract, GE-P, and GE-L, were prepared by the Taiwan Herbal Biopharma Co., Ltd., which is a TCM Good Manufacturing Practice manufacturer certified in Taiwan. GEG was comprised of the following medicinal herbs: *Testudinis Plastrum*, *Cornu Cervi*, *Lycii Fructus*, and *Ginseng Radix* at a weight proportion of 10:5:1.3:1, sequentially. According to the well-documented TCM formula described in a TCM book known as "The Golden Mirror of Medicine." GE-P was prepared by stewing *Testudinis Plastrum* and *Cornu Cervi* for 7 days, after which, *Lycii Fructus* and *Radix Ginseng* were added to the mixture, filtered, and a concentrated paste was formed. GE-L was prepared by conventional hot-water reflux extraction concentrated under reduced pressure; 1 kg of GE-P was dissolved in 5 L of double-distilled water and extracted with hot water (70 °C) after 8–9 h. The impurity-free solutions were stored at − 80 °C until use. The working concentrations of GE-P and GE-L were determined by calculating the initial weight of the raw materials (g) and the final vehicle volume (mL). High-performance liquid chromatography was used to detect the contents in the GE-P samples at 255 ± 19 mg/mL for Putrescine, 6.0 ± 0.8 mg/mL for Scopoletin, and 83 ± 5.3 mg/mL for Ginsenoside Re, respectively. The three compounds were deduced by comparing the individual peak retention times with those of the authentic reference substances. GE-L was also adjusted to the quality (standard effective components) of GE-P in order to prepare the same working concentration for the treatments.

Osteoarthritis surgery and experimental groups

9-week-old mice were anesthetized with Zoletil, and the anterior cruciate ligament was surgically transected to induce mechanical destabilization on the right knee, causing joint instability and post-traumatic OA. All surgical procedures were performed using a stereoscopic microscope (SMZ1000, Nikon, Tokyo, Japan). 4 weeks after ACLT surgery to restore, all tested mice were forced to run on a treadmill at a speed of 16 m/min every day for 30 consecutive days to achieve the histological progression of the knee OA. Sham operations were conducted by making a capsular incision and subjecting the mice to the treadmill run. The mice were randomized into the following groups: group 1 ($n = 10$), animals underwent sham operations and were orally treated with PBS; group 2 ($n = 10$), animals underwent ACLT surgery with oral vehicle treatment; and group 3 ($n = 10$), animals underwent ACLT surgery and were orally treated with celecoxib (10 mg/kg/day); group 4 ($n = 10$), animals underwent ACLT surgery and were orally treated with GE-P (100 mg/kg/day); group 5 ($n = 10$), animals underwent ACLT surgery and were orally treated with GE-P (300 mg/kg/day); group 6 ($n = 10$), animals underwent ACLT surgery and were orally treated with GE-L (100 mg/kg/day); and group 7 ($n = 10$), animals underwent ACLT surgery and were orally treated with GE-L (300 mg/kg/day). The oral administrations were performed for 28 consecutive days. Celecoxib, a COX-2 selective NSAID, was used as a positive control to evaluate the analgesic and anti-inflammatory roles in OA. The operated mice were sacrificed after the last treatment; at least six mice were used at each time-point for every set of experiments. Body weight was recorded regularly at 0, 2, and 4 weeks after the treatments.

Tactile sensitivity testing

Prior to pain testing, the mice were habituated to the testing chambers (plexiglass cubicles with a mesh floor) 1 week prior to baseline readings. Subsequently, the animals were acclimated for 30 min on a wire grid platform in individual chambers, before the von Frey testing. Mechanical sensitivity was measured by determining the hind paw withdrawal threshold using a set of 17 von Frey filaments (Somedic SenseLab, Sösdala, Skåne län, Sverige) with ascending force intensities. The force required to buckle the monofilament increases from 0.026 g in the first handle of the set to 110 g in the last (corresponding to a pressure range from 5 g/mm^2 to 178 g/mm^2). For optimum accuracy, each case was equipped with a thermo- or hygrometer. Mice were assessed three times at each time-point, and percent changes from baseline readings were reported. A positive response was defined as a rapid withdrawal of the hind paw when the stimulus was applied, and the number of positive responses for each stimulus was recorded. Tactile threshold was defined as a withdrawal response to a given stimulus intensity in 5 of 10 trials. This threshold was calculated once per animal.

Open-field behavioral testing

Quantitative motor testing was performed to find out whether the nerve pain had resulted from knee OA or from peripheral neuropathy in the mice. Thus, the ambulatory activity was measured using an OFT. All mice were allowed to adapt to the environment for 1 h prior to testing. Mice were placed individually in the center of a square open field ($50 \times 50 \times 50$ cm) with white plexiglass walls and were observed for 10 min under normal lighting. Movements and trajectories of the mice were videotaped and analyzed by the TM-01 Animal Video Behavior System (Diagnostic & Research Instruments Co., Ltd., Taiwan), which is a versatile video tracking system for automatically recording and analyzing animal activity, movement, and behavior. All data of given parameters such as motion tracking trajectory and mean velocity (MV) in all four 10×10 cm^2 corners were recorded and calculated by the same TM-01 Video Tracking Software program.

Radiographic assessments

After 4 weeks of administration, the animals that underwent sham operation or ACLT surgery were anesthetized, and X-rays were taken using a Faxitron Specimen Radiography System (Field Emission Corp., McMinnville, OR). The mice were radiographed at the same exposure for accurate comparisons of the hind legs; lateral radiographs were taken for both experimental and sham groups. The radiographs were analyzed for the presence of bony lesions, fracture callus, and bone remodeling. To facilitate congruency between radiographs, the mice were placed in a prone position with hips in abduction, causing external rotation of the tibia and creating a lateral position. Standardized radiographs of the entire skeleton of the mice were collected at 32 kV with an exposure time of 48 s on manual mode.

RNA isolation and quantitative real-time PCR analysis

RNA from articular cartilage tissues was isolated using a Phenol-Free Total RNA Purification Kit (Solon, IA, USA), and cDNA was synthesized using iScript reverse transcriptase kit (Bio-Rad Laboratories, Hercules, CA, USA). Quantitative real-time PCR (qPCR) was performed using the Applied Biosystems® 7500 Real-Time PCR Systems (Thermo Fisher Scientific Inc.). The resulting cDNAs were used to assay gene expression using the following primers: IL-6, (Plus: 5'-CAAATTCGGTACAT CCTCGAC-3'/Minus:5'-CTACGTTATTGGTGGGGAC TG-3'); IL-1β (Plus: 5'-TCA AAG CAA TGT GCT

GGT GC-3'/Minus: 5'-ACC TAG CTG TCA ACG TGT GG-3'); TNF-α (Plus: 5'-CGC GGA TCA TGC TTT CTG TG-3'/Minus: 5'-GGA CTA GCC AGG AGG GAG AA-3'); and the housekeeping gene GAPDH (Plus: 5'-GAG CTA CGT GCA CCC GTA AA-3'/ Minus: 5'-CAA AAA TGA GGC GGG TCC AA-3'). All reactions were performed using qPCR™ Core Kit for SYBR Green I®. Data were analyzed using the $2^{-\Delta\Delta Ct}$ method followed by its validation. Each experiment was performed in triplicate and repeated at least three times.

Western blotting analysis

Western blotting was used to evaluate the IL-1β and TNF-α protein expression. Proteins from each articular cartilage were extracted by using lysis buffer [50 mm Tris–HCl, pH 6.8; 10% sodium dodecyl sulfate (SDS)] and homogenized. After 30 min of incubation at 4 °C, the lysates were heated at 100 °C during 5 min and were centrifuged at 10 000×g for 30 min at 4 °C. Lysates containing equal amounts of proteins (100 μg) were resolved on 8.5% SDS-polyacrylamide gel electrophoresis. Rainbow-colored protein molecular weight standards obtained from Amersham were used for the estimation of molecular size. The proteins were blotted to a hybond-enzyme chemio luminiscence (ECL) nitrocellulose membrane that was probed and washed according to the instructions for the enhanced chemiluminescence western blotting detection system (Amersham Pharmacia Biotech, Little Chalfont, UK), with transfer buffer (pH 8.3) containing 20% methanol (v/v) using an Hoefer miniEV electrotransfer unit (Amersham Pharmacia Biotech). The membrane with transferred proteins was blocked with 5% serum albumin in tris-buffered saline (TBS) containing 0.1% Tween 20 (TBST) for 1 h at room temperature and incubated with the first antibody diluted in TBST for 1 h at room temperature. After blocking, membranes were incubated for 1 h at room temperature in wash buffer with either anti-IL-1β antibody (1:1000) and anti-TNF-α antibody (1:1000) followed by four times 10 min washing. Horse radish peroxidase-conjugated anti-rabbit and anti-mouse IgG antibody was diluted to 1:5000 in washed buffer and incubated with blots for 1 h at room temperature. For measuring immunoreactive expression of IL-1β and TNF-α proteins from kidney, finally joins HRP to assume the stain (Reagent A + Reagent B by 1: 1 proportion) on NC membrane under the room temperature responded 1 min develops again using the cold light image analyzer (FUJIFILM LAS-3,000). For quantification of immunoblots, relative intensities of bands were quantified by densitometry using image master image analysis software (Amersham Pharmacia Biotech). Control for loading and transfer was obtained by probing with anti-β-actin.

Histological evaluation

The mice were sacrificed and the knees were excised; samples were harvested and fixed in 4% paraformaldehyde, decalcified in 9% formic acid for 3–5 days, and embedded in paraffin. The formalin-fixed tissues were sliced into 5-μm-thick sections using a Microtome RM2135 (Leica Microsystems Inc., Bannockburn, IL, USA), placed on to silane-coated slides and immersed in tris-buffered saline, pH 7.4. After rehydration in graded ethanol solutions, the samples were dried overnight at 37 °C, and stored at room temperature. Serial sections of the knees were stained with HE (Sakura Finetek, Tokyo, Japan) and Safranin-O with fast green counterstain. HE staining of OA cartilage (pale blue color) generally indicates extensive cartilage destruction and calcification of the cartilage tissue. A necessary constraint on the validity of this scoring system is the consistency with which cartilage lesions are classified by HE staining. The 14-point Mankin score for evaluation of OA cartilage has also been used for the grading of animal cartilage. Safranin-O, an indicator of cell chondrogenesis, is a cationic dye that stains acidic proteoglycan present in the cartilage tissues. Safranin-O binds to glycosaminoglycan and appears orange-red in color, enabling the assessment of the structural integrity of the cell–extracellular matrix in cartilaginous tissue. Each sample was also stained with Safranin-O/fast green for the histopathological classification of cartilage degeneration during OA progression. The OA grade is defined as an index of the severity or biologic progression of the OA lesion based on the extent of pathology in the cartilage and the destabilization of the medial meniscus. The values range from 0 (surface intact) to 24(full-thickness loss of cartilage and bone deformation) on the OARSI score [31]. Lastly, the slides were examined using a Motic BA 400 microscope with Motic Advance 3.0 software (Motic Co., Fujian, China).

Theory/calculation

All results are presented as the mean ± standard deviation (SD). Differences between groups were evaluated by analysis of variance and post hoc comparisons with Bonferroni step-down (Holm) correction. Statistical analysis was performed using SigmaPlot software (version 10.0; SPSS Inc., USA). Post hoc testing of behavioral data utilized a two-tailed Welch's test. Post hoc testing of biochemical data utilized a regression analysis. Each value represents the mean ± SD from 10 mice. p values less than 0.05 were considered statistically significant. $^{*}p < 0.05$, $^{**}p < 0.01$, and $^{***}p < 0.001$ represent significant differences from the sham group (no ACLT). $^{#}p < 0.05$, $^{##}p < 0.01$, and $^{###}p < 0.001$ represent significant differences from the saline group (ACLT).

Results

GE extracts attenuate joint pain without affecting motor activity in OA mice

The progression of OA is accompanied by secondary clinical symptoms, with pain being the most prominent. In von Frey testing, a non-noxious stimulus was used to measure the response evoked by a mechanical stimulus. We estimated the effects of the GEG extracts GE-P and GE-L on pain following ACLT surgeries in mice using the von Frey filament assay (Fig. 1). Paw withdrawal threshold (PWT) was significantly reduced in the saline-treated ACLT mice when compared with the sham-operated controls ($^{**}p < 0.01$), with a hind paw pressure of 2.3 g below baseline. At 4 weeks after treatment, both GE-P (300 mg/kg/day) and GE-L (300 mg/kg/day) decreased secondary allodynia ($^{##}p < 0.01$ and $^{##}p < 0.01$, respectively) more than celecoxib (10 mg/kg/day) did ($^{#}p < 0.05$) when compared with the saline group. The open-field test (OFT) revealed no significant differences in representative traveling patterns and total ambulatory distance (locomotion) between the low dose of GEG-treated, high dose GEG-treated, celecoxib-treated, and saline-treated mice (Fig. 2). The results also implied that ACLT-induced pain behavior in OA mice mainly resulted from tactile hypersensitivity of the paw, but motor dysfunction of the hidden legs

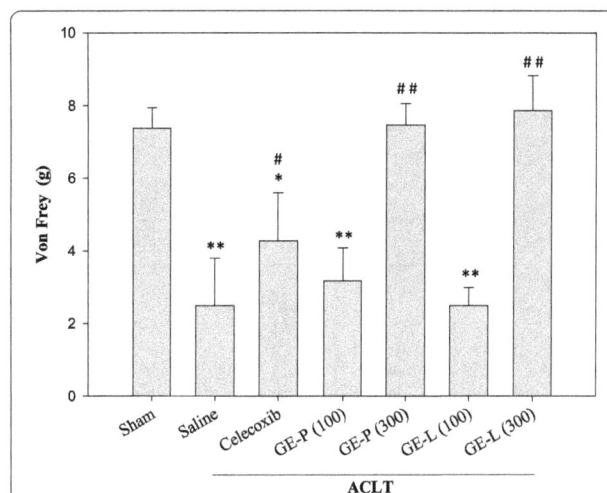

Fig. 1 Tactile sensitivity in ACLT-induced OA-related allodynia. Von Frey testing was used to measure the response evoked by mechanical stimulus in the groups treated with GE-P (100 and 300 mg/kg/day), GE-L (100 and 300 mg/kg/day), and celecoxib (10 mg/kg/day) when compared to the saline group. Mechanical hyperalgesia was tested by observing the changes in tactile sensitivity (pain behavior) on day 28, before sacrifice. Paw withdrawal threshold (PWT) was significantly reduced in the saline-treated ACLT mice ($^{**}p < 0.01$) when compared with the vehicle controls. Each value represents the mean values obtained from 10 mice in two different experimental sets. $^{*}p < 0.05$ and $^{**}p < 0.01$ denote significant differences when compared with the vehicle control (sham). $^{#}p < 0.05$ and $^{##}p < 0.01$ denote significant differences when compared with the saline-treated (ACLT) mice

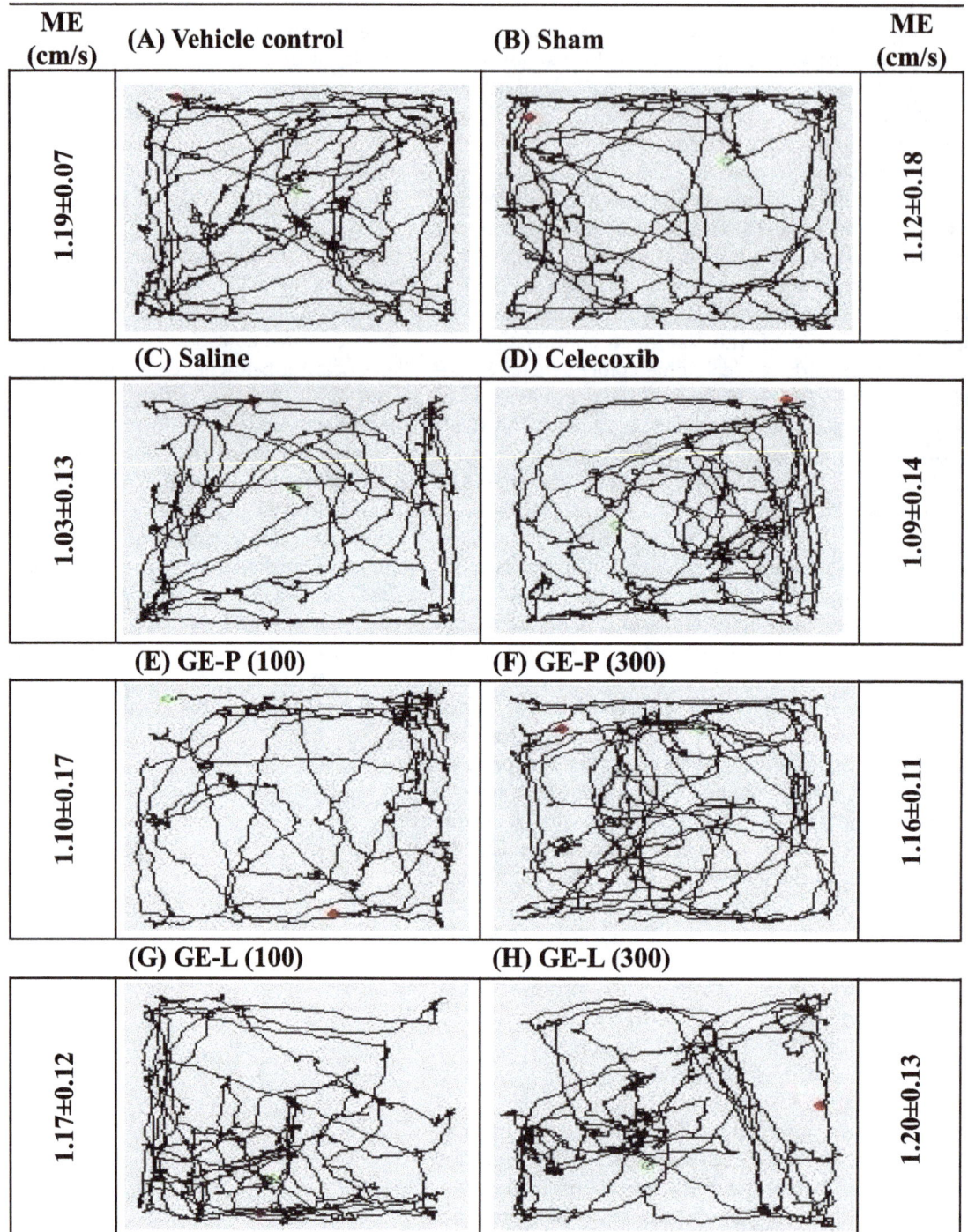

Fig. 2 Exploratory assessments in ACLT-induced OA-related pain behavior. There was no ACLT surgery in vehicle control (**a**) and sham (**b**) group. The effects of GE-P (100 mg/kg/day, **e**), GE-P (300 mg/kg/day, **f**), GE-L (100 mg/kg/day, **g**), GE-L (300 mg/kg/day, **h**), and celecoxib (10 mg/kg/day, **d**) when compared with the saline group (**c**) were analyzed by the open-field test (OFT) on day 28, before sacrifice. Each mouse was placed in the corner of an "open field" and allowed to roam the field. Movements were automatically recorded within 10 min via a TM-01 Animal Video Behavior System. Representative images (motion tracking behavior) showing the mouse traveling patterns were obtained and total ambulatory distance during the 10 min were measured by mean velocity (MV). Each value/error bar is expressed as the mean ± SD of 10 mice

was mostly unchanged between the sham-operated control and the experimental controls; the nerve pain could be relieved following treatment with the GEG extracts.

GE extracts minimize osteolytic lesions in knee joints (radiographic evaluation)

Radiographic analysis was performed to observe the abnormal bone architecture and soft bone loss of between the femur and tibia subchondral bone. The plain radiographs in the sham-operated controls demonstrated relatively preserved architecture of the femur and tibia in mice 4 weeks after sham surgery (Fig. 3a), however. The saline-treated group can be detected radiographically, indicated by bony lesions and evident with prominent bone formation extending into the soft tissue (Fig. 3b). In ACLT-induced OA mice, these radiographic findings also confirmed that administration of GE-P (100 and 300 mg/kg/day) and GE-L (100 and 300 mg/kg/day) did significantly and dose-dependently (Fig. 3d–g) reduce the decrease in osteolytic lesions and bone spur formation compared to saline group (Fig. 3b). This radiographic appearance is quite similar to that of the sham-operated control, GE-L (300 mg/kg/day) had the better improving effect than celecoxib did (Fig. 3c) on the inhibition of the subchondral bone formation and the decrease of cartilage loss while improperly formed joints in ACLT-induced OA mice.

GE extracts inhibit cytokines mRNA and protein expression of periarticular tissues

In order to understand the mechanisms underlying the effects of GEG extracts on articular cartilage integrity, we examined the expression of genes encoding proteins with functions closely related to cartilage homeostasis. IL-1β, IL-6, and TNF-α are considered to be the main pro-inflammatory cytokines involved in the pathophysiology of OA. qPCR results showed that relative mRNA levels of IL-1β (Fig. 4a), IL-6 (Fig. 4b), and TNF-α (Fig. 4c) were significantly elevated in the saline-treated group ($^{**}p < 0.01$) when compared with the sham-operated controls. GE-P (300 mg/kg/day) treatment significantly reduced the mRNA levels of IL-1β, IL-6, and TNF-α in the articular cartilage of the ACLT-induced OA mice when compared with the saline-treated mice ($^{##}p < 0.01$, $^{##}p < 0.01$, and $^{###}p < 0.001$, respectively). Interestingly, GE-L (100 mg/kg/day) treatment also significantly decreased the mRNA levels of IL-1β, IL-6, and TNF-α when compared to celecoxib treatment in the ACLT-induced OA mice. Furthermore, IL-6 mRNA levels were significantly reduced in the GE-L (300 mg/kg/day) group ($^{###}p < 0.001$ vs saline-treated) when compared with the celecoxib group ($^{##}p < 0.01$ vs saline-treated) in the articular cartilages of the ACLT-induced OA mice. Consistently, a significant decrease in IL-1β and TNF-α protein

expression was observed in the celecoxib treatment and GE-L (300 mg/kg/day) compared with the saline-treated mice ($^{#}p < 0.05$, $^{#}p < 0.05$, and $^{#}p < 0.05$, $^{##}p < 0.01$, respectively). Interestingly, we also found that GE-L (300 mg/kg/day) treatment had dramatically decreased the levels of IL-1β and TNF-α expression than the GE-P (300 mg/kg/day) treatment did ($^{#}p < 0.05$ and $^{#}p > 0.05$, respectively) (Fig. 5). These data suggested that the GE-L had an anti-inflammatory effect in vivo by decreasing the gene and protein expressions of proinflammatory cytokines.

GE extracts improve cartilage degeneration in the knee joint (histopathologic evaluation)

The beneficial effects of GEG extracts on articular cartilage and subchondral bone in OA mice were evaluated by staining the bone sections with HE and visualizing the cartilaginous tissue. HE staining (pale blue color) indicated the smooth surface, intact superficial layer, and normal chondrocyte population in the upper zone of the cartilage in the sham-operated control mice (Fig. 6a); conversely, erosion, clefting, chondrocyte degeneration, matrix changes, and typical chondrocyte clustering with apparent hypocellularity were noted in the saline group (Fig. 6b). For the histopathological classification of the severity of osteoarthritic lesions (denudation or deformation) in the cartilage, the Mankin score was used based on the OA grade levels of cartilage structure and cell distribution (Fig. 6h). Our results indicated that similarly to that of the celecoxib group (Fig. 6c, h, $^{#}p < 0.05$), the administration of 100 and 300 mg/kg/day of GE-P and GE-L attenuated cartilage destruction, with uneven surfaces and chondrocyte degeneration in the superficial layer in a dose-dependent manner (Fig. 6d–g). The Mankin scores were significantly reduced ($^{#}p < 0.05$, $^{##}p < 0.01$ and $^{#}p < 0.05$, $^{###}p < 0.001$) when compared with the saline-treated group (Fig. 6b, h, $^{***}p < 0.001$ vs sham-operated control).

We next determined the efficacy of Guilu Erxian Glue (GEG) extracts on ACLT-induced OA progression, the structural integrity of the articular cartilage was examined by microscopy after Safranin-O staining and OARSI evaluation. Safranin-O staining (a sensitive indicator of proteoglycan content) revealed serious OA lesions in the cartilage and meniscus in the saline-treated group 28 days after ACLT in mice; the mice exhibited moderate pathological osteoarthritic changes characterized by degeneration of articular cartilage, including proteoglycan loss, cartilage fibrillation, cartilage erosion, and an average OARSI of 10.7 ± 0.9 score (Fig. 7b, f, $^{***}p < 0.001$), compared to sham-operated control (Fig. 7a, f). In contrast, the cartilage of knee joints in GE-P (300 mg/kg/day) and GE-L (300 mg/kg/day)-treated mice exhibited less Safranin-O loss, no cartilage erosion, and significant cartilage degradation with a significantly lower OARSI score

(A) Sham

ACLT

(B) Saline

(C) Celecoxib

(D) GE-P (100)

(E) GE-P (300)

(F) GE-L (100)

(G) GE-L (300)

Fig. 3 Determination of osteolytic lesions on knee joints in OA mice by radiography. On the 28th day before sacrifice, the mouse was placed in a lying position with the legs spread out in order to quantify subchondral bone thickening associated with post-traumatic OA by X-ray evaluation of the knee joints. The saline-treated group (ACLT, **b**) presented with osteolytic lesions and evidence of prominent bone formation extending into the soft tissue when compared with the vehicle control (sham, **a**). The architecture of both femur and tibia were relatively well preserved. Radiographs from the mice treated with GE-P (100 mg/kg/day, **d**), GE-P (300 mg/kg/day, **e**), GE-L (100 mg/kg/day, **f**), GE-L (300 mg/kg/day, **g**), and celecoxib (10 mg/kg/day, **c**) presented with areas of minimal subchondral thickness when compared with those in the saline group. The arrow denotes an area of increased subchondral bone thickness or prominent bone formation on the femur/tibia

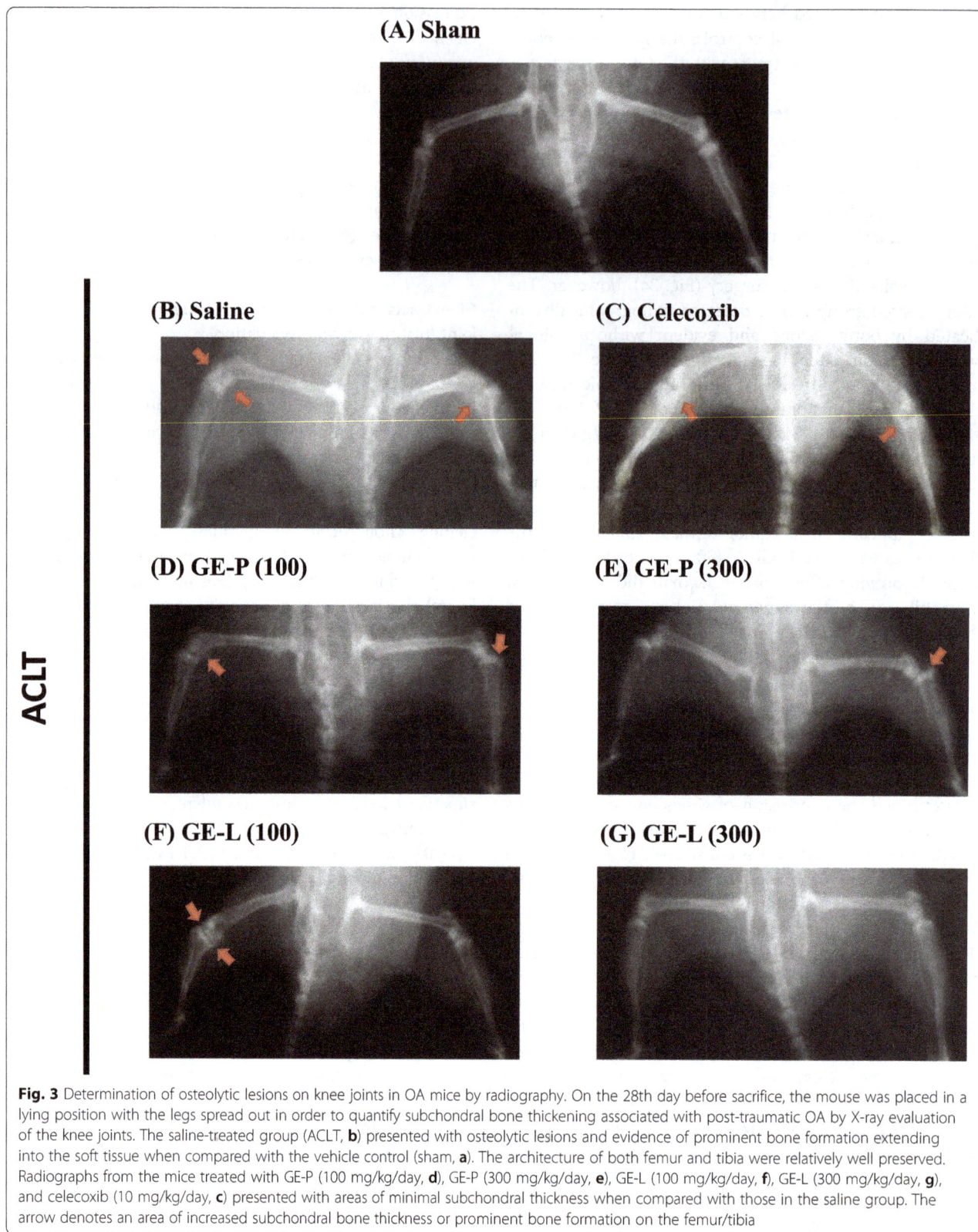

$(6.7 \pm 0.5$ and 5.8 ± 0.4, respectively; $^{\#\#}p < 0.01$, $^{\#\#\#}p < 0.001)$ compared to that in saline-treated group (Fig. 7d–f). Moreover, Safranin-O staining and OARSI evaluation demonstrated sufficient articular chondrocytes, retention of proteoglycan, and decreased thickness of calcified cartilage zone in GE-P (300 mg/kg/day) and GE-L

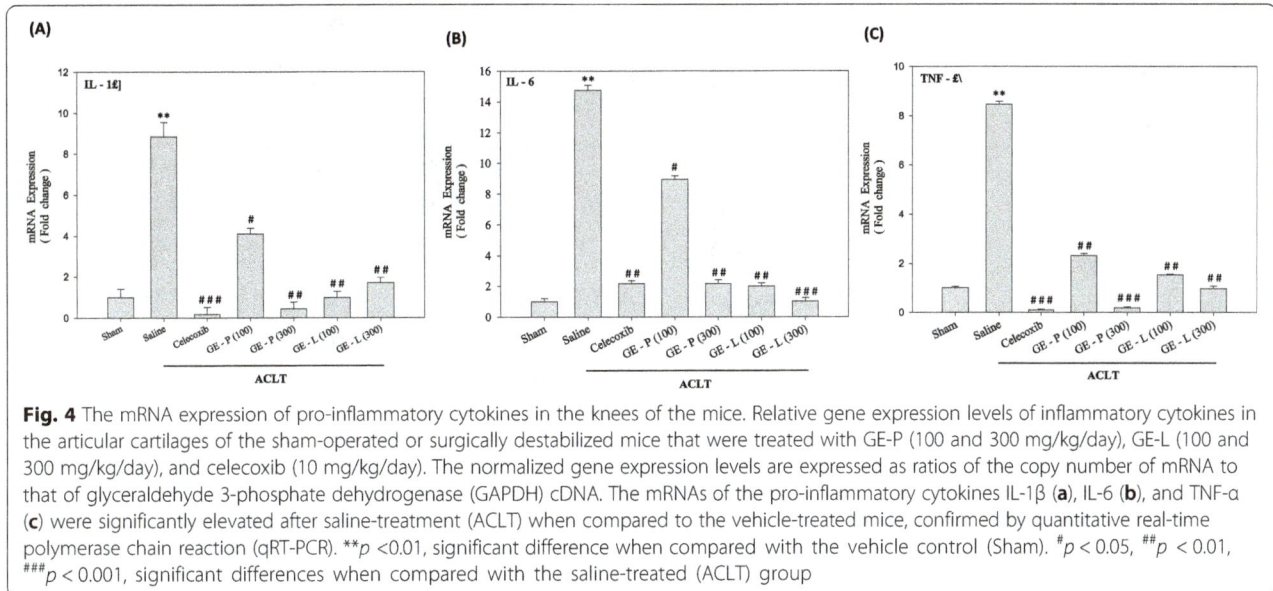

Fig. 4 The mRNA expression of pro-inflammatory cytokines in the knees of the mice. Relative gene expression levels of inflammatory cytokines in the articular cartilages of the sham-operated or surgically destabilized mice that were treated with GE-P (100 and 300 mg/kg/day), GE-L (100 and 300 mg/kg/day), and celecoxib (10 mg/kg/day). The normalized gene expression levels are expressed as ratios of the copy number of mRNA to that of glyceraldehyde 3-phosphate dehydrogenase (GAPDH) cDNA. The mRNAs of the pro-inflammatory cytokines IL-1β (**a**), IL-6 (**b**), and TNF-α (**c**) were significantly elevated after saline-treatment (ACLT) when compared to the vehicle-treated mice, confirmed by quantitative real-time polymerase chain reaction (qRT-PCR). **$p < 0.01$, significant difference when compared with the vehicle control (Sham). #$p < 0.05$, ##$p < 0.01$, ###$p < 0.001$, significant differences when compared with the saline-treated (ACLT) group

(300 mg/kg/day)-treated mice relative to celecoxib group (Fig. 7c, f). Collectively, these results indicate that GE-G extracts would attenuate cartilage degeneration in OA development.

Discussion

OA is a widespread chronic joint disease characterized by articular cartilage destruction accompanied with pain and disability [32, 33]. In the present study, we used a post-traumatic OA mouse model to test whether GE-G could slow the progression of OA and relieve both pain as well as OA-associated inflammation. The present study compared the anti-nociceptive, anti-inflammatory, and anti-arthritic activities of GE-P and GE-L prepared from GE-G extracts in ACLT-induced OA mice. The major findings of this study included inhibition of paw/joint pain, prevention of cytokine-induced inflammatory response, and suppression of certain osteoarthritis parameters (such as narrowing of joint space and osteophyte formation) by both GEG extracts. Moreover, the

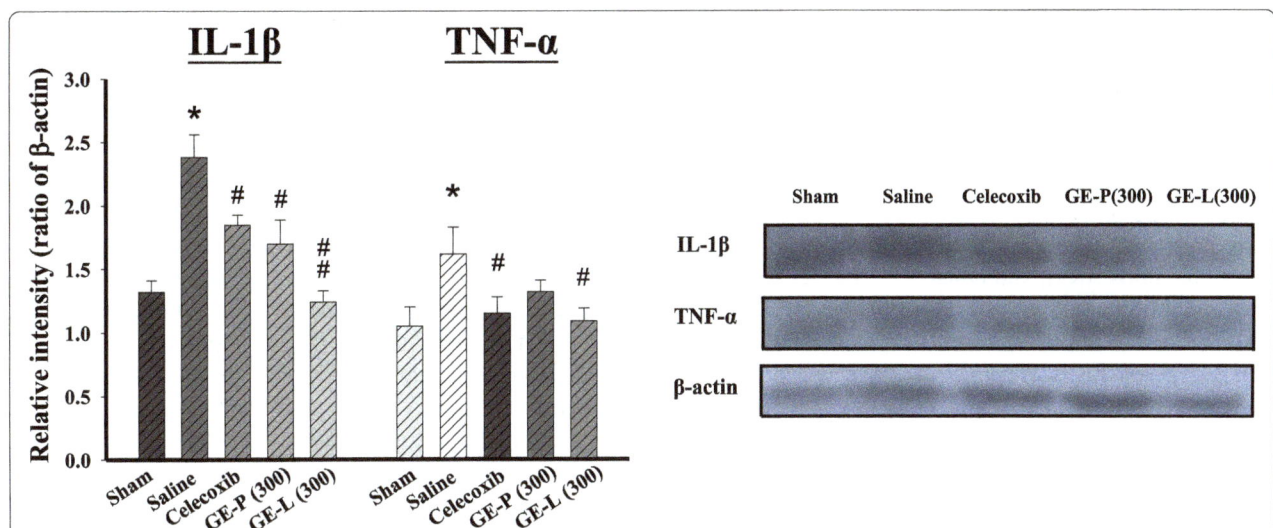

Fig. 5 The proteins expression of pro-inflammatory cytokines in the knees of the mice. Relative protein expression levels of inflammatory cytokines in the articular cartilages of the sham-operated or surgically destabilized mice that were treated with GE-P (300 mg/kg/day), GE-L (300 mg/kg/day) and celecoxib (10 mg/kg/day). Expression levels of the IL-1β, TNF-α and β-actin proteins were determined by western blot and quantitated by microcomputer image device (MCID) image analysis. The β-actin levels were evaluated as a loading control, and the data are expressed as the IL-1β/β-actin and TNF-α/β-actin ratios, respectively. Each value represents the mean ± SE of three replicate experiments. *$p < 0.01$, significant difference when compared with the vehicle control (Sham). #$p < 0.05$, significant differences when compared with the saline-treated (ACLT) group

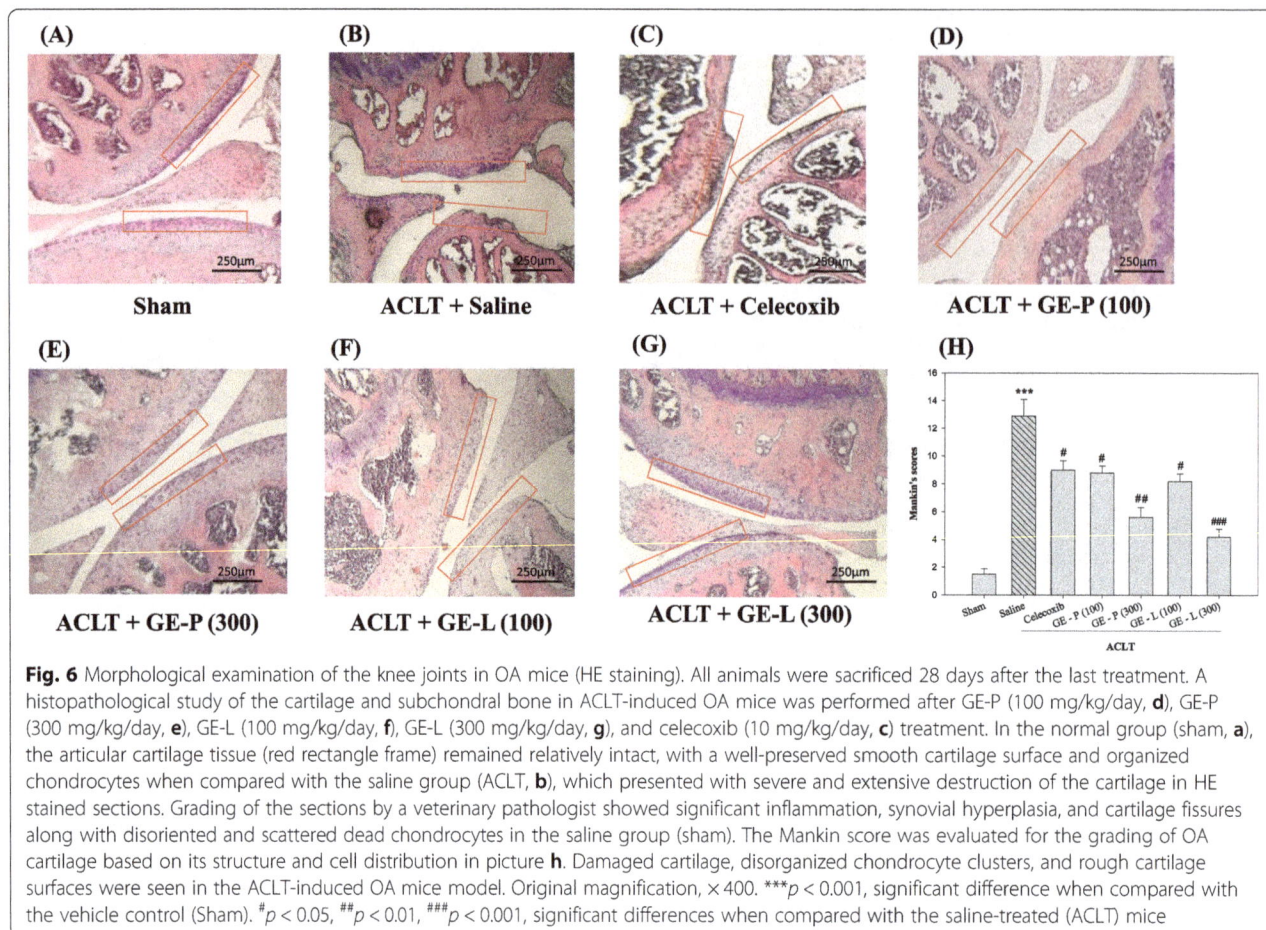

Fig. 6 Morphological examination of the knee joints in OA mice (HE staining). All animals were sacrificed 28 days after the last treatment. A histopathological study of the cartilage and subchondral bone in ACLT-induced OA mice was performed after GE-P (100 mg/kg/day, **d**), GE-P (300 mg/kg/day, **e**), GE-L (100 mg/kg/day, **f**), GE-L (300 mg/kg/day, **g**), and celecoxib (10 mg/kg/day, **c**) treatment. In the normal group (sham, **a**), the articular cartilage tissue (red rectangle frame) remained relatively intact, with a well-preserved smooth cartilage surface and organized chondrocytes when compared with the saline group (ACLT, **b**), which presented with severe and extensive destruction of the cartilage in HE stained sections. Grading of the sections by a veterinary pathologist showed significant inflammation, synovial hyperplasia, and cartilage fissures along with disoriented and scattered dead chondrocytes in the saline group (sham). The Mankin score was evaluated for the grading of OA cartilage based on its structure and cell distribution in picture **h**. Damaged cartilage, disorganized chondrocyte clusters, and rough cartilage surfaces were seen in the ACLT-induced OA mice model. Original magnification, × 400. ***$p < 0.001$, significant difference when compared with the vehicle control (Sham). #$p < 0.05$, ##$p < 0.01$, ###$p < 0.001$, significant differences when compared with the saline-treated (ACLT) mice

results demonstrate that both GE-P and GE-L exert similar effects on articular cartilage degeneration and subchondral bone deterioration when compared with celecoxib, and present with substantially lower Mankin and OARSI scores in the ACLT-induced OA mice.

Pain is the chief complaint of OA patients; however, due to the nature of the clinical studies and the limitation of the animal studies conducted so far, only a few have linked functional impairment and behavioral changes to cartilage loss and histopathology in OA animal models [34–36]. The findings of the present study demonstrate that GE-P and GE-L exhibited anti-nociceptive properties against mechanical stimuli in the paw, consistent with a state of chronic pain without causing motor impairment. Thus, we believe that the GEG extracts may be used as a clinically relevant aid in the treatment of chronic pain, possibly by acting as a good replacement for celecoxib during OA development. Recent reports have suggested that several TCMs are currently available for the treatment of chronic pain, especially neuropathic pain, which may have clinical relevance and open new possibilities for the development of new anti-hyperalgesic and anti-arthritic agents [37, 38].

OA is the most prevalent disease of the articular joints and is characterized by joint pain, narrowing of the joint space on the X-ray, and loss of joint function through progressive cartilage degradation and intermittent synovial inflammation [39, 40]. Compelling studies report the presence of empty lacunae and hypocellularity in the cartilage with OA progression, suggesting that chondrocyte cell death occurs and participates in OA development [41, 42]. In the current study, radiographic analyses of the knee joints confirmed that administration of GE-P (100 and 300 mg/kg/day) and GE-L (100 and 300 mg/kg/day) significantly and dose-dependently attenuated the narrowing of the joint space, osteophyte formation, and other features of osteoarthritis in the ACLT-induced OA mice. Meanwhile, nociception in the knee is complex, and the nociceptive stimuli are related to but fundamentally different from those producing cartilage loss [43]. As indicated in a previous study, daily treatment with celecoxib does not prevent cartilage degradation or osteophyte formation during OA development in the mouse model [44]. Consistently, significant inhibition of joint space narrowing and osteophyte formation was achieved with GE-L (300 mg/kg/day)

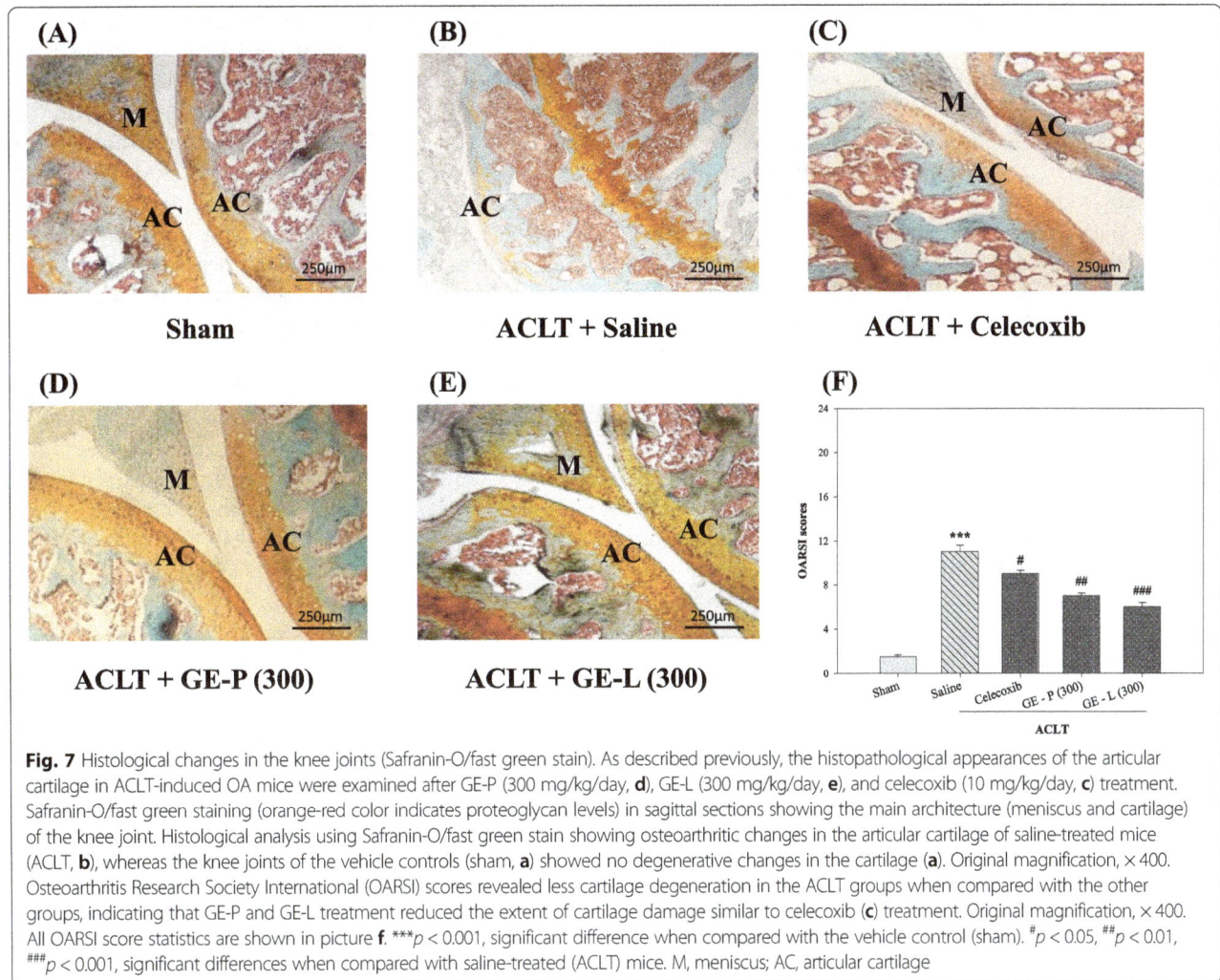

Fig. 7 Histological changes in the knee joints (Safranin-O/fast green stain). As described previously, the histopathological appearances of the articular cartilage in ACLT-induced OA mice were examined after GE-P (300 mg/kg/day, **d**), GE-L (300 mg/kg/day, **e**), and celecoxib (10 mg/kg/day, **c**) treatment. Safranin-O/fast green staining (orange-red color indicates proteoglycan levels) in sagittal sections showing the main architecture (meniscus and cartilage) of the knee joint. Histological analysis using Safranin-O/fast green stain showing osteoarthritic changes in the articular cartilage of saline-treated mice (ACLT, **b**), whereas the knee joints of the vehicle controls (sham, **a**) showed no degenerative changes in the cartilage (**a**). Original magnification, × 400. Osteoarthritis Research Society International (OARSI) scores revealed less cartilage degeneration in the ACLT groups when compared with the other groups, indicating that GE-P and GE-L treatment reduced the extent of cartilage damage similar to celecoxib (**c**) treatment. Original magnification, × 400. All OARSI score statistics are shown in picture **f**. ***$p < 0.001$, significant difference when compared with the vehicle control (sham). #$p < 0.05$, ##$p < 0.01$, ###$p < 0.001$, significant differences when compared with saline-treated (ACLT) mice. M, meniscus; AC, articular cartilage

treatment. These favorable effects were confirmed histologically in the same groups of animals, thus revealing the protective action of GE-P (300 mg/kg/day) and GE-L (300 mg/kg/day) against destruction and degeneration of cartilage in the mouse OA model.

Synovial inflammation is a frequently observed phenomenon in osteoarthritic joints and contributes to the pathogenesis of OA by the formation of various catabolic and pro-inflammatory mediators, which alter the balance between cartilage matrix degradation and repair [45]. Secreted inflammatory molecules such as pro-inflammatory cytokines are among the critical mediators of the disturbed processes implicated in OA pathophysiology [46]. Recent evidence has implicated cytokines including IL-1, IL-6, and TNF-α in the promotion of articular cartilage extracellular matrix protein degradation; they are also known to synergize with other cytokines to amplify and accelerate cartilage destruction [47, 48]. Most importantly, many of these cytokines have been implicated in causing synovial tissue activation, damage to subchondral bone and alterations in cartilage

homeostasis in spontaneously occurring or surgically induced animal models of OA [49, 50]. The primary role of these cytokines is to modulate the expression of matrix metalloproteinases and cartilage extracellular matrix (ECM) proteins; in addition, they have been implicated in the development OA and could be therapeutically targeted in the future [51]. Interleukin-1 beta (IL-1β) is a potent pro-inflammatory cytokine that is capable of inducing chondrocytes and synovial cells to synthesize matrix metalloproteinases (MMPs), and acts as a key mediator of the degeneration of articular cartilage in OA [52]. IL-1β could also play a role in the early progression or initiation of OA as evidenced in many in vitro studies [53]. Induction of IL-1β expression in the TMJs of adult mice led to pathologic development, dysfunction, and related pain in the joints [54, 55].

Tumor necrosis factor alpha (TNF-α) is generally considered to be involved in the dysregulation of bone and cartilage remodeling in chondrodestructive diseases, especially osteoarthritis, in several in vitro and in vivo models [56, 57]. Recently, oral consumption of a hydrolyzed type 1 collagen preparation has been reported to reduce pain in human OA, and the supplemented mice also displayed reduced synovial hyperplasia that paralleled a reduction in TNF-α mRNA suggesting an anti-inflammatory effect [58]. Furthermore, the use of IL-1 and/or TNF-α inhibitors in experimental models of inflammatory arthritis and OA has provided strong support for the role of IL-1 in the regulation of catabolic events and inflammatory processes in degenerative joint diseases [59]. It is generally accepted that IL-1 is the pivotal cytokine during the early and late stages, while TNF-α is primarily involved during the onset of arthritis, and IL-6 is released during the inflammatory process in an OA joint [60]. In chondrocytes and cartilage explants, IL-6 treatment can stimulate chondrocyte calcification and reduce proteoglycan content with increased production of MMP-3 and MMP-13 [61]. IL-6 gene knock out in male mice resulted in the development of advanced OA suggesting its role as a crucial mediator in the biomechanical control of cartilage destruction and bone remodeling in OA [62, 63]. Our qPCR results showed that the mRNA levels of IL-1β, IL-6, and TNF-α in the articular cartilage were partially reversed by GE-L (100 mg/kg/day) treatment similar to the effects of celecoxib (10 mg/kg/day), whereas GE-L (300 mg/kg/day) treatment exerted maximum inhibition on the IL-6 mRNA levels resulting in amelioration of OA progression in the mice. In this study, a significant decrease in IL-1β and TNF-α protein expression was observed in the celecoxib treatment and GE-L (300 mg/kg/day) more than the GE-P (300 mg/kg/day) treatment did as compared to the saline-treated mice. These data suggested that the GE-L had an anti-inflammatory effect in vivo is consistent with those from previous studies where treatment with celecoxib (5 mg/kg) was effective in decreasing the elevated levels of IL-1β and TNF-α, inhibiting synovial thickening and balancing MMPs levels, thus resulting in the preservation of ECM in a posttraumatic OA mouse model [64, 65].

Several recent experimental studies performed in animal models of OA sustained the previously held view that the magnitude of behavioral changes was directly correlated with higher OARSI histological scores of OA, synovitis in the knee joints, cartilage volume loss, and osteophyte formation [66, 67]. Loss of articular cartilage is a crucial event in OA and is characterized by a disturbance in the regulation of synthetic (anabolic) and resorptive (catabolic) activities of the resident chondrocytes, which results in net loss of the cartilage matrix components and deterioration in the structural and functional properties of the cartilage [68, 69]. In the present study, histological analysis demonstrated progressive joint degeneration, as measured by a modified Mankin scale and an OARSI score, with significantly less

cartilage destruction and proteoglycan loss in the articular cartilage after GE-L (300 mg/kg/day) administration compared to that of GE-P (300 mg/kg/day) while GE-L (100 mg/kg/day) and GE-P (100 mg/kg/day) had the same treatment effectiveness. Observations from HE and Safranin-O staining suggest that GE-P (300 mg/kg/day) rather than GE-L (300 mg/kg/day) can protect the mice chondrocytes from degeneration and normalize the altered cartilage matrix remodeling/degradation via catabolic reactions caused by the cytokines (IL-1β and TNF-α). These morphological data also suggest that the potency of GE-L is remarkably similar to GE-P, even the high dose (300 mg/kg/day) of GE-L can exert greater chondroprotective effect in an attempt to reduce inflammation in vivo, alleviates synovitis, retards the senescence of chondrocytes and suppresses structural changes while reducing the number of catabolic enzymes in the knee cartilage in OA.

Conclusions

This study demonstrates that the anti-arthritic effects of GE-L (a novel substitute for GE-P, which is not convenient for oral administration) were better than those of celecoxib. Dose-dependent increases in the narrowing of joint space, and in cartilage area, as well as the proteoglycan matrix, are blocked early during the osteoarthritic process and sustained through the course of the disease, partially through nociceptive and inflammatory responses. These results may highlight the need to develop new therapeutic TCM in order to improve the management of patients with OA, which currently lack general therapeutic principles.

Abbreviations

ACLT: Anterior cruciate ligament; COX-2: Cyclooxygenase-2; ECM: Extracellular matrix; GAPDH: Glyceraldehyde 3-phosphate dehydrogenase; GEG: Guilu Erxian Glue; GE-L: Guilu Erxian Liquid; GE-P: Guilu Erxian Paste; HE: Hematoxylin-eosin; IL-1β: Interleukin-1β; MMPs: Matrix metalloproteinases; MV: Mean velocity; NSAIDs: Non-steroidal anti-inflammatory drugs; OA: Osteoarthritis; OARSI: Osteoarthritis Research Society International; OFT: Open-field test; PWT: Paw withdrawal threshold; qPCR: Quantitative real-time PCR; SD: Standard deviation; TCM: Traditional Chinese medicine; TNF-α: Tumor necrosis factor-alpha

Acknowledgements

The study was financially supported by En Chu Kong Hospital Research Grant (no. ECKH10307 and no. ECKH10411) and MacKay Memorial Hospital Research Grant (no. MMH10406). The funding sources had no involvement in the study design; in the collection, analysis, and interpretation of data; in the writing of the report; or in the decision to submit the paper for publication.

Funding

The study was financially supported by En Chu Kong Hospital Research Grant (no. ECKH10307 and no. ECKH10411) and MacKay Memorial Hospital Research Grant (no. MMH10406).

Authors' contributions

Y-JC and J-JC wrote the paper. Y-JC, Y-HC, and C-MC performed the experiments. Y-JP analyzed the data. C-HC contributed reagents/materials/analysis tools. H-WL conceived and designed the experiments. All authors read and approved the final paper.

Competing interests

The authors declare that they have no competing interests.

Author details

¹Department of Traditional Chinese Medicine, MacKay Memorial Hospital, Taipei City, Taiwan. ²Department of Life Science, Fu Jen Catholic University, New Taipei City, Taiwan. ³Graduate Institute of Applied Science and Engineering, Fu Jen Catholic University, No. 510, Zhongzheng Rd., Xinzhuang Dist., New Taipei City 24205, Taiwan. ⁴Department of Biotechnology, College of Engineering, Southern Taiwan University, Tainan City, Taiwan. ⁵Department of Pathology, Tri-Service General Hospital, National Defense Medical Center, Taipei City, Taiwan. ⁶Department of Cosmetic Science, Chang Gung University of Science and Technology, Tao-Yuan City, Taiwan. ⁷Department of Traditional Chinese Medicine, En Chu Kong Hospital, New Taipei City 237, Taiwan.

References

1. Egloff C, Hügle T, Valderrabano V. Biomechanics and pathomechanisms of osteoarthritis. Swiss Med Wkly. 2012;142:w13583. https://doi.org/10.4414/smw.2012.13583.
2. Ratneswaran A, LeBlanc EA, Walser E, Welch I, Mort JS, Borradaile N, Beier F. Peroxisome proliferator-activated receptor δ promotes the progression of posttraumatic osteoarthritis in a mouse model. Arthritis Rheum. 2015;67(2):454–64. https://doi.org/10.1002/art.38915.
3. Huskisson EC. Applying the evidence in osteoarthritis: strategies for pain management. Clin Drug Investig. 2007;27(Suppl 1):23–9. https://doi.org/10.2165/00044011-200727001-00005.
4. Yu SP, Hunter DJ. Emerging drugs for the treatment of knee osteoarthritis. Expert Opin Emerg Drugs. 2015;20(3):361–78. https://doi.org/10.1517/14728214.2015.1037275 Epub 2015 Jul 3.
5. Veje K, Hyllested JL, Østergaard K. Osteoarthritis. Pathogenesis, clinical features and treatment. Ugeskr Laeger. 2002;164(24):3173–9.
6. Waung JA, Bassett JH, Williams GR. Adult mice lacking the type 2 iodothyronine deiodinase have increased subchondral bone but normal articular cartilage. Thyroid. 2015;25(3):269–77. https://doi.org/10.1089/thy.2014.0476 Epub 2015 Feb 3.
7. Veronesi F, Della Bella E, Cepollaro S, Brogini S, Martini L, Fini M. Novel therapeutic targets in osteoarthritis: narrative review on knock-out genes involved in disease development in mouse animal models. Cytotherapy. 2016;18(5):593–612. https://doi.org/10.1016/j.jcyt.2016.02.001.
8. Welch ID, Cowan MF, Beier F, Underhill TM. The retinoic acid binding protein CRABP2 is increased in murine models of degenerative joint disease. Arthritis Res Ther. 2009;11(1):R14. https://doi.org/10.1186/ar2604 Epub 2009 Jan 28.
9. Dong Y, Liu H, Zhang X, Xu F, Qin L, Cheng P, Huang H, Guo F, Yang Q, Chen A. Inhibition of SDF-1α/CXCR4 Signalling in subchondral bone attenuates post-traumatic osteoarthritis. Int J Mol Sci. 2016;17(6). https://doi.org/10.3390/ijms17060943.
10. Felson DT. The sources of pain in knee osteoarthritis. Curr Opin Rheumatol. 2005;17(5):624–8.
11. Sutton S, Clutterbuck A, Harris P, Gent T, Freeman S, Foster N, Barrett-Jolley R, Mobasheri A. The contribution of the synovium, synovial derived inflammatory cytokines and neuropeptides to the pathogenesis of osteoarthritis. Vet J. 2009;179(1):10 24 Epub 2007 Oct 29.
12. da Silva Arrigo J, Balen E, Júnior UL, da Silva Mota J, Iwamoto RD, Barison A, Sugizaki MM, Leite Kassuya CA. Anti-nociceptive, anti-hyperalgesic and anti-arthritic activity of amides and extract obtained from Piper amalago in rodents. J Ethnopharmacol. 2016;179:101–9. https://doi.org/10.1016/j.jep.2015.12.046 Epub 2015 Dec 23.
13. Mabey T, Honsawek S. Cytokines as biochemical markers for knee osteoarthritis. World J Orthop. 2015;6(1):95–105. https://doi.org/10.5312/wjo.v6.i1.95. eCollection 2015 Jan 18.
14. Kapoor M, Martel-Pelletier J, Lajeunesse D, Pelletier JP, Fahmi H. Role of proinflammatory cytokines in the pathophysiology of osteoarthritis. Nat Rev Rheumatol. 2011;7(1):33–42. https://doi.org/10.1038/nrrheum.2010.196 Epub 2010 Nov 30.
15. Melo Júnior JM, Damasceno MB, Santos SA, Barbosa TM, Araújo JR, Vieira-Neto AE, Wong DV, Lima-Júnior RC, Campos AR. Acute and neuropathic orofacial antinociceptive effect of eucalyptol. Inflammopharmacology. 2017;25(2):247–54. https://doi.org/10.1007/s10787-017-0324-5 Epub 2017 Feb 16.
16. Cho H, Walker A, Williams J, Hasty KA. Study of osteoarthritis treatment with anti-inflammatory drugs: cyclooxygenase-2 inhibitor and steroids. Biomed Res Int. 2015;2015:595273. https://doi.org/10.1155/2015/595273 Epub 2015 Apr 27.
17. Khayyal MT, El-Ghazaly MA, El-Hazek RM, Nada AS. The effects of celecoxib, a COX-2 selective inhibitor, on acute inflammation induced in irradiated rats. Inflammopharmacology. 2009;17(5):255–66. https://doi.org/10.1007/s10787-009-0014-z Epub 2009 Oct 2.
18. Lou Y, Wang C, Zheng W, Tang Q, Chen Y, Zhang X, Guo X, Wang J. Salvianolic acid B inhibits IL-1β-induced inflammatory cytokine production in human osteoarthritis chondrocytes and has a protective effect in a mouse osteoarthritis model. Int Immunopharmacol. 2017;46:31–7. https://doi.org/10.1016/j.intimp.2017.02.021 Epub 2017 Feb 27.
19. Wang Z, Huang J, Zhou S, Luo F, Xu W, Wang Q, Tan Q, Chen L, Wang J, Chen H, Chen L, Xie Y, Du X. Anemonin attenuates osteoarthritis progression through inhibiting the activation of IL-1β/NF-κB pathway. J Cell Mol Med. 2017. https://doi.org/10.1111/jcmm.13227.
20. Li X, Yang J, Liu D, Li J, Niu K, Feng S, Yokota H, Zhang P. Knee loading inhibits osteoclast lineage in a mouse model of osteoarthritis. Sci Rep. 2016; 6:24668. https://doi.org/10.1038/srep24668.
21. Moreira DRM, Santos DS, Espírito Santo RFD, Santos FED, de Oliveira Filho GB, Leite ACL, Soares MBP, Villarreal CF. Structural improvement of new thiazolidinones compounds with antinociceptive activity in experimental chemotherapy-induced painful neuropathy. Chem Biol Drug Des. 2017;90(2):297–307. https://doi.org/10.1111/cbdd.12951 Epub 2017 Feb 22.
22. Li L, Liu H, Shi W, Liu H, Yang J, Daohua X, Huang H, Longhuo W. Insights into the action mechanisms of traditional Chinese medicine in osteoarthritis. Evid Based Complement Alternat Med. 2017 ; Article ID 5190986:13. https://doi.org/10.1155/2017/5190986.
23. Tsai CC, Chou YY, Chen YM, Tang YJ, Ho HC, Chen DY. Effect of the herbal drug guilu erxian jiao on muscle strength, articular pain, and disability in elderly men with knee osteoarthritis. Evid Based Complement Alternat Med. 2014;2014:297458. https://doi.org/10.1155/2014/297458 Epub 2014 Sep 16.
24. Wang J, Wei DN, Zhang WP, Ran R, Xu K, Gao JW, Lin SY. Adjuvant function of guilu erxian glue cataplasm in treating carcinoma of the large intestine patients with myelosuppression after chemotherapy: a clinical observation. Zhongguo Zhong Xi Yi Jie He Za Zhi. 2014;34(8):947–51.
25. Wang P-H, Li Y-C, Wu Y-H, Chen J-L, Qiu J-T, Yang S-H. Clinical evaluation of Guilu Erxian Jiao in treating perimenopausal syndrome. J Chin Med. 2012;23(2):165–81.
26. Mao C, Zhang Y, Yan W, Zheng X. Effects of serum containing oral liquid of Guilu-Erxian on the therapy of osteoporosis at the cellular level. Sheng Wu Yi Xue Gong Cheng Xue Za Zhi. 2008;25(4):897–902.
27. Zhang Y, Mao C, Yan W, Zheng X. Application of cell engineering of herbal medicine treating bone resorption of osteoclasts. Conf Proc IEEE Eng Med Biol Soc. 2005;5:4958–61.
28. Patterson-Buckendahl P, Sowinska A, Yee S, Patel D, Pagkalinawan S, Shahid M, Shah A, Franz C, Benjamin DE, Pohorecky LA. Decreased sensory responses in osteocalcin null mutant mice imply neuropeptide function. Cell Mol Neurobiol. 2012;32(5):879–89. https://doi.org/10.1007/s10571-012-9810-x Epub 2012 Feb 17.
29. Furman BD, Strand J, Hembree WC, Ward BD, Guilak F, Olson SA. Joint degeneration following closed intraarticular fracture in the mouse knee: a model of posttraumatic arthritis. J Orthop Res. 2007;25(5):578–92.

30. Lorenz J, Grässel S. Experimental osteoarthritis models in mice. Methods Mol Biol. 2014;1194:401–19. https://doi.org/10.1007/978-1-4939-1215-5_23.

31. Pritzker KP, Gay S, Jimenez SA, Ostergaard K, Pelletier JP, Revell PA, Salter D, van den Berg WB. Osteoarthritis cartilage histopathology: grading and staging. Osteoarthr Cartil. 2006;14:13–29.

32. Uchimura T, Foote AT, Smith EL, Matzkin EG, Zeng L. Insulin-like growth factor II (IGF-II) inhibits IL-1β-induced cartilage matrix loss and promotes cartilage integrity in experimental osteoarthritis. J Cell Biochem. 2015; 116(12):2858–69. https://doi.org/10.1002/jcb.25232.

33. Veronesi F, Giavaresi G, Maglio M, Scotto d'Abusco A, Politi L, Scandurra R, Olivotto E, Grigolo B, Borzì RM, Fini M. Chondroprotective activity of N-acetyl phenylalanine glucosamine derivative on knee joint structure and inflammation in a murine model of osteoarthritis. Osteoarthr Cartil. 2017; 25(4):589–99. https://doi.org/10.1016/j.joca.2016.10.021 Epub 2016 Nov 9.

34. Ruan MZ, Patel RM, Dawson BC, Jiang MM, Lee BH. Pain, motor and gait assessment of murine osteoarthritis in a cruciate ligament transection model. Osteoarthr Cartil. 2013;21(9):1355–64. https://doi.org/10.1016/j.joca.2013.06.016.

35. Säämänen AM, Vuorio E. Generation and use of transgenic mice as models of osteoarthritis. Methods Mol Med. 2004;101:1–23.

36. Bendele A, McComb J, Gould T, McAbee T, Sennello G, Chlipala E, Guy M. Animal models of arthritis: relevance to human disease. Toxicol Pathol. 1999;27(1):134–42.

37. Abdelaziz DM, Abdullah S, Magnussen C, Ribeiro-da-Silva A, Komarova SV, Rauch F, Stone LS. Behavioral signs of pain and functional impairment in a mouse model of osteogenesis imperfecta. Bone. 2015;81:400–6. https://doi.org/10.1016/j.bone.2015.08.001 Epub 2015 Aug 13.

38. Vachon P, Millecamps M, Low L, Thompsosn SJ, Pailleux F, Beaudry F, Bushnell CM, Stone LS. Alleviation of chronic neuropathic pain by environmental enrichment in mice well after the establishment of chronic pain. Behav Brain Funct. 2013;9:22. https://doi.org/10.1186/1744-9081-9-22.

39. Brewster M, Lewis EJ, Wilson KL, Greenham AK, Bottomley KM. Ro 32-3555, an orally active collagenase selective inhibitor, prevents structural damage in the STR/ORT mouse model of osteoarthritis. Arthritis Rheum. 1998;41(9):1639–44.

40. Qin L, Han T, Zhang Q, Cao D, Nian H, Rahman K, Zheng H. Antiosteoporotic chemical constituents from Er-Xian decoction, a traditional Chinese herbal formula. J Ethnopharmacol. 2008;118(2):271–9. https://doi.org/10.1016/j.jep.2008.04.009 Epub 2008 Apr 15.

41. Charlier E, Relic B, Deroyer C, Malaise O, Neuville S, Collée J, Malaise MG, De Seny D. Insights on molecular mechanisms of chondrocytes death in osteoarthritis. Int J Mol Sci. 2016;17(12). https://doi.org/10.3390/ijms17122146.

42. Fernández-Criado C, Martos-Rodríguez A, Santos-Alvarez I, García-Ruíz JP, Delgado-Baeza E. The fate of chondrocyte in osteoarthritic cartilage of transgenic mice expressing bovine GH. Osteoarthr Cartil. 2004;12(7):543–51.

43. Fukai A, Kamekura S, Chikazu D, Nakagawa T, Hirata M, Saito T, Hosaka Y, Ikeda T, Nakamura K, Chung UI, Kawaguchi H. Lack of a chondroprotective effect of cyclooxygenase 2 inhibition in a surgically induced model of osteoarthritis in mice. Arthritis Rheum. 2012;64(1):198–203. https://doi.org/10.1002/art.33324.

44. Puljak L, Marin A, Vrdoljak D, Markotic F, Utrobicic A, Tugwell P. Celecoxib for osteoarthritis. Cochrane Database Syst Rev. 2017;5:CD009865. https://doi.org/10.1002/14651858.CD009865.pub2.

45. Chen L, Li DQ, Zhong J, Wu XL, Chen Q, Peng H, Liu SQ. IL-17RA aptamer-mediated repression of IL-6 inhibits synovium inflammation in a murine model of osteoarthritis. Osteoarthr Cartil. 2011;19(6):711–8. https://doi.org/10.1016/j.joca.2011.01.018 Epub 2011 Feb 22.

46. Chevalier X, Mugnier B, Bouvenot G. Targeted anti-cytokine therapies for osteoarthritis. Bull Acad Natl Med. 2006;190(7):1411–20 discussion 1420, 1475–7.

47. Malemud CJ. Anticytokine therapy for osteoarthritis: evidence to date. Drugs Aging. 2010;27(2):95–115. https://doi.org/10.2165/11319950-000000000-00000.

48. Malemud CJ. Cytokines as therapeutic targets for osteoarthritis. BioDrugs. 2004;18(1):23–35.

49. Zheng W, Tao Z, Chen C, Zhang C, Zhang H, Ying X, Chen H. Plumbagin prevents IL-1β-induced inflammatory response in human osteoarthritis chondrocytes and prevents the progression of osteoarthritis in mice. Inflammation. 2017;40(3):849–60. https://doi.org/10.1007/s10753-017-0530-8.

50. Jacques C, Gosset M, Berenbaum F, Gabay C. The role of IL-1 and IL-1Ra in joint inflammation and cartilage degradation. Vitam Horm. 2006;74:371–403.

51. Sheu SY, Ho SR, Sun JS, Chen CY, Ke CJ. Arthropod steroid hormone (20-Hydroxyecdysone) suppresses IL-1β-induced catabolic gene expression in cartilage. BMC Complement Altern Med. 2015;15:1. https://doi.org/10.1186/s12906-015-0520-z.

52. Mohamed-Ali H. Influence of interleukin-1 beta, tumour necrosis factor alpha and prostaglandin E2 on chondrogenesis and cartilage matrix breakdown in vitro. Rheumatol Int. 1995;14(5):191–9.

53. Blasioli DJ, Kaplan DL. The roles of catabolic factors in the development of osteoarthritis. Tissue Eng Part B Rev. 2014;20(4):355–63. https://doi.org/10.1089/ten.TEB.2013.0377 Epub 2013 Dec 11.

54. Ricks ML, Farrell JT, Falk DJ, Holt DW, Rees M, Carr J, Williams T, Nichols BA, Bridgewater LC, Reynolds PR, Kooyman DL, Seegmiller RE. Osteoarthritis in temporomandibular joint of Col2a1 mutant mice. Arch Oral Biol. 2013;58(9): 1092–9. https://doi.org/10.1016/j.archoralbio.2013.02.008 Epub 2013 Mar 19.

55. Lai YC, Shaftel SS, Miller JN, Tallents RH, Chang Y, Pinkert CA, Olschowka JA, Dickerson IM, Puzas JE, O'Banion MK, Kyrkanides S. Intraarticular induction of interleukin-1beta expression in the adult mouse, with resultant temporomandibular joint pathologic changes, dysfunction, and pain. Arthritis Rheum. 2006;54(4):1184–97.

56. Lago R, Gomez R, Otero M, Lago F, Gallego R, Dieguez C, Gomez-Reino JJ, Gualillo O. A new player in cartilage homeostasis: adiponectin induces nitric oxide synthase type II and pro-inflammatory cytokines in chondrocytes. Osteoarthr Cartil. 2008;16(9):1101–9. https://doi.org/10.1016/j.joca.2007.12.008 Epub 2008 Feb 7.

57. Wang Y, Xu J, Zhang X, Wang C, Huang Y, Dai K, Zhang X. TNF-α-induced LRG1 promotes angiogenesis and mesenchymal stem cell migration in the subchondral bone during osteoarthritis. Cell Death Dis. 2017;8(3):e2715. https://doi.org/10.1038/cddis.2017.129.

58. Dar QA, Schott EM, Catheline SE, Maynard RD, Liu Z, Kamal F, Farnsworth CW, Ketz JP, Mooney RA, Hilton MJ, Jonason JH, Prawitt J, Zuscik MJ. Daily oral consumption of hydrolyzed type 1 collagen is chondroprotective and anti-inflammatory in murine posttraumatic osteoarthritis. PLoS One. 2017; 12(4):e0174705. https://doi.org/10.1371/journal.pone.0174705.

59. Klatt AR, Klinger G, Neumüller O, Eidenmüller B, Wagner I, Achenbach T, Aigner T, Bartnik E. TAK1 downregulation reduces IL-1beta induced expression of MMP13, MMP1 and TNF-alpha. Biomed Pharmacother. 2006; 60(2):55–61 Epub 2005 Dec 27.

60. Goldring MB. The role of cytokines as inflammatory mediators in osteoarthritis: lessons from animal models. Connect Tissue Res. 1999;40(1):1–11.

61. Latourte A, Cherifi C, Maillet J, Ea HK, Bouaziz W, Funck-Brentano T, Cohen-Solal M, Hay E, Richette P. Systemic inhibition of IL-6/Stat3 signalling protects against experimental osteoarthritis. Ann Rheum Dis. 2017;76(4):748–55. https://doi.org/10.1136/annrheumdis-2016-209757 Epub 2016 Oct 27.

62. Hooge AS, van de Loo FA, Bennink MB, Arntz OJ, de Hooge P, van den Berg WB. Male IL-6 gene knock out mice developed more advanced osteoarthritis upon aging. Osteoarthr Cartil. 2005;13(1):66–73.

63. Ryu JH, Yang S, Shin Y, Rhee J, Chun CH, Chun JS. Interleukin-6 plays an essential role in hypoxia-inducible factor 2α-induced experimental osteoarthritic cartilage destruction in mice. Arthritis Rheum. 2011;63(9): 2732–43. https://doi.org/10.1002/art.30451.

64. Tang J, Dong Q. Knockdown of TREM-1 suppresses IL-1β-induced chondrocyte injury via inhibiting the NF-κB pathway. Biochem Biophys Res Commun. 2017; 482(4):1240–5. https://doi.org/10.1016/j.bbrc.2016.12.019 Epub 2016 Dec 5.

65. Sanchez C, Gabay O, Salvat C, Henrotin YE, Berenbaum F. Mechanical loading highly increases IL-6 production and decreases OPG expression by osteoblasts. Osteoarthr Cartil. 2009;17(4):473–81. https://doi.org/10.1016/j.joca.2008.09.007 Epub 2008 Oct 29.

66. Okura T, Matsushita M, Mishima K, Esaki R, Seki T, Ishiguro N, Kitoh H. Activated FGFR3 prevents subchondral bone sclerosis during the development of osteoarthritis in transgenic mice with achondroplasia. J Orthop Res. 2017. https://doi.org/10.1002/jor.23608.

67. Zheng W, Feng Z, You S, Zhang H, Tao Z, Wang Q, Chen H, Wu Y. Fisetin inhibits IL-1β-induced inflammatory response in human osteoarthritis chondrocytes through activating SIRT1 and attenuates the progression of osteoarthritis in mice. Int Immunopharmacol. 2017;45:135–47. https://doi.org/10.1016/j.intimp.2017.02.009 Epub 2017 Feb 16.

68. Chambers MG, Bayliss MT, Mason RM. Chondrocyte cytokine and growth factor expression in murine osteoarthritis. Osteoarthr Cartil. 1997;5(5):301–8.

69. Prasadam I, Zhou Y, Shi W, Crawford R, Xiao Y. Role of dentin matrix protein 1 in cartilage redifferentiation and osteoarthritis. Rheumatology (Oxford). 2014; 53(12):2280–7. https://doi.org/10.1093/rheumatology/keu262 Epub 2014 Jul 1.

21

Comparison of collum femoris-preserving stems and ribbed stems in primary total hip arthroplasty

Mingqing Li, Can Xu, Jie Xie, Yihe Hu and Hua Liu[*]

Abstract

Background: This retrospective study investigated the relative benefits of using a collum femoris-preserving prosthesis or ribbed stem during total hip arthroplasty (THA).

Methods: The clinical results were compared of patients who underwent THA, between January 2010 and December 2012, with either a CFP prosthesis or a ribbed stem (66 and 75 patients, respectively, aged 43.4 ± 10.8 and 42.3 ± 9.8 years). Patients were assessed using the Harris Hip Score (HHS), Western Ontario and McMaster University Osteoarthritis Index (WOMAC), 12-Item Short Form Health Survey (SF-12), and physical component summary (PCS) score. Intraoperative and postoperative complications and leg-length differences were noted.

Results: The mean follow-up times of the CFP and ribbed groups were 67.2 ± 7.5 and 68.3 ± 7.2 months, respectively. The HHS, SF-12 MCS, SF-12 PCS, and WOMAC scores of the two groups were similar. The rates of periprosthetic femoral fractures and leg-length differences > 10 mm in the CFP group (10.6% and 13.6%, respectively) were significantly higher than those in the ribbed group (1.3% and 2.7%). The groups were similar regarding complications of osteolysis, ectopic ossification, dislocation, deep infection, deep venous thrombosis, thigh pain, and aseptic loosening. The survival rates of the CFP and ribbed groups were comparable (98.5% and 97.8%).

Conclusion: The clinical results of the CFP and ribbed prostheses in young patients given THA were similar for Chinese patients. However, the CFP stem should be used with caution, given the high incidence of technical problems associated with implantation especially for Chinese patients.

Keywords: Total hip arthroplasty, Collum femoris preservation, Hip surgery, Implantation

Background

Increasing numbers of patients are undergoing total hip arthroplasty (THA) because of highly successful rates and good clinical results [1]. The femoral neck is the most solid structure of the proximal femur and the center of stress distribution for the hip joint. Retention of the femoral neck preserves the trabecular systems of the metaphyseal cancellous bone, which allows a more even distribution of the physiological load along the diaphysis. Furthermore, protecting the blood supply to the femoral neck permits increased bone ingrowth [2, 3].

The collum femoris-preserving (CFP) short-stem prosthesis (Waldemar Link GmbH, Hamburg, Germany) is a cementless implant, especially appropriate for younger patients. Although there have been many reports of good early-to-midterm results with the CFP prosthesis [4–8], few studies have compared it with those that are more commonly used, in particular prostheses with a ribbed anatomical stem that require excision of the femoral neck for implantation [9, 10]. Burchard et al. [11] concluded from a virtual model that the CFP prosthesis has a stress-shielding effect and thus is harmful for bone remodeling. Thus, the question remains whether femoral neck-preserving hip prostheses perform better than traditional neck implants that require resection.

The present retrospective study compared the clinical results and complications of 66 patients who underwent THA with a CFP prosthesis, relative to 75 patients given a ribbed stem.

* Correspondence: xyzhwk@163.com
Department of Orthopedics, Xiangya Hospital, Central South University, Changsha, Hunan 410008, People's Republic of China

Methods

Patients and implants

Our Institutional Review Board approved this retrospective observational study.

The study comprised two cohorts. One cohort received a CFP short-stem prosthesis, and the other received a ribbed stem (both from Waldemar Link GmbH, Hamburg, Germany). Both stems are anatomical S-shaped stems; the principal difference being that the CFP short-stem prosthesis allows retention of the femoral neck. Patients were selected for either treatment by simple randomization.

From January 2010 to December 2012, 78 patients underwent THA by an experienced surgeon (the corresponding author) using the CFP stems. Eight patients with bilateral THAs were excluded from this study. An additional four patients were lost to follow-up. The remaining 66 were included in the study cohort.

The 66 patients who received CFP stems during THA were individually matched by age, gender, body mass index, and calendar year of the operation to 75 patients who underwent primary unilateral THA with ribbed stems (Table 1). The 75 patients were identified through the longitudinal registry as patients who underwent THA using ribbed stems. Thus, the patient demographics and clinical profiles of the two cohorts are similar.

Surgical data

All surgeries were performed by an experienced surgeon (the corresponding author) using a posterolateral approach after general anesthesia. All procedures were discussed by more than three experienced orthopedic surgeons and preoperatively planned according to the clinical manifestation and radiological inspections. A T.O.P. press-fit porous-coated TiAl6V4 acetabular cup (Waldemar Link GmbH) was used in both groups. Screws (Waldemar Link GmbH) were placed when the surgeon believed they would be helpful for acetabular fixation, based on the patient's age and bone quality.

Table 1 Demographics and preoperative diagnoses of patients undergoing primary THA

	CFP stems	Ribbed stems	P value
Total subjects, n	66	75	–
Gender, m/f	38/30	41/34	0.90
Age, years	43.4 ± 10.8	42.3 ± 9.8	0.52
Body mass index, kg/m^2	25.3 ± 4.5	24.4 ± 3.9	0.20
Preoperative diagnosis			
Osteoarthritis	28 (42.4%)	60 (44.4%)	0.78
Avascular necrosis	30 (45.5%)	64 (47.4%)	0.79
Other	8 (12.1%)	11 (8.2%)	0.36
Follow-up, months	67.2 ± 7.5	68.3 ± 7.2	0.32

Postoperatively, all patients received an intravenous antibiotic to prevent postoperative infection. All patients received standard-of-care treatment. Low-molecular-weight heparin was given, and a lower-extremity venous pump was used for about 30 min, twice a day, to prevent thromboembolic incidents. Patients were instructed regarding hip exercises, and all therapy was supervised. Patients were mobilized as tolerated, starting with a walker and progressing to a cane. All patients were able to accomplish stair climbing before discharge from the hospital.

Clinical evaluation

All patients agreed to enter the arthroplasty registry and were followed clinically and radiographically at 3 and 6 months postoperatively, and then annually. At each follow-up visit, patients completed the 12-Item Short Form Health Survey (SF-12) [12] (including mental and physical components) and the Western Ontario and McMaster University Osteoarthritis Index (WOMAC) [13, 14]. The evaluators also completed the Harris Hip Score (HHS) forms and documented the range of motion of the operative hip.

Radiological evaluation

Standard anteroposterior radiographs of the pelvis and lateral radiographs of the hip, including the length of the total prosthesis, were obtained at regular follow-up intervals. Two qualified reviewers evaluated the radiographs for osteolysis and radiolucent lines > 1 mm using the zones of DeLee and Charnley [15] for the acetabulum and Gruen et al. [16] for the femur.

Complications, revisions, and implant failures were recorded. Leg length and offset was evaluated before and after surgery by tape measure [17, 18]. Offset was based on the contralateral hip; an offset difference ≤ 5 mm was considered a good result. For the purposes of this study, we compared the mean offset difference and percentage of hips with an offset difference ≤ 5 mm between the two cohorts. A tape was used to measure leg-length discrepancy, as the difference in lengths from the anterior spina to inner malleolus, between the operated and contralateral side.

Any patient who underwent a second surgery (i.e., femoral head or stem) was considered a survivorship failure.

Statistical analysis

The HHS, WOMAC, and the Physical Composite Scale (PCS) and Mental Health Composite Scale (MCS) scores of the SF-12 were tested for improvement at the final follow-up, using an independent sample t test if the data had a normal distribution. A nonparametric test (Mann-Whitney U test) was used if the data had a skewed distribution. The chi-squared or Fisher's exact test was used to determine if the incidence of complications was different between the two groups. A two-sided value of $P < 0.05$ was considered statistically significant. The statistical power of this study was 80%.

Results

Follow-ups of > 5 years were completed in both the CFP and ribbed stem groups. In both groups, at 1 year after THA and at each follow-up, the scores of the following were significantly improved relative to before surgery: HHS, WOMAC, SF-12 MCS, and SF-12 PCS (Table 2 and Fig. 1). At 1-year follow-up, the HHS, SF-12 MCS, and SF-12 PCS scores of the CFP group were significantly higher than that of the ribbed group. However, the mean WOMAC score of the CFP group was significantly less than that of the ribbed group ($P = 0.01$). At the other follow-up times, the scores of the two groups were comparable (HHS, WOMAC, SF-12 MCS, and SF-12 PCS).

In the CFP group, there were seven (10.6%) intraoperative fractures of the lateral femoral diaphysis at the tip of the stem, whereas only one (1.3%) occurred in the ribbed stem group (Fig. 2). No patient required additional treatment. At 5 days after surgery, all of the patients were allowed partial load-bearing (20 kg), and by 3 months, a gradual increase to full weight bearing. During this time, patients were asked to walk with the aid of crutches to assist with partial weight bearing. The fractures in all patients were healed at postoperative 8 months.

In the CFP group, radiological analysis showed that two (3.0%) patients developed periprosthetic osteolytic hips (both in Gruen zone 7). In the ribbed stem group, there were three (4%) osteolytic cases (one in Gruen zone 1, two in Gruen zone 7). A representative case is shown in Fig. 3. The difference in the incidence of osteolysis in the two groups was not statistically significant ($P > 0.05$).

Periarticular ossification was observed in seven hips: three (4.5%) in the CFP group and four (5.3%) in the ribbed stem group ($P > 0.05$). At the final follow-up, one (1.5%) hip dislocation had occurred in the CFP group (because of a tumble) and three (4%) had occurred in

the ribbed group (two because of a tumble, the other because of acetabular cup malposition). The groups were statistically similar regarding rates of complications of deep infection, deep venous thrombosis, thigh pain, and aseptic loosening (all $P > 0.05$). Two hips required revision in the ribbed stem group, one because of recurrent dislocation, and the other because of deep infection; the latter was subsequently revised with two-stage reimplantation. Only one revision was performed in the CFP group (due to recurrent dislocation). The survival rate of the CFP group (98.5%) was similar to that of the ribbed group (97.3%; $P > 0.05$; Table 3).

The results of leg-length differences are shown in Table 4. In the ribbed group, the majority of patients (65.3%) had equal leg length (≤ 5 mm), compared to 40.9% in the CFP group ($P = 0.004$). The percentage of patients with a leg-length difference > 10 mm in the CFP group (13.6%) was higher than that in the ribbed group (2.7%; $P = 0.025$).

Discussion

The CFP and ribbed stem are both anatomically S-shaped stems. The main difference between them is that the ribbed stem requires that femoral neck be cut, while the CFP does not. To investigate the relative benefits and suitability of the CFP and ribbed stem prostheses during THA for non-elderly patients, we retrospectively compared the clinical results of 66 patients given a CFP prosthesis during THA, with those of 75 patients given a ribbed stem. All the patients were followed for more than 5 years. The clinical and radiographic results suggest that both the CFP and ribbed prostheses perform well. We found that the use of the CFP stems did not improve the HHS, WOMAC, or SF-12 scores above that of the ribbed stems. On the contrary, use of the CFP stems was associated with an increase in the incidence of periprosthetic femoral fractures during surgery, and postoperative leg-length discrepancy, compared with the ribbed stems. Whether the CFP prosthesis is better than the ribbed stem for patients is still unknown, but the present study found that the CFP had no advantage over the ribbed stem.

Table 2 Results of HHS, WOMAC score, and SF-12 in the two groups

	HHS			WOMAC			SF-12 MCS			SF-12 PCS		
	CFP	Ribbed	P	CFP	Ribbed	P	CFP	Ribbed	P	CFP	Ribbed	P
Preoperative	50 ± 10	51 ± 11	0.53	62 ± 19	61 ± 18	0.72	50 ± 8	49 ± 9	0.44	33 ± 6	32 ± 7	0.32
1 year	86 ± 15	90 ± 11	0.03	11 ± 7	8 ± 7	0.01	54 ± 9	55 ± 10	0.49	45 ± 8	49 ± 9	0.00
2 year	90 ± 16	92 ± 18	0.44	7 ± 6	8 ± 5	0.21	54 ± 8	55 ± 10	0.48	48 ± 9	49 ± 8	0.43
3 year	92 ± 19	91 ± 18	0.72	7 ± 3	8 ± 6	0.20	54 ± 8	55 ± 9	0.44	48 ± 7	49 ± 7	0.34
4 year	93 ± 18	92 ± 10	0.61	7 ± 5	8 ± 4	0.13	54 ± 9	55 ± 8	0.43	49 ± 8	49 ± 10	1
Last follow-up	93 ± 15	92 ± 19	0.71	7 ± 4	8 ± 5	0.16	54 ± 7	55 ± 9	0.43	49 ± 9	49 ± 8	1

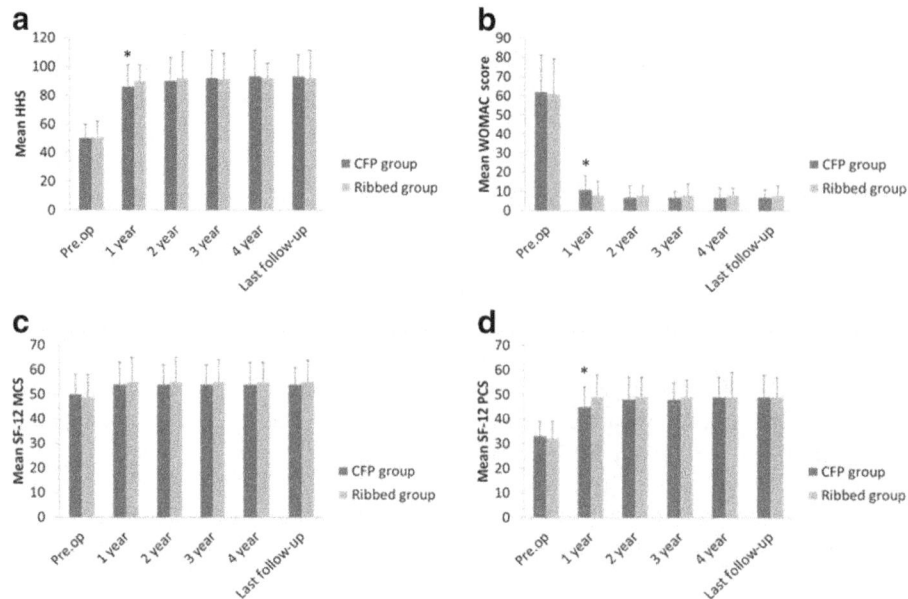

Fig. 1 Histograms showing the mean HHS (**a**), WOMAC score (**b**), SF-12 MCS (**c**), and SF-12 PCS (**d**). The asterisk indicates a statistically significant difference between the CFP group and the ribbed group

Overall, the patients in the CFP group experienced seven intraoperative fractures of the lateral femoral diaphysis at the tip of the stem and six of these involved an exaggerated neck-shaft angle. The CFP prosthesis is designed in accordance with the normal anatomy of the femur, with two neck-shaft angles (126° and 117°); Jiang et al. [19] reported that the mean neck-shaft angle in a Chinese Han population was 133°. They also showed that adults younger than 60 years had a significantly higher neck-shaft angle. Hoaglund and Low [20] found the average neck-shaft angle in Hong Kong Chinese was 135°. The reasons for the differences in neck-shaft angle

between these ethnicities are not known. All these results show that the average neck-shaft angle in Chinese people is larger than that in the CFP prosthesis. The compressive and tensile stresses surrounding the prosthesis are higher when the CFP prosthesis is used in patients with a smaller neck-shaft angle, and these stresses eventually lead to a fracture [21]. Thus, we concluded that the design of the CFP prosthesis may not be suitable for Chinese people.

The current study found that the incidence of intraoperative fractures with the CFP prosthesis was higher than that when the ribbed system is applied. There are few

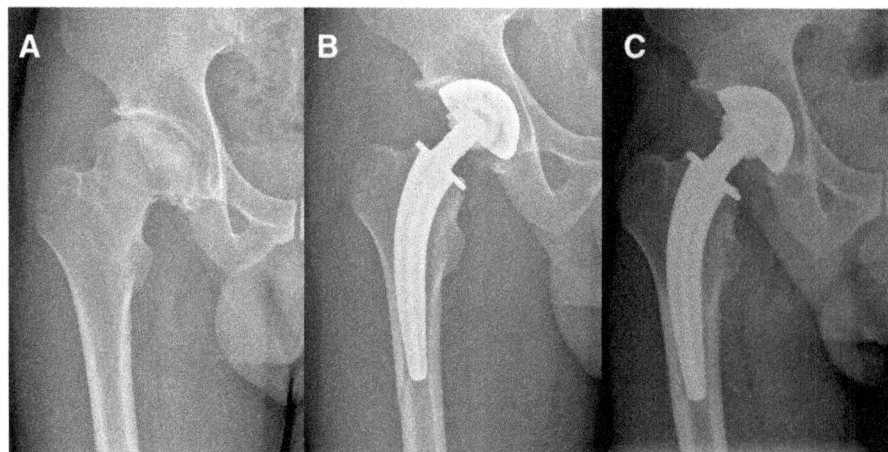

Fig. 2 Preoperative anteroposterior radiograph of a 30-year-old man showing femoral head osteonecrosis of the right hip (**a**). Anteroposterior radiograph after THA using CFP stem showing PPF of the lateral femoral diaphysis (**b**). Anteroposterior radiograph at 1-year follow-up showing healing fracture (**c**)

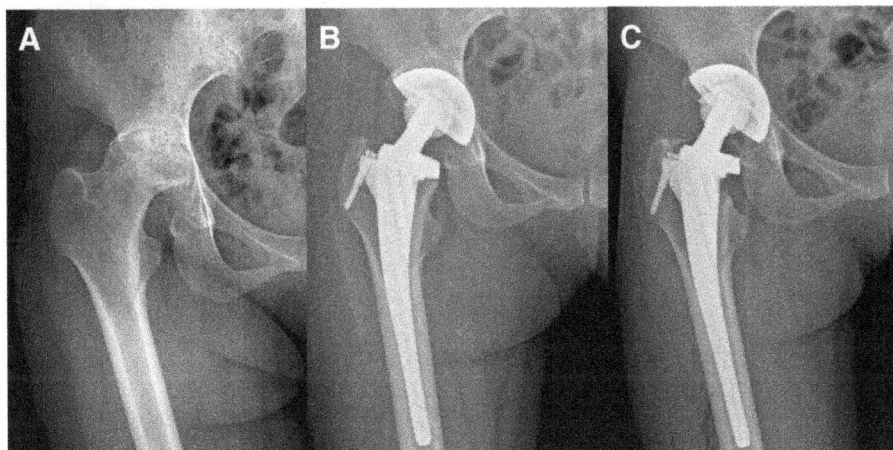

Fig. 3 Preoperative anteroposterior radiograph of a 36-year-old woman showing femoral head osteonecrosis of the right hip (**a**). Anteroposterior radiograph 3 weeks after THA using a ribbed stem (**b**). Anteroposterior radiograph at 2-year follow-up showing osteolysis in Gruen zone 7 (**c**)

relevant articles regarding why intraoperative fractures occur when using either the CFP or ribbed stem prostheses, but such fractures were associated with the minimally invasive technique, press-fit cementless stems, female gender, metabolic bone disease, bone diseases that lead to altered morphology such as Paget's disease, or intraoperative technical errors [22].

A difference in leg lengths is a well-recognized and common complication after THA [23, 24]. It is generally believed that differences of more than 1.5 cm can cause lower back pain, gait disorders, and general dissatisfaction [25]. However, it was determined that leg-length discrepancy was not associated with patients' outcomes [25]. In the current study, the percentage of patients with a leg-length discrepancy of > 5 mm was higher in the CFP group than in the ribbed group. We consider that this is mainly because the operated femoral neck, with the length of the prosthesis neck in addition to the remaining patient's neck, is longer than the patient's original, or it can be due to the use of longer-neck femoral heads. However, other factors also influence leg-length discrepancy [26].

Radiographic evidence of osteolysis was detected in both the CFP and ribbed groups. Both the stems are collared prostheses, which can effectively prevent the subsidence of the stem, and may also lead to osteolysis in Gruen zone 7 due to stress shielding [27]. Another reason is the generation of wear particles [28], depending on implant design and manufacturing materials. Previous studies have shown that alumina-on-alumina articulations minimize osteolysis [29, 30].

The CFP prosthesis is designed especially for young (non-elderly) patients. According to the data we found, the CFP prosthesis failed to exhibit any advantages over the ribbed prosthesis. Whether the CFP prosthesis is more suitable for young patients is still unknown. Randomized controlled trials are warranted before the benefits of the CFP prosthesis are confirmed.

This study had several limitations. Firstly, the number of cases in the study was insufficient for good statistical power. Secondly, the study is retrospective, and all of the patients were from our hospital, constituting selection bias. Thirdly, we used only clinical measurements for the leg length, and these apparent assessments can differ from the more accurate radiographic evidence.

Table 3 Intra- and postoperative complications of the CFP and ribbed stem patient groups, n (%)

	CFP	Ribbed	P
PPFF	7 (10.6%)	1 (1.3%)	0.026
Osteolysis or lucent lines	2 (3.0%)	3 (4%)	1.0
Ectopic ossification	3 (4.5%)	4 (5.3%)	1.0
Dislocation	1 (1.5%)	3 (4%)	0.623
Deep infection	0	1 (1.3%)	1.0
Deep venous thrombosis	0	2 (2.7%)	0.498
Thigh pain	0	1 (1.3%)	1.0
Aseptic loosening	0	0	–
Survival rate	98.5%	97.3%	1.0

PPFF periprosthetic femoral fracture

Table 4 Limb length discrepancies of the CFP and ribbed stem patient groups

	CFP	Ribbed	P
0–5 mm	40.9% (27/66)	65.3% (49/75)	0.004
5–10 mm	45.5% (30/66)	32% (24/75)	0.101
>10 mm	13.6% (9/66)	2.7% (2/75)	0.025

Conclusions

The results indicate that both the CFP prosthesis and ribbed prosthesis significantly improved the preoperative HHS, WOMAC, and SF-12 PCS scores. However, differences between the two stems were insignificant, and the CFP prosthesis failed to exhibit any advantages over the ribbed prosthesis for Chinese patients. In addition, the CFP prosthesis is more prone to causing periprosthetic femoral fractures, so surgeons need to take preventive measures, especially for Chinese patients. Whether the clinical effect of the CFP prosthesis with femoral neck preservation is better than the ribbed stem with femoral neck truncation requires further study.

Abbreviations

CFP: Collum femoris-preserving; HHS: Harris Hip Score; PCS: Physical component summary; SF-12: Item Short Form Health Survey; THA: Total hip arthroplasty; WOMAC: Western Ontario and McMaster University Osteoarthritis Index

Acknowledgements
None.

Funding
None.

Authors' contributions

MQL, CX, JX, YHH, and HL designed the study. MQL, CX, and JX collected and analyzed the data. MQL drafted and wrote the manuscript. YHH and HL revised the manuscript critically for intellectual content. All authors gave intellectual input to the study and approved the final version of the manuscript.

Competing interests

The authors declare that they have no competing interests.

References

1. Kuijpers MFL, Hannink G, van Steenbergen LN, et al. Total hip arthroplasty in young patients in the Netherlands: trend analysis of >19,000 primary hip replacements in the Dutch Arthroplasty Register. J Arthroplast. 2018. https://doi.org/10.1016/j.arth.2018.08.020.
2. Kress AM, Schmidt R, Nowak TE, et al. Stress-related femoral cortical and cancellous bone density loss after collum femoris preserving uncemented total hip arthroplasty: a prospective 7-year follow-up with quantitative computed tomography. Arch Orthop Trauma Surg. 2012;132:1111–9.
3. Molfetta L, Capozzi M, Caldo D. Medium term follow up of the biodynamic neck sparing prosthesis. Hip Int. 2011;21:76–80.
4. Briem D, Schneider M, Bogner N, et al. Mid-term results of 155 patients treated with a collum femoris preserving (CFP) short stem prosthesis. Int Orthop. 2011;35:655–60.
5. Ghera S, Bisicchia S. The collum femoris preserving stem: early results. Hip Int. 2013;23:27–32.
6. Li M, Hu Y, Xie J. Analysis of the complications of the collum femoris preserving (CFP) prostheses. Acta Orthop Traumatol Turc. 2014;48:623–7.
7. Nowak M, Nowak TE, Schmidt R, et al. Prospective study of a cementless total hip arthroplasty with a collum femoris preserving stem and a trabeculae oriented pressfit cup: minimun 6-year follow-up. Arch Orthop Trauma Surg. 2011;131:549–55.
8. Van Oldenrijk J, Schafroth MU, Rijk E, et al. Learning curve analysis of the Collum Femoris preserving total hip surgical technique. Hip Int. 2013;23:154–61.
9. Hu K, Zhang X, Zhu J, et al. Periprosthetic fractures may be more likely in cementless femoral stems with sharp edges. Ir J Med Sci. 2010;179:417–21.
10. Zhang Q, Liu M, Chai W, et al. Total hip arthroplasty with double-tapered cementless femoral stem for hip bony. Zhongguo Xiu Fu Chong Jian Wai Ke Za Zhi. 2013;27:278–82.
11. Burchard R, Braas S, Soost C, et al. Bone preserving level of osteotomy in short-stem total hip arthroplasty does not influence stress shielding dimensions - a comparing finite elements analysis. BMC Musculoskelet Disord. 2017;18:343.
12. Ware J Jr, Kosinski M, Keller SD. A 12-item short-form health survey: construction of scales and preliminary tests of reliability and validity. Med Care. 1996;34:220–33.
13. Bellamy N, Buchanan WW, Goldsmith CH, et al. Validation study of WOMAC: a health status instrument for measuring clinically important patient relevant outcomes to antirheumatic drug therapy in patients with osteoarthritis of the hip or knee. J Rheumatol. 1988;15:1833–40.
14. Hawker G, Melfi C, Paul J, et al. Comparison of a generic (SF-36) and a disease specific (WOMAC) (Western Ontario and McMaster Universities Osteoarthritis Index) instrument in the measurement of outcomes after knee replacement surgery. J Rheumatol. 1995;22:1193–6.
15. DeLee JG, Charnley J. Radiological demarcation of cemented sockets in total hip replacement. Clin Orthop Relat Res. 1976;121:20–32.
16. Gruen TA, McNeice GM, Amstutz HC. "Modes of failure" of cemented stem-type femoral components: a radiographic analysis of loosening. Clin Orthop Relat Res. 1979;141:17–27.
17. Aguilar EG, Dominguez AG, Pena-Algaba C, et al. Distance between the malleoli and the ground: a new clinical method to measure leg-length discrepancy. J Am Podiatr Med Assoc. 2017;107:112–8.
18. Badii M, Wade AN, Collins DR, et al. Comparison of lifts versus tape measure in determining leg length discrepancy. J Rheumatol. 2014;41:1689–94.
19. Jiang N, Peng L, Al-Qwbani M, et al. Femoral version, neck-shaft angle, and acetabular anteversion in Chinese Han population: a retrospective analysis of 466 healthy adults. Medicine (Baltimore). 2015;94:e891.
20. Hoaglund FT, Low WD. Anatomy of the femoral neck and head, with comparative data from Caucasians and Hong Kong Chinese. Clin Orthop Relat Res. 1980;152:10–6.
21. Capello WN, D'Antonio JA, Naughton M. Periprosthetic fractures around a cementless hydroxyapatite-coated implant: a new fracture pattern is described. Clin Orthop Relat Res. 2014;472:604–10.
22. Davidson D, Pike J, Garbuz D, et al. Intraoperative periprosthetic fractures during total hip arthroplasty. Evaluation and management. J Bone Joint Surg Am. 2008;90:2000–12.
23. Kitada M, Nakamura N, Iwana D, et al. Evaluation of the accuracy of computed tomography-based navigation for femoral stem orientation and leg length discrepancy. J Arthroplast. 2011;26:674–9.
24. Kurtz WB. In situ leg length measurement technique in hip arthroplasty. J Arthroplast. 2012;27:66–73.
25. Whitehouse MR, Stefanovich-Lawbuary NS, Brunton LR, et al. The impact of leg length discrepancy on patient satisfaction and functional outcome following total hip arthroplasty. J Arthroplast. 2013;28:1408–14.
26. Kersic M, Dolinar D, Antolic V, et al. The impact of leg length discrepancy on clinical outcome of total hip arthroplasty: comparison of four measurement methods. J Arthroplast. 2014;29:137–41.
27. Schaller G, Black J, Asaad A, et al. Primary collared uncemented total hip arthroplasties in the elderly: a safe and reliable treatment option. J Arthroplast. 2015;30:407–10.
28. Lazarinis S, Mattsson P, Milbrink J, et al. A prospective cohort study on the short collum femoris-preserving (CFP) stem using RSA and DXA. Primary stability but no prevention of proximal bone loss in 27 patients followed for 2 years. Acta Orthop. 2013;84:32–9.
29. Kim YH, Choi Y, Kim JS. Cementless total hip arthroplasty with ceramic-on-ceramic bearing in patients younger than 45 years with femoral-head osteonecrosis. Int Orthop. 2010;34:1123–7.

22

Efficacy of intravenous acetaminophen in multimodal management for pain relief following total knee arthroplasty: a meta-analysis

Song-bo Shi, Xing-bo Wang, Jian-min Song, Shi-fang Guo, Zhi-xin Chen and Yin Wang*

Abstract

Background: The efficacy of intravenous acetaminophen in multimodal pain management in patients undergoing total knee arthroplasty (TKA) is controversial. The purpose of this meta-analysis was to compare the efficacy of intravenous acetaminophen versus placebo in TKA.

Methods: Randomized controlled trials (RCTs) or retrospective cohort studies (RCSs) concerning related topics were retrieved from PubMed (1996–June 2018), Embase (1980–June 2018), and the Cochrane Library (CENTRAL June 2018). Any studies comparing intravenous acetaminophen with a placebo were included in this meta-analysis. Meta-analysis results were collected and analyzed by Stata 12.0. Subgroup analysis was performed according to the general characteristics of the patients.

Results: In total, the patients from six studies met the inclusion criteria. Our meta-analysis results indicated that compared with a control group, intravenous acetaminophen was associated with reductions in total morphine consumption and visual analogue scale (VAS) score at postoperative day (POD) 3. However, there was no significant difference in morphine consumption at POD 1 or in VAS at POD 1 or POD 2. Moreover, there was no significant difference in the length of hospital stay.

Conclusions: Based on our results, intravenous acetaminophen in multimodal management has shown better efficacy in pain relief at POD 3 and has morphine-sparing effects. High-quality studies with more patients are needed in the future.

Keywords: Acetaminophen, Pain control, Total knee arthroplasty, Meta-analysis

Background

Total knee arthroplasty (TKA) is being widely used for end-stage osteoarthritis (OA) or rheumatoid arthritis (RA) [1]. However, over 80% of TKA patients experience severe to moderate postoperative pain [2]. Inadequate pain management may result in dissatisfaction, complications, stunted postoperative functional recovery, and longer hospital stays [3, 4]. Conventionally, multimodal pain management is widely recommended and accepted [5, 6]. Multimodal pain management usually includes two or more analgesics, such as opioids, nonsteroidal anti-inflammatory medications, steroid hormones, and epinephrine [7]. It has been reported that rebounding pain in patients treated with multimodal pain management after 24 h postoperatively remains a real problem for surgeons [8, 9]. Furthermore, the use of opioids is frequently associated with some side effects, including gastrointestinal symptoms, autonomic nervous system symptoms, and central nervous system symptoms, among others [10, 11]. Thus, adjunctive pain management medication is needed.

Recently, combination therapy with intravenous (IV) acetaminophen has been used to reduce postoperative pain, and opioid use across a variety of surgical procedures has also been applied to the TKA [12–14]. Kelly et al. [15]

---
* Correspondence: 246771930@qq.com
Orthopaedics Department, Gansu Provincial Hospital, Lanzhou 730000, Gansu, China

drew the conclusion that IV acetaminophen did not significantly decrease postoperative opioid use in patients who underwent surgical knee procedures. Studies conducted by Blank et al. [16] and Nwagbologu et al. [17] presented similar conclusions. However, O'Neal et al. [18] reported that neither IV nor oral acetaminophen provided better analgesia in patients undergoing TKA. Similar results were reported by subsequent studies [19]. Thus, conclusions concerning the use of IV acetaminophen in reducing postoperative pain and opioid consumption have been inconsistent. Several studies have reported that IV acetaminophen has a beneficial role in reducing pain intensity and morphine consumption after TKA [19, 20]. However, some other studies suggest that the use of acetaminophen in multimodal pain management does not result in improved safety or reduced opioid utilization in hip or knee arthroplasty [17, 21].

Therefore, it is necessary to investigate whether IV acetaminophen as an adjunctive pain management medication provides better analgesic effects, as well as whether it reduces opioid consumption in patients after TKA. The purpose of the current meta-analysis was to compare results concerning the efficacy of IV acetaminophen for pain control in patients undergoing TKA.

Methods
Search strategy
We manually searched randomized controlled trials (RCTs), retrospective cohort studies (RCSs), and cohort studies through PubMed (1996–June 2018), Embase (1980–June 2018), and the Cochrane Library (CENTRAL, June 2018). We also searched trials from related references and reviews. The key words and MeSH terms were "total knee arthroplasty," "total knee replacement," "TKA," "TKR," "Arthroplasty, Replacement, Knee" [MeSH], and "acetaminophen." These key words or MeSH terms were combined using the Boolean operators "AND" or "OR." The search results are presented in Fig. 1.

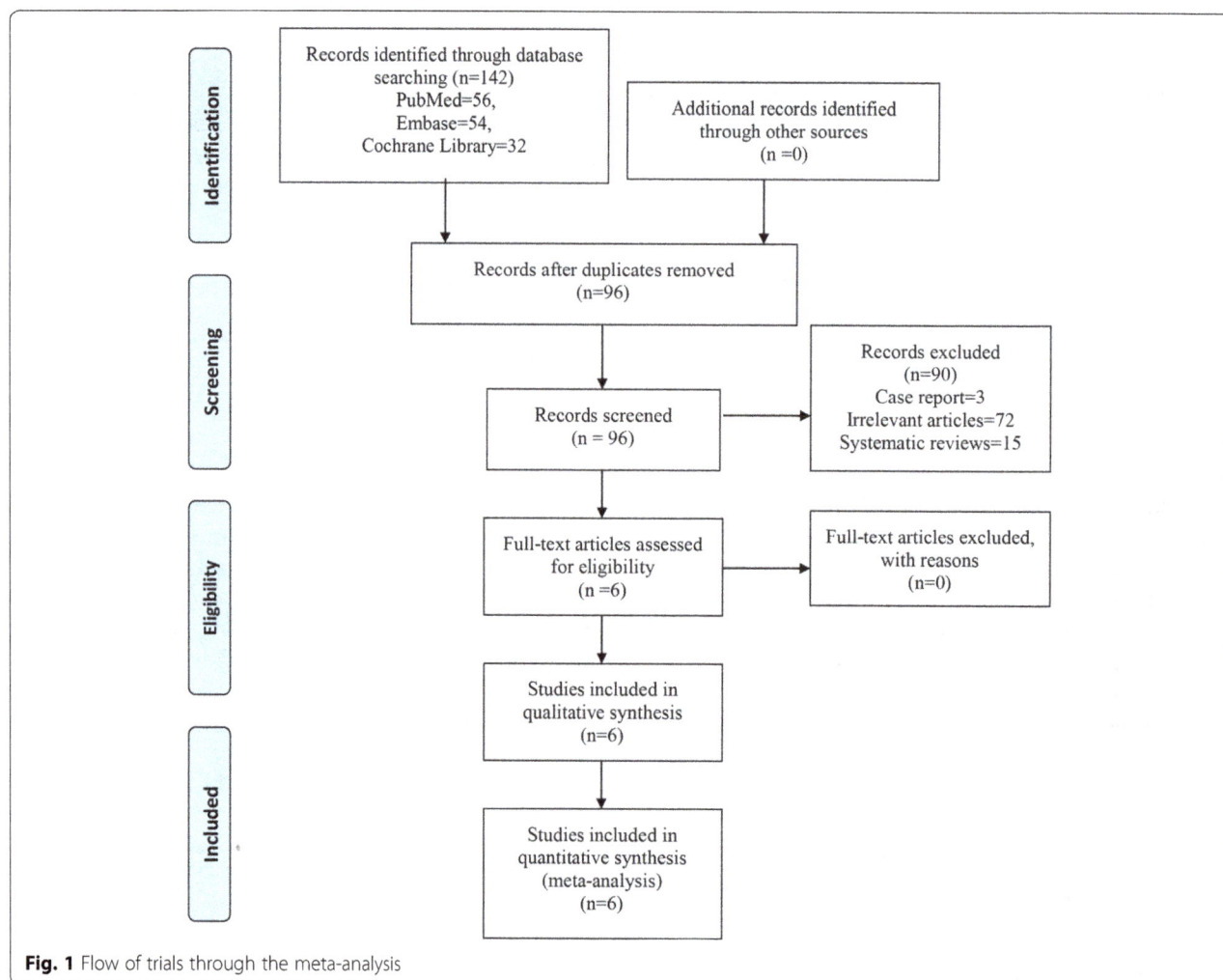

Fig. 1 Flow of trials through the meta-analysis

Table 1 General characteristic of the included studies

Author	Country	Age (year)	Study	Dose of acetaminophen	Control	Follow-up	Anesthesia
Kelly [15]	America	63.9/65.3	RCS	1000 mg/day	Placebo	NS	NS
Nwagbologu [17]	Mexico	61/63.9	RCS	1000 mg/day	Placebo	3 days	NS
O'Neal [18]	America	68/70	RCT	1000 mg/day	Placebo	NS	SA
Murata-Ooiwa [19]	Japan	73.6/75.3	RCT	1000 mg/day	Placebo	3 days	SA
Ciummo [23]	America	NS	RCS	NS	Placebo	NS	NS
Huang [21]	America	71.3/71.6	RCS	4000 mg/day	Placebo	3 days	SA/GA

RCT randomized controlled trials, *RCS* retrospective controlled studies, *NS* not stated, *SA* spinal anesthesia, *GA* general anesthesia

Inclusion criteria

Studies were included in our meta-analysis provided that they satisfied the condition of meeting the PICOS (patients, intervention, comparator, outcomes, and study design) study quality assurance guidelines. Other inclusion criteria included the following: (1) Patients had undergone TKA. (2) The intervention was intravenous acetaminophen. (3) The comparator was non-intravenous administration of acetaminophen or placebo. (4) The outcomes included morphine equivalent consumption at POD 1, total morphine equivalent consumption, VAS score at 24, 48, and 72 h and length of hospital stay.

Data extraction

Two reviewers extracted available data from the included studies independently. Extracted data included first author, publication data, participants, age, gender, body mass index, and study design. The primary outcome of our meta-analysis consisted of morphine equivalent consumption at POD 1, total morphine consumption, and VAS score at 24, 48, and 72 h

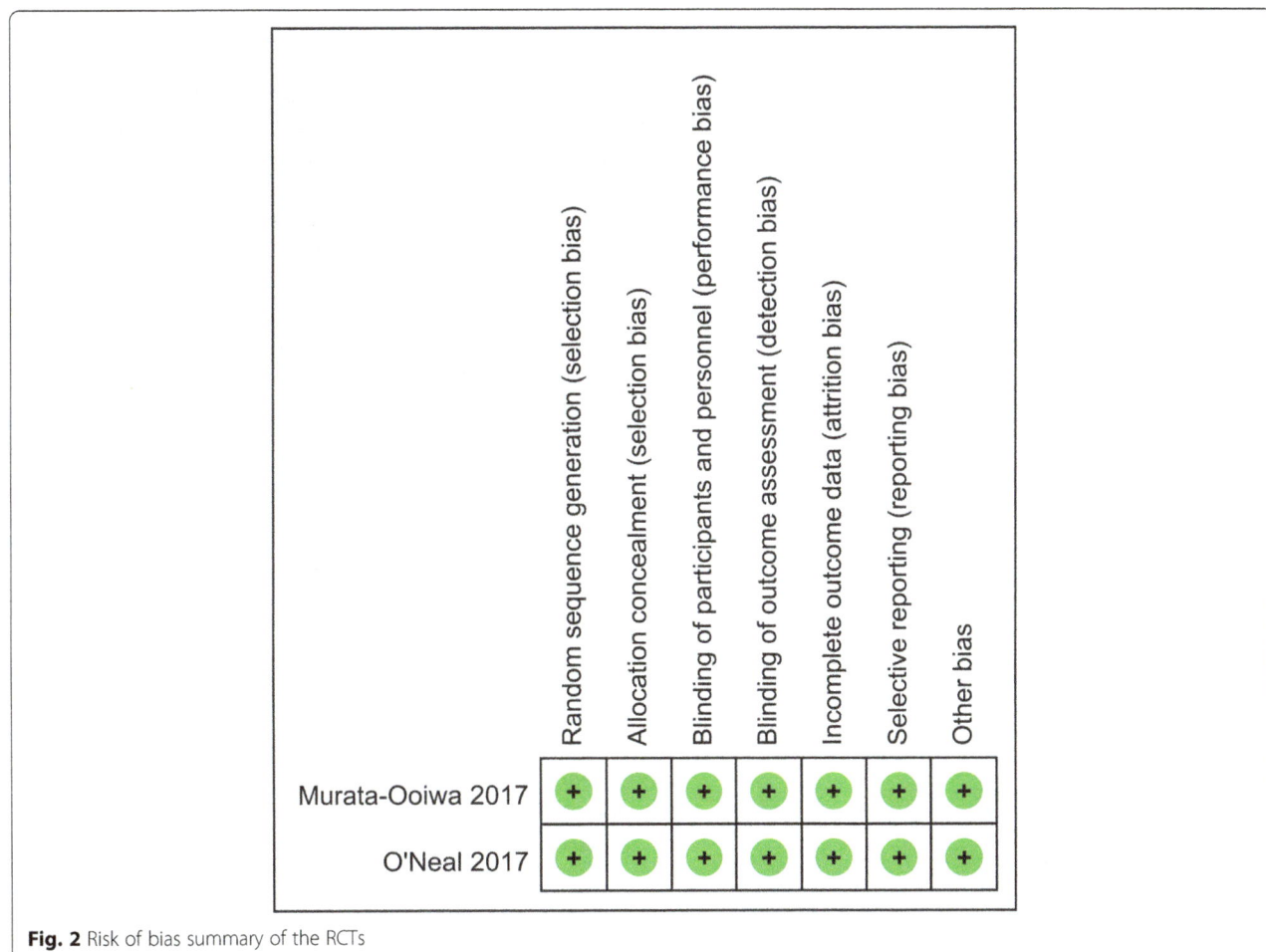

Fig. 2 Risk of bias summary of the RCTs

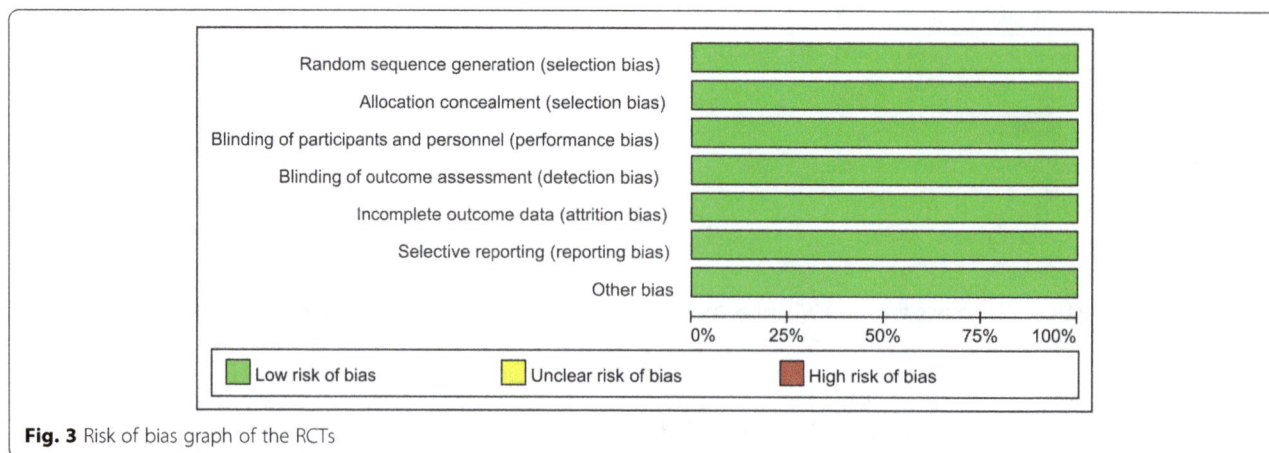

Fig. 3 Risk of bias graph of the RCTs

postoperatively. Secondary outcomes consisted of length of hospital stay. We tried emailing the corresponding authors of the studies that used graphical data or had incomplete data. Any disagreement between the two reviewers was resolved by a third reviewer.

Quality assessment

Quality assessment for RCTs was performed according to the Cochrane Handbook for Systematic Reviews of Interventions. Two authors independently evaluated the risk of bias of the included RCTs based on the following items: random sequence generation, allocation concealment, blinding, incomplete outcome data, selective reporting, and other sources of bias. For non-RCTs, we used the Newcastle-Ottawa scale to evaluate the risk of bias [22]. We considered a study to be of high quality for non-RCTs when a study achieved a score on the Newcastle-Ottawa scale of more than six points.

Statistical analysis

Stata 12.0 was applied for our meta-analysis. For continuous outcomes, mean difference (MD) with a 95% confidence interval (CI) was used to weigh the effect intervals. We judged the statistical heterogeneity by the P value derived using the standard chi-square test. Values of $I^2 > 50\%$ were thought to have significant heterogeneity of the outcomes, and a random-effect model was applied for assessment; for others, such as for extracted data, a fixed-effect model was used. We performed subgroup analysis by omitting studies in turn. Subgroup analysis was done according to the study type, anesthesia, allocation concealment, and dose of acetaminophen.

Results

Search results and general characteristics

A total of 142 relevant studies were identified by our search strategies. After duplicates were removed, there were 96 studies left to review. After reading the title and abstract, 90 studies were excluded. Finally, 6 studies [15, 17–19, 21, 23] were included in our meta-analysis after full-text reading. Among them, there were 2 RCTs [18, 19] and 4 RCSs [15, 17, 21, 23]. General characteristics of the included RCTs can be seen in Table 1. All of the studies were published in 2014. The ages of the TKA patients ranged from 61 to 75.3 years. Four studies [15, 17–19] administered acetaminophen at a dose of 1000 mg/day, and one study administered acetaminophen at a dose of 4000 mg/day [21].

Quality assessment of the included studies

The risk of bias summary and the risk of bias graph for the RCTs can be seen in Figs. 2 and 3, respectively. The two RCTs were both determined to be of high quality. The quality assessments of the non-RCTs can be seen in Table 2. Total scores of NOS ranged from 6 to 8.

Meta-analysis results

Total morphine equivalent consumption

Four studies, having a total of 398 patients, reported equivalent total morphine consumptions. Compared with the control group, the IV acetaminophen group

Table 2 Newcastle-Ottawa scale for the non-RCTs

Author	Selection	Comparability	Outcomes	Total score
Kelly [15]	***	**	**	7
Nwagbologu [17]	**	**	**	6
Ciummo [23]	***	**	***	8
Huang [21]	**	**	**	6

* represent 1 score

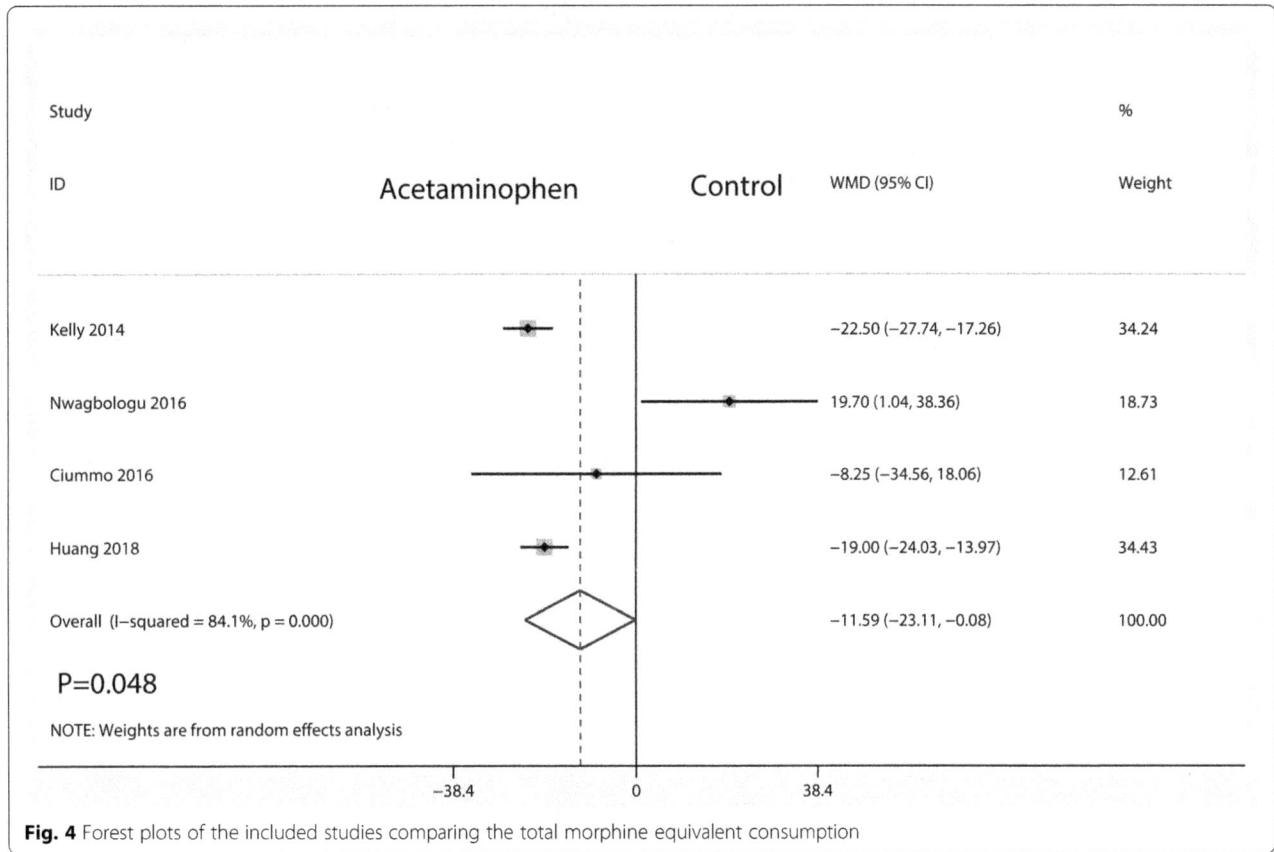

Fig. 4 Forest plots of the included studies comparing the total morphine equivalent consumption

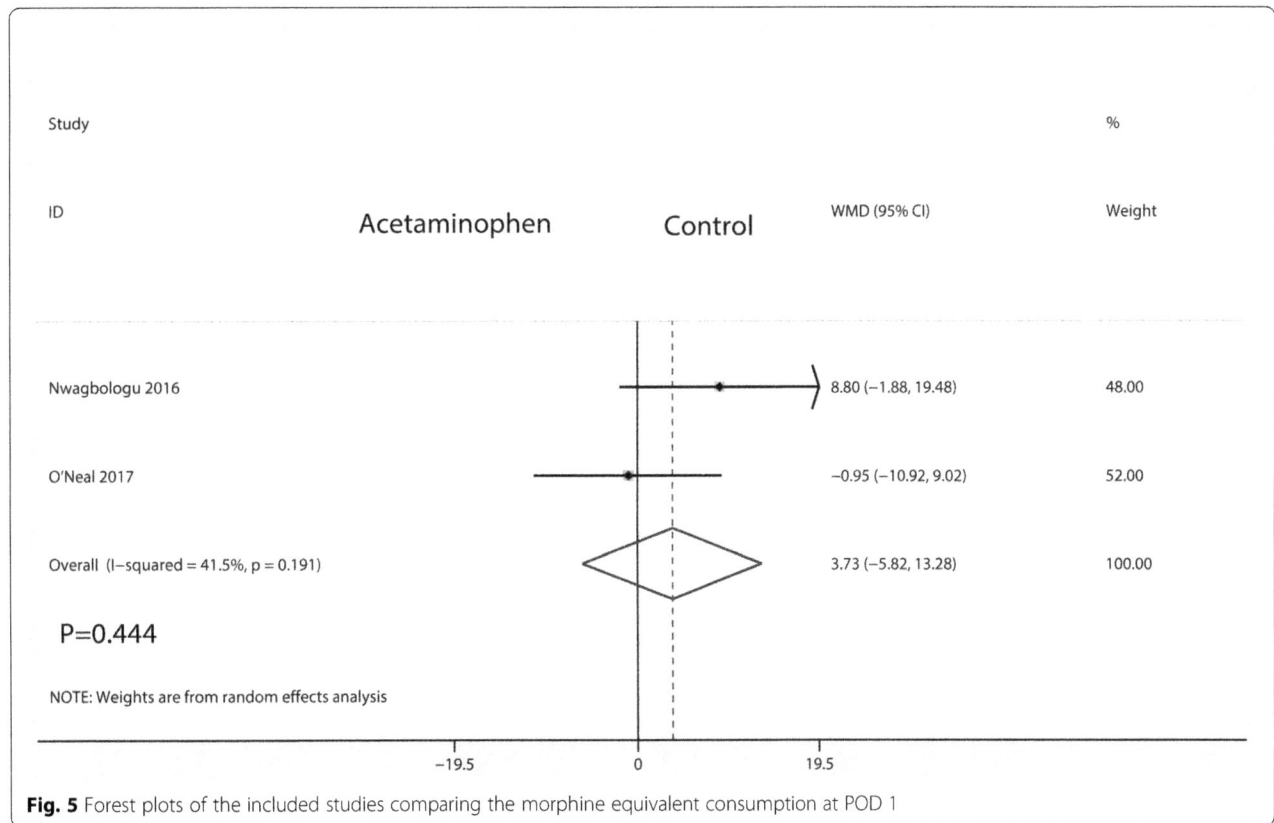

Fig. 5 Forest plots of the included studies comparing the morphine equivalent consumption at POD 1

was associated with a reduction in total morphine consumption of approximately 11.59 mg (WMD = − 11.59; 95%CI, [− 23.11, − 0.08]; $P = 0.048$; $I^2 = 84.1\%$, Fig. 4).

Morphine equivalent consumption at POD 1

Data from 2 studies, including 264 patients, reported equivalent morphine consumption at POD 1. There were no significant differences between the IV acetaminophen group and control group in terms of morphine consumption at POD 1 (WMD = 3.73; 95%CI, [− 5.82, 13.28]; $P = 0.444$; $I^2 = 41.5\%$, Fig. 5).

Visual analogue scale at POD 1

The visual analogue scale score at POD 1 was measured in 4 studies, having a total of 216 patients. We did not find any significant difference between the IV acetaminophen and control groups (WMD = − 4.24; 95%CI, [− 20.24, 11.75]; $P = 0.603$; $I^2 = 95.2\%$, Fig. 6).

Visual analogue scale at POD 2

The visual analogue scale score at POD 2 was measured in 3 studies, having a total of 216 patients. There was no significant difference between IV acetaminophen and control groups in terms of the VAS score at POD 2 (WMD = − 0.26; 95%CI, [− 0.57, 0.05]; $P = 0.105$; $I^2 = 0.0\%$, Fig. 7).

Visual analogue scale at POD 3

The visual analogue scale score at POD 3 was reported in 4 studies, having a total of 331 patients. Compared with the control group, the IV acetaminophen group was associated with a reduction in VAS score at POD 3 (WMD = − 0.34; 95%CI, [− 0.68, − 0.01]; $P = 0.045$; $I^2 = 0.0\%$, Fig. 8).

Length of hospital stay

We extracted length of hospital stay data from 4 studies, involving 398 patients. There were no significant differences between the IV acetaminophen and control groups in terms of the length of hospital stay (WMD = − 0.09; 95%CI, [− 0.23, 0.05]; $P = 0.226$; $I^2 = 58.1\%$, Fig. 9).

Sensitivity analysis and subgroup analysis

The sensitivity analysis can be seen in Additional file 1: Figure S1. The results showed that after omitting each study in turn, the overall effects were in the upper CI limit and lower CI limit.

Subgroup analysis results can be seen in Table 3. The findings of decreased total morphine consumption were consistent in all subgroup analyses except for the allocation concealment and anesthesia subgroups.

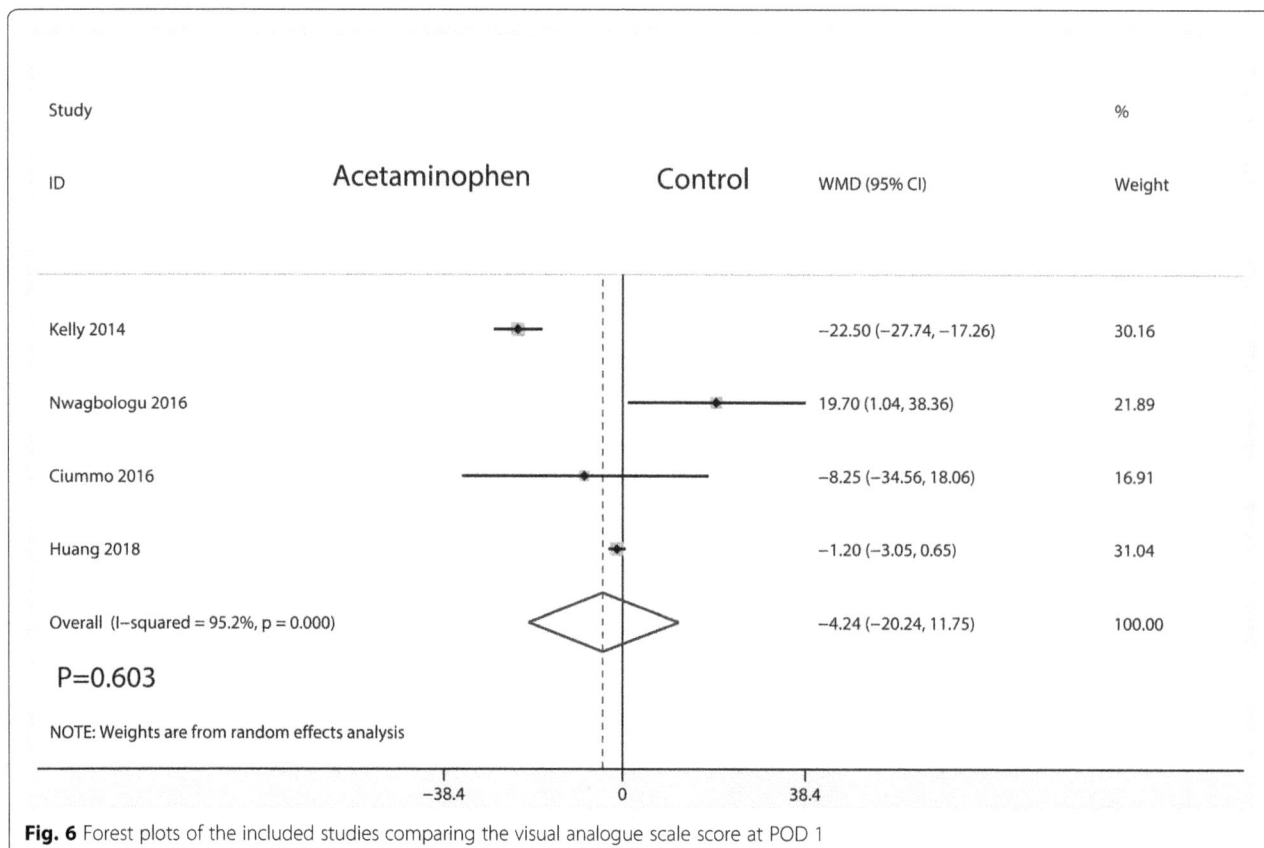

Fig. 6 Forest plots of the included studies comparing the visual analogue scale score at POD 1

Efficacy of intravenous acetaminophen in multimodal management for pain relief following total knee...

193

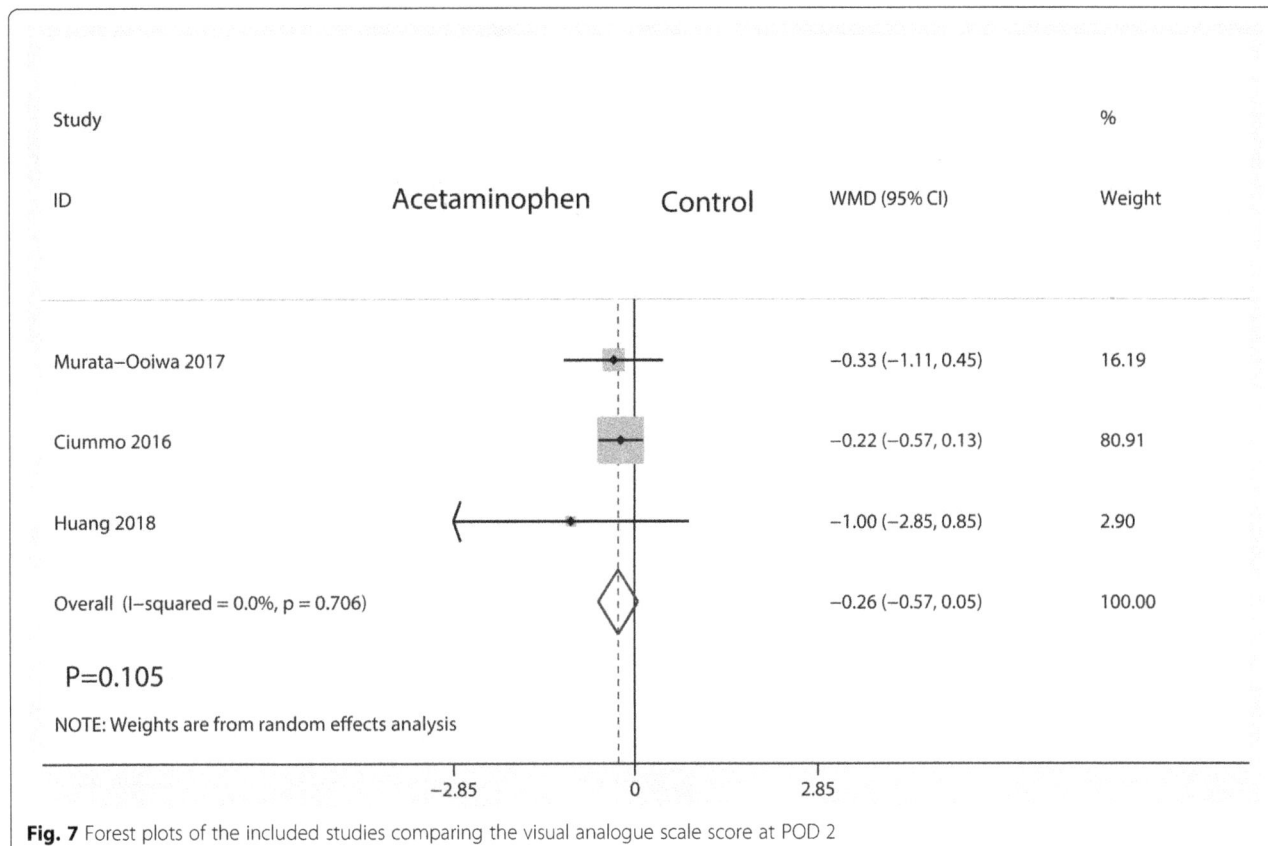

Fig. 7 Forest plots of the included studies comparing the visual analogue scale score at POD 2

Study ID / Acetaminophen / Control / WMD (95% CI) / % Weight:

- Murata–Ooiwa 2017 — −0.33 (−1.11, 0.45) — 16.19
- Ciummo 2016 — −0.22 (−0.57, 0.13) — 80.91
- Huang 2018 — −1.00 (−2.85, 0.85) — 2.90
- Overall (I–squared = 0.0%, p = 0.706) — −0.26 (−0.57, 0.05) — 100.00

P=0.105

NOTE: Weights are from random effects analysis

−2.85 / 0 / 2.85

Discussion

The current meta-analysis indicated that compared with a control group, intravenous acetaminophen was associated with reductions in total morphine consumption and VAS score at POD 3. There was no significant difference in morphine consumption at POD 1 or in VAS score at POD 1 or 2. Moreover, there was no significant difference in length of hospital stay between the intravenous acetaminophen group and the control group.

Inadequate pain management following TKA may influence the functional recovery, increase opioid consumption, and contribute to several complications [24]. Recently, multimodal pain management has been widely applied in TKA [25]. Multimodal pain management usually includes two or more medications with different mechanisms, such as opioids, nonsteroidal anti-inflammatory medications, steroids, and epinephrine. It is worth noting that the usage of opioids is frequently associated with side effects, such as nausea, vomiting, and pruritus [26]. Moreover, it has been reported that the pain score became worse at 24 h after TKA. The rebounding pain of multimodal pain management after POD 1 remains an important issue in patients who have received TKA [9]. More recently, multimodal pain management with IV acetaminophen for postoperative pain management has generated much discussion [27].

It was reported that opioid consumption was reduced from 29 to 39% in patients who received IV acetaminophen compared to a placebo in orthopedic procedures [28]. IV acetaminophen has been shown to have efficacy for reducing the consumption of opioids [15]. Murata-Ooiwa et al. [19] demonstrated that the VAS score was significantly better in the intravenous acetaminophen group than the placebo group at day 1 after TKA, with no significant differences in terms of the rate of complications between the groups. They drew the conclusion that intravenous acetaminophen provided better pain relief for patients undergoing unilateral TKA.

However, recently, other studies have reported different conclusions [18, 23]. In the O'Neal et al. study [18], the VAS scores of IV acetaminophen and placebo groups were compared, as well as total the morphine consumption, among other parameters. No significant differences were found between all groups for any outcome. Nwagbologu et al. [17] reported that the use of IV acetaminophen was not associated with a decrease in opioid use, opioid-related side effects, or any other outcomes in patients who received TKA. The current meta-analysis indicated that IV acetaminophen was associated with a statistically significant reduction in total morphine consumption by approximately 11.59 mg compared with a control group.

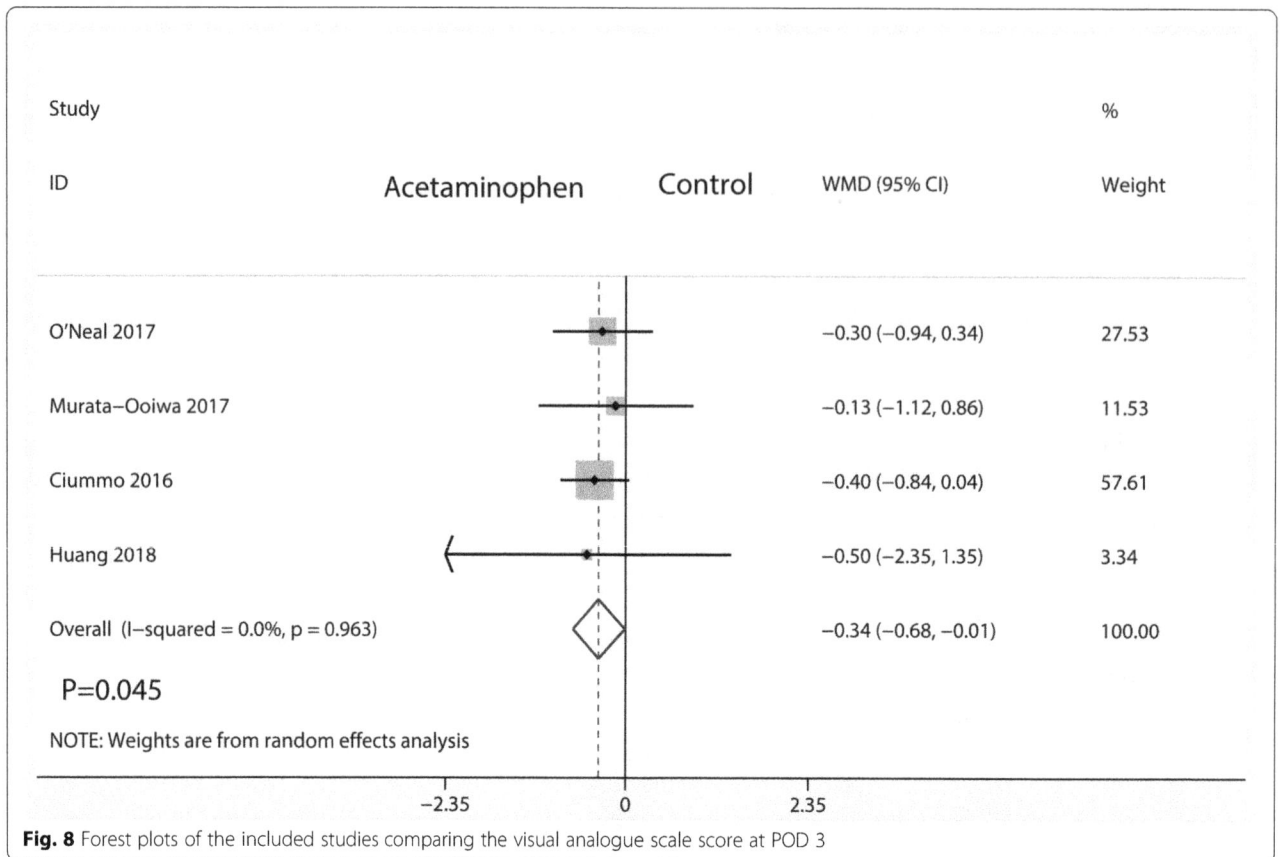

Fig. 8 Forest plots of the included studies comparing the visual analogue scale score at POD 3

There was significantly heterogeneity between the included studies (I^2 = 84.1%). Despite performing sensitivity analysis to diminish the impact of heterogeneity, the effect of heterogeneity still could not be eliminated completely. In the sensitivity analysis, we found that the study of Nwagbologu et al. [17] was the source of this heterogeneity. Nwagbologu et al. [17] recorded that the IV acetaminophen group and placebo group received similar doses of total morphine equivalents at 24 and 48 h postoperatively. We analyze the reason as follows: (1) this was a retrospective cohort study and may have had a selection bias; (2) this study comprised two doses of acetaminophen (1000 mg/day and 2000 mg/day), so opioid-sparing effects may be related to the amount of IV acetaminophen received; (3) this study simply added onto other pain medication orders without any organized or concerted effort to use a multimodal pain regimen to reduce opioid consumption.

VAS score was also an important result in our meta-analysis. Current meta-analysis indicated that IV acetaminophen only has a beneficial role in reducing VAS score at POD 3. Murata-Ooiwa et al... [19] reported that the VAS score at 17:00 1 day after TKA was significantly better in the intravenous acetaminophen group than the placebo group. In contrast, some published studies have recently reported that IV acetaminophen has no effects on pain relief [18]. O'Neal et al. [18] reported that no significant differences were found between the IV acetaminophen and placebo groups regarding the VAS score. Similarly, Ciummo et al. [23] declared that there was no statistically significant difference in average daily postoperative VAS score.

Similar findings were reported by Murata-Ooiwa et al. [19]. In Murata-Ooiwa et al.'s study [19], there were no significant differences in the rate of complications. With regard to LOS, Ciummo et al. [23] reported that no significant differences were found. Kelly et al. [15] reported that the median length of LOS for both the IV acetaminophen and placebo groups was 3 days. In the Nwagbologu et al. study [17], the LOS in IV acetaminophen and control groups were 3.7 days and 3.9 days, respectively. These results were consistent with our meta-analysis. Therefore, we concluded that IV acetaminophen was not associated with a reduction in the length of hospital stay in patients who received TKA.

Our meta-analysis has several limitations: (1) Only six studies were included in our meta-analysis. The statistical efficacy of our results would be more reliable if more studies had been included. (2) Only English publications were included in our meta-analysis; therefore, publication bias was unavoidable. (3) Outcomes such as range of motion of the knee and knee society score were not analyzed due

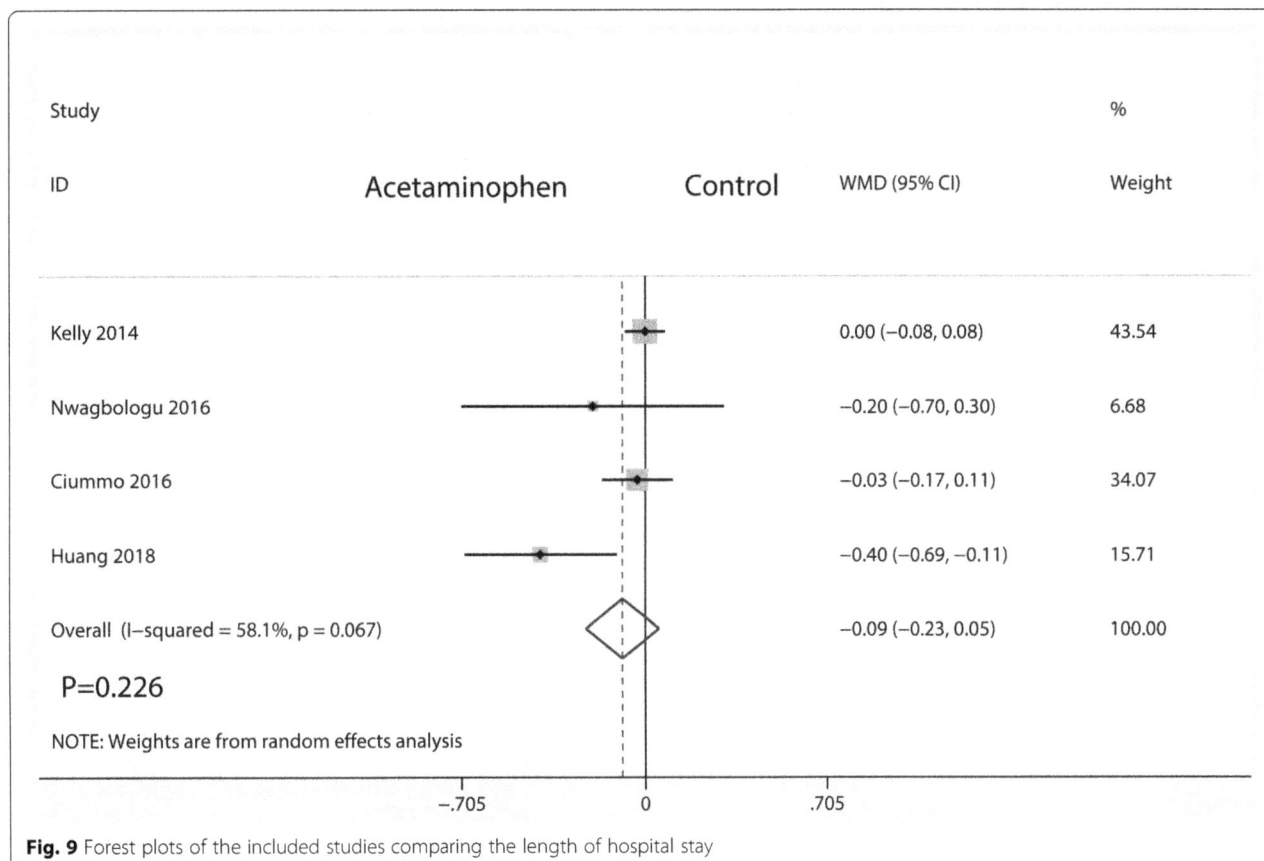

Fig. 9 Forest plots of the included studies comparing the length of hospital stay

to insufficient data. (4) Follow-ups of these studies were relatively short, and long-term follow-ups are needed to identify the knee function between these two groups. (5) There was substantial heterogeneity between included outcomes. We performed subgroup analysis and sensitivity analysis to decrease the heterogeneity; however, the overall heterogeneity was not changed after subgroup

analysis or after sensitivity analysis. Thus, the results of this meta-analysis should be carefully interpreted.

Conclusion

In conclusion, based on our results, IV acetaminophen in multimodal management has shown better efficacy than a control for pain relief at POD 3 and has morphine-sparing

Table 3 Subgroup analysis of the total morphine consumption

Subgroups	No. of studies	Mean difference [95% CI]	P value	I^2 (%)	Between subgroup significance
Total morphine consumption					
Allocation concealment					
Adequate	2	− 2.39 (− 43.70, 38.92)	0.910	94.5	0.002
Unclear	2	− 18.62 (− 23.56, − 0.08)	0.000	0	
Study type					
RCT	1	− 19.70 (− 22.35, − 15.43)	0.029	0	0.124
RCS	3	− 20.45 (− 24.04, − 16.85)	0.038	0	
Acetaminophen dose					
1000 mg/day	3	− 4.42 (− 33.04, 24.20)	0.762	89.4	0.139
4000 mg/day	1	− 19.00 (− 24.03, − 13.97)	0.000		
Anesthesia					
GA	2	− 2.39 (− 43.70, 38.92)	0.910	94.5	0.048
SA	2	− 18.62 (− 23.56, − 13.68)	0.000		

GA general anesthesia, *SA* spinal anesthesia, *RCT* randomized controlled trials, *RCS* retrospective controlled studies

effects. We identified six studies; in the future, the multi-modal pain management protocol after TKA may change when more studies are published and included in the meta-analysis. Due to the limited studies and participants, further high-quality studies with more patients are needed to validate the optimal dose of IV-acetaminophen.

Abbreviations
CI: Confidence interval; IV: Intravenous; NOS: Newcastle-Ottawa Quality Assessment Scale; OA: Osteoarthritis; POD: Postoperative day; RA: Rheumatoid arthritis; RCS: Retrospective cohort studies; RCTs: Randomized controlled trials; RR: Risk ratio; TKA: Total knee arthroplasty; VAS: Visual analogue scale; WMD: Weighted mean difference

Funding
There is no funding for this article.

Authors' contributions
SBS and XBW conceived the study design. JMS performed the study, collected the data, and contributed to the study design. SFG and ZXC prepared the manuscript. YW edited the manuscript. All authors read and approved the final manuscript.

Competing interests
The authors declare that they have no competing interests.

References
1. Sun X, Su Z. A meta-analysis of unicompartmental knee arthroplasty revised to total knee arthroplasty versus primary total knee arthroplasty. J Orthop Surg Res. 2018;13(1):158.
2. Dong P, Tang X, Cheng R, Wang J. Comparison of the efficacy of different analgesia treatments for total knee arthroplasty: a network meta-analysis. Clin J Pain. 2018;34(11):1047–60.
3. Li C, Qu J, Pan S, Qu Y. Local infiltration anesthesia versus epidural analgesia for postoperative pain control in total knee arthroplasty: a systematic review and meta-analysis. J Orthop Surg Res. 2018;13(1):112.
4. Mont MA, Beaver WB, Dysart SH, Barrington JW, Del Gaizo DJ. Local infiltration analgesia with liposomal bupivacaine improves pain scores and reduces opioid use after total knee arthroplasty: results of a randomized controlled trial. J Arthroplast. 2018;33(1):90–6.
5. Suarez JC, Al-Mansoori AA, Kanwar S, Semien GA, Villa JM, McNamara CA, Patel PD. Effectiveness of novel adjuncts in pain management following total knee arthroplasty: a randomized clinical trial. J Arthroplast. 2018;33(7s): S136–s141.
6. Gaffney CJ, Pelt CE, Gililland JM, Peters CL. Perioperative pain management in hip and knee arthroplasty. Orthop clin North Am. 2017; 48(4):407–19.
7. Brooks E, Freter SH, Bowles SK, Amirault D. Multimodal pain management in older elective arthroplasty patients. Geriatric orthop surg rehabilitation. 2017;8(3):151–4.
8. Tsukada S, Wakui M, Hoshino A. Postoperative epidural analgesia compared with intraoperative periarticular injection for pain control following total knee arthroplasty under spinal anesthesia: a randomized controlled trial. J Bone Joint Surg Am. 2014;96(17):1433–8.
9. Tsukada S, Wakui M, Hoshino A. The impact of including corticosteroid in a periarticular injection for pain control after total knee arthroplasty: a double-blind randomised controlled trial. bone joint j. 2016;98-b(2):194–200.
10. Dahl JB, Rosenberg J, Dirkes WE, Mogensen T, Kehlet H. Prevention of postoperative pain by balanced analgesia. Br J Anaesth. 1990;64(4): 518–20.
11. Cancienne JM, Patel KJ, Browne JA, Werner BC. Narcotic use and total knee arthroplasty. J Arthroplast. 2018;33(1):113–8.
12. Saurabh S, Smith JK, Pedersen M, Jose P, Nau P, Samuel I. Scheduled intravenous acetaminophen reduces postoperative narcotic analgesic demand and requirement after laparoscopic roux-en-Y gastric bypass. Surg Obes Relat Dis. 2015;11(2):424–30.
13. Mont MA, Lovelace B, Pham AT, Hansen RN, Chughtai M, Gwam CU, Khlopas A, Barrington JW. Intravenous acetaminophen may be associated with reduced odds of 30-day readmission after total knee arthroplasty. j knee surg. 2018.
14. Subramanyam R, Varughese A, Kurth CD, Eckman MH. Cost-effectiveness of intravenous acetaminophen for pediatric tonsillectomy. Paediatr Anaesth. 2014;24(5):467–75.
15. Kelly JS, Opsha Y, Costello J, Schiller D, Hola ET. Opioid use in knee arthroplasty after receiving intravenous acetaminophen. Pharmacotherapy. 2014;34(Suppl 1):22s–6s.
16. Blank JJ, Berger NG, Dux JP, Ali F, Ludwig KA, Peterson CY. The impact of intravenous acetaminophen on pain after abdominal surgery: a meta-analysis. J Surg Res. 2018;227:234–45.
17. Nwagbologu N, Sarangarm P, D'Angio R. Effect of intravenous acetaminophen on postoperative opioid consumption in adult orthopedic surgery patients. Hosp Pharm. 2016;51(9):730–7.
18. O'Neal JB, Freiberg AA, Yelle MD, Jiang Y, Zhang C, Gu Y, Kong X, Jian W, O'Neal WT, Wang J. Intravenous vs oral acetaminophen as an adjunct to multimodal analgesia after total knee arthroplasty: a prospective, randomized, double-blind clinical trial. J Arthroplast. 2017; 32(10):3029–33.
19. Murata-Ooiwa M, Tsukada S, Wakui M. Intravenous acetaminophen in multimodal pain management for patients undergoing total knee arthroplasty: a randomized, double-blind, placebo-controlled trial. J Arthroplast. 2017;32(10):3024–8.
20. Apfel C, Jahr JR, Kelly CL, Ang RY, Oderda GM. Effect of i.v. acetaminophen on total hip or knee replacement surgery: a case-matched evaluation of a national patient database. Am J Health Syst Pharm. 2015;72(22):1961–8.
21. Huang PS, Gleason SM, Shah JA, Buros AF, Hoffman DA. Efficacy of intravenous acetaminophen for postoperative analgesia in primary total knee arthroplasty. J Arthroplast. 2018;33(4):1052–6.
22. Hartling L, Ospina M, Liang Y, Dryden DM, Hooton N, Krebs Seida J, Klassen TP. Risk of bias versus quality assessment of randomised controlled trials: cross sectional study. BMJ (Clinical research ed). 2009;339:b4012.
23. Ciummo F, Cheon E, Samide J, Habib H, Abraham T, Tischler H. 1570: multimodal pain management in total knee replacement with or without intravenous acetaminophen. Crit Care Med. 2016;44(12):468.
24. Laoruengthana A, Rattanaprichavej P, Rasamimongkol S, Galassi M. Anterior vs posterior periarticular multimodal drug injections: a randomized, controlled trial in simultaneous bilateral total knee arthroplasty. J Arthroplast. 2017;32(7):2100–4.
25. Parvizi J, Miller AG, Gandhi K. Multimodal pain management after total joint arthroplasty. J Bone Joint Surg Am. 2011;93(11):1075–84.
26. Jiang J, Teng Y, Fan Z, Khan MS, Cui Z, Xia Y. The efficacy of periarticular multimodal drug injection for postoperative pain management in total knee or hip arthroplasty. J Arthroplast. 2013;28(10):1882–7.
27. Politi JR, Davis RL 2nd, Matrka AK. Randomized prospective trial comparing the use of intravenous versus oral acetaminophen in total joint arthroplasty. J Arthroplast. 2017;32(4):1125–7.
28. Sinatra RS, Jahr JS, Reynolds LW, Viscusi ER, Groudine SB, Payen-Champenois C. Efficacy and safety of single and repeated administration of 1 gram intravenous acetaminophen injection (paracetamol) for pain management after major orthopedic surgery. Anesthesiology. 2005;102(4):822–31.

23

Tibial plateau fractures in elderly people: an institutional retrospective study

Qi-fang He[1†], Hui Sun[1†], Lin-yuan Shu[2], Yu Zhan[1], Chun-yan He[3], Yi Zhu[1], Bin-bin Zhang[1] and Cong-feng Luo[1*] ⓘ

Abstract

Background: Tibial plateau fractures are the most common intra-articular fractures, which require careful evaluation and preoperative planning. The treatment of tibial plateau fractures in elderly patients is challenging, and the comprehension of epidemiology and morphology can be helpful. This study described the characteristics of geriatric tibial plateau fractures.

Methods: A total of 327 (23.24%) patients aged ≥60 years were reviewed in our level one trauma center over a 4-year period (from January 2013 to November 2016). The following parameters were collected and evaluated: (1) demographic data, (2) injury mechanisms and (3) fracture classifications.

Results: Females accounted for 60.86% in all included elderly patients. Electric-bike accidents were the cause of 32. 42% of all these injuries, and 39.62% of these led to high-energy injuries. The most common type of fracture was Schatzker II (54.74%). According to the three-column classification, single lateral column fracture (28.75%) and four-quadrant fracture (involving lateral, medial, posterolateral and posteromedial fractures) (23.24%) were the two most frequent patterns. In all cases, 67.58% involved the posterior column, and the prevalence of posterolateral and posteromedial fractures were 62.69% and 37.92% respectively. Isolated posterior column fractures accounted for 12. 54% of patients in total, which mostly consisted of posterolateral fracture in older females (85.37%).

Conclusions: The majority of elderly patients with tibial plateau fractures are females, and Electric-bike accidents are an important cause of injury. Geriatric tibial plateau fractures have unique distribution in classification.

Keywords: Classification, Epidemiology, Geriatric fractures, Morphology, Tibial plateau fractures

Introduction

Tibial plateau fractures (TPFs) are relatively common, accounting for approximately 1% of all fractures, and the population-based incidence of TPFs has been reported as 10.3–13.3 per 100,000 people annually [1, 2]. Cases of TPFs were most common between the ages of 30 years and 60 years [3, 4]. However, with improved life expectancy, incidences of TPFs in elderly patients are probably rising [5, 6]. Comprehension of the epidemiology and morphology can be helpful to manage the fractures, but there is little epidemiological information available and to date virtually none about the morphology of TPFs focusing on the elderly population [6, 7]. This current study reports the basic epidemiology and morphological classification of TPFs in elderly patients in a level one trauma center, including incidence, injury mechanisms, combined injuries, and fracture classifications.

In the literature, the AO/OTA and Schatzker classifications were the most frequently used to assess the morphology and severity of TPFs. Because both classifications provide only two-dimensional information of the fracture, a CT-based three-column classification (TCC) would be a good supplement for evaluation [8]. There were already numerous studies which indicated that implementation of the three-column classification (TCC) might improve the surgical outcome of cases of TPFs [9, 10]. This is the first time that the TCC has been used to evaluate the morphological features of tibial plateau fractures in a large sample size of elderly patients.

---

* Correspondence: Congfengl@outlook.com
†Qi-fang He and Hui Sun contributed equally to this work.
[1]Department of Orthopaedic Surgery, Shanghai Jiao Tong University
Affiliated Sixth People's Hospital, 600 YiShan Road, Shanghai 200233, China
Full list of author information is available at the end of the article

Materials and methods

Patients

The approval of our institution's ethical review board was obtained prior to initiation of the study. The study included all patients treated for TPFs over a 4-year period (from January 2013 to November 2016) in the trauma center of our hospital, which is a level one trauma center. Patients were excluded based on the following criteria: (1) isolated avulsion fracture of tibial plateau, such as tibial avulsion fractures of anterior or posterior cruciate ligament, Segond fractures; (2) suspected fractures which could not be confirmed by X-ray radiographs or computerized tomography (CT) scans; (3) fractures in children and skeletally immature adolescents; and (4) pathological or old fractures, namely, the fractures for more than 3 weeks. Finally, 1407 patients with TPFs were included and 327 elderly patients aged ≥ 60 years (23.24%) were isolated for further analysis.

Epidemiology

The following parameters of patients aged ≥ 60 years were collected and evaluated: (1) demographic data, (2) injury mechanism, (3) combined injuries, and (4) fracture classification. According to local conditions and lifestyles, we subdivided traffic accidents into the car, E-bike, and bicycle accidents and differentiated falls as being from height (more than 2 m), from medium height (less than 2 m), or on the ground. Other causes of injury included industrial and agricultural-related accidents, sport-related, and fighting-induced accidents.

Fracture classification

The images of normal X-ray and CT scans of enrolled patients were obtained from Picture Archiving and Communication System (PACS) workstations. Both the X-ray-based Schatzker classification and CT-based TCC were all applied to evaluate the fractures' morphology. Based on the TCC, the tibial plateau is divided into three relatively independent columns, individually defined as the lateral, medial, and posterior columns as observed on the images of the CT axial plane and three-dimensional reconstructions. An articular depression alone without cortical splitting is defined as a "zero-column (ZC)" fracture. The fractures involving the cortex of lateral and medial columns are renamed as anterolateral (AL) and anteromedial (AM) pattern fractures. A fracture involving the cortex of

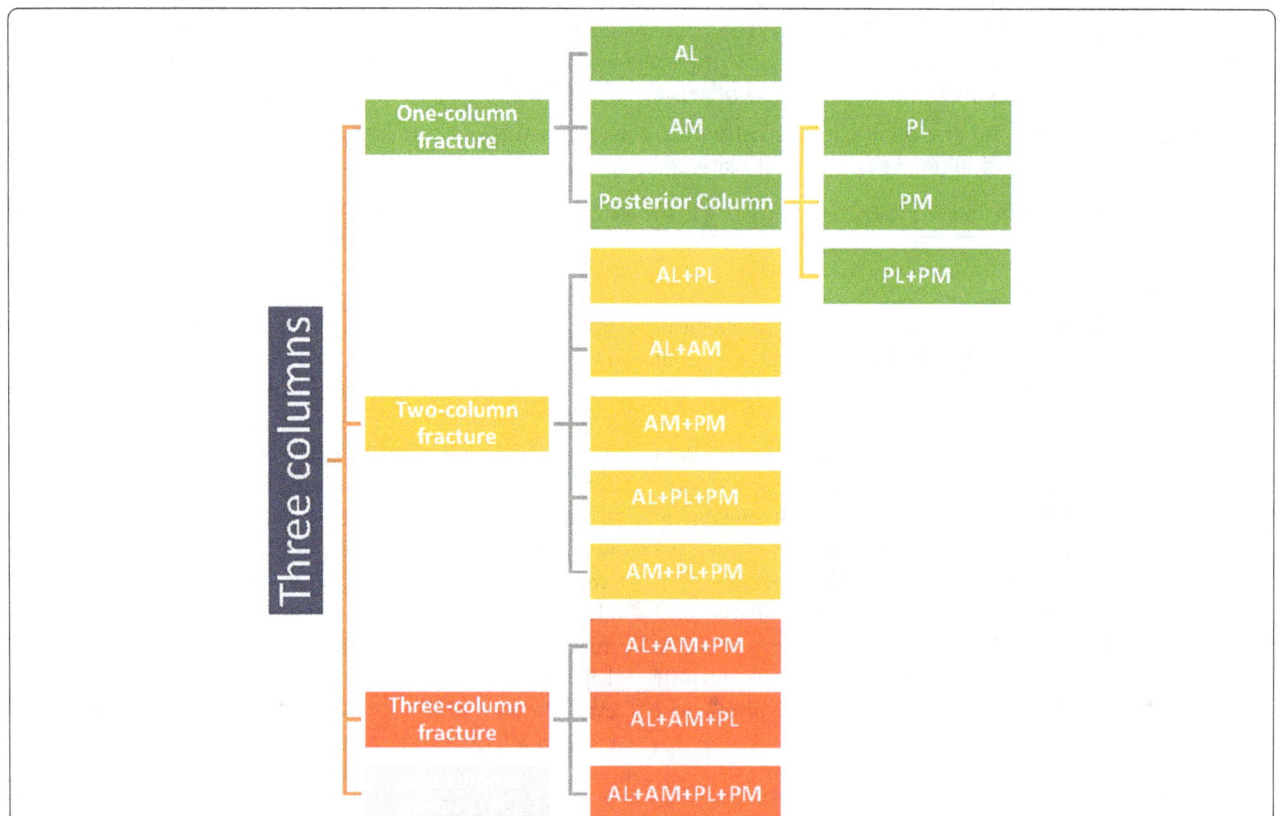

Fig. 1 The subdivision of TPFs by TCC. According to the three-column classification (TCC), the tibial plateau is divided into three columns, including the lateral (anterolateral), medial (anteromedial), and posterior columns. The posterior column is then subdivided into two sub-columns, the posterolateral and posteromedial sub-columns. The fractures could be divided into 14 patterns, in which four different quadrants of the tibial plateau might be involved. AL, anterolateral column; AM, anteromedial column; PL, posterolateral sub-column; PM, posteromedial sub-column

the posterior column is further divided into posterolateral (PL) and posteromedial (PM) pattern fractures. The reason for this division is based on different injury mechanisms and a distinct operation plan including the choice of surgical approaches and fixation strategies [11, 12]. The subdivision of tibial plateau fracture by TCC is summarized in Fig. 1.

The classifications of all fractures were executed by a research team consisting of a chief surgeon, an attending surgeon of orthopedic trauma, and two resident surgeons. The chief surgeon (C-F L) and attending surgeon (Hui S) were the original contributors to the TCC system, and the other surgeons were trained and familiar with both classification systems (the Schatzker classification and TCC). The consensus of classification for each fracture was made among all members of the team to achieve an accurate evaluation.

Statistics

Continuous variables were presented as the mean and range values, and categorical data as frequencies and percentages. The chi-square test was used to compare the differences between male and female, injury mechanisms, and fracture types. SPSS 19.0 software (Statistical Package for Social Sciences, Inc., Chicago, IL, USA) was used for all analysis. $P < 0.05$ was considered statistically significant.

Results

Epidemiology

Most of the elderly patients were aged between 60 and 70 years (Fig. 2). The average age of all elderly patients with TPFs was 66.4 years (range 60–94 years), and males (mean age 65.5 years; range 60–81 years) were younger than females (mean age 67.00 years; range 60–94 years) ($P = 0.013$). Of these patients, 60.86% (199/327) were females and the number of female patients was increasing (Fig. 3). Among the 327 elderly patients, 277 suffered from a single injury, and 37 patients (11.31%) had injuries that were combined with additional injuries. The distal femoral (10 cases) and upper extremity fractures (9 cases) were the most frequently combined injuries. The majority of injury mechanisms were traffic accidents, especially involving an electric bike (E-bike) (106/327, 32.42%) (Table 1).

Schatzker classification

According to the Schatzker classification, type II accounted for more than half of all fractures (179/327, 54.74%), followed by type V (47/327, 14.37%), type VI (45/327,13.76%), type III (29/327, 8.87%), type VI (22/327, 6.73%), and type I (5/327, 1.53%). Schatzker type I TPFs only occurred to males, while females tended to have a higher incidence of Schatzker type II TPFs and a lower incidence of type VI fractures compared with males ($P < 0.05$).

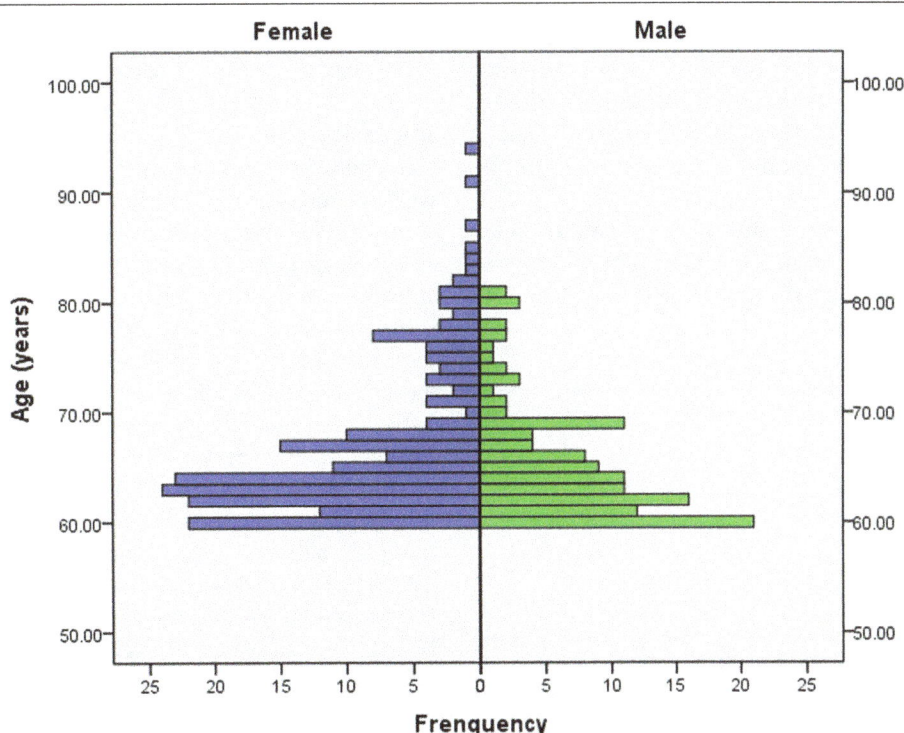

Fig. 2 The age distribution of elderly patients with TPFs between females and males. Most of the elderly patients were aged between 60 and 70 years

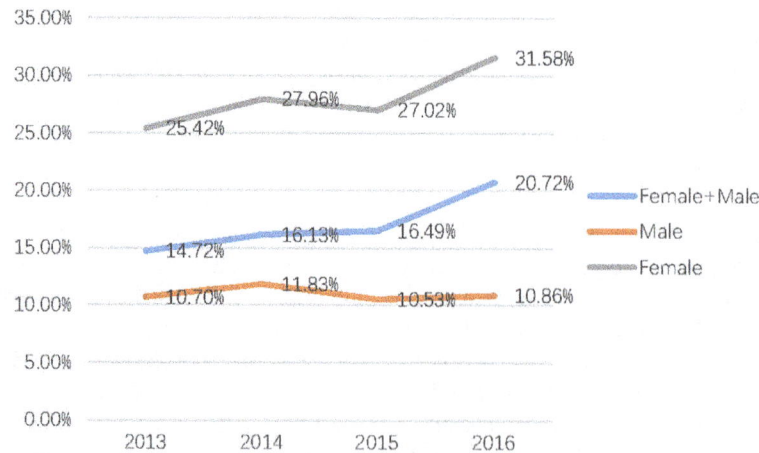

Fig. 3 The incidence of geriatric TPFs from 2013 to 2016. The number of elderly patients with TPFs, especially female patients, presented an increasing trend

There was no significant gender difference in Schatzker type I, III, IV, and V fractures ($P > 0.05$).

The relationship between Schatzker classification and injury mechanism is demonstrated in Fig. 4. Injuries from E-bike use caused 62 cases of Schatzker type II (58.49%) fractures and 42 cases (39.62%) of severe injuries, including Schatzker type IV, V, and VI fractures.

Three-column classification (TCC)

On the basis of TCC, the incidences of different fracture patterns were analyzed in elderly patients. The one-column fractures were the most commonly occurring injuries (66.67%), followed by the two-column (32.72%), and three-column fractures (23.85%). Compared with male patients, female patients had a higher incidence of one-column fractures (44.2% vs 39.06%, $P < 0.05$) and a lower incidence of three-column fractures (22.61% vs 25.78%, $P < 0.05$).

The AL fractures were the most frequent (94, 28.75%), followed by the four quadrants fracture of three columns (AL + AM + PL + PM pattern) (76, 23.24%) and the AL +

PL pattern fracture of two columns (65, 19.88%). The least common types were PM (0), PL + PM (1, 0.31%), AL + AM+PM (1, 0.31%), AL + AM+PL (1, 0.31%). The gender difference for TCC is shown in Fig. 5. Compared with males, female patients had a significantly higher proportion of PL pattern (17.59% vs 3.91%, $P < 0.05$).

The posterior column of the tibial plateau was involved in 67.58% of all elderly patients, and the prevalence of PL and PM were 62.69% and 37.92% respectively. The morbidity of PL alone pattern fracture accounted for 12.23%, and the majority occurred in females (35/5). (details are shown in Table 2). There were four cases(3 males, 1 female) of ZC pattern, which were hardly detected from X-ray, only seen from CT slices.

Discussion

Incidences of TPFs are a complex spectrum of intra-articular fractures around the knee joint which are still of great challenge to treat [13]. Epidemiological and morphological studies of TPFs have been reported to improve the concept and surgical techniques of the treatment [2, 3, 14, 15]. Previously, almost all TPFs-centred studies have analyzed the patients of different age groups as a whole, which possibly confounded the distinctions among age groups [16, 17]. Because of different injury mechanisms and age-related structural variation in bone tissue, the management of TPFs in the elderly population should be very different from that in younger patients and might be more challenging [18–21]. Thus, we isolated an elderly population with TPFs based on age and the epidemiological and morphological characteristics of TPFs in these patients were evaluated and summarized.

In the study, patients aged ≥ 60 years accounted for 23.24% of all consecutively registered patients with TPFs. Among these older patients, females account for 60.86%,

Table 1 Distribution of injury mechanisms

Injury mechanisms	Females	Males	Total (percent)
Traffic injuries			
Car accidents	21	19	40 (12.23%)
E-bike accidents	69	37	106(32.42%)
Bicycle	28	13	41(12.54%)
Fall injuries			
From height	13	22	35(10.7%)
From medium height	42	26	68(20.80%)
On ground	17	7	24(7.34%)
Others	9	4	13(3.98%)

E-bike electric-bike

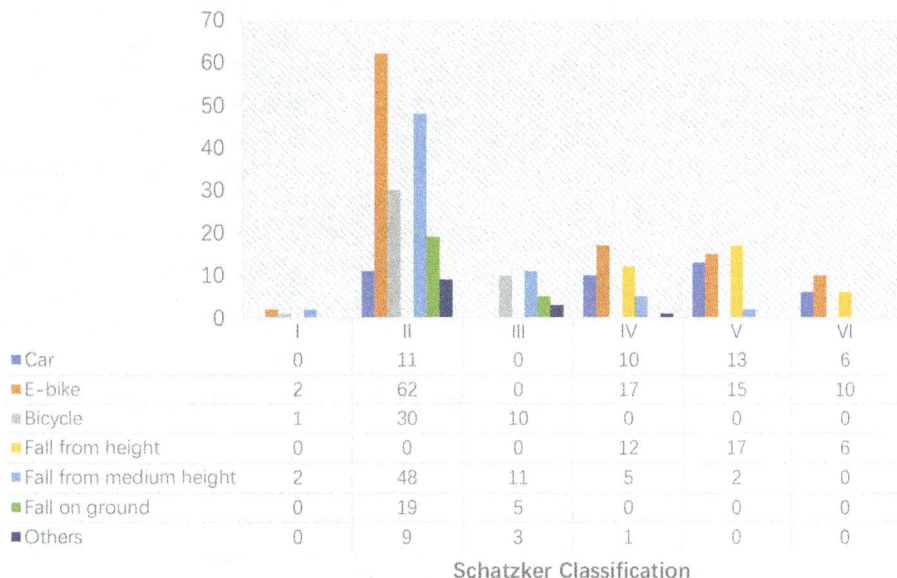

Fig. 4 The distribution of injury mechanism according to the Schatzker classification in elderly patients. Females tended to have a higher incidence of Schatzker type II TPFs and a lower incidence of type VI fractures when compared with males. There is no significant gender difference in Schatzker type I, III, IV, and V fractures

	I	II	III	IV	V	VI
Car	0	11	0	10	13	6
E-bike	2	62	0	17	15	10
Bicycle	1	30	10	0	0	0
Fall from height	0	0	0	12	17	6
Fall from medium height	2	48	11	5	2	0
Fall on ground	0	19	5	0	0	0
Others	0	9	3	1	0	0

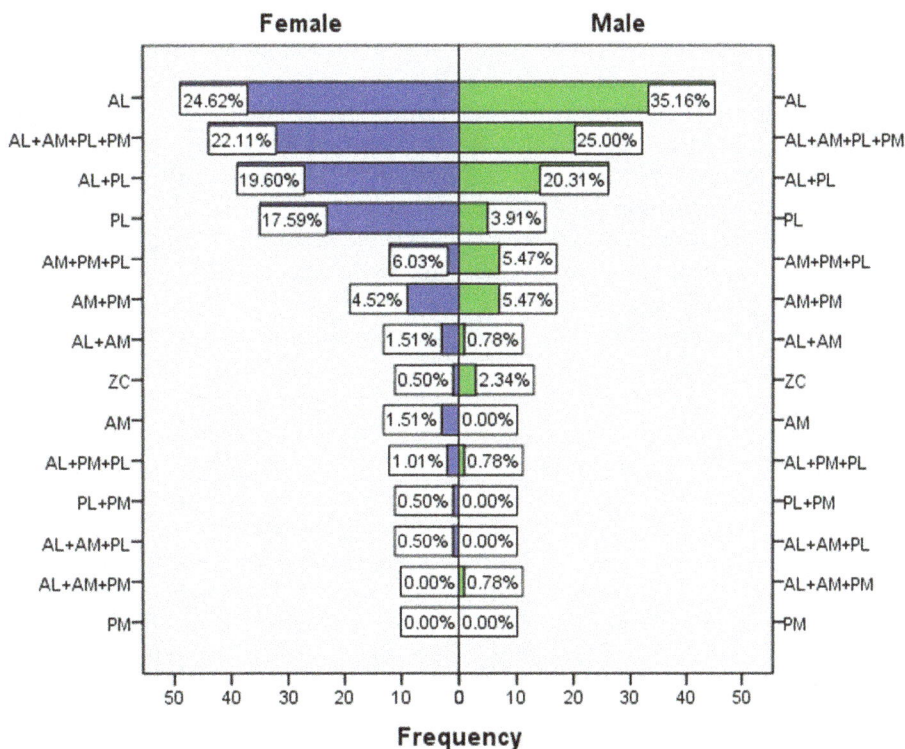

Fig. 5 The distribution of fracture patterns based on the TCC in elderly patients between females and males. Compared with males, females had a higher incidence of PL pattern fractures and a lower incidence of AL fractures. The morbidity of complex AL + AM+PL + PM pattern fractures was significantly higher in the male patients

Table 2 Distribution of posterior column injuries in elderly patients

Posterior column injuries	Gender		Total
	Female	Male	
PL	35	5	40(12.23%)
PM	0	0	0
PL + PM	1	0	1
AL + PL	39	26	65
AM+PM	9	7	16
AM+PM + PL	12	7	19
AL + PM + PL	2	1	3
AL + AM+PM	0	1	1
AL + AM+PL	1	0	1
AL + AM+PL + PM	44	32	76
PL involved	134 (67.34%)	71 (55.47%)	205 (62.69%)
PM involved	76 (38.19%)	48 (37.5%)	124 (37.92%)
Posterior column involved	142 (71.36%)	79 (61.72%)	221 (67.58%)

TCC three-column classification, *AL* anterolateral column, *AM* anteromedial column, *PL* posterolateral sub-column, *PM* posteromedial sub-column

which is higher than previously reported in younger patients. This is in accordance with the gender trend of fractures, in which men younger than 50 years have a higher incidence of fractures, but after the age of 50 years, the incidence increases markedly in women and decreases in men [2, 6]. Older female patients often are at high risk of osteoporosis [22, 23]. Decreased bone quality leads to more low-energy traumatic fractures, and this study demonstrated a higher incidence of Schatzker type I, II, and III fractures and one-column fractures in elderly patients than that reported in the literature for younger patients [3, 15]. It is well known that osteoporotic fractures are a frequent and important cause of disability and rising medical costs worldwide; however, researchers on osteoporotic or senile fractures have usually concentrated on the classic fragility fractures of the proximal humerus, distal radius, and proximal femur [23, 24]. Although only 7.34% (24/327) of fractures in this study were due to falling on the ground and can be accurately categorized as fragile fractures, it is obvious that the influence of age or estrogen-related bone structural changes in this group of patients cannot be ignored.

The injury mechanisms may vary between different areas and populations. Among all injury causes of TPFs, traffic accidents range from 35.49 to 54.4%. In elderly patients, more than half of TPFs (57.19%) were due to traffic accidents and E-bike accidents played an important part (32.42%), with 39.62% of them leading to high-energy injuries. Use of E-bikes is a major traffic mode in the plains area of China [25, 26]. Nevertheless, it is not only an important issue in China, because many

reports have referred to the global prevalence of the E-bike and its related injuries [27–29]. Tenenbaum et al. [28] reported that 65% of injured E-bike riders sustained orthopedic injuries, and the tibia was the most fractured bone (19.2%) in all E-bike-related fractures. Too fast a speed, carrying passengers, and traffic rule violations are the major reasons for E-bike accidents [29–31]. Importantly, age could be the most important risk factor for E-bike injuries according to a traffic report [32]. In a review according to the Groningen bicycle accident database [33], the average age of injured E-bike riders was 65 years, which is very close to the average age of 66.4 years in our study. Considering that more than one third of TPFs in the elderly were caused by E-bike injuries, related preventive measures would be of benefit to decrease the numbers of these injuries.

According to the CT-based TCC, the pattern of TPFs in elderly patients presented a bipolar model as a whole. The AL fracture alone and the most complicated four quadrants fracture were the two most frequent patterns in the elderly population. Low-energy injury to the knee joint, which might be a valgus injury, always leads to a high frequency of the lateral plateau fracture, including the single-column AL fractures alone or the two-column AL + PL fractures, while the total plateau consisting of three columns and four quadrants might be all related to high-energy trauma due to age-related bone fragility.

In the past decade, posterior column injuries of TPFs have drawn more and more attention. There is growing evidence that posterior tibial plateau fractures affect the functional outcome [17, 34]. The reported incidence of posterior tibial plateau fractures ranges from 28.8 to 70.7% [9, 15]. The results of this study found a clear indication that the posterior column fracture was also associated with high morbidity in elderly patients (67.58%), and the PL sub-column (62.69%) was more often involved than the PM sub-column (37.92%). According to the updated TCC protocol, a ruptured posterolateral wall often needs to be exposed and buttressed [14]. However, because the access to the PL fracture is hindered by the fibula and peroneal nerve to the anterior and by the popliteal neurovascular structures to the posterior, the risk of iatrogenic damage to these adjacent structures during exposure and fixation is high [35–37]. Subsequently, the exposure of the posterolateral articular surface is still insufficient due to the popliteus and strong posterior capsule. To date, although various approaches and fixation patterns have been developed to surgically treat the PL fractures, there are still many defects with these posterolateral approaches [37–40].

Isolated posterior column fractures are uncommon [41, 42]. This type of fracture more frequently occurred in our study compared with our another related study (regardless of age) (12.54% vs 7.8%) [15]. In particular, most isolated posterior column fractures we found were single PL fractures involving female patients (85.37%, 35/41). This single PL fracture was caused by low-energy valgus injury mechanisms in different degrees of knee flexion, which was characterized by a main articular depression or split fragment limited to the posterior half of the lateral column [43]. Yu reported a similar frequency of 11.4% (15/132) in patients with the average age of 53.3 years and indicated that this low-energy posterolateral fracture was highly associated with E-bike injury (8/15 cases) and mostly involved male patients [44]. In our study, we did not investigate further whether this fracture pattern was related to E-bike injury but we found that it mostly occurred in females rather than males in the older population. Another type to be noted is secluded ZC fracture exist in geriatric TPFs. CT scan is necessary when X-ray knee is suspicious.

There are several limitations to this study. First, this is a single-center research study which only represents a regional epidemiology of this population. Second, this remains a qualitative, not quantitative morphological study which is mainly based on the TCC system. Third, there were no clinical features and treatment outcomes for a number of reasons. Different treatment concepts were held by several different treatment teams in our trauma center; therefore, different treatment choices (conservation vs surgery, various surgical approaches and fixation styles, internal fixation vs arthroplasty) might be selected for the TPFs in elderly patients and the follow-up data could not be collected uniformly. Thus, valuable clinical outcome data became difficult to obtain. Further prospective investigations with measurable parameters or refined clinical outcomes are needed for a more accurate assessment and to reveal the full extent of TPFs in the elderly.

Conclusion
The majority of elderly patients with tibial plateau fractures are females, and the population involved was increasing. Electric-bike accidents are an important cause of injury. Geriatric tibial plateau fractures have unique distribution in classification.

Abbreviations
AL: Anterolateral; CT: Computerized tomography; E-bike: Electric-bike; PL: Posterolateral; PM: Anteromedial; PM: Posteromedial; TCC: Three-column classification; TPFs: Tibial plateau fractures; ZC: Zero-column

Acknowledgments
The authors gratefully thank Kanchan Kumar Sabui of Medical College Kolkata for advice and literature support.

Funding
No funds were received in support of this study.

Authors' contributions
Y-Z, Y-Z, and BB-Z performed the data collection and analysis. CF-L, QF-H, H-S, CY-H, and LY-S performed the database setup and statistical analysis, which include analysis of epidemiology and fracture classification. CF-L, QF-H, and H-S participated in the study design and manuscript writing. All of the authors have read and approved the final manuscript.

Competing interests
No benefits in any form have been or will be received from a commercial party related directly or indirectly to the subject of this article. The authors declare that they have no competing interests.

Author details
[1]Department of Orthopaedic Surgery, Shanghai Jiao Tong University Affiliated Sixth People's Hospital, 600 YiShan Road, Shanghai 200233, China. [2]Department of Emergency, Shanghai Jiao Tong University Affiliated Sixth People's Hospital, 600 YiShan Road, Shanghai 200233, China. [3]Chongqing Health Center for Women and Children, 64 Jintang Street, Yuzhong District, Chongqing 400013, China.

References
1. Court-Brown CM, Caesar B. Epidemiology of adult fractures: a review. Injury. 2006;37(8):691–7.
2. Elsoe R, Larsen P, Nielsen NP, Swenne J, Rasmussen S, Ostgaard SE. Population-based epidemiology of tibial plateau fractures. Orthopedics. 2015;38(9):e780–6.
3. Albuquerque RP, Hara R, Prado J, Schiavo L, Giordano V, do Amaral NP. Epidemiological study on tibial plateau fractures at a level I trauma center. Acta Orto Bras. 2013;21(2):109–15.
4. Schulak DJ, Gunn DR. Fractures of tibial plateaus. A review of the literature. Clin Orthop Relat Res. 1975;109:166–77.
5. Court-Brown CM, Clement ND, Duckworth AD, Aitken S, Biant LC, McQueen MM. The spectrum of fractures in the elderly. Bone Joint J. 2014;96-b(3):366–72.
6. Court-Brown CM, McQueen MM. Global forum: fractures in the elderly. J Bone Joint Surg Am Vol. 2016;98(9):e36.
7. Rozell JC, Vemulapalli KC, Gary JL, Donegan DJ. Tibial plateau fractures in elderly patients. Geriatr Orthop Surg Rehabil. 2016;7(3):126–34.
8. Luo CF, Sun H, Zhang B, Zeng BF. Three-column fixation for complex tibial plateau fractures. J Orthop Trauma. 2010;24(11):683–92.
9. van den Berg J, Reul M, Nunes Cardozo M, Starovoyt A, Geusens E, Nijs S, Hoekstra H. Functional outcome of intra-articular tibial plateau fractures: the impact of posterior column fractures. Int Orthop. 2017. https://doi.org/10.1007/s00264-017-3566-3.
10. Prat-Fabregat S, Camacho-Carrasco P. Treatment strategy for tibial plateau fractures: an update. EFORT Open Rev. 2016;1(5):225–32.
11. Sohn HS, Yoon YC, Cho JW, Cho WT, Oh CW, Oh JK. Incidence and fracture morphology of posterolateral fragments in lateral and bicondylar tibial plateau fractures. J Orthop Trauma. 2015;29(2):91–7.
12. El-Alfy B, Ali KA, El-Ganiney A. Bicondylar tibial plateau fractures involving the posteromedial fragment: morphology based fixation. Acta Orthop Belg. 2016;82(2):298–304.
13. Reul M, Nijs S, Rommens PM, Hoekstra H. Intra-articuliar tibial plateau fractures. Z Orthop Unfall. 2017;155(3):352–70.
14. Wang Y, Luo C, Zhu Y, Zhai Q, Zhan Y, Qiu W, Xu Y. Updated three-column concept in surgical treatment for tibial plateau fractures - a prospective cohort study of 287 patients. Injury. 2016;47(7):1488–96.
15. Yang G, Zhai Q, Zhu Y, Sun H, Putnis S, Luo C. The incidence of posterior tibial plateau fracture: an investigation of 525 fractures by using a CT-based classification system. Arch Orthop Trauma Surg. 2013;133(7):929–34.
16. Chen P, Shen H, Wang W, Ni B, Fan Z, Lu H. The morphological features of different Schatzker types of tibial plateau fractures: a three-dimensional computed tomography study. J Orthop Surg Res. 2016;11(1):94.

17. Jiwanlal A, Jeray KJ. Outcome of posterior tibial plateau fixation. J Knee Surg. 2016;29(1):34–9.

18. Luria S, Liebergall M, Elishoov O, Kandel L, Mattan Y. Osteoporotic tibial plateau fractures: an underestimated cause of knee pain in the elderly. Am J Orthop (Belle Mead, NJ). 2005;34(4):186–8.

19. Krappinger D, Struve P, Smekal V, Huber B. Severely comminuted bicondylar tibial plateau fractures in geriatric patients: a report of 2 cases treated with open reduction and postoperative external fixation. J Orthop Trauma. 2008; 22(9):652–7.

20. Shimizu T, Sawaguchi T, Sakagoshi D, Goshima K, Shigemoto K, Hatsuchi Y. Geriatric tibial plateau fractures: clinical features and surgical outcomes. J Orthop Sci. 2016;21(1):68–73.

21. Su EP, Westrich GH, Rana AJ, Kapoor K, Helfet DL. Operative treatment of tibial plateau fractures in patients older than 55 years. Clin Orthop Relat Res. 2004;421:240–8.

22. Alswat KA. Gender disparities in osteoporosis. J Clin Med Res. 2017;9(5):382–7.

23. Boschitsch EP, Durchschlag E, Dimai HP. Age-related prevalence of osteoporosis and fragility fractures: real-world data from an Austrian menopause and osteoporosis clinic. Climacteric. 2017;20(2):157–63.

24. Yoo JH, Moon SH, Ha YC, Lee DY, Gong HS, Park SY, Yang KH. Osteoporotic fracture: 2015 position statement of the Korean Society for Bone and Mineral Research. J Bone Metabol. 2015;22(4):175–81.

25. Zhou SA, Ho AFW, Ong MEH, Liu N, Pek PP, Wang YQ, Jin T, Yan GZ, Han NN, Li G, et al. Electric bicycle-related injuries presenting to a provincial hospital in China: a retrospective study. Medicine. 2017;96(26):e7395.

26. Li X, Yun Z, Li X, Wang Y, Yang T, Zheng L, Qian J. Orthopedic injury in electric bicycle-related collisions. Traffic Injury Prev. 2017;18(4):437–40.

27. Siman-Tov M, Radomislensky I, Israel Trauma G, Peleg K. The casualties from electric bike and motorized scooter road accidents. Traffic Inj Prev. 2017; 18(3):318–23.

28. Tenenbaum S, Weltsch D, Bariteau JT, Givon A, Peleg K, Thein R. Orthopaedic injuries among electric bicycle users. Injury. 2017. https://doi. org/10.1016/j.injury.2017.08.020.

29. Weber T, Scaramuzza G, Schmitt KU. Evaluation of e-bike accidents in Switzerland. Accid Anal Prev. 2014;73:47–52.

30. Wu C, Yao L, Zhang K. The red-light running behavior of electric bike riders and cyclists at urban intersections in China: an observational study. Accid Anal Prev. 2012;49:186–92.

31. Yang J, Hu Y, Du W, Powis B, Ozanne-Smith J, Liao Y, Li N, Wu M. Unsafe riding practice among electric bikers in Suzhou, China: an observational study. BMJ Open. 2014;4(1):e003902.

32. Hu F, Lv D, Zhu J, Fang J. Related risk factors for injury severity of e-bike and bicycle crashes in Hefei. Traffic Inj Prev. 2014;15(3):319–23.

33. Poos H, Lefarth TL, Harbers JS, Wendt KW, El Moumni M, IHF R. E-bikers are more often seriously injured in bicycle accidents: results from the Groningen bicycle accident database. Ned Tijdschr Geneeskd. 2017;161(0): D1520.

34. Molenaars RJ, Mellema JJ, Doornberg JN, Kloen P. Tibial plateau fracture characteristics: computed tomography mapping of lateral, medial, and bicondylar fractures. J Bone Joint Surg Am. 2015;97(18):1512–20.

35. Sun H, Luo CF, Yang G, Shi HP, Zeng BF. Anatomical evaluation of the modified posterolateral approach for posterolateral tibial plateau fracture. Eur J Orthop Surg Traumatol. 2013;23(7):809–18.

36. Heidari N, Lidder S, Grechenig W, Tesch NP, Weinberg AM. The risk of injury to the anterior tibial artery in the posterolateral approach to the tibia plateau: a cadaver study. J Orthop Trauma. 2013;27(4):221–5.

37. Pierrie SN, Harmer LS, Karunakar MA, Angerame MR, Andrews EB, Sample KM, Hsu JR. Limited added value of the posterolateral approach. J Knee Surg. 2016;29(1):21–7.

38. Solomon LB, Stevenson AW, Lee YC, Baird RP, Howie DW. Posterolateral and anterolateral approaches to unicondylar posterolateral tibial plateau fractures: a comparative study. Injury. 2013;44(11):1561–8.

39. Garner MR, Warner SJ, Lorich DG. Surgical approaches to posterolateral tibial plateau fractures. J Knee Surg. 2016;29(1):12–20.

40. Cho JW, Samal P, Jeon YS, Oh CW, Oh JK. Rim plating of posterolateral fracture fragments (PLFs) through a modified anterolateral approach in tibial plateau fractures. J Orthop Trauma. 2016;30(11):e362–8.

41. Chang SM, Zheng HP, Li HF, Jia YW, Huang YG, Wang X, Yu GR. Treatment of isolated posterior coronal fracture of the lateral tibial plateau through posterolateral approach for direct exposure and buttress plate fixation. Arch Orthop Trauma Surg. 2009;129(7):955–62.

42. Tao J, Hang DH, Wang QG, Gao W, Zhu LB, Wu XF, Gao KD. The posterolateral shearing tibial plateau fracture: treatment and results via a modified posterolateral approach. Knee. 2008;15(6):473–9.

43. Chen HW, Chen CQ, Yi XH. Posterior tibial plateau fracture: a new treatment-oriented classification and surgical management. Int J Clin Exp Med. 2015;8(1):472–9.

44. Yu GR, Xia J, Zhou JQ, Yang YF. Low-energy fracture of posterolateral tibial plateau: treatment by a posterolateral prone approach. J Trauma Acute Care Surg. 2012;72(5):1416–23.

24

Incidence and risk factors of neurological complications during posterior vertebral column resection to correct severe post-tubercular kyphosis with late-onset neurological deficits

Wenbin Hua, Xinghuo Wu, Yukun Zhang, Yong Gao, Shuai Li, Kun Wang, Xianzhe Liu, Shuhua Yang and Cao Yang[*]

Abstract

Background: Severe post-tubercular kyphosis with late-onset neurological deficits is difficult to treat, with high risk of neurological complications. This study retrospectively evaluates the efficacy and safety of posterior vertebral column resection (PVCR) for treating severe post-tubercular kyphosis with late-onset neurological deficits.

Methods: From January 2012 to December 2015, 13 patients with severe post-tubercular kyphosis underwent PVCR. All these patients were of late-onset neurological deficits. The operative time, blood loss, preoperative and postoperative kyphotic angles, sagittal vertical axis (SVA), neurological status, and complications were recorded. The preoperative and postoperative Oswestry Disability Index (ODI) scores and visual analog scale (VAS) scores for back pain were compared. The American Spinal Injury Association (ASIA) grading system was used to evaluate neurological function.

Results: The mean postoperative follow-up period was 28.6 months. The mean operative time was 388 ± 46 min. The mean blood loss was 2554 ± 1459 ml. The mean preoperative and postoperative kyphotic angles were $93.7 \pm 14.4°$ and $31.7 \pm 7.3°$, respectively, with a mean correction of $62.0 \pm 13.8°$. The mean preoperative and postoperative SVA were 43.2 ± 44.4 mm and 17.8 ± 16.2 mm, respectively. The mean ODI score improved from 56.3 ± 5.1 preoperatively to 18.3 ± 18.5 at last follow-up. The mean VAS score improved from 6.4 ± 1.8 preoperatively to 1.8 ± 0.8 at last follow-up. Two cases had spinal cord injuries, including one complete paraplegia and one incomplete paraplegia, and a total neurological complication rate of 15.4%. The risk factors for neurological complications were summarized.

Conclusions: Severe post-tubercular kyphosis with late-onset neurological deficits can be corrected by PVCR carefully and properly to prevent neurological complications. In many cases with stenosis adjacent to the angular kyphosis, sufficient decompression of the spinal cord at the segments with stenosis is necessary before correcting the kyphosis.

Keywords: Post-tubercular kyphosis, Kyphosis, Late-onset neurological deficits, Posterior vertebral column resection, Neurological complication

* Correspondence: yangcao1971@sina.com
Department of Orthopaedics, Union Hospital, Tongji Medical College,
Huazhong University of Science and Technology, Wuhan 430022, China

Background

Tuberculosis (TB) of the spine is one of the most common causes of kyphosis [1–3]. Although anti-tuberculosis drugs are highly effective for controlling tubercular infection, 3–5% of patients with this condition have severe progression of the disease, with a kyphotic angle greater than 60°, leading to "buckling collapse" [2, 4]. Severe kyphosis results in back pain, spinal cord compression, cardiopulmonary dysfunction, costopelvic impingement, and cosmetic concerns [1].

The major complications of spinal tuberculosis are kyphosis, neurological deficits, or paraplegia. Neurological deficits can be caused by tuberculosis infection and the progression of post-tubercular kyphosis [1]. Early-onset neurological deficits or paraplegia is usually found in the active stages of tuberculosis, which should be treated with chemotherapy and surgery [5]. Late-onset neurological deficits or paraplegia usually develops due to the progression of kyphosis, which can be prevented with early stabilization surgery or a combined anterior-posterior procedure or posterior three-column osteotomy [5, 6]. Besides, late-onset neurological deficits may be related to a lesion cephalad or caudal from the kyphosis [7].

In cases with severe kyphosis, osteotomies are essential to reconstruct the sagittal alignment. Various techniques have been described for correcting post-tubercular kyphosis, including pedicle subtraction osteotomy [8], closing-opening wedge osteotomy [9, 10], and vertebral column resection [11–18]. Due to the complexity of severe post-tubercular kyphosis and accompanying late-onset neurological deficits, posterior vertebral column resection (PVCR) seems to be the most effective surgery that allows for sufficient correction of the deformity and decompression of the spinal cord [12–14, 16, 17].

Even though excellent correction of the kyphosis could be achieved with PVCR [12–14, 16, 17], it may be of high risk of neurological complications in cases of severe post-tubercular kyphosis with late-onset neurological deficits. To the best of our knowledge, there is a rare study about PVCR for correcting severe post-tubercular kyphosis with late-onset neurological deficits. Besides, severe post-tubercular kyphosis with late-onset neurological deficits caused by stenosis adjacent to the angular kyphosis is also rarely reported. In the present study, we summarized the clinical efficacy, incidence, and risk factors for neurological complications of PVCR to correct severe post-tubercular kyphosis with late-onset neurological deficits.

Methods

Patient population

From January 2012 to December 2015, 13 patients (9 male, 4 female; mean age 40.7 years, range 31–54 years) with severe post-tubercular kyphosis (kyphotic angle > 60°) underwent PVCR in our department. This study was conducted in accordance with the guidelines of the Declaration of Helsinki and was approved by the ethics committee of our hospital. Written informed consents were obtained from all the patients. Each patient included had a history of spinal tuberculosis in childhood or adolescence and was treated by chemotherapy. Each patient included had back pain and late-onset neurological deficits, with preoperative neurologic symptoms, including leg weakness (13 cases) and additional leg pain (4 cases). One case (No. 8) must walk with a cane. No case was found with sphincter dysfunction. Details of preoperative deformity and neurologic status of included patients were summarized in Tables 1 and 2. Patients with active tuberculosis, congenital kyphosis, kyphosis caused by other diseases, or early-onset neurological deficits were excluded.

Radiographic assessment

Full-length spine radiographs (i.e., those that included the whole spine and pelvis) of patients standing in a neutral, unsupported position were taken preoperatively, immediately postoperatively, and at the last follow-up. Computed tomography (CT) was used to assess deformity and stenosis adjacent to the angular kyphosis. Magnetic resonance imaging (MRI) was used to assess deformity and stenosis adjacent to the angular kyphosis, evaluate the status of the spinal cord, and exclude intraspinal lesions.

The kyphotic angle was defined as the angle between the superior endplate of the first normal vertebrae above the collapsed segments and the inferior endplate of the first normal vertebrae below the collapsed segments [12]. The postoperative kyphotic angle was measured at the same segments. Sagittal vertical axis (SVA) was defined as the distance between the C7 plumb line (C7PL) and the posterior-superior corner of S1, and defined as positive if the C7PL was anterior to the posterior-superior corner of S1, or negative if the C7PL was posterior to the posterior-superior corner of S1 [19, 20]. Thoracic kyphosis and lumbar lordosis were not used to evaluate the sagittal balance of the whole group because of the destruction of the thoracolumbar junction in most cases.

Surgical technique

PVCR was performed in each case to correct the deformity and improve the neurologic status. The osteotomy should be performed at the apex of the deformity. Spinal cord function was continuously monitored with somatosensory-evoked potentials (SEP) and motor-evoked potentials (MEP). Wake-up tests should be performed in necessary.

After administering general anesthesia, the patients were placed in prone position. A midline incision was made to expose the vertebrae to be fixed as far as the transverse processes. Transpedicular screws were implanted at least

Table 1 Details of the deformity and osteotomy

Patient no.	Age (years)	Gender	Time between first TB infection and surgery (years)	Affected segments	Number of affected segments	Deformity sites	Resected segments	Number of resected segments	Instrumented segments
1	47	Male	42	T9-L3	7	Thoracolumbar	T12-L1	2	T7–9, L3-L4
2	40	Female	23	T7-T9	3	Thoracic	T8	1	T5-T6, T10-T11
3	45	Male	31	T10-L1	4	Thoracolumbar	T11-T12	2	T8-T10, L2-L4
4	47	Male	29	T8-T10	3	Thoracic	T9	1	T7-T8, T10-T11
5	42	Male	32	T3-T7	5	Thoracic	T5	1	C6,T1-T3, T8–11
6	37	Male	34	T5-T10	6	Thoracic	T7-T8	2	T2-T5, T10-L1
7	50	Male	45	T10-L2	5	Thoracolumbar	T11-L1	3	T8-T10, L3, L4
8	54	Female	53	T8-L2	7	Thoracolumbar	T11-T12	2	T6-T9, L2-L4
9	32	Male	21	T8-T10	3	Thoracic	T9	1	T5-T7, T11-L1
10	53	Female	49	T11-L2	4	Thoracolumbar	T12	1	T9-T11, L2-L4
11	42	Male	27	T6-T9	4	Thoracic	T7-T8	2	T4-T6, T9-T11
12	35	Male	30	T9-T12	4	Thoracolumbar	T10-T11	2	T6-T8, L1-L3
13	31	Female	15	T10-T12	3	Thoracolumbar	T12	1	T9-T11, L1-L2
Mean	40.7 ± 11.0	–	–	–	4.5 ± 1.4	–	–	1.6 ± 0.6	–

TB tuberculosis

two segments above and below the resected segments. After performing facetectomy and laminectomy at the osteotomy sites, the spinal cord was sufficiently exposed and decompressed. The costal heads were transected together with the costotransverse joints, with the pleura carefully protected [9]. Two temporary titanium rods were applied on the opposite sides to maintain spinal stability when performing osteotomy and the following correcting procedures. The deformity was corrected step-by-step with one of the rods fixed. Sagittal alignment was restored by moderately compressing the posterior column and distracting the anterior column. Thoracic nerve roots at the osteotomy segments were sacrificed by ligation. Meanwhile, the spinal cord and nerve roots were examined carefully to avoid excessive spinal cord tension, shrinkage, or compression near the osteotomy sites. The prevertebral vessels were protected by S-shaped retractor. The bleeding from the intravertebral venous plexus could be controlled by fluid gelatin. In cases with stenosis at the adjacent segments of the apex, the segments with stenosis should be decompressed before correcting the deformity. After performing the correcting procedures, the temporary rods were replaced by permanent rods. A titanium cage with autogenous iliac crest bone inside was applied to support the vertebral column and

Table 2 Details of late-onset neurological deficits

Patient no.	Angular kyphosis	Intervertebral disc degeneration	Calcification of ligamentum flavum	ASIA grade		
				Pre-op	Immediate post-op	Last follow-up
1	+	+ (T8/9)	+ (T8/9)	D	A	A
2	+	–	–	D	D	E
3	+	–	–	D	D	D
4	+		+ (T7/8, T10/11)	D	D	E
5	+	–	–	D	D	E
6	+	–	–	D	C	D
7	+	+ (T10/11)	+ (T10/11)	D	D	E
8	+	–	+(T10/11)	C	C	D
9	+	–	–	D	D	E
10	+	–	–	D	D	E
11	+	–	–	D	D	D
12	+	+ (T9/10)	+ (T9/10)	D	D	D
13	+	–	–	D	D	E

ASIA American Spinal Injury Association, *pre-op* pre-operation, *post-op* post-operation

prevent excessive shortening of the spine. Posterolateral allograft (Aorui, China) was applied to achieve posterior column fusion of the spine. The wound was closed in layers over drains.

Data collection

Serial radiographs were obtained, and clinical examination was performed at 3, 6, 12, and 24 months postoperatively. Each patient underwent at least 24 months follow-up. The preoperative and postoperative kyphotic angles and SVA were documented. The Oswestry Disability Index (ODI) scores and visual analog scale (VAS) scores for back pain were used to assess the back pain before surgery and at follow-up visits. Intraoperative and postoperative neurological complications and general complications were recorded. The American Spinal Injury Association (ASIA) grading system was used to evaluate neurological function.

Statistical analysis

SPSS version 22.0 (SPSS Inc., Chicago, IL, USA) was used for statistical analysis. All data were presented as the mean ± standard deviation. The Wilcoxon signed-rank test was used to compare preoperative and postoperative data. A P value less than 0.05 was considered statistically significant.

Results

Clinical outcome

The baseline demographic details of the deformity and osteotomy of these patients are summarized in Table 1 (Fig. 1). Details of late-onset neurological deficits, including preoperative status and postoperative improvement, are summarized in Table 2 (Fig. 2).

The mean postoperative follow-up period was 28.6 months (range, 24–48 months). The mean operative time was 388 ± 46 min (range, 300–450 min). The mean blood loss was 2554 ± 1459 ml (range, 800–6800 ml). The mean kyphotic angle improvement is summarized in Table 3. The mean SVA improvement is summarized in Table 3. Details of the improvement of clinical measurements, including ODI score and VAS score, are summarized in Table 4.

Neurological complications

Five cases had SEP or MEP changes during surgery. Two of them were confirmed to be spinal cord injuries (15.4%), of which one developed permanent complete paraplegia (ASIA grade A), the other developed incomplete paraplegia (ASIA grade C) and recovered (ASIA grade D) at the 6-month follow-up after surgery. Another three cases had temporary SEP or MEP changes during surgery without spinal cord injuries. The neurological function of the remaining cases improved during follow-up (Table 2).

For the two cases of spinal cord injuries, the possible causes were investigated. In the first case, SEP and MEP disappeared during surgery, with permanent complete spinal cord injury after surgery. Accompanying stenosis at the segments adjacent to the angular kyphosis was confirmed by preoperative MRI scanning, but the stenosis was not decompressed before correcting the kyphosis. Then, the spinal cord was compressed further at the segment with stenosis during the correcting procedures. In the later four cases with stenosis adjacent to the angular kyphosis, similar spinal cord injuries were avoided by sufficient decompression of the stenosis before correcting the deformity. Another case of stationary SEP and no MEP was found with weakened muscle strength of one leg after surgery. This may be resulted from over-correction of the kyphosis. As a result, such cases should be moderately corrected to prevent neurological complications.

Discussion

Due to the multiple fused vertebral bodies and severe spinal cord compression in cases of severe post-tubercular kyphosis, the destroyed anterior column should be completely resected [13]; therefore, PVCR should be performed to achieve adequate correction. By using PVCR, the mean kyphotic angle of post-tubercular kyphosis can be improved significantly, with a mean correction ranged between 40.5 and 80° (57.3–82.3%) in the sagittal plane [12–14, 16, 17]. In the present study, a mean correction of 62.0° (66.2%) was achieved. Because of preexisting severe spinal cord compression or distraction before surgery, all these patients included were of late-onset neurological deficits; complete correction of post-tubercular kyphosis is unnecessary and associated with a high risk of neurological complications. Therefore, nearly 50% improvement of the kyphotic angle may be relatively safe during the correction of post-tubercular kyphosis [12].

Even though PVCR is effective in restoring alignment of the whole spine in patients with severe kyphosis, PVCR has a high risk of neurological complications because of the aggressiveness of the procedure and its high technical demands [12–14, 16, 17, 21–24]. According to the literature, Cobb angle of the main curve, sharp and angulated deformity, dural buckling, compression of the spinal cord, preexisting neurologic dysfunction, spinal cord ischemia during the surgery, levels of osteotomy, and subluxation of the spinal column contribute to the high risk of neurological complications when correcting severe spinal deformities by PVCR [21–24].

Performing PVCR in patients with severe post-tubercular kyphosis seems to be more challenging because of the additional risk factors involved; indeed, Tuli [25] reported that worse prognosis and higher incidence of postoperative paraplegia were observed in tuberculosis patients with

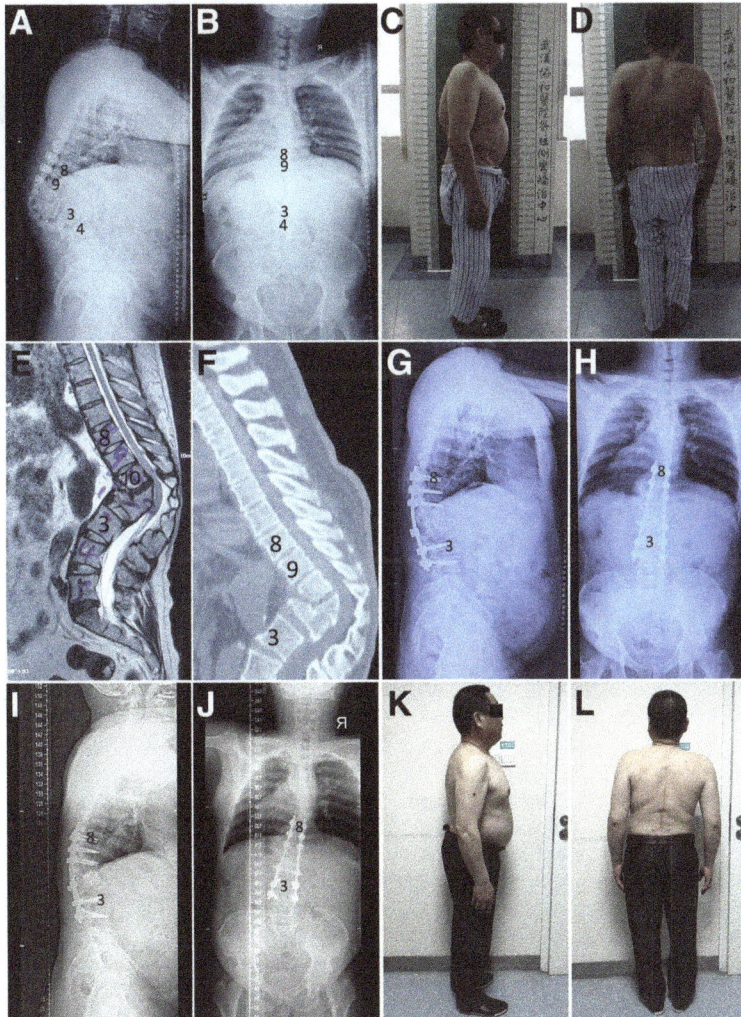

Fig. 1 Standing radiographs and images of a 50-year-old male patient with severe post-tubercular kyphosis. **a, b** Preoperative lateral and antero-posterior radiographs, demonstrating severe angular kyphosis, with preoperative kyphotic angle 86° and sagittal vertical axis 45 mm. **c, d** Preoperative appearance in side and posterior view. **e** Preoperative magnetic resonance imaging scanning demonstrates stenosis adjacent to the angular kyphosis and severe spinal compression. **f** Preoperative computed tomography scanning demonstrates severe angular kyphosis and "buckling collapse." **g, h** Postoperative lateral and antero-posterior radiographs, showing correction of thoracolumbar kyphosis after PVCR of T11, T12, and L1, with postoperative kyphotic angle 27° and sagittal vertical axis 33 mm. **i, j** Postoperative lateral and antero-posterior radiographs, showing excellent correction of thoracolumbar angular kyphosis and osteotomy site fusion at the 24-month follow-up, with kyphotic angle 29° and sagittal vertical axis 42 mm. **k, l** Postoperative appearance in side and posterior view

kyphotic angle larger than 60°. Multiple fused vertebral bodies, post-infectious fusion masses, and tethered dural sacs were common in most cases of severe post-tubercular kyphosis [6]. Healed bony bars, calcified caseous material, tissue fibrosis, and increased kyphosis may aggravate the compression and distraction, contributing to ischemia and atrophy of the spinal cord [7]. Due to long-term compression, the spinal cord is already at the limit of its tolerance; therefore, patients with late-onset neurological deficits may suffer further spinal cord injuries and have relatively poorer prognosis than those without neurological deficits during osteotomy [7].

According to previous studies, the rate of neurological complications after PVCR, including paraplegia and incomplete spinal cord injury, ranged between 0 and 17.1% [22, 24, 26–32]. However, the incidence of neurological complications for severe post-tubercular kyphosis after PVCR is 0–11.1% [12–14, 16, 17]. In the present study, the neurological complication rate after PVCR is higher than that in the literature. As a result, much more attention should be paid to the risk factors of neurological complications during the correction of severe post-tubercular kyphosis with late-onset neurological deficits.

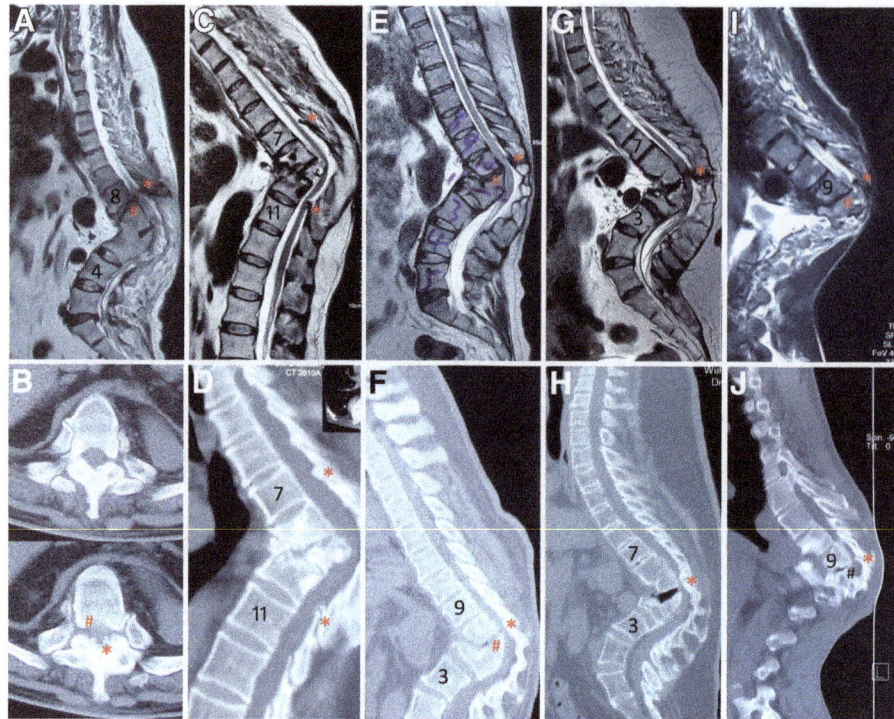

Fig. 2 Causes of late-onset neurological deficits according to the lesions. **a, b** Preoperative magnetic resonance image (MRI) and computed tomography (CT) scanning demonstrate severe angular kyphosis, "buckling collapse" from T9 to L3, intervertebral disc herniation and calcified ligamentum flavum at T8/9, and severe spinal cord compression. **c, d** Preoperative MRI and CT scanning demonstrate severe angular kyphosis from T8 to T10, calcified ligamentum flavum at T7/8 and T10/11, and severe spinal cord compression. **e, f** Preoperative MRI and CT scanning demonstrate severe angular kyphosis, "buckling collapse" from T10 to L2, intervertebral disc herniation and calcified ligamentum flavum at T10/11, and severe spinal cord compression. **g, h** Preoperative MRI and CT scanning demonstrate severe angular kyphosis, "buckling collapse" from T8 to L2, calcified ligamentum flavum at T10/11, and severe spinal cord compression. **i, j** Preoperative MRI and CT scanning demonstrate severe angular kyphosis, intervertebral disc herniation and calcified ligamentum flavum at T9/10, and severe spinal cord compression. *Calcified ligamentum flavum at the segments adjacent to the angular kyphosis; #disc herniation at the segments adjacent to the angular kyphosis

Table 3 Details of the correction of kyphotic angle and sagittal vertical axis

Patient no.	Kyphotic angle/°					SVA/mm				
	Pre-op	Immediate post-op	Correction	Last follow-up	Loss of correction	Pre-op	Immediate post-op	Correction	Last follow-up	Loss of correction
1	90	33	57	35	2	45	21	24	25	4
2	75	25	50	27	2	31	10	21	12	2
3	102	38	64	41	3	69	15	44	16	1
4	80	39	41	42	3	14	42	−28	36	−6
5	85	22	63	23	1	42	39	3	51	12
6	106	45	61	55	10	−5	31	−36	62	31
7	86	27	59	29	2	45	33	12	42	9
8	98	24	74	30	6	118	5	113	−28	−33
9	86	36	50	40	4	44	12	30	17	5
10	94	28	66	33	5	60	11	49	19	8
11	107	40	67	43	3	43	14	29	20	6
12	128	30	98	36	6	109	18	91	22	4
13	81	25	56	28	3	−54	−19	35	8	27
Mean	93.7 ± 14.4	31.7 ± 7.3*	62.0 ± 13.8	35.5 ± 8.6*	3.8 ± 2.4	43.2 ± 44.4	17.8 ± 16.2#	29.8 ± 40.9	23.2 ± 22.2#	5.4 ± 15.3

SVA sagittal vertical axis, *pre-op* pre-operation, *post-op* post-operation. *P = 0.001 compared with pre-op; #P > 0.05 compared with pre-op

Table 4 Details of the improvement of clinical measurements

Patient no.	ODI score		VAS score	
	Pre-op	Last follow-up	Pre-op	Last follow-up
1	52	78	7	3
2	54	8	4	1
3	54	24	6	3
4	46	10	4	1
5	60	12	8	2
6	56	20	7	2
7	52	10	4	1
8	66	18	9	3
9	60	12	8	1
10	54	12	6	2
11	60	14	9	2
12	58	10	5	2
13	60	10	6	1
Mean	56.3 ± 5.1	18.3 ± 18.5*	6.4 ± 1.8	1.8 ± 0.8#

ODI Oswestry Disability Index, *VAS* visual analog scale, *pre-op* pre-operation, *post-op* post-operation. *$P = 0.002$ compared with pre-op; #$P = 0.001$ compared with pre-op

In typical cases of severe post-tubercular kyphosis, two or more vertebrae are destroyed, leading to shortening or "buckling collapse" of the anterior column, without collapse of the posterior column height [4, 10]. Because of the accompanying severe spinal cord compression and distraction, preexisting neurologic dysfunction, and the high risk of potential neurological deficits, sufficient decompression of the spinal cord at the segments of angular kyphosis and the adjacent segments with stenosis may be necessary. The main goal in treating severe post-tubercular kyphosis should be to improve neurologic deficits, prevent further neurological lesions, moderately correct severe kyphosis, and restore alignment and stability of the whole spine.

Stretching or kinking of the spinal cord could occur during opening or closing wedge osteotomy [3, 9]. Besides, subluxation of the spinal column may occur during the correction procedures [16]. Therefore, two temporary titanium rods are essential to maintain the stability of the spine and prevent sudden subluxation of the spine after resection of the apical vertebrae. Moreover, a titanium cage is necessary to support the anterior column, maintain the stability of the spine, and prevent over-shortening of the spine and spinal cord. A balance between the amount of anterior column height restoration and posterior column shortening is essential to avoid spinal cord damage.

Stenosis adjacent to the angular kyphosis, which may be an important reason of late-onset neurological deficits and risk factor for neurological complications during PVCR, can be caused by intervertebral disc degeneration and/or calcification of ligamentum flavum at the adjacent segments. Mechanical stress may be the cause for intervertebral disc degeneration and calcification of ligamantum flavum at the adjacent segments [33]. Luk and Krishna [34] reported two cases with late-onset neurological deficits caused by spinal stenosis above healed tubercular kyphosis. Chen et al. [35] found ossification of the ligamentum flavum at segments adjacent to the kyphotic apex in six patients with thoracic tuberculosis. Ha et al. [7] reported ten cases with late-onset neurological deficits, including ossified ligament flavum (four), spinal stenosis (four), and intervertebral disc herniation (two). In the present study, five cases with late-onset neurological deficits were confirmed with stenosis at the segments adjacent to the apex of angular kyphosis (Table 2, Fig. 2).

Additional risk factors for neurological complications include affected segments, number of resected segments, and intraoperative hypotension, among others. Zeng et al. [13] reported that preoperative neurological function was worse in the thoracic group, and this may be related to higher sensitivity of spinal cord to either direct compression or tension over the kyphotic deformity in the thoracic segments. In the present study, two cases with multilevel PVCR were found with spinal cord injuries. Intraoperative hypotension must be prevented to minimize the risk of spinal cord ischemia. A mean blood pressure higher than 80 mmHg should be recommended to ensure the adequate perfusion of the spinal cord [16, 36].

Spinal cord monitoring is essential to ensure safety of the correction osteotomy during PVCR [16, 36, 37]. Therefore, any preoperative SEP and MEP changes during surgery should be paid attention to.

However, this study is limited by its relatively small sample size; more studies with a large patient group are necessary to evaluate the neurological complications after treatment of severe post-tubercular kyphosis with late-onset neurological deficits by PVCR.

Conclusions

Even though PVCR is effective to restore alignment of the whole spine, our findings suggest that it is nevertheless associated with a high risk for neurological complications following its use in the management of severe post-tubercular kyphosis with late-onset neurological deficits.

Abbreviations
ASIA: American Spinal Injury Association; C7PL: C7 plumb line; CT: Computed tomography; MEP: Motor-evoked potentials; MRI: Magnetic resonance imaging; ODI: Oswestry Disability Index; PVCR: Posterior vertebral column resection; SEP: Somatosensory-evoked potentials; SVA: Sagittal vertical axis; TB: Tuberculosis; VAS: Visual analog scale

Acknowledgements
Not applicable.

Funding

This work was supported by the National Key Research and Development Program of China (2018YFB1105700) and the National Natural Science Foundation of China (Grant nos. 81772401 and U1603121).

Authors' contributions

WH and CY participated in the design of this study and drafted the manuscript. WH, XW, YZ, and YG carried out the study and collected important background information. SL, KW, and XL collected the clinical data and performed the statistical analysis. SY and CY supervised this study. All authors read and approved the final manuscript.

Competing interests

The authors declare that they have no competing interests.

References

1. Jain AK. Tuberculosis of the spine: a fresh look at an old disease. J Bone Joint Surg Br. 2010;92(7):905–13.
2. Rajasekaran S. The natural history of post-tubercular kyphosis in children. Radiological signs which predict late increase in deformity. J Bone Joint Surg Br. 2001;83(7):954–62.
3. Rajasekaran S. Kyphotic deformity in spinal tuberculosis and its management. Int Orthop. 2012;36(2):359–65.
4. Rajasekaran S. Buckling collapse of the spine in childhood spinal tuberculosis. Clin Orthop Relat Res. 2007;460:86–92.
5. Moon MS, Moon YW, Moon JL, Kim SS, Sun DH. Conservative treatment of tuberculosis of the lumbar and lumbosacral spine. Clin Orthop Relat Res. 2002;398:40–9.
6. Boachie-Adjei O, Papadopoulos EC, Pellise F, Cunningham ME, Perez-Grueso FS, Gupta M, Lonner B, Paonessa K, King A, Sacramento C, Kim HJ, Mendelow M, Yazici M. Late treatment of tuberculosis-associated kyphosis: literature review and experience from a srs-gop site. Eur Spine J. 2013; 22(Suppl 4):641–6.
7. Ha KY, Kim YH. Late onset of progressive neurological deficits in severe angular kyphosis related to tuberculosis spondylitis. Eur Spine J. 2016;25(4): 1039–46.
8. Kalra KP, Dhar SB, Shetty G, Dhariwal Q. Pedicle subtraction osteotomy for rigid post-tuberculous kyphosis. J Bone Joint Surg Br. 2006;88(7):925–7.
9. Rajasekaran S, Vijay K, Shetty AP. Single-stage closing-opening wedge osteotomy of spine to correct severe post-tubercular kyphotic deformities of the spine: a 3-year follow-up of 17 patients. EurSpine J. 2010;19(4):583–92.
10. Rajasekaran S, Rishi Mugesh Kanna P, Shetty AP. Closing-opening wedge osteotomy for severe, rigid, thoracolumbar post-tubercular kyphosis. Eur Spine J. 2011;20(3):343–8.
11. Pappou IP, Papadopoulos EC, Swanson AN, Mermer MJ, Fantini GA, Urban MK, Russell L, Cammisa FP Jr, Girardi FP. Pott disease in the thoracolumbar spine with marked kyphosis and progressive paraplegia necessitating posterior vertebral column resection and anterior reconstruction with a cage. Spine (Phila Pa 1976). 2006;31(4):E123–7.
12. Wang Y, Zhang Y, Zhang X, Wang Z, Mao K, Chen C, Zheng G, Li G, Wood KB. Posterior-only multilevel modified vertebral column resection for extremely severe Pott's kyphotic deformity. Eur Spine J. 2009;18(10):1436–41.
13. Zeng Y, Chen Z, Qi Q, Guo Z, Li W, Sun C, White AP. Clinical and radiographic evaluation of posterior surgical correction for the treatment of moderate to severe post-tuberculosis kyphosis in 36 cases with a minimum 2-year follow-up. J Neurosurg Spine. 2012;16(4):351–8.
14. Zhang HQ, Li JS, Liu SH, Guo CF, Tang MX, Gao QL, Lin MZ, Yin XH, Wang YX, Deng A. The use of posterior vertebral column resection in the management of severe posttuberculous kyphosis: a retrospective study and literature review. Arch Orthop Trauma Surg. 2013;133(9):1211–8.
15. Liu X, Yuan S, Tian Y, Wang L, Zheng Y, Li J. Expanded eggshell procedure combined with closing-opening technique (a modified vertebral column resection) for the treatment of thoracic and thoracolumbar angular kyphosis. J Neurosurg Spine. 2015;23(1):42–8.
16. Lu G, Wang B, Li Y, Li L, Zhang H, Cheng I. Posterior vertebral column resection and intraoperative manual traction to correct severe post-tubercular rigid spinal deformities incurred during childhood: minimum 2-year follow-up. Eur Spine J. 2015;24(3):586–93.
17. Liu C, Lin L, Wang W, Lv G, Deng Y. Long-term outcomes of vertebral column resection for kyphosis in patients with cured spinal tuberculosis: average 8-year follow-up. J Neurosurg Spine. 2016;24(5):777–85.
18. Zhou T, Li C, Liu B, Tang X, Su Y, Xu Y. Analysis of 17 cases of posterior vertebral column resection in treating thoracolumbar spinal tuberculous angular kyphosis. J Orthop Surg Res. 2015;10:64.
19. Glassman SD, Bridwell K, Dimar JR, Horton W, Berven S, Schwab F. The impact of positive sagittal balance in adult spinal deformity. Spine (Phila Pa 1976). 2005;30(18):2024–9.
20. Hua WB, Zhang YK, Gao Y, Liu XZ, Yang SH, Wu XH, Wang J, Yang C. Analysis of sagittal parameters in patients undergoing one- or two-level closing wedge osteotomy for correcting thoracolumbar kyphosis secondary to ankylosing spondylitis. Spine (Phila Pa 1976). 2017;42(14):E848–54.
21. Suk SI, Kim JH, Kim WJ, Lee SM, Chung ER, Nah KH. Posterior vertebral column resection for severe spinal deformities. Spine (Phila Pa 1976). 2002; 27(21):2374–82.
22. Suk SI, Chung ER, Kim JH, Kim SS, Lee JS, Choi WK. Posterior vertebral column resection for severe rigid scoliosis. Spine (Phila Pa 1976). 2005; 30(14):1682–7.
23. Lenke LG, O'Leary PT, Bridwell KH, Sides BA, Koester LA, Blanke KM. Posterior vertebral column resection for severe pediatric deformity: minimum two-year follow-up of thirty-five consecutive patients. Spine (Phila Pa 1976). 2009;34(20):2213–21.
24. Lenke LG, Sides BA, Koester LA, Hensley M, Blanke KM. Vertebral column resection for the treatment of severe spinal deformity. Clin Orthop Relat Res. 2010;468(3):687–99.
25. Tuli SM. Severe kyphotic deformity in tuberculosis of the spine. Int Orthop. 1995;19(5):327–31.
26. Wang Y, Zhang Y, Zhang X, Huang P, Xiao S, Wang Z, Liu Z, Liu B, Lu N, Mao K. A single posterior approach for multilevel modified vertebral column resection in adults with severe rigid congenital kyphoscoliosis: a retrospective study of 13 cases. Eur Spine J. 2008;17(3):361–72.
27. Hamzaoglu A, Alanay A, Ozturk C, Sarier M, Karadereler S, Ganiyusufoglu K. Posterior vertebral column resection in severe spinal deformities: a total of 102 cases. Spine (Phila Pa 1976). 2011;36(5):E340–4.
28. Kim SS, Cho BC, Kim JH, Lim DJ, Park JY, Lee BJ, Suk SI. Complications of posterior vertebral resection for spinal deformity. Asian Spine J. 2012;6(4):257–65.
29. Xie J, Wang Y, Zhao Z, Zhang Y, Si Y, Li T, Yang Z, Liu L. Posterior vertebral column resection for correction of rigid spinal deformity curves greater than 100 degrees. J Neurosurg Spine. 2012;17(6):540–51.
30. Xie JM, Zhang Y, Wang YS, Bi N, Zhao Z, Li T, Yang H. The risk factors of neurologic deficits of one-stage posterior vertebral column resection for patients with severe and rigid spinal deformities. Eur Spine J. 2014;23(1): 149–56.
31. Papadopoulos EC, Boachie-Adjei O, Hess WF, Sanchez Perez-Grueso FJ, Pellise F, Gupta M, Lonner B, Paonessa K, Faloon M, Cunningham ME, Kim HJ, Mendelow M, Sacramento C, Yazici M. Early outcomes and complications of posterior vertebral column resection. Spine J. 2015;15(5):983–91.
32. Wang S, Aikenmu K, Zhang J, Qiu G, Guo J, Zhang Y, Weng X. The aim of this retrospective study is to evaluate the efficacy and safety of posterior-only vertebral column resection (PVCR) for the treatment of angular and isolated congenital kyphosis. Eur Spine J. 2017;26(7):1817–25.
33. Fukuyama S, Nakamura T, Ikeda T, Takagi K. The effect of mechanical stress on hypertrophy of the lumbar ligamentum flavum. J Spinal Disord. 1995; 8(2):126–30.
34. Luk KD, Krishna M. Spinal stenosis above a healed tuberculous kyphosis. A case report. Spine (Phila Pa 1976). 1996;21(9):1098–101.
35. Chen Y, Lu XH, Yang LL, Chen DY. Ossification of ligamentum flavum related to thoracic kyphosis after tuberculosis: case report and review of the literature. Spine (Phila Pa 1976). 2009;34(1):E41–4.
36. Ferguson J, Hwang SW, Tataryn Z, Samdani AF. Neuromonitoring changes in pediatric spinal deformity surgery: a single-institution experience. J Neurosurg Pediatr. 2014;13(3):247–54.
37. Cho SK, Lenke LG, Bolon SM, Kang MM, Zebala LP, Pahys JM, Cho W, Koester LA. Progressive myelopathy patients who lack spinal cord monitoring data have the highest rate of spinal cord deficits following posterior vertebral column resection surgery. Spine Deform. 2015;3(4):352–9.

25

Preliminary experience in treating thoracic spinal tuberculosis via a posterior modified transfacet debridement, instrumentation, and interbody fusion

Yun-Peng Huang[1], Jian-Hua Lin[1], Xiao-Ping Chen[2], Gui Wu[1] and Xuan-Wei Chen[1*]

Abstract

Background: Posterior transfacet approach has been proved to be a safe and effective access to treat thoracic disc herniation. However, the therapeutic effect and safety of modified transfacet approach for treating thoracic spinal tuberculosis (TST) has not been reported in the clinical literature. In this study, the clinical efficacy and safety of a single-stage posterior modified transfacet debridement, posterior instrumentation, and interbody fusion for treating TST were retrospectively evaluated.

Patients and methods: From 2009 to 2014, 37 patients with TST underwent a posterior modified transfacet debridement, interbody fusion following posterior instrumentation, under the cover of 18 months of antituberculosis chemotherapy. The patients were evaluated preoperatively and postoperatively in terms of Frankel Grade, visual analog scale (VAS) pain score, kyphotic Cobb angle, and bony fusion.

Results: The follow-up time was 39.8 ± 5.1 months (29–50 months). No postoperative complication or recurrence of spinal tuberculosis was observed. Definitive bony fusion was achieved in all patients. At the final follow-up, 2 cases were rated as Frankel grade D, 35 as grade E. VAS was recovered from 8.4 ± 1.0 cm to 0.4 ± 0.8 cm. The kyphotic angles were corrected from 29.4 ± 10.9° to 17.6 ± 6.3°. Using the Kirkaldy-Willis criteria, functional outcome was excellent in 29 patients, good in 7, and fair in 1.

Conclusions: Our preliminary results showed that single-stage posterior modified transfacet debridement, posterior instrumentation, and interbody fusion are effective and safe surgical options for treating TST.

Keywords: Focal debridement, Modified transfacet approach, Surgical treatment, Thoracic spine tuberculosis

Background

The incidence of tuberculosis (TB) is rising. In China, spinal TB is the most common form of extrapulmonary tuberculosis and remains a severe public health threat. According to the World Health Organization, 1.4 million new cases of TB occur annually in China, with spinal TB found in approximately 1% of all affected patients [1]. Thoracic spine tuberculosis (TST) is the most common spinal tuberculosis (TB), leading to local pain, paralysis, kyphotic deformity, and even death [2]. Although

antituberculosis chemotherapy is the mainstay in the management of the disease, surgical treatment is indicated for patients with cold abscess, neurologic lesion, spinal instability, kyphosis, and/or failure of conservative treatment [3]. The primary goals of a surgical approach are to completely debride the lesion, restore nerve function, and correct and avoid spinal deformity progression. Various surgical approaches have been developed, including anterior, posterior, and combined antero-posterior approaches. Selection of the optimum surgical approach remains controversial [4–6]. Anterior or combined antero-posterior approaches are associated with a high rate of major mobility and mortality [4, 7, 8]. On the other hand, posterior approaches such as posterolateral [3], transpedicular [9], or

* Correspondence: spine2018@sina.com
[1]Department of Spine Surgery, The First Affiliated Hospital of Fujian Medical University, 20 Chazhong Road, Fuzhou City 350005, Fujian Province, China
Full list of author information is available at the end of the article

the transforaminal approach [7] have been favored due to their simple anatomical demands and a lower rate of complications. However, even these approaches require a relatively extensive bone dissection and tissue disruption to provide adequate exposure of the lesion via removal of the proximal rib, costotransverse articulations, and posterior elements (including spinous process, lamina, facet joints and transverse process) linked to complications including pneumothorax and postoperative pain, particularly in multilevel TST [3, 7, 10].

The posterior transfacet approach and its variations have been shown to be a safe and effective method for the treatment of thoracic disc herniation (TDH) with relatively low morbidity [11, 12]. Furthermore, the posterior approach can provide a better correction of the kyphosis which most frequently occurs with TST. Anatomically, there is lesion of the intervertebral disk space in TST [13, 14], which is similar to that in TDH. Therefore, the authors believe that TST patients can be managed adequately by the posterior modified transfacet approach. The aim of this study was to validate the efficacy and safety of posterior modified transfacet debridement, instrumentation, and interbody fusion for the treatment of TST.

Methods

This study was approved by the Ethics Committee of the Hospital. Between 2009 and 2014, the authors treated 37 consecutive patients with TST via a modified transfacet approach. All patients were treated by the same surgical team though the team treated other patients (non-participants) with other approaches during the study period. The cohort was comprised of 22 males and 15 females, with an average age of 43.1 ± 17.3 years. The diagnosis of TST was based on clinical presentation, plain radiographs, computed tomography (CT), magnetic resonance imaging (MRI), hematologic tests, and pathological examinations from CT-guided biopsy. Twenty-three were confirmed radiologically as multilevel TST. Of these, 5 were non-contiguous multifocal TST. Twenty-five were accompanied with paraspinal abscess. Eleven cases had bilateral paraspinal abscess and 4 had large abscess. One patient had abdominal draining sinuses before surgery. Twenty-six patients had a neurological deficit of grade B, C, or D according to the Frankel Grade, including motor weakness, sensory change, and radiating pain to the lower limbs. Eleven cases had combined pulmonary tuberculosis. Patients rated their pain intensity on a visual analog scale (VAS), from "no pain" (0 cm) to "maximal pain" (10 cm). The mean preoperative VAS score of the cohort was 8.4 ± 1.0 cm (range 5.4–9.8 cm).

Preoperative procedure

Patients were treated with the standard regimen of isoniazid (H), rifampin (R), ethambutol (E), and pyrazinamide

(Z) (HREZ) chemotherapy regimen [11], consisting of isoniazid (300 mg/d), rifampicin (450 mg/d), ethambutol (750 mg/d), and pyrazinamide (750 mg/d) for at least 4 weeks before surgery. The erythrocyte sedimentation rate (ESR) was 44.7 ± 23.3 mm/h; the kyphosis angle was 29.4 ± 10.9°. When the ESR had significantly decreased (< 40 mm/h), surgery was carried out. The preoperative anti-TB treatment reduces Mycobacterium tuberculosis in lesions and increases surgical safety [15]. Preoperative clinical and radiological characteristics are shown in Tables 1 and 2.

Surgical technique

The modified transfacet approach was similar to that described by Bransford et al. [12] for approaching protruded thoracic discs. Under general anesthesia, patients were placed in prone position and a linear, midline incision was made. The spinous process, lamina, facet joints, and transverse processes were exposed (subperiosteal dissection). Pedicle screws were inserted at least two levels above and below the level of involvement (outlined in Table 1). Pedicle screws were placed in the affected vertebrae if the vertebrae were not destroyed by infection. For thoracic spine, a unilateral or bilateral facet complex and parts of the lamina were removed, exposing the affected disc space (lateral one-third), granulation tissue, lateral aspect of dural sac, and exiting nerve root. When required, the upper and lower transverse processes were partially excised to increase the exposure (Fig. 1a, b). No rib or thoracic nerve root was removed in any patient. When there was a large paraspinal abscess, a catheter was inserted deep into the abscess cavity to flush the abscess until no pus outflowed. The annulus was opened with a blade, and debridement in the affected intervertebral space was subsequently performed with rongeurs and curettes until the sclerotic bone, disc, pus, and granulation tissue were completely removed through to healthy bleeding bone (working in a lateral to medial direction to create a central cavity). Granulation tissue adherent to the ventral aspect of the dural tube was pushed downward into the central cavity with curettes and was then removed piecemeal (Fig. 1c). Anterior spinal cord decompression was obtained. Multi-affected intervertebral spaces were chosen for focal debridement if there was involvement of a long segment [4]. Tricortical harvested from the iliac crest was implanted for posterior fusion in the intervertebral space that underwent focal debridement (Fig. 1d). Two pre-bent titanium rods were fixed to correct the local deformity, and screws were compressed to achieve bone-to-bone contact at the anterior column. Finally, after irrigation by sterile physiologic saline, 0.5 g streptomycin was embedded in the pathological intervertebral space [3]. Two drainage tubes were inserted routinely,

Table 1 Patient demographics, operative information, and disease characteristics

No.	Gender	Age (years)	Levels	Focal debridement	Operative time (min)	Blood loss (ml)	Follow-up (months)	Bone fusion (months)	Complications
1	F	39	T10–11	T10–11	210	500	42	6	
2	F	62	T7–9	T7–8	230	300	45	9	
3	M	52	T5–6.	T5–6	208	200	36	6	
4	F	75	T5–7	T5–6	230	700	47	12	
5	M	65	T6–7	T6–7	220	250	45	6	
6	M	27	T11–L1	T11–12	160	200	36	6	Pain at the donor site
7	F	39	T11–12	T11–12	180	300	39	6	
8	M	48	T1–2, T5–6	T5–6	230	300	35	6	
9	M	64	T10–12	T10–11, T11–12	290	600	38	9	
10	M	64	T8–9	T8–9	215	400	38	6	
11	F	24	T4–L2	T6–7, T11–12	410	1800	29	12	Hypoproteinemia
12	F	81	T10–11	T10–11	240	500	40	6	
13	F	59	T8–9	T8–9	152	100	45	6	
14	F	39	T10–L2	T10–11	230	450	43	6	
15	M	31	T11–L1	T11–12	200	400	36	6	
16	M	64	T10–12	T10–11	195	600	39	6	
17	F	76	T8–9	T8–9	202	500	37	6	
18	M	24	T8–L2	T9–10, T11–12	310	800	40	9	
19	M	55	T10–L2	T11–12	230	300	33	6	
20	M	21	T4–12	T6–7, T9–10	360	1500	43	9	Water–electrolyte imbalance
21	M	33	T6–L1	T8–9, T11–12	320	1000	48	9	
22	F	40	T10–L2	T11–12	220	450	33	6	
23	F	23	T8–L3	T9–10, T12–L1	355	1300	41	12	
24	M	30	T8–L1	T9–10	190	300	48	6	
25	M	36	T11–L2	T11–12	210	700	42	6	
26	M	23	T10–L4	T10–11	180	200	50	6	
27	M	28	T11–L1	T11–12	110	200	31	6	
28	M	42	T8–10	T8–9	270	500	40	6	
29	M	39	T7–9	T8–9	160	300	36	6	
30	M	31	T7–L1	T9–10, T10–11	240	600	37	6	
31	M	26	T5–11	T6–7, T9–10	290	1200	46	9	
32	M	44	T6–7	T6–7	190	200	40	6	
33	F	60	T8–9	T8–9	180	300	42	9	Pain at the donor site
34	M	23	T5–6	T5–6	200	350	33	6	
35	F	48	T9–10	T9–10	130	200	38	6	
36	F	25	T7–8	T7–8	170	300	35	6	
37	F	34	T6–8	T7–8	160	300	46	6	

M male, *F* female, *T* thoracic spine, *L* lumbar spine

and the incision was closed. The material debrided was sent for culturing and histopathologic examination.

Postoperative procedure

The postural drain was usually removed when drainage volume is < 50 ml/24 h. For patients with large paraspinal abscess, percutaneous drainage was performed under sonographic or CT guidance [16]. Patients continued with the oral HREZ chemotherapy post-operatively. Six months later, pyrazinamide was discontinued. Patients then received a 12-month regimen of HRE chemotherapy [11]. Frankel Grade, VAS, and ESR were evaluated monthly,

Table 2 Summary of clinical and radiological data

No.	Kyphosis (°)			Frankel grade			ESR (mm/h)			VAS (mm)		Kirkaldy-Willis criteria
	Preop	Postop	FFU	Preop	Postop	FFU	Preop	Postop	FFU	Preop	FFU	
1	19.5	13.7	14.5	E	E	E	9	12	10	9.8	0	Excellent
2	38.3	28.8	30.1	D	D	E	49	7	6	8.9	0	Excellent
3	23.7	15.9	16.3	E	E	E	26	11	10	7.8	0	Excellent
4	23.2	17.3	19.1	D	D	E	40	10	7	8.3	0	Excellent
5	25.4	16.7	18.0	E	E	E	117	36	10	9.1	0	Excellent
6	13.7	6.1	7.2	E	E	E	95	22	4	6.8	2	Good
7	11.9	9.1	9.2	E	E	E	51	13	11	8.4	0	Excellent
8	35.7	27.7	29.5	B	C	D	26	9	7	8.9	3.5	Fair
9	25.2	17.5	19.1	E	E	E	16	11	12	7.5	0	Excellent
10	17.6	9.8	9.8	C	D	D	67	15	5	7.7	1	Good
11	38.2	35.1	35.1	E	E	E	52	19	7	7.4	0	Excellent
12	15.9	11.7	12.0	C	E	E	19	6	8	6.3	0	Excellent
13	20.2	16.3	16.9	D	D	E	45	12	9	8.2	0	Excellent
14	17.0	9.2	9.0	E	E	E	83	14	11	9.0	0	Excellent
15	29.3	17.5	20.1	C	E	E	32	12	9	8.6	0	Excellent
16	27.2	18.8	19.2	D	E	E	36	9	8	9.3	0	Excellent
17	32.5	20.2	19.7	C	E	E	26	12	15	7.6	1	Good
18	25.5	12.5	13.2	D	E	E	79	15	7	9.1	0	Excellent
19	28.3	17.7	18.4	D	E	E	55	9	11	8.4	0	Excellent
20	49.0	23.6	24.3	D	E	E	47	12	15	7.8	0	Excellent
21	45.8	21.3	23.6	C	D	E	87	25	12	9.0	2	Good
22	26.3	13.4	14.5	D	E	E	39	15	14	8.2	0	Excellent
23	33.1	19.5	20.7	D	D	E	24	13	9	9.3	0	Excellent
24	17.9	7.1	9.8	E	E	E	33	7	10	8.8	0	Excellent
25	31.4	18.8	19.4	D	E	E	45	12	9	9.6	2.6	Good
26	28.3	13.4	14.2	D	E	E	23	10	13	9.4	0	Excellent
27	22.0	10.4	11.6	E	E	E	51	11	9	7.8	0	Excellent
28	37.5	19.5	19.7	B	D	E	18	10	10	5.4	1	Good
29	39.7	18.6	19.3	E	E	E	43	10	7	9.7	0	Excellent
30	36.3	20.4	21.7	C	D	E	30	19	10	7.9	0	Excellent
31	65.4	23.4	26.4	B	C	E	51	20	13	8.8	1	Good
32	36.5	16.3	19.1	D	E	E	49	21	9	8.2	0	Excellent
33	28.2	8.8	10.9	C	D	E	39	9	9	8.0	0	Excellent
34	30.4	13.9	17.4	D	E	E	41	12	10	9.5	0	Excellent
35	17.5	9.9	10.7	D	E	E	26	8	6	7.6	0	Excellent
36	33.1	11.3	13.6	C	D	E	47	10	10	7.9	0	Excellent
37	42.4	14.6	17.3	D	E	E	38	9	7	9.4	0	Excellent

The reference value of ESR in our hospital is as follows: < 20 mm/h (male), < 15 mm/h (female)

Preop preoperative, *Postop* postoperative 3 months, *FFU* final follow-up, *ESR* erythrocyte sedimentation rate, *VAS* visual analog scale

and X-ray was examined every 3–6 months. CT and/or MRI scan were taken at the 18-month or final follow-up (Table 1). Bony spinal fusion was assessed according to the criteria defined by Lee et al. [6, 17]. Functional outcome was assessed by Frankel Grade and the Kirkaldy-Willis criteria [18]. Using SPSS 19.0 software (SPSS, Inc., Chicago, IL, USA), VAS, ESR, Frankel Grade, and kyphosis angles were statistically analyzed by paired *t* test pre- and post-operatively and final follow-up. Using R software (version 3.2.2, 2015), the *P* values of paired *t* test

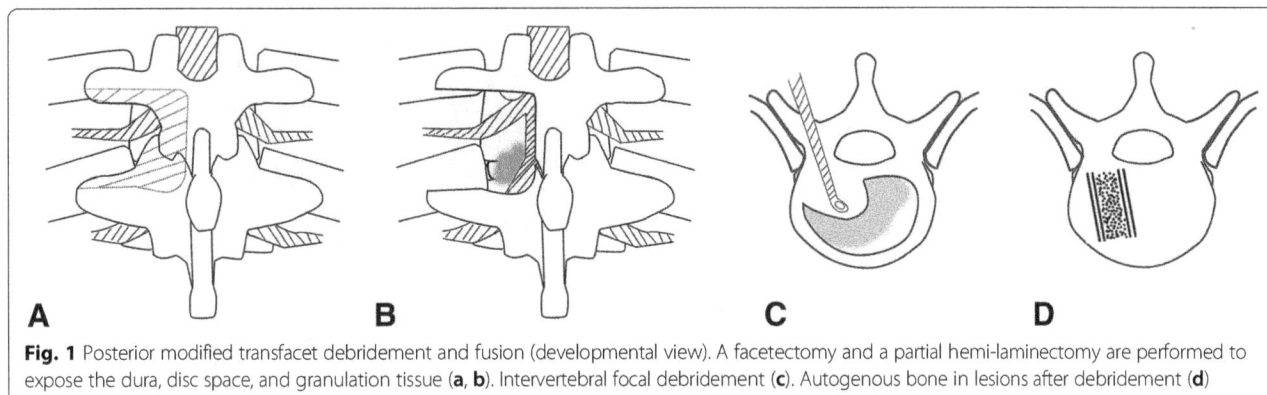

Fig. 1 Posterior modified transfacet debridement and fusion (developmental view). A facetectomy and a partial hemi-laminectomy are performed to expose the dura, disc space, and granulation tissue (**a**, **b**). Intervertebral focal debridement (**c**). Autogenous bone in lesions after debridement (**d**)

were adjusted for multiple comparison by BH (Benjamini & Hochberg, 1995) method [19]. $P < 0.05$ was considered significant.

Results

For all cases, the mean follow-up time was 39.8 ± 5.1 months (29–50 months). The mean operative time, blood loss, and duration of hospital stay were presented in Table 1. No severe operation-related complications including sinus formation, dural tear, wound infection, or pneumothorax were observed (Table 2). During the period, no clinical or radiological relapse was found. At the final follow-up, all patients showed satisfactory clinical, laboratory, and imaging basis eradication of the infection. All patients achieve definitive bony fusion with an average time of 7.1 ± 1.9 months [17]. The average VAS pain score dropped to 0.4 ± 0.8 cm (range 0.0–3.5 cm) at the final follow-up ($P < 0.01$). ESR returned to normal (13.2 ± 5.9 mm/h) within 3 months after surgery ($P < 0.01$). The mean kyphotic angle before and after surgery and at the final follow-up was $29.4 \pm 10.9°$, $16.4 \pm 6.2°$, and $17.6 \pm 6.3°$, respectively. The pre- and post-operative differences were statistically significant ($P < 0.01$), as were the post-operative and final ($P < 0.01$) Cobb angles. At the final follow-up visit, the neurologic status of 2 patients with preoperative neurologic deficit improved by three grades, 7 by two grades, and 16 by one grade (Table 2). Using the Kirkaldy-Willis criteria [18], functional outcomes were denoted as excellent in 29 patients, good in 7, and fair in 1. The typical cases are shown in Figs. 2 and 3.

Discussions

TST accounts for the largest proportion (30.3–55.8%) of spinal tuberculosis cases [2]. Anti-TB chemotherapy and surgery are currently the standard methods for treating TST. Surgical approaches for TST have evolved over time, including anterior, posterior, and combined antero-posterior approaches. Anterior and combined approaches are often associated with higher morbidities and mortality, although they grant direct access to

debridement and strut grafts [20]. Conversely, the posterior approach is simple and associated with a low risk of morbidity [7, 10]. However, the posterior approach for TST has its own risk profile, owing to its special anatomical characteristics and positioning. For most cases of TST, the anterior and middle columns are difficult to operate from the back. On the other hand, the thoracic spinal canal allows little room for intraoperative manipulation and the spinal cord is vulnerable to damage. Therefore, the posterior approach and its variants require proximal rib and costotransverse articulation resection in order to offer direct exposure to lateral aspects of the diseased vertebral bodies [3, 10]. Additionally, total laminectomy is required to achieve decompression. In sum, the complications of posterior surgery are not minimal and are usually related to the surgical outcomes.

A simpler operation with fewer risks is desirable, especially for the high-risk patient. A posterior transfacet approach was described initially by Stillerman et al. [11] and modified by other authors [12, 21]. This procedure for the treatment of TDH has yielded excellent results. The essence of the transfacet approach is to provide safe and effective access for the removal of herniated discs with relatively low morbidity [11, 22]. The anatomical characteristics of TDH are similar to those of TST since *Mycobacterium tuberculosis* is also prone to affect the anterior column including the intervertebral disc and its upper and lower adjoining vertebral bodies (peridiscal) [14, 23]. In light of this, we used a posterior transfacet approach for the treatment of TST, as described for the treatment for TDH. In this study, we modified this approach to allow for the safe debridement and interbody fusion via complete facetectomy and partial hemilaminectomy to minimize tissue disruption and preserve ribs and the partial posterior element of the thoracic spine [12]. In our study, all patients obtained satisfactory results with respect to pain relief, neurologic function, kyphosis correction, bone fusion, and laboratory findings. No relapse was detected in our patients by the time of the last follow-up visit.

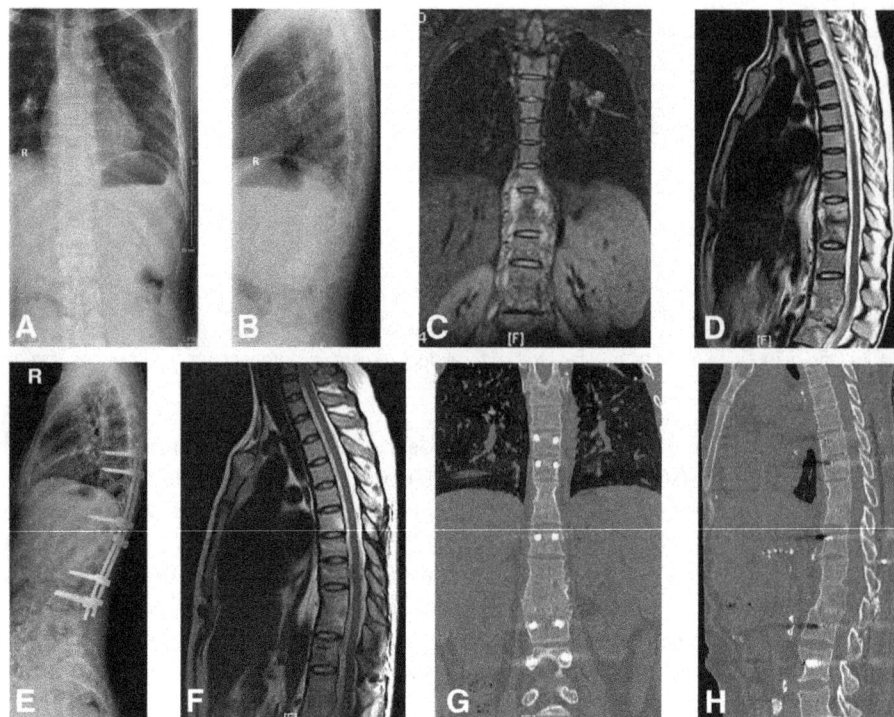

Fig. 2 Preoperative radiography (**a**, **b**) and MRI (**c**, **d**) of a 23-year-old female patient with tuberculosis at T8–L3 with extensive paravertebral abscesses. Radiography (**e**), MRI (**f**), and CT (**g** and **h**) at the final follow-up showed definitive interbody bone fusion was achieved at T9–10 and T12–L1. MRI: magnetic resonance image; CT: computed tomography scan

Compared with conventional posterior approaches, our approach has a limited view. Clinically, our preliminary experience showed that the posterior modified transfacet approach provides an adequate exposure and acceptable access for effective focal debridement. The reasons may be attributed to the following. First, resection of one or both sides of thoracic facet joint and partial hemi-laminectomy offers an oblique visualization and posterolateral manipulations facilitate effective focal debridement in the affected intervertebral space and limit "around-the-corner" or blind-spot dissection [12]. Additionally, partial removal of the upper and lower transverse processes enlarges the exposure to focal lesions and increases the window for posterolateral manipulation. Third, during focal debridement, the sclerotic bone, dead osteons, pus, granulation tissue, and disc were completely removed, reaching the subnormal substance of bones between normal cancellous bones and pathologic bones [3, 5, 24, 25]. Fourth, for multilevel TST, the affected foci were chosen to perform debridement separately since it is unnecessary to achieve debridement in each lesion as radical debridement is relative in any surgical approach [3, 5, 9]. Finally, anti-TB chemotherapy, rest, and nutritional improvement are still the most basic methods of TB treatment [3, 13].

The posterior approach has become popular, but potential operation-related complications and morbidity remain a serious concern. Luo et.al [26] described a pneumonia rate of 16.2%, a cerebrospinal fluid (CSF) leakage rate of 5.4%, and a thrombosis rate of 2.7% in 37 cases treated with a posterior transpedicular approach. Yin et.al [3] reported that 5 of 31 patients operated via a posterior approach with costotransversectomy experienced complications including pneumothoraxic, CSF leakage, sinus formation, and wound infection. The purpose of posterior modified transfacet approach is minimizing the surgical impact. Owing to its simple anatomy, this approach minimizes the intraoperative and postoperative complications that may occur with the posterolateral, transpedicular, or transforaminal approach. In our study, no severe complication was noted.

The following are the major advantages of this approach. First, posterolateral manipulation during focal debridement produces a "cavitation" of the intervertebral space to allow the granulation tissue be completely pushed without any retraction of the dura sac [12], which minimizes the risks of dura tears, CSF leakages, or worsening of neurological deficiencies. Second, this approach allows for simultaneous debridement and stabilization of the spine via a single posterior midline incision, compared with the posterolateral [3] or transforaminal approaches [7]. Third, bone removal and soft-tissue disruption are minimal since the modified transfacet approach obviates the need for dissecting the proximal rib and exposing the lateral aspects of the infected vertebral bodies. Thus, it eliminates the risk of

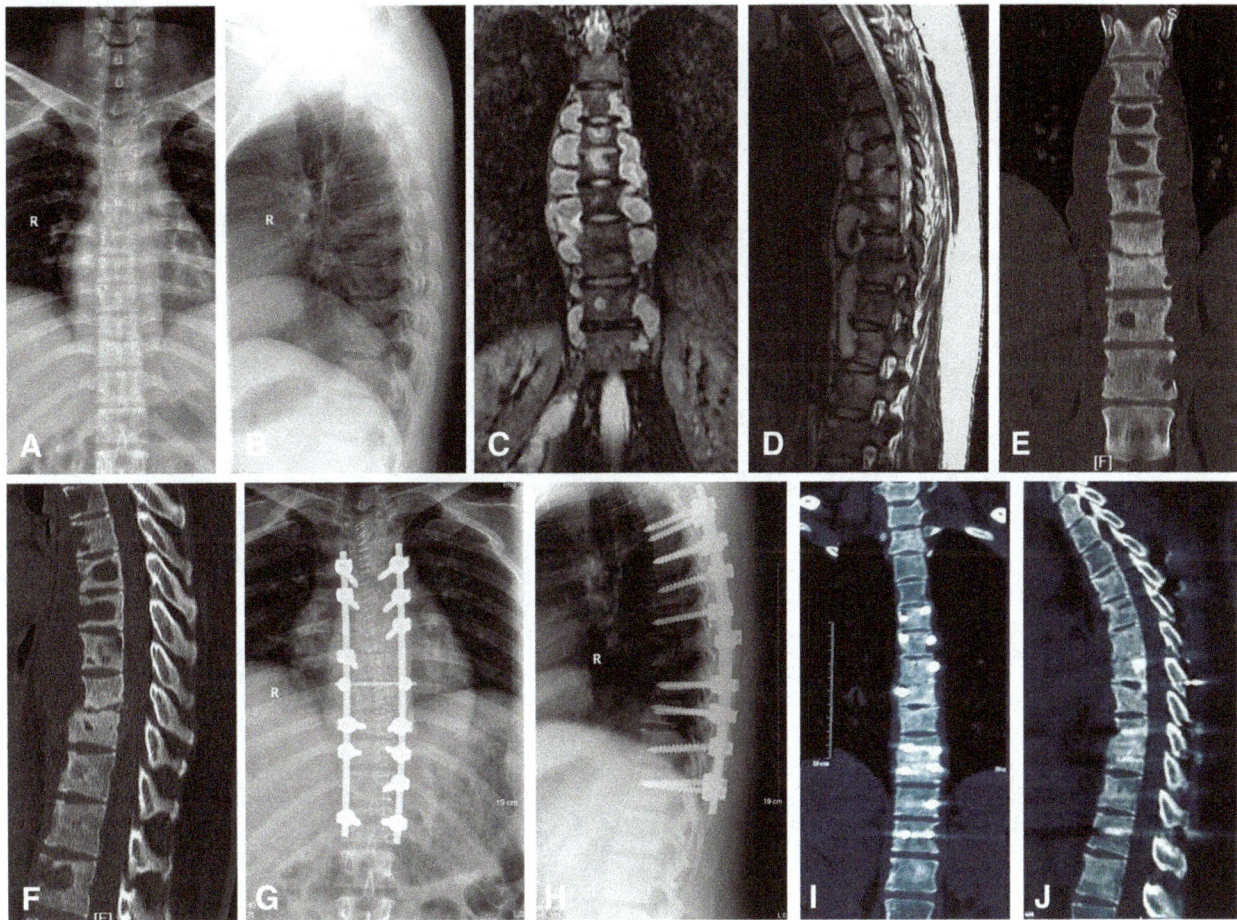

Fig. 3 Preoperative radiography (**a** and **b**), MRI (**c** and **d**), and CT (**e** and **f**) of a 24-year-old female patient with tuberculosis at T4–L2 with extensive paravertebral abscesses. Radiography (**g**, **h**) and CT (**i**, **j**) at the final follow-up showed definitive interbody bone fusion was achieved at T6–7 and T9–10 (**e–h**). MRI: magnetic resonance image; CT: computed tomography scan (**i–j**)

pneumothoraxic complications and diminishes long-term localized pain. Fourth, compared with total laminectomy, facetectomy and partial hemilaminectomy have been reported to lead to reduced operation time, bone loss, and tissue disruption, especially for patients with multilevel disease. Lastly, a single posterior midline incision and the minimal amount of bone removal and tissue dissection result in decreased intraoperative anesthetic, shorter operative time, less blood loss, shorter hospital stays, and less time off normal activities. Due to the small sample and single site study, the above findings should be validated in expanded and comparative method studies.

The main limitation to this study was the relatively small series of patients enrolled in a single institution. Nonetheless, patient data continues to be accumulated including clinical follow-up of patients. Additionally, no comparative treatment group was available to the transfacet approach such as anterior, posterior, or combined anterior and other posterior approaches. Finally, the transfacet approach has its potential limits which should

be comprehensively discussed. All things considered, the author considers that the following indications are inappropriate for this approach: (1) lesions confined to the anterior vertebral column, (2) > 50% collapse of the vertebral body, and (3) severe segment kyphosis.

Conclusions

Our experience suggests that posterior modified transfacet approach for the treatment of TST is safe and effective, providing adequate exposure for intervertebral focal debridement, posterior instrumentations, and interbody fusion. The results using this technique were excellent. The risk of operation-related complications was minimized, likely owing to the simple anatomy, minimal bone dissection, and tissue disruption of the technique. This approach may become the procedure of choice in the surgical management of all TST. Future studies should attempt to reproduce the results of this study with larger number of patients and longer follow-up times.

Abbreviations

ASIA: The American Spinal Injury Association; CSF: Cerebrospinal fluid; CT: Computed tomography; ESR: Erythrocyte sedimentation rate; FFU: Final follow-up; HREZ: The standard regimen of isoniazid (H), rifampin (R), ethambutol (E), and pyrazinamide (Z); MRI: Magnetic resonance imaging; Postop: Postoperative; Preop: Preoperative; TB: Tuberculosis; TDH: Thoracic disc herniation; TST: Thoracic spine tuberculosis; VAS: Visual analog scale

Acknowledgements

We thank the support from the colleague in our department.

Funding

This study was supported by a grant from the Department of Public Health Bureau, Fujian, P.R.C (No. 2013-ZQN-ZD-19); by a grant from the key Clinical Specialty Discipline Construction Program of Fujian, P.R.C.; by a grant from National Natural Science Foundation of China (NSFC) (11601083); a grant from Natural Science Foundation of Fujian Province, China (2016J05002); and a grant from Probability and Statistics: Theory and Application (IRTL1704).

Authors' contributions

YPH, JHL, and XWC contributed to the study conception and design. YPH, JHL, GW, XPC, and XWC contributed to the acquisition of data. YPH, XPC, and GW analyzed and interpreted the data. YPH, JHL, and XWC drafted the manuscript. YPH, JHL, XWC, and GW critically revised the manuscript. All authors read and approved the final manuscript.

Competing interests

The authors declare that they have no competing interests.

Author details

[1]Department of Spine Surgery, The First Affiliated Hospital of Fujian Medical University, 20 Chazhong Road, Fuzhou City 350005, Fujian Province, China. [2]School of Mathematics and Informatics, Fujian Normal University, Fuzhou City 350117, Fujian Province, China.

References

1. Yao Y, Song W, Wang K, Ma B, Liu H, Zheng W, et al. Features of 921 patients with spinal tuberculosis: a 16-year investigation of a general hospital in Southwest China. Orthopedics. 2017;40(6):e1017–23.
2. Yao Y, Zhang H, Liu M, Liu H, Chu T, Tang Y, et al. Prognostic factors for recovery of patients after surgery for thoracic spinal tuberculosis. World neurosurgery. 2017;105:327–31.
3. Yin XH, Liu SH, Li JS, Chen Y, Hu XK, Zeng KF, et al. The role of costotransverse radical debridement, fusion and postural drainage in the surgical treatment of multisegmental thoracic spinal tuberculosis: a minimum 5-year follow-up. Eur Spine J. 2016;25(4):1047–55.
4. Zhang HQ, Guo CF, Xiao XG, Long WR, Deng ZS, Chen J. One-stage surgical management for multilevel tuberculous spondylitis of the upper thoracic region by anterior decompression, strut autografting, posterior instrumentation, and fusion. J Spinal Disord Tech. 2007;20(4):263–7.
5. Shi JD, Wang ZL, Geng GQ, Niu NK. Intervertebral focal surgery for the treatment of non-contiguous multifocal spinal tuberculosis. Int Orthop. 2012;36(7):1423–7.
6. Li L, Xu J, Ma Y, Tang D, Chen Y, Luo F, et al. Surgical strategy and management outcomes for adjacent multisegmental spinal tuberculosis: a retrospective study of forty-eight patients. Spine (Phila Pa 1976). 2014;39(1):E40–8.
7. Zhang HQ, Lin MZ, Shen KY, Ge L, Li JS, Tang MX, et al. Surgical management for multilevel noncontiguous thoracic spinal tuberculosis by single-stage posterior transforaminal thoracic debridement, limited

8. decompression, interbody fusion, and posterior instrumentation (modified TTIF). Arch Orthop Trauma Surg. 2012;132(6):751–7.
8. Li M, Du J, Meng H, Wang Z, Luo Z. One-stage surgical management for thoracic tuberculosis by anterior debridement, decompression and autogenous rib grafts, and instrumentation. Spine J. 2011;11(8):726–33.
9. Chacko AG, Moorthy RK, Chandy MJ. The transpedicular approach in the management of thoracic spine tuberculosis: a short-term follow up study. Spine (Phila Pa 1976). 2004;29(17):E363–7.
10. Pang X, Shen X, Wu P, Luo C, Xu Z, Wang X. Thoracolumbar spinal tuberculosis with psoas abscesses treated by one-stage posterior transforaminal lumbar debridement, interbody fusion, posterior instrumentation, and postural drainage. Arch Orthop Trauma Surg. 2013;133(6):765–72.
11. Stillerman CB, Chen TC, Day JD, Couldwell WT, Weiss MH. The transfacet pedicle-sparing approach for thoracic disc removal: cadaveric morphometric analysis and preliminary clinical experience. J Neurosurg. 1995;83(6):971–6.
12. Bransford R, Zhang F, Bellabarba C, Konodi M, Chapman JR. Early experience treating thoracic disc herniations using a modified transfacet pedicle-sparing decompression and fusion. J Neurosurg Spine. 2010; 12(2):221–31.
13. Garg RK, Somvanshi DS. Spinal tuberculosis: a review. The journal of spinal cord medicine. 2011;34(5):440–54.
14. Zeng H, Zhang P, Shen X, Luo C, Xu Z, Zhang Y, et al. One-stage posterior-only approach in surgical treatment of single-segment thoracic spinal tuberculosis with neurological deficits in adults: a retrospective study of 34 cases. BMC Musculoskelet Disord. 2015;16:186.
15. Yang L, Liu Z. Analysis and therapeutic schedule of the postoperative recurrence of bone tuberculosis. J Orthop Surg Res. 2013;8:47.
16. Pieri S, Agresti P, Altieri AM, Ialongo P, Cortese A, Alma MG, et al. Percutaneous management of complications of tuberculous spondylodiscitis: short- to medium-term results. La Radiologia medica. 2009;114(6):984–95.
17. Lee JS, Moon KP, Kim SJ, Suh KT. Posterior lumbar interbody fusion and posterior instrumentation in the surgical management of lumbar tuberculous spondylitis. J Bone Joint Surg Br. 2007;89(2):210–4.
18. Kirkaldy-Willis WH, Paine KW, Cauchoix J, McIvor G. Lumbar spinal stenosis. Clin Orthop Relat Res. 1974;99:30–50.
19. Benjamini Y, Hochberg. Controlling the false discovery rate: a practical and powerful approach to multiple testing. J R Stat Soc Ser B Methodol. 1995; 57(1):289–300.
20. Yin XH, Zhou ZH, Yu HG, Hu XK, Guo Q, Zhang HQ. Comparison between the antero-posterior and posterior only approaches for treating thoracolumbar tuberculosis (T10-L2) with kyphosis in children: a minimum 3-year follow-up. Childs Nerv Syst. 2016;32(1):127–33.
21. Nishimura Y, Thani NB, Tochigi S, Ahn H, Ginsberg HJ. Thoracic discectomy by posterior pedicle-sparing, transfacet approach with real-time intraoperative ultrasonography: clinical article. J Neurosurg Spine. 2014;21(4):568–76.
22. Stillerman CB, Chen TC, Couldwell WT, Zhang W, Weiss MH. Experience in the surgical management of 82 symptomatic herniated thoracic discs and review of the literature. J Neurosurg. 1998;88(4):623–33.
23. Yin XH, Zhang HQ, Hu XK, Li JS, Chen Y, Zeng KF. Treatment of pediatric spinal tuberculosis abscess with percutaneous drainage and low-dose local antituberculous therapy: a preliminary report. Child's nervsyst. 2015;31(7):1149–55.
24. Khandan A, Karamian E, Bonakdarchian M. Mechanochemical synthesis evaluation of nanocrystalline bone-derived bioceramic powder using for bone tissue engineering. Dental Hypotheses. 2014;5(4):155–61.
25. Karamian E, Motamedi MRK, Khandan A, Soltani P, Maghsoudi S. An in vitro evaluation of novel NHA/zircon plasma coating on 316L stainless steel dental implant. Progress in Natural Science: Materials International. 2014; 24(2):150–6.
26. Luo C, Wang X, Wu P, Ge L, Zhang H, Hu J. Single-stage transpedicular decompression, debridement, posterior instrumentation, and fusion for thoracic tuberculosis with kyphosis and spinal cord compression in aged individuals. Spine J. 2016;16(2):154–62.

26

Effect of pedicle screw augmentation with a self-curing elastomeric material under cranio-caudal cyclic loading—a cadaveric biomechanical study

Werner Schmoelz[1*†] (iD), Alexander Keiler[1†], Marko Konschake[2], Richard A Lindtner[1] and Alessandro Gasbarrini[3]

Abstract

Background: Pedicle screws can be augmented with polymethylmethacrylate (PMMA) cement through cannulated and fenestrated pedicle screws to improve screw anchorage. To overcome the drawbacks of PMMA, a modified augmentation technique applying a self-curing elastomeric material into a balloon-created cavity prior to screw insertion was developed and evaluated. The aim of the study was to compare the effect of the established and novel augmentation technique on pedicle screw anchorage in a biomechanical in vitro experiment.

Methods: In ten lumbar vertebral bodies, the right pedicles were instrumented with monoaxial cannulated and fenestrated pedicle screws and augmented in situ with 2 ml PMMA. The left pedicles were instrumented with monoaxial cannulated pedicle screws. Prior to left screw insertion, a balloon cavity was created and filled with 3 ml of self-curing elastomer (silicone). Each screw was subjected to a cranio-caudal cyclic load starting from − 50 to 50 N while the upper load was increased by 5 N every 100 load cycles until loosening or 11,000 cycles (600 N). After cyclic loading, a pullout test of the screws was conducted.

Results: The mean cycles to screw loosening were 9824 ± 1982 and 7401 ± 1644 for the elastomer and PMMA group, respectively ($P = 0.012$). The post-cycling pullout test of the loosened screws showed differences in the failure mode and failure load, with predominantly pedicle/vertebrae fractures in the PMMA group (1188.6 N ± 288.1) and screw pullout through the pedicle (671.3 N ± 332.1) in the elastomer group.

Conclusion: The modified pedicle screw augmentation technique involving a balloon cavity creation and a self-curing elastomeric silicone resulted in a significantly improved pedicle screw anchorage under cyclic cranio-caudal loading when compared to conventional in situ PMMA augmentation.

Keywords: Pedicle screw anchorage, Screw augmentation, PMMA, Silicone, Elastoplasty, In situ screw augmentation

Background

Posterior implant systems are used for stabilization and fixation of the human thoracic and lumbar spine if the load-bearing capacity is lost by injury, disease, or degeneration [1]. In selected cases, such as patients with reduced bone quality or in revision spine surgery, anchorage and load bearing of pedicle screws are diminished [2], and augmentation of transpedicular screws is recommended [2–7]. In general, pedicle screws can be augmented with two different techniques. The so-called in situ augmentation applies a specifically designed cannulated and fenestrated pedicle screw and carries out augmentation through the cannulated pedicle screw after screw placement. Alternatively, the augmentation can be conducted prior to screw placement with a standard pedicle screw being placed in the non-cured augmentation material. In order to better control the flow of the augmentation material, a cavity may be created by cutting a screw thread or

---

* Correspondence: Werner.schmoelz@i-med.ac.at
[†]Werner Schmoelz and Alexander Keiler contributed equally to this work.
[1]Department of Trauma Surgery, Medical University of Innsbruck, Anichstraße 35, 6020 Innsbruck, Austria
Full list of author information is available at the end of the article

by kyphoplasty balloon inflation prior to augmentation [5, 8–10].

Although polymethylmethacrylate (PMMA) has been used for many years—at the beginning for reconstructive surgery, more recently as augmentation material in several conditions—the application can have negative side effects. Due to its exothermic curing behavior, the temperature at the interface increases substantially, and concerns for thermal bone necrosis were raised [11–13]. Other drawbacks include the lack of osteoconductivity [14–16], the limited time frame for processing [17], and the still not entirely investigated interaction between PMMA and the surrounding tissue, as in some cases a toxic property of the monomer (methyl methacrylate) has been reported in the literature [18–22]. Bone cements are extensively employed in orthopedics for joint arthroplasty. However, implant failure in the form of aseptic loosening is known to occur after long-term use [23]. Laboratory studies showed a decrease in molecular weight and hydrolysis of PMMA associated with long-term implantation [24] while the stress-strain behavior of the PMMA/bone composite is affected by the polymerization shrinkage during curing [25]. Because PMMA was already in clinical use when the FDA gained regulatory authority over medical devices, its approval was grandfathered by the FDA. Current testing of PMMA is conducted in its fully cured state and not in the state of the application to the human body (ASTM standard) [26].

Consequently, the emphasis was put on the development of alternative augmentation materials—for example, calcium-phosphate cement, calcium-sulfate cement, or silicone. Calcium-based cements are osteoconductive and osteoinductive [27] but have drawbacks such as long curing time or early resorption [28]. The use of silicones in the medical field has constantly increased since the 1960s, and nowadays, they are a thoroughly tested and important biomaterial with well-documented biocompatible and biodurable properties [29, 30].

With the development of a medical grade, injectable, self-curing elastomeric polymer with silicone basis, a new alternative material is available for vertebral augmentation. The silicone is intended to be osteoconductive and non-hazardous to the surrounding tissue, showing a non-exothermic curing [31]. Although silicones have been used and tested in the medical field for some decades, the augmentation of implants with silicones has not been investigated yet and represents the application of a well-known material in a new field [29].

The purpose of the present study was to compare the fixation strength of in situ PMMA-augmented fenestrated pedicle screws with that of standard pedicle screws inserted in a balloon-created cavity filled with an injectable silicone-based polymer. We hypothesized that the number of cranio-caudal load cycles until screw loosening

does not differ between in situ PMMA-augmented screws and balloon cavity-augmented silicone screws.

Methods

Ten lumbar vertebrae (L1–L5) from human donors were used for biomechanical testing. The bodies were donated by people who had given their informed consent for their use for scientific and educational purposes prior to death [32–34]. The specimens were double shrink-wrapped and frozen at – 20 °C. Prior to testing, a quantitative computed tomography (LightSpeed VCT 64; GE Healthcare, Waukesha, WI) was performed to rule out bony pathologies and to determine the bone mineral density via a European Forearm Phantom calibration. Specimens had an average age of 77.7 ± 8.7 years and an average BMD of 92.1 ± 33.6 mg/cm^3. Specimens were thawed overnight at 6 °C, prepared, and implanted at room temperature. Monoaxial pedicle screws of identical size and thread geometry were used for the left to right comparison (S^4, BBraun, Milan, Italy). For in situ PMMA augmentation, the screws were cannulated and fenestrated, while for balloon cavity augmentation, the screws were only cannulated (Fig. 1a. b).

Left pedicle screws were augmented with medical silicone (VK100, BONWRx, Lansing, MI, USA) using the kyphoplasty technique (inflatable balloon 15 mm, Tsunami SRL, Medolla, Italy) to create a cavity which was filled with 3 ml of silicone prior to screw placement. After this, a cannulated pedicle screw was inserted into the cured silicone.

Into the right pedicles, cannulated and fenestrated pedicle screws were implanted and in situ augmented with 2 ml of PMMA cement (Osteofix, Tsunami SRL, Medolla, Italy).

Isolated single vertebral bodies were embedded in PMMA (Technovit 3040, Heraeus Kulzer GmbH, Wehrheim, Germany) for fixation purpose in the testing machine, and an axial X-ray was taken to document the cement distribution.

Cyclic loading in cranio-caudal direction was conducted in a servohydraulic biaxial material testing machine (858 Mini Bionix II, MTS, Eden Prairie, MN, USA). Specimens were fixed on an x-y plane-bearing table, and a straight rod (Ø 5.5 mm) was connected to the pedicle screw. Axial loading was conducted with a lever arm of 15 mm to the pedicle screw head [35]. A 3D motion analysis system (Zebris, Winbiomechanics, Isny, Germany) was mounted to the pedicle screw and to the base plate to measure the relative motion of the pedicle screw head to the fixed vertebra (Fig. 2).

Each pedicle screw was initially cycled with 50 N in tension and 50 N in compression (speed 5 mm/s), with an increase of compressive load by 5 N every 100th cycle for a total of 11,000 cycles (600 N compressive loading). The cyclic protocol was terminated after 10 mm axial displacement of the machine crosshead.

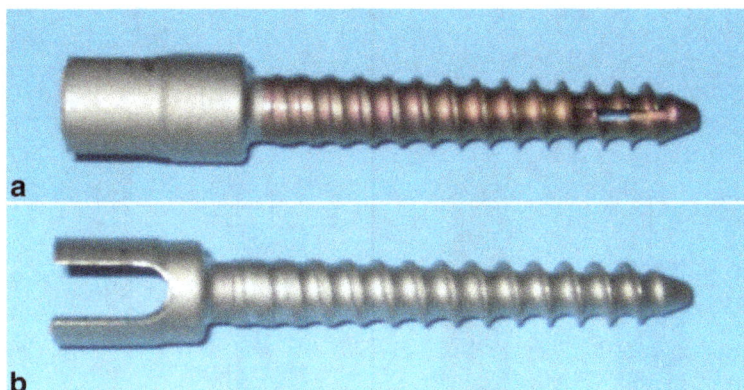

Fig. 1 Screw types used. **a** 5.5 × 35 mm cannulated and fenestrated monoaxial screw. **b** 5.5 × 35 mm monoaxial cannulated screw

For post-test data analysis, the motion of the screw head relative to the vertebra was evaluated. Screw loosening was defined as an absolute angular tilt of more than 8° or an increase in angular motion of more than 1° within one load step (100 cycles).

After cyclic loading, each pedicle screw was subjected to a pullout test in the direction of the screw axis. Pullout testing was conducted in a material testing machine (858 Mini Bionix II, MTS, Eden Prairie, MN, USA) with a speed of 10 mm/min. During all testing, the displacement and force at the actuator were recorded with 100 Hz.

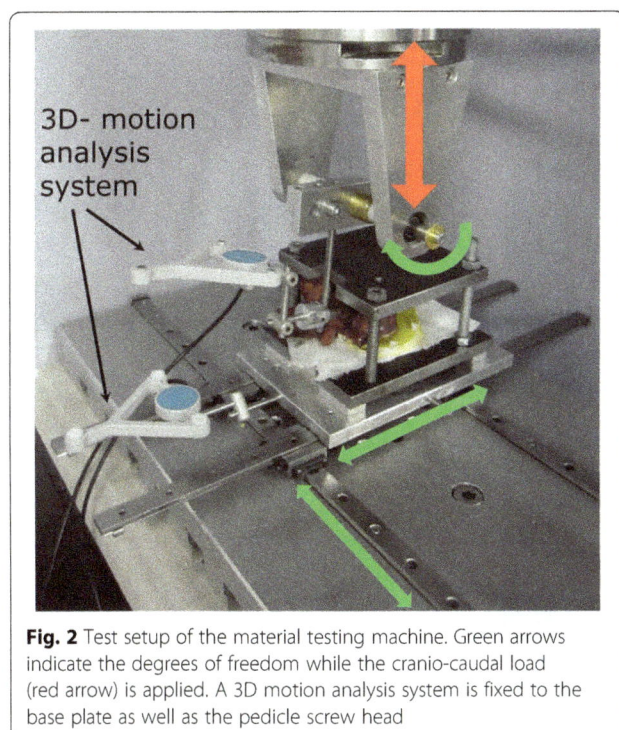

Fig. 2 Test setup of the material testing machine. Green arrows indicate the degrees of freedom while the cranio-caudal load (red arrow) is applied. A 3D motion analysis system is fixed to the base plate as well as the pedicle screw head

Statistical analysis

Statistical analysis was carried out using SPSS software package (version 21.0, SPSS, Chicago, IL, USA). Data are given as mean ± SD. Paired t tests were applied for comparisons between the two augmentation techniques (screws inserted into the left pedicles (silicone) vs. screws inserted into the right pedicles (PMMA)). Level of significance was set to a value of $P < 0.05$.

Results

One in situ augmented pedicle screw placed in an L1 vertebra breached the pedicle after implantation. Therefore, this vertebra was excluded from the data analysis resulting in a total of nine vertebrae with left-right comparisons of the two augmentation techniques.

Cyclic loading

All in situ PMMA-augmented screws loosened by caudal screw cutout through the pedicle. In the balloon cavity silicone-augmented group, only two screws loosened by caudal screw cutout through the pedicle. Two screws showed a loosening of the screw inside the intact pedicle, and five screws did not reach the predefined failure criteria.

The mean number of load cycles until loosening was 7401 ± 1645 for the in situ PMMA-augmented screws and 9824 ± 1982 for the balloon cavity silicone-augmented screws ($P = 0.012$). With the stepwise increasing load magnitude, these cycle numbers correspond to a mean load level of 420 ± 82 N for in situ PMMA-augmented screws and 542 ± 99 N for balloon cavity silicone-augmented screws (Fig. 3).

In seven out of nine vertebrae, the screws augmented with silicone outperformed the screws augmented with PMMA in terms of load cycles and load magnitude until loosening.

Pullout test

The mean maximum pullout force after loosening was 1189 ± 288 N for in situ PMMA-augmented screws and

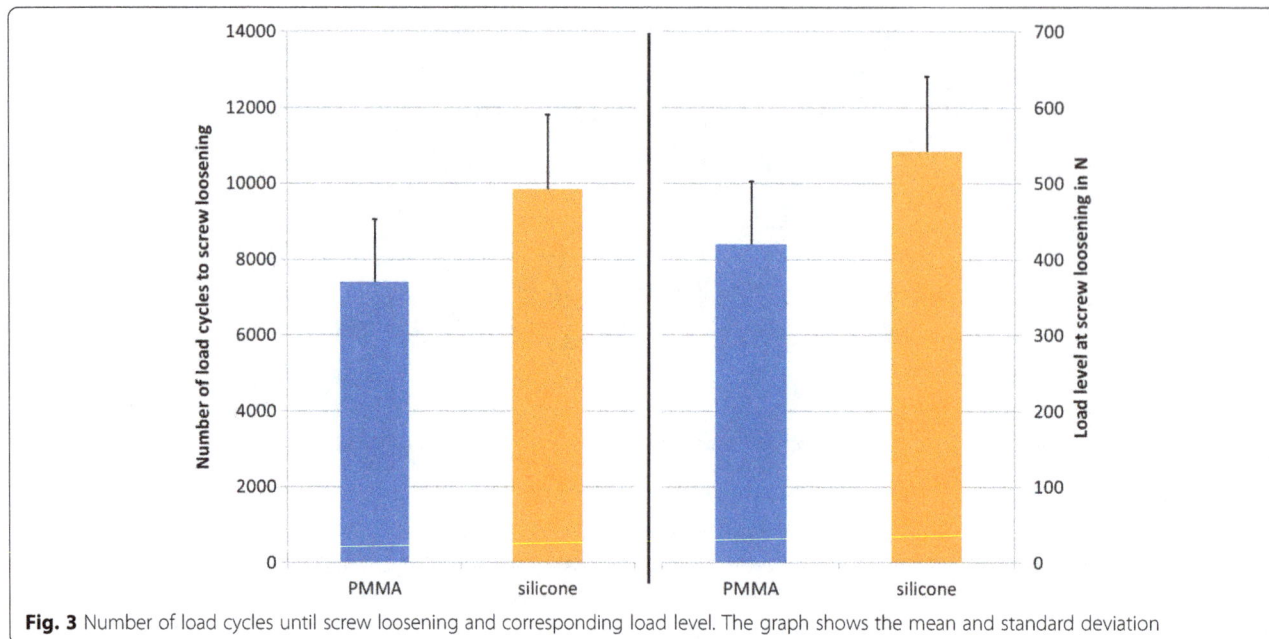

Fig. 3 Number of load cycles until screw loosening and corresponding load level. The graph shows the mean and standard deviation

671 ± 332 N for balloon cavity silicone-augmented screws (P = 0.003) (Fig. 4). The mean displacement at which maximal pullout force was recorded was 12.3 ± 2.2 mm for PMMA-augmented screws and 5.9 ± 4.6 mm for silicone-augmented screws (P = 0.002).

For balloon cavity silicone-augmented screws, the main failure mode (seven of nine) during the pullout test was axial pullout of the screw with the silicone cloud still bonded to the trabecular structure while only two specimens failed by pedicle fracture. For in situ

PMMA-augmented screws, the main failure mode (eight of nine) during pullout testing was pedicle fracture with the PMMA cement cloud still attached to the screw while only one specimen failed by axial screw pullout.

Discussion

Several biomechanical studies have shown that, compared to standard non-augmented pedicle screws, augmentation of the screw with PMMA cement can significantly improve screw anchorage in patients with

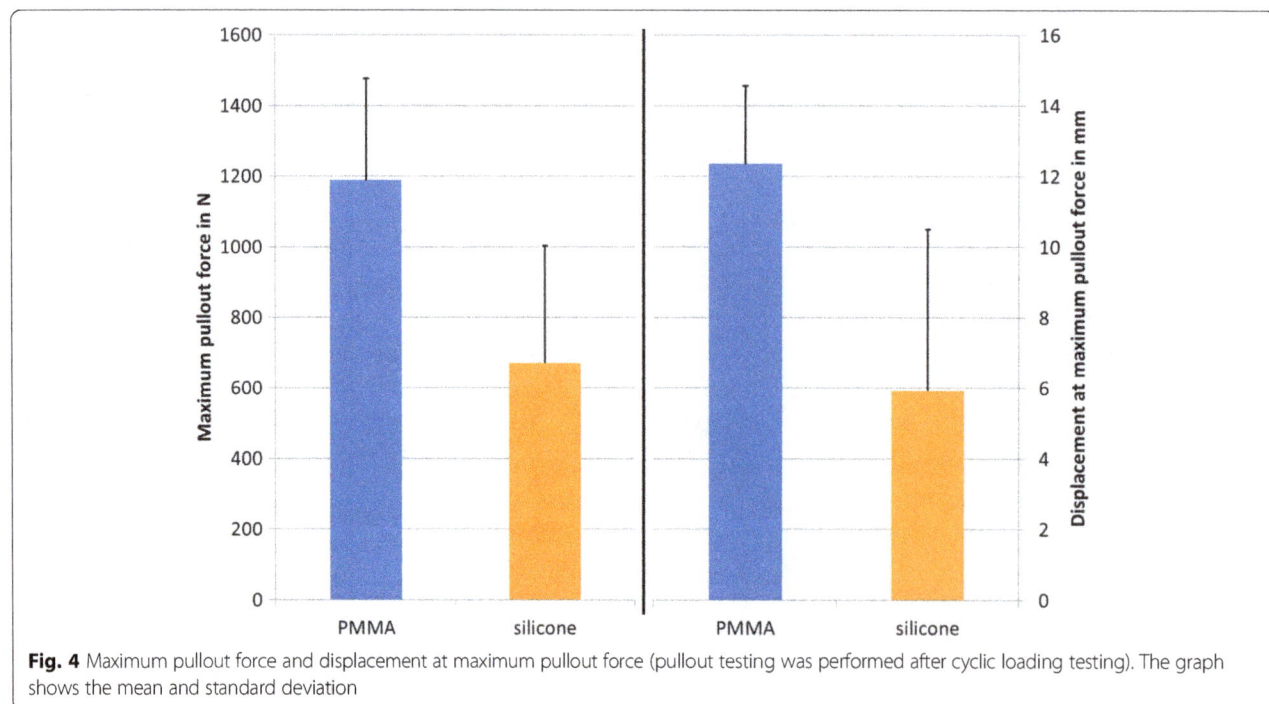

Fig. 4 Maximum pullout force and displacement at maximum pullout force (pullout testing was performed after cyclic loading testing). The graph shows the mean and standard deviation

reduced bone quality, independent of the augmentation technique [5, 35, 36]. Therefore, the hypothesis of the present study was that the novel silicone augmentation with prior balloon cavity creation will be non-inferior to in situ augmentation using PMMA cement, which is currently regarded as the gold standard for the improvement of pedicle screw anchorage in several countries [37–39]. Under physiological cyclic loading in cranio-caudal direction, the novel silicone augmentation sustained a significantly higher number of load cycles and load magnitude until loosening than standard PMMA augmentation. In the pullout test after the cyclic loading, the predominant failure mode of in situ PMMA-augmented screws was a fracture of the pedicle with the cement still attached to the screw. In contrast to this, balloon cavity silicone-augmented screws predominantly failed by the pullout of the screw through the pedicle with the augmentation material still attached to the trabecular bone.

The test setup and loading protocol used in the present study consisted of a cyclic cranio-caudal loading with a superimposed bending moment and thus resembles the physiological loading of pedicle screws reported in "in vivo" measurements of patients with an instrumented internal fixator [40–42] much more closely than a pullout test. The cyclic load protocol with a stepwise increasing load magnitude was designed to investigate implant anchorage in reduced bone quality and enables the investigation of implant anchorage for a wide stiffness range in reduced bone quality under cyclic loading [35, 43, 44].

For "in vivo" measurements with an instrumented internal fixator, Rohlmann et al. showed that pedicle screws are mainly loaded axially in cranio-caudal direction and can be superimposed with a small bending moment. In daily activities of the patients, the peak axial forces were reported to range from 100 to 250 N [41, 42]. Using a setup and load protocol similar to that of the present study, Bostelmann et al. reported pedicle screw loosening loads for three different PMMA augmentation techniques ranging from 415 to 453 N, while the non-augmented control only reached 239 N [35]. Hence, they noted that in patients with reduced bone quality, pedicle screws might be loaded during daily activity beyond their loosening threshold. However, with screw augmentation, the load-bearing capacity of pedicle screws can be increased well beyond the load magnitudes occurring during daily activities. The findings of the present study for the in situ PMMA augmentation (420 N) are comparable to the loosening load magnitude reported by Bostelmann et al. for different PMMA augmentation techniques [35], while the balloon cavity silicone augmentation even outperformed the in situ PMMA augmentation.

The post-cycling pullout force of silicone-augmented screws was lower than that of PMMA-augmented screws but was still of higher magnitude than the values reported by Liu et al. for non-augmented and non-cycled screws in osteoporotic (528 N) and severely osteoporotic (358 N) vertebrae [45]. The post-cycling pullout force of PMMA augmented, however, was comparable to the ones reported by Liu et al. for PMMA augmentation (2 ml) without prior cyclic loading [45]. This indicates that the high pullout forces after PMMA augmentation can be attributed to the extensive structural damage caused by pulling the screw with the PMMA still attached through the pedicle, no matter whether the screw is loose or not.

A limitation of this study is that two different augmentation techniques and two different augmentation materials were used. Therefore, it is not possible to decisively attribute the better performance of the balloon cavity silicone augmentation to the material or the technique. Most likely, it is a combination of both. Another limitation is that the study was conducted on cadaver specimens and therefore cannot take account of any biological factors such as bone remodeling and osteointegration, as well as PMMA aging and volumetric shrinkage.

In a comparative study on PMMA screw augmentation techniques, Becker et al. reported no difference in screw anchorage between the augmentation techniques, vertebroplasty, kyphoplasty, and in situ augmentation technique [5]. The present experiment compared two different strategies to enhance pedicle screw anchorage. These two strategies encompassed two different augmentation materials and two different augmentation techniques. Both materials were applied with the technique that best highlights its mechanical properties. The stiffness of PMMA is higher than that of the bone, and during in situ augmentation, the material interdigitates with the trabecular structure and thereby reinforces and interlocks with the trabecular structure [46]. In contrast to that, the stiffness of the self-curing elastomer (VK100) was engineered to resemble the bulk stiffness of trabecular bone and not the stiffness of a single trabecula. Therefore, a cavity was created and filled with silicone in order to benefit from its material properties.

Conclusion

Pedicle screw augmentation with balloon cavity creation and self-curing elastomeric silicone represents a valuable alternative to PMMA augmentation and resulted in superior pedicle screw anchorage under cyclic cranio-caudal loading. Pullout forces after cyclic loading were higher for in situ PMMA-augmented screws and showed a different failure mode. Using an alternative silicone-based augmentation material, however, might also necessitate a modification of the conventional in situ augmentation technique.

Acknowledgements

The authors wish to thank the individuals who donated their bodies and tissues for the advancement of education and research. Laboratory costs of the study were supported by BBraun, Italy, by institutional grants.

Funding

There is no funding source. The laboratory costs were supported by an institutional grant by BBraun, Italy, to the first authors' institution.

Authors' contributions

WS reviewed the literature; contributed to the conception and design, acquisition of data, analysis and interpretation of data, drafting of the manuscript, and statistical analysis; and obtained funding. AK reviewed the literature and contributed to the conception and design, acquisition of data, analysis and interpretation of data, drafting of the manuscript, and critical revision of the manuscript. MK contributed to the conception and design and critical revision of the manuscript. RL reviewed the literature and contributed to the conception and design, acquisition of data, analysis and interpretation of data, drafting of the manuscript, and critical revision of the manuscript. AG contributed to the drafting and critical revision of the manuscript. All authors read and approved the final manuscript.

Competing interests

Werner Schmoelz has received an institutional research grant of BBraun, Italy, for laboratory costs. All other authors declare that they have no conflict of interests.

Author details

[1]Department of Trauma Surgery, Medical University of Innsbruck, Anichstraße 35, 6020 Innsbruck, Austria. [2]Department of Anatomy, Histology and Embryology, Medical University of Innsbruck, Innsbruck, Austria. [3]Instituto Orthopedic Rizzoli, Bologna, Italy.

References

1. Keiler A, Schmoelz W, Erhart S, Gnanalingham K. Primary stiffness of a modified transforaminal lumbar interbody fusion cage with integrated screw fixation: cadaveric biomechanical study. Spine. 2014;39:E994–E1000. https://doi.org/10.1097/BRS.0000000000000422.
2. Burval DJ, McLain RF, Milks R, Inceoglu S. Primary pedicle screw augmentation in osteoporotic lumbar vertebrae: biomechanical analysis of pedicle fixation strength. Spine. 2007;32:1077–83. https://doi.org/10.1097/01.brs.0000261566.38422.40.
3. Bullmann V, Schmoelz W, Richter M, Grathwohl C, Schulte TL. Revision of cannulated and perforated cement-augmented pedicle screws: a biomechanical study in human cadavers. Spine. 2010;35:E932–9. https://doi.org/10.1097/BRS.0b013e3181c6ec60.
4. Choma TJ, Frevert WF, Carson WL, Waters NP, Pfeiffer FM. Biomechanical analysis of pedicle screws in osteoporotic bone with bioactive cement augmentation using simulated in vivo multicomponent loading. Spine. 2011;36:454–62. https://doi.org/10.1097/BRS.0b013e3181d449ec.
5. Becker S, Chavanne A, Spitaler R, Kropik K, Aigner N, Ogon M, Redl H. Assessment of different screw augmentation techniques and screw designs in osteoporotic spines. European Spine Journal. 2008;17:1462–9. https://doi.org/10.1007/s00586-008-0769-8.
6. Pfeifer BA, Krag MH, Johnson C. Repair of failed transpedicle screw fixation. A biomechanical study comparing polymethylmethacrylate, milled bone, and matchstick bone reconstruction. Spine. 1994;19:350–3.
7. Sarzier JS, Evans AJ, Cahill DW. Increased pedicle screw pullout strength with vertebroplasty augmentation in osteoporotic spines. J Neurosurg. 2002;96:309–12.
8. Kueny RA, Kolb JP, Lehmann W, Püschel K, Morlock MM, Huber G. Influence of the screw augmentation technique and a diameter increase on pedicle screw fixation in the osteoporotic spine: pullout versus fatigue testing. Eur Spine J. 2014;23:2196–202. https://doi.org/10.1007/s00586-014-3476-7.
9. McKoy BE, An YH. An injectable cementing screw for fixation in osteoporotic bone. J Biomed Mater Res. 2000;53:216–20.
10. Paré PE, Chappuis JL, Rampersaud R, Agarwala AO, Perra JH, Erkan S, Wu C. Biomechanical evaluation of a novel fenestrated pedicle screw augmented with bone cement in osteoporotic spines. Spine. 2011;36:E1210–4. https://doi.org/10.1097/BRS.0b013e318205e3af.
11. Belkoff SM, Molloy S. Temperature measurement during polymerization of polymethylmethacrylate cement used for vertebroplasty. Spine. 2003;28:1555–9.
12. Jefferiss CD, Lee AJ, Ling RS. Thermal aspects of self-curing polymethylmethacrylate. The Journal of Bone and Joint Surgery British. 1975;57:511–8.
13. Stańczyk M, van Rietbergen B. Thermal analysis of bone cement polymerisation at the cement-bone interface. J Biomech. 2004;37:1803–10. https://doi.org/10.1016/j.jbiomech.2004.03.002.
14. Freeman MA, Bradley GW, Revell PA. Observations upon the interface between bone and polymethylmethacrylate cement. The Journal of Bone and Joint Surgery British. 1982;64:489–93.
15. Fukuda C, Goto K, Imamura M, Neo M, Nakamura T. Bone bonding ability and handling properties of a titania-polymethylmethacrylate (PMMA) composite bioactive bone cement modified with a unique PMMA powder. Acta Biomater. 2011;7:3595–600. https://doi.org/10.1016/j.actbio.2011.06.006.
16. Shinzato S, Nakamura T, Kokubo T, Kitamura Y. PMMA-based bioactive cement: effect of glass bead filler content and histological change with time. J Biomed Mater Res. 2002;59:225–32.
17. Breusch SJ, Kühn K-D. Bone cements based on polymethylmethacrylate. Der Orthopade. 2003;32:41–50. https://doi.org/10.1007/s00132-002-0411-0.
18. Ciapetti G, Granchi D, Cenni E, Savarino L, Cavedagna D, Pizzoferrato A. Cytotoxic effect of bone cements in HL-60 cells: distinction between apoptosis and necrosis. J Biomed Mater Res. 2000;52:338–45.
19. Goodman SB, Huie P, Song Y, Lee K, Doshi A, Rushdieh B, Woolson S, Maloney W, Schurman D, Sibley R. Loosening and osteolysis of cemented joint arthroplasties. A biologic spectrum. Clin Orthop Relat Res. 1997;337:149–63.
20. Granchi D, Stea S, Ciapetti G, Savarino L, Cavedagna D, Pizzoferrato A. In vitro effects of bone cements on the cell cycle of osteoblast-like cells. Biomaterials. 1995;16:1187–92.
21. Kalteis T, Lüring C, Gugler G, Zysk S, Caro W, Handel M, Grifka J. Acute tissue toxicity of PMMA bone cements. Z Orthop Ihre Grenzgeb. 142:666–72. https://doi.org/10.1055/s-2004-832317.
22. Leggat PA, Smith DR, Kedjarune U. Surgical applications of methyl methacrylate: a review of toxicity. Arch Environ Occup Health. 2009;64:207–12. https://doi.org/10.1080/19338240903241291.
23. Ayre WN, Denyer SP, Evans SL. Ageing and moisture uptake in polymethyl methacrylate (PMMA) bone cements. J Mech Behav Biomed Mater. 2014;32:76–88. https://doi.org/10.1016/j.jmbbm.2013.12.010.
24. Hughes KF, Ries MD, Pruitt LA. Structural degradation of acrylic bone cements due to in vivo and simulated aging. J Biomed Mater Res A. 2003;65:126–35. https://doi.org/10.1002/jbm.a.10373.
25. Kinzl M, Boger A, Zysset PK, Pahr DH. The mechanical behavior of PMMA/bone specimens extracted from augmented vertebrae: a numerical study of interface properties, PMMA shrinkage and trabecular bone damage. J Biomech. 2012;45:1478–84. https://doi.org/10.1016/j.jbiomech.2012.02.012.
26. ASTM. ASfTM standard specifications for acrylic bone cement, ASTM standard F451-99a. In: Annual book of ASTM standards. West Conshohocken: ASTM; 2007.
27. Larsson S, Bauer TW. Use of injectable calcium phosphate cement for fracture fixation: a review. Clin Orthop Relat Res. 2002;395:23–32.
28. Elder BD, Lo SF, Holmes C, Goodwin CR, Kosztowski TA, Lina IA, Locke JE, Witham TF. The biomechanics of pedicle screw augmentation with cement. Spine J. 2015;15:1432–45. https://doi.org/10.1016/j.spinee.2015.03.016.

29. Colas A, Curtis J (2004) Silicone biomaterials: history and chemistry.

30. Thomas X. Silicones in medical applications. In: Gleria RDJM, editor. Inorganic Polymers. New York: Nova Science Publishers (www. novapublishers.com); 2007.

31. Song W, Seta J, Eichler MK, Arts JJ, Boszczyk BM, Markel DC, Gasbarrini A, Ren W. Comparison of in vitro biocompatibility of silicone and polymethyl methacrylate during the curing phase of polymerization. J Biomed Mater Res B Appl Biomater. 2018. https://doi.org/10.1002/jbm.b.34086.

32. McHanwell S, Brenner E, Chirculescu ARM, Drukker J, van Mameren H, Mazzotti G, Pais D, Paulsen F, Plaisant O, Caillaud MM, Laforet E, Riederer BM, Sanudo JR, Bueno-Lopez JL, Donate-Oliver F, Sprumont P, Teofilovski-Parapid G, BJ M. The legal and ethical framework governing Body Donation in Europe - a review of current practice and recommendations for good practice. Eur J Anat. 2008;12:1–24.

33. Riederer BM, Bolt S, Brenner E, Bueno-Lopez JL, Circulescu ARM, Davies DC, DeCaro R, Gerrits PO, McHanwell S, Pais D, Paulsen F, Sendemir E, Stabile I, BJ M. The legal and ethical framework governing Body Donation in Europe – 1st update on current practice. Eur J Anat. 2012;16:1–21.

34. Konschake M, Brenner E. "Mors auxilium vitae"--causes of death of body donors in an Austrian anatomical department. Ann Anat. 2014;196:387–93. https://doi.org/10.1016/j.aanat.2014.07.002.

35. Bostelmann R, Keiler A, Steiger HJ, Scholz A, Cornelius JF, Schmoelz W. Effect of augmentation techniques on the failure of pedicle screws under cranio-caudal cyclic loading. European Spine Journal. 2015. https://doi.org/10.1007/s00586-015-3904-3.

36. Renner SM, Lim T-H, Kim W-J, Katolik L, An HS, Andersson GBJ. Augmentation of pedicle screw fixation strength using an injectable calcium phosphate cement as a function of injection timing and method. Spine. 2004;29:E212–6.

37. Gonschorek O, Hauck S, Weiss T, Buhren V. Fractures of the thoracic and lumbar spine. Chirurg. 2015;86:901–14; quiz 915-906. https://doi.org/10.1007/s00104-015-0045-5.

38. Pesenti S, Blondel B, Peltier E, Adetchessi T, Dufour H, Fuentes S. Percutaneous cement-augmented screws fixation in the fractures of the aging spine: is it the solution? Biomed Res Int. 2014;2014:610675. https://doi.org/10.1155/2014/610675.

39. Krappinger D, Kastenberger TJ, Schmid R. Augmented posterior instrumentation for the treatment of osteoporotic vertebral body fractures. Oper Orthop Traumatol. 2012;24:4–12. https://doi.org/10.1007/s00064-011-0098-7.

40. Rohlmann A, Bergmann G, Graichen F. Loads on an internal spinal fixation device during walking. J Biomech. 1997;30:41–7.

41. Rohlmann A, Graichen F, Bergmann G. Influence of load carrying on loads in internal spinal fixators. J Biomech. 2000;33:1099–104.

42. Rohlmann A, Bergmann G, Graichen F. Loads on internal spinal fixators measured in different body positions. European Spine Journal. 1999;8:354–9.

43. Unger S, Erhart S, Kralinger F, Blauth M, Schmoelz W. The effect of in situ augmentation on implant anchorage in proximal humeral head fractures. Injury. 2012;43:1759–63. https://doi.org/10.1016/j.injury.2012.07.003.

44. Windolf M, Maza ER, Gueorguiev B, Braunstein V, Schwieger K. Treatment of distal humeral fractures using conventional implants. Biomechanical evaluation of a new implant configuration. BMC Musculoskelet Disord. 2010; 11:172. https://doi.org/10.1186/1471-2474-11-172.

45. Liu D, Zhang B, Xie QY, Kang X, Zhou JJ, Wang CR, Lei W, Zheng W. Biomechanical comparison of pedicle screw augmented with different volumes of polymethylmethacrylate in osteoporotic and severely osteoporotic cadaveric lumbar vertebrae: an experimental study. Spine J. 2016;16:1124–32. https://doi.org/10.1016/j.spinee.2016.04.015.

46. Windolf M. Biomechanics of implant augmentation. Unfallchirurg. 2015;118: 765–71. https://doi.org/10.1007/s00113-015-0050-7.

Minimally invasive treatment for anterior pelvic ring injuries with modified pedicle screw-rod fixation: a retrospective study

Chun-Chi Hung[1], Jia-Lin Wu[2,3], Yuan-Ta Li[1], Yung-Wen Cheng[1], Chia-Chun Wu[1], Hsain-Chung Shen[1] and Tsu-Te Yeh[1*]

Abstract

Background: Pelvic ring injuries constitute only 2 to 8% of all fractures; however, they occur in 20% of polytrauma patients. High-energy pelvic fractures often result in mechanical instability of the pelvic ring. Successful treatment of unstable pelvic ring fractures remains a challenge for orthopedic surgeons. This study presents a novel internal fixation method for stabilizing unstable anterior pelvic ring fractures using a minimally invasive modified pedicle screw-rod fixation (MPSRF) technique.

Methods: This retrospective study included six patients with unstable pelvic ring injuries who underwent MPSRF, with or without posterior fixation. Intraoperative parameters such as blood loss, operative time, complications, and quality of reduction (Matta criteria) were recorded and evaluated by a blinded reviewer.

Results: In the present clinical series, the mean operative times and mean blood loss for unilateral versus bilateral anterior ring fixations were 176.0 min versus 295.6 min, and 153.3 mL versus 550.0 mL, respectively. No iatrogenic neuropraxia of the lateral femoral cutaneous nerve or femoral nerve palsy occurred. The reduction quality, graded by the Matta criteria, was excellent in five patients and good in one patient.

Conclusions: There were no infections, delayed unions, nonunions, or loss of reductions during the follow-up period. Only one patient suffered from a broken rod at 4 months postoperatively. The modified technique represents a novel, minimally invasive procedure for the treatment of anterior pelvic ring fractures and offers a reliable and effective alternative to currently available surgical techniques.

Keywords: Pelvic ring, Minimally invasive treatment, Modified pedicle screw-rod fixation (MPSRF)

Background

Pelvic ring injuries constitute only 2 to 8% of all fractures but occur in 20% of polytrauma patients [1]. High-energy pelvic fractures often result in mechanical instability of the pelvic ring. Pelvic fixation has traditionally been divided into posterior and anterior fixation, and although pelvic stability is mainly sustained by the posterior ring, the anterior ring provides 30% of pelvic stability [2]. Thus,

to acquire better reduction of unstable pelvic fractures, a combination of anterior and posterior fixation is needed.

Stabilization of anterior pelvic ring fractures can be achieved via multiple techniques, including external fixation [3], open reduction and internal fixation with plating, or percutaneous trans ramus screw fixation [4]. External fixation is helpful for initial hemodynamic stabilization, and it involves lower operating time and blood loss than does open surgery. However, there are limitations to this treatment, including pin tract infections, aseptic loosening, hindrance to surgical abdominal access, and difficulties in nursing care [5, 6]. Open reduction has the potential disadvantage of an extensive exposure,

* Correspondence: tsutey@gmail.com
[1]Department of Orthopedic Surgery, Tri-Service General Hospital and National Defense Medical Center, 325 Cheng-Kung Road, Section 2, Taipei 114, Taiwan
Full list of author information is available at the end of the article

which includes muscle stripping, and the risk of damage to neurovascular structures [7].

With the aim of improving patient comfort and minimizing the complications associated with traditional treatment techniques, minimally invasive techniques have been widely used for anterior pelvic ring fixation. The potential benefits include minimal soft tissue dissection, diminished surgical site infections, and faster patient rehabilitation with better pain control. These procedures comprise subcutaneous implants fixed into the ilium with or without fixation into the parasymphyseal region (reported as the pelvic bridge) [8], the occipitocervical spinal plate-rod technique [9], and an anterior subcutaneous pedicle screw-rod internal fixator (INFIX) [10–12]. However, iatrogenic lateral femoral cutaneous nerve (LFCN) palsy is a common complication of these procedures and is reported in 30 to 48.3% of patients [13, 14]. The placement of pedicle screws in the supra-acetabular region, as in external fixation, and of INFIX, requires incisions directly over the anterior inferior iliac spine (AIIS) with pedicle screws placed in a high-risk zone for LFCN [15].

Inspired by the pelvic bridge with the plate-rod fixator and INFIX techniques, we designed a new method in which a submuscular pedicle screw-rod device was placed through small incisions over the iliac wing and the pubic region. We modified the pedicle screw position from the AIIS to being over the inner table of the iliac bone and the ipsilateral or contralateral superior pubic ramus, which was dependent on the fracture pattern, fixed with connecting rods. We aimed to evaluate the clinical application of this minimally invasive modified pedicle screw-rod fixation (MPSRF) technique for the treatment of anterior pelvic ring fractures.

Methods

This retrospective clinical series included patients who presented to the Tri-Service General Hospital, a level 1 trauma center in Taiwan, between October 2014 and October 2016. Six patients with unstable pelvic ring injuries underwent anterior fixation using the MPSRF technique, with or without posterior fixation. If posterior ring instability was present, it was first operated on using standard techniques of reduction and fixation methods, such as percutaneous iliosacral screws, percutaneous transiliac plates, or spinal pelvic fixations. The exclusion criteria were (1) hemodynamically unstable patients, (2) infections or soft tissue defects, (3) patients < 16 years old, and (4) insufficiency fractures in elderly patients. Included patients were two men and four women with an average age of 37.6 (range, 28–44) years, four cases of type B (two of type B2 and two of type B3) and two cases of type C (two of type C2) fractures using the Marvin Tile classification [3]. Among

them, fracture mechanisms included traffic accidents ($n = 1$), falls from heights ($n = 4$), and crush injuries ($n = 1$). Preoperatively, all patients received a detailed neurological examination and a complete radiological evaluation, including anteroposterior (AP), pelvic inlet, and outlet views, and computed tomography (CT) scans of the pelvis to evaluate the displaced pelvic ring comprehensively. The surgery was scheduled as soon as the patients' physiological condition was stable, with an average duration of 6.8 (range, 1–14) days from injury to surgery (Table 1).

Surgical technique

All surgical operations were performed by one surgeon with the patients under general anesthesia. Patients were positioned on a radio-transparent operation table in the supine position. The skin was prepared and draped from above the umbilicus to the lower extremities to facilitate the reduction technique. The lateral window of the ilioinguinal approach started at 1 cm proximal to the anterior superior iliac spine (ASIS) and the posterior window extended along the iliac crest with approximately 4- to 5-cm-long curves (Fig. 1a). The origins of the abdominal and iliacus muscles at the iliac crest were sharply elevated within a limited area. The iliacus muscle from the inner table of the iliac wing was elevated using a blunt dissection, which continued medially to the superior pubic ramus. Flexing the hip was also helpful for relaxing the iliopsoas muscle when small sub-muscular tunnels were being created. Once the two appropriate entry points, 3 to 4 cm apart, were identified, the cortex was opened using a 2.5-mm drill bit at approximately 4 cm medial to ASIS for establishing the bony corridors. Two 4.0-mm-diameter Axon Spine System (Depuy Synthes, Switzerland) polyaxial pedicle screws were inserted in the same direction (Fig. 1b). The length of the screws varied from 12 to 20 mm, depending on the habitus of the patient. The procedure was repeated for the contralateral hemipelvis if bilateral anterior pelvic fractures were present.

Another transverse Pfannenstiel incision began at one fingerbreadth proximal to the pubic symphysis and was extended laterally for approximately 4 to 5 cm (Fig. 1a). Sharp dissection was performed on the anterior rectus fascia, and the subcutaneous fatty layer was elevated away from the rectus fascia. The rectus abdominis muscle was split along the linea alba, and the transversalis fascia was opened just proximal to the pubic symphysis to allow access to the retropubic space of Retzius. The bladder was mobilized bluntly from the anterior pelvic ring. The insertion of the rectus abdominis muscle was left intact on the anterior aspect of the pubic rami but was released on the superior border of the pubic rami and symphysis. A sub-muscular plane was created using a blunt dissection along the cranial surface of the

Table 1 Patient characteristics

Patient	Age (years)	Sex	Tile type	Surgical procedures (anterior + posterior fixation)	Implant site of anterior ring	Time from injury to surgery (days)	Operation time (min)	Blood loss (mL)	Injury mechanism	Matta criteria	Complications
1	39	F	B2	MPSRF + PIS + SPF	U	14	151	200	Fall	Excellent	
2	44	F	B3	MPSRF + SPF	B	8	312	600	Fall	Good	
3	28	F	B2	MPSRF + PTP	U	8	194	100	Fall	Excellent	
4	37	F	C2	MPSRF + PTP + SPF	B	8	292	350	Fall	Excellent	
5	36	M	C2	MPSRF + PIS + SPF	U	2	183	160	Crush	Excellent	Rod breakage
6	42	M	B3	MPSRF	B	1	283	700	Traffic	Excellent	

Patient data as abbreviated terms, *F* female, *M* male, *MPSRF* modified pedicle screw-rod fixation, *PIS* percutaneous iliosacral screw, *PTP* percutaneous transiliac plate, *SPF* spinal pelvic fixation, *U* unilateral, *B* bilateral

superior ramus to the iliac wing where the sub-muscular tunnel from both incisions connected. The placement of the pedicle screws on the ipsilateral or contralateral pubic ramus was determined by the fracture pattern. If pubic symphysis diastasis occurred or the residual fragment of the ipsilateral pubic ramus was not large enough for the placement of the two pedicle screws, screw anchoring to the contralateral pubic ramus was necessary. After the two starting points on the superior plane of the superior ramus were confirmed radiographically, the cortex was opened with a 2.5-mm drill bit to establish the bony corridor towards the inferior ramus. Next, two 3.5-mm-diameter polyaxial pedicle screws were inserted (Fig. 1b), and safe placement of screw positions was confirmed using the pelvic inlet view. The screw length varied from 20 to 40 mm.

Once both side screws were in place and an acceptable reduction had been achieved, a rod template was placed on the pedicle screws through the submuscular tunnel to estimate its length and curvature. Next, the contoured rod (3.5 mm diameter) was gently inserted in the submuscular tunnel from the incision at the pubic ramus to the iliac wing below the iliacus and psoas muscles. The rod was connected to pedicle screw heads, whose caps

were loosely secured to maintain the rod in place. At this point, reduction tools were used to manipulate the fracture site into an appropriate reduction, and the screw caps were locked with a torque screwdriver to maintain the reduction. Radiographs of typical cases are provided to illustrate the preoperative and postoperative changes (Figs. 2 and 3). Suitable reduction and implant position were confirmed on the C-arm fluoroscopic AP, inlet, and outlet views. Prophylactic intravenous antibiotics were administered until 24 h postsurgery to prevent infections.

Postoperative management and follow-up

Non-weight-bearing functional exercises of the lower limbs and joints were initiated on the postoperative day 1. Patients were allowed to sit on the bedside at 1 week, and crutch-assisted partial weight bearing was allowed from 6 weeks, postoperatively. They were allowed to walk with full weight-bearing at 8 weeks, postoperatively.

Routine follow-ups for clinical and radiological assessment were scheduled for postoperative weeks 4 and 8; months 3, 6, and 9; and at 1 year. Radiographic images at each follow-up visit included a three-view pelvis series (AP, inlet, and outlet). At all visits, thorough neurological

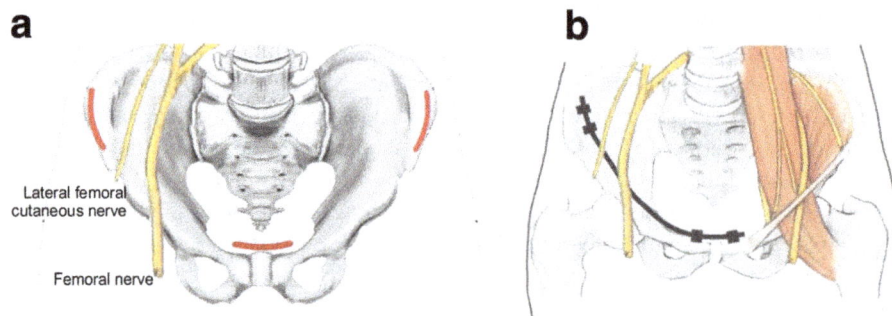

Fig. 1 a Incisions for minimally invasive modified pedicle screw-rod fixation (MPSRF). This includes a curved incision over 1 cm proximal to the anterior inferior iliac spine (AIIS) and a transverse incision one fingerbreadth superior to the pubic symphysis. Lateral femoral cutaneous nerve coursing medially and inferiorly to the iliac incision. Red line: skin incisions, yellow line: lateral femoral cutaneous nerve (LFCN) and femoral nerve. **b** The final construct of MPSRF with the pedicle screws placed over the iliac wing and superior pubic ramus. Rod was placed submuscularly under the major neurovascular bundles. There are at least a few centimeters between the screw and LFCN, to prevent compression through this region

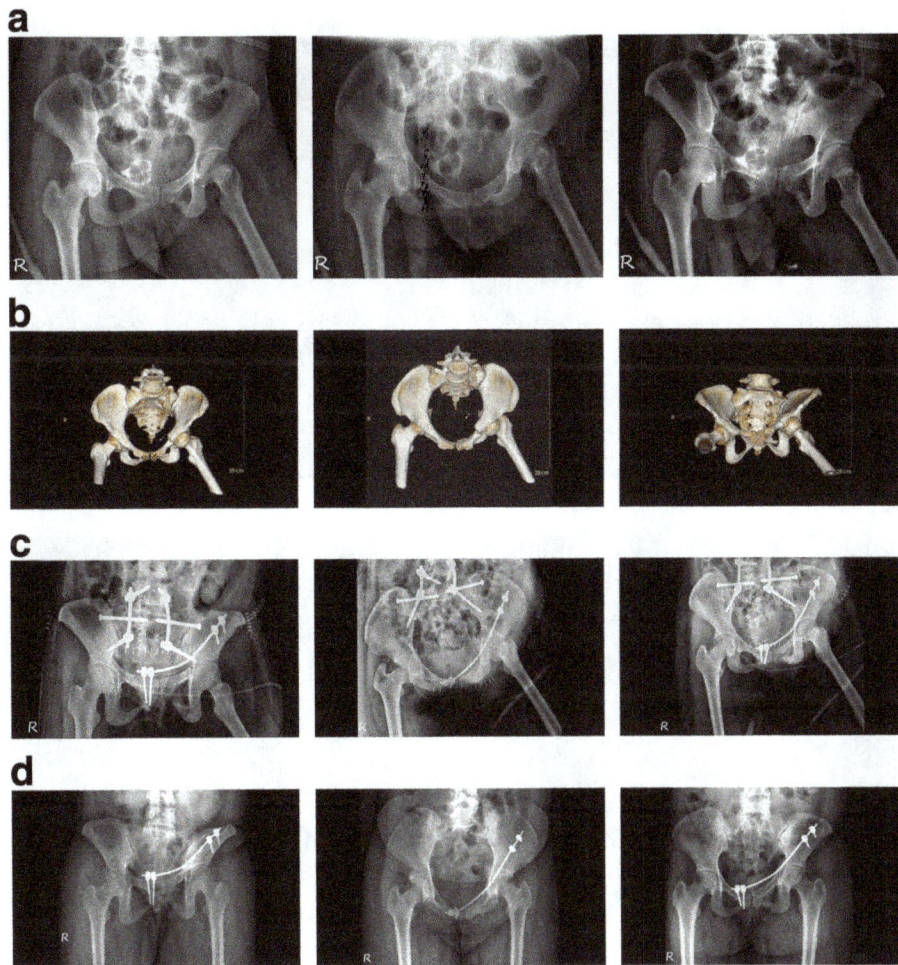

Fig. 2 A 39-year-old woman with anterior and posterior pelvic ring injuries caused by a fall. **a** Preoperative pelvic radiology series (AP, inlet, outlet view) demonstrating left superior and inferior pubic ramus fractures combined with a sacral fracture. **b** Preoperative 3D reconstructed CT images (AP, inlet, outlet view). **c** Postoperative pelvic radiology series (AP, inlet, outlet view) demonstrating percutaneous iliosacral screws, spinal pelvic fixation, and the modified pedicle screw-rod fixation. **d** Postoperative pelvic radiology series (AP, inlet, outlet view) at 22 months follow-up, demonstrating bone union

examinations focused on LFCN and the femoral nerves, physical examinations focused on pelvic stability, and local irritation of the implants was performed.

Outcome measures

Outcome measures were total operation time, blood loss, complications, reduction achieved from surgery, and fracture healing time. Radiographs were assessed by a specialist surgeon with experience in pelvic surgery, who was blinded to all identifiable patient information. The results of fracture reduction were graded based on published criteria [16] as excellent (0–5 mm), good (5–10 mm), fair (10–20 mm), and poor (> 20 mm), according to the maximal residual displacement of the fracture site in the three-view pelvis series. Fracture healing was determined by the progression of callus formation until radiographic union and by the ability of the patient to

bear weight without pain. Failure of fixation was assessed by implant breakage, uncoupling of the instruments, or by loosening at the screw-bone interface.

Specific complications for our technique included injuries of LFCN, the femoral artery, femoral vein, femoral nerve, and the round ligament in women or the spermatic cord in men. Moreover, other general complications included infections, erosion of the soft tissue overlying the implant, loss of fracture reduction, implant failure, nonunion, and heterotopic ossification.

Results

In our series, one patient underwent anterior fixation using MPSRF alone and five patients underwent both anterior and posterior fixations. These five patients included two patients with percutaneous iliosacral screws and spinal pelvic fixations, one patient with a percutaneous

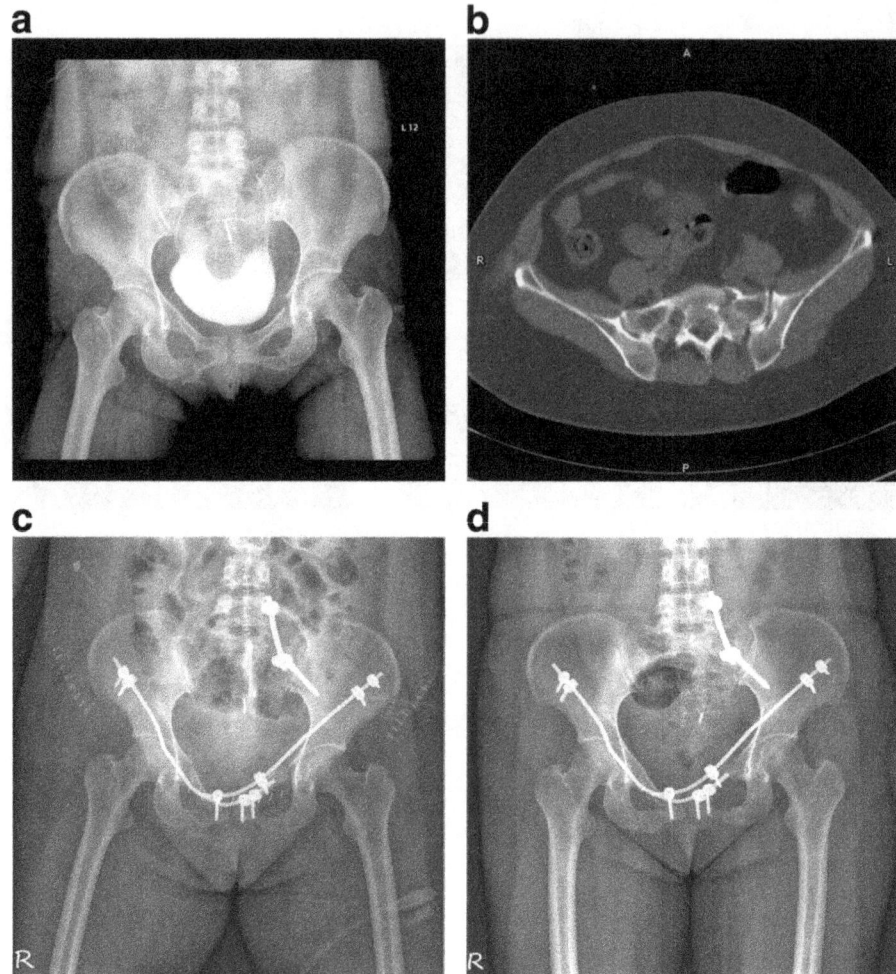

Fig. 3 A 44-year-old woman with anterior and posterior pelvic ring injuries caused by a fall. **a** Preoperative radiology plain images showing bilateral pubic rami fracture. **b** Preoperative axial computed tomography scan image showing a left side sacral fracture. **c** Postoperative radiology plain images showing good reduction with the modified pedicle screw-rod fixation technique for the anterior ring and spinal pelvic fixation for the sacral fracture. **d** Radiology plain image showing fracture healing at 8 months postoperatively

transiliac plate and spinal pelvic fixation, one patient with a percutaneous transiliac plate, and one patient with spinal pelvic fixation. Three patients underwent unilateral anterior ring fixation, and the other three patients underwent bilateral fixation. The average operative time and mean intraoperative blood loss for unilateral anterior ring fixation were 176.0 (range, 151–194) min and 153.3 (range, 100–200) mL, and 295.6 (range, 282–312) min and 550.0 (range, 350–700) mL for bilateral anterior ring fixation. The mean time of injury-to-surgery was 1 day in the patient who underwent anterior pelvic ring fixation alone and 8 (range, 2–14) days in patients who underwent both anterior and posterior fixation (Table 1).

No iatrogenic neuropraxia of LFCN or femoral nerve palsy occurred after the surgeries. No intraabdominal hollow organ injury or urinary bladder injury was observed in relation to screw insertion. In addition, no

patient experienced postoperative complications such as hemorrhagic shock, deep venous thrombosis, or wound infections.

All patients were followed up for an average of 26.7 (range, 14–40) months, and no one died or was lost to follow-up. During the follow-up period, healing was achieved in all pelvic fractures at a mean postoperative period of 4 (range, 3–6) months. Fracture reduction was excellent in five patients and good in one patient, postoperatively (Table 1). No loss of reduction, delayed osseous union, nonunion, malunion, loss of fixation, loosening of implant, or heterotopic ossification was observed in physical and radiographic examinations during the follow-up period. One patient suffered from a broken connecting rod at 4 months postsurgery, but complete fracture healing without discomfort was noted.

All the patients could sit normally, stand, squat, and lie in the prone position or on either side and were reintegrated into society without any restrictions. The implant was removed in one patient, 8 months postoperatively, at the patient's request. Five patients preferred to retain the device and have reported no problems to date.

Discussion

Successful management of unstable pelvic fractures remains challenging for orthopedic surgeons, and the optimal fixation technique remains controversial. To combine the advantages of the pedicle screw-rod system and the pelvic bridge techniques for treating unstable anterior pelvic ring fractures, we designed a new form of minimally invasive pelvic fixation using pedicle screw-rod fixators, which were applied submuscularly from the iliac wing to the superior pubic ramus. This method can be used for patients with residual instability in the anterior ring after the posterior pelvis has either been fixed or verified to be stable by stressing the pelvis intraoperatively under fluoroscopy.

The concept of minimally invasive plate osteosynthesis in pelvic fractures has recently been introduced. Yu et al. introduced a minimally invasive plate osteosynthesis technique for pubic ramus fracture treatment [17]. Owing to the lack of direct visualization, some anatomic structures, including LFCN, the femoral artery, femoral vein, femoral nerve, and the round ligament in women or the spermatic cord in men, are theoretically at risk of injury during implant placement. LFCN irritation is the most prevalent iatrogenic neurovascular complication during surgical treatment of anterior ring fractures. Temporary LFCN neuropraxia was observed by Vaidya et al. [18] in up to 30% of the 91 patients included in their study. A previous study verified that placement of implants over AIIS could be complicated with LFCN injury and hip joint capsule violation [19]. Furthermore, INFIX pedicle screw placement requires deep dissection in the space between the sartorius and the tensor fasciae latae muscles where LFCN is vulnerable. Hence, we changed the pedicle screw positions of the ilium from the AIIS, a high-risk zone for LFCN, to the inner table of the iliac wing medial to the ASIS level, which is further away from LFCN (Fig. 1b). Theoretically, the selected locations of the pedicle screws were relatively safe areas for surgical dissection, implant application, and removal. However, with a 2.9 to 4% incidence of unusual superolateral course, the nerve may be endangered during dissection over the anterior aspect of the iliac wing when the attachment of the pelvic bridge construct is contemplated [8, 15]. To avoid potential impingement on LFCN, medial and lateral fixation of the implant

should be performed under direct visualization and after careful dissection [20].

In previous bridge techniques, the subcutaneous corridor was created directly from the iliac crest to the pubic tubercle with a high risk of neurovascular injury and abdominal perforation. The connecting rods of the pedicle screws in the MPSRF technique were fixed through the submuscular tunnel, below the vital neurovascular bundles, as mentioned above. Alternatively, Hoskins et al. [21] attributed traction-induced neuropraxia to the large size of lumbar pedicle screws but the implants used in the MPSRF technique are small cervical pedicle screws. Unlike other studies, there were no cases of postoperative temporary LFCN neuropraxia in our series; this might be explained by the changes in screw positions, the application method of the connecting rod, the smaller diameter of screws, and our meticulous approach during dissection because of our awareness of this complication based on previous studies.

A cadaveric study found that the femoral nerve is at the greatest risk of compression by the rod [22]. In the MPSRF technique, the connecting rod was placed under the muscular and neurovascular structure; therefore, the compression force of the femoral nerve could be minimized, thus decreasing the risk of femoral nerve injury. In our series, no femoral nerve palsy was noted during the follow-up period. Theoretically, the MPSRF technique is relatively protective of nerves compared to other subcutaneous techniques for anterior pelvic ring injuries. One of the limitations of our study was the small sample size and the limited follow-up duration, which might explain the absence of neurovascular complications. Future studies with larger sample sizes and longer follow-up periods may reveal the actual incidences of the complications related to the MPSRF technique.

In the INFIX technique, large-diameter lumbar spinal pedicle screws, ranging from 6.5 to 7.5 mm, were used for fixation [23]. In the MPSRF technique, we used small-diameter pedicle screws, ranging from 3.5 to 4.0 mm, which are used in cervical spinal surgery. While Owen et al. [24] reported fixation failure with small-diameter screws salvaged by larger screws in morbidly obese patients, we increased the number of screws in the MPSRF technique for fixation of the anterior pelvic ring. Two to three pedicle screws were used in the INFIX technique, while four screws were used in MPSRF. The thinner screw head of smaller pedicle screws not only prevented soft tissue irritation, it also preserved more space for adjacent screw placement. Although Vigdorchik et al. pointed out that anterior neutralization plate fixation is stiffer than INFIX for fracture stability at the pubic symphysis [25], the lack of a biomechanical study that compared fixation stability between MPSRF and plate osteosynthesis limited our study. Based on our results, we believe that smaller-diameter and more pedicle screws could provide suitable and acceptable fixation stability in anterior pelvic ring fractures without loss of reduction, osseous nonunion, or loosening of screws during the follow-up period, although biomechanical testing is required for verification.

The type of pedicle screw determines the performance of fixation stability, with monoaxial screws providing significantly greater stiffness than polyaxial screws [26]. However, the polyaxial screws used in the MPSRF technique reduced the difficulty of rod manipulation. The use of a monoaxial screw by an inexperienced surgeon may be challenging because the accurate placement of screws is mandatory for precise positioning of the connecting rod. Conversely, polyaxial screws allow inaccuracies in their placement. Further biomechanical studies on the MPSRF fixation device are necessary to verify our results.

Previous studies have shown that subcutaneous devices are typically palpable in the lower abdominal fold, and surgeons recommend implant removal at a mean postoperative period of 1.5 to 9.4 months once the patient's injuries have healed and their symptoms have plateaued [27]. However, the submuscular device in the MPSRF technique was not palpable and did not require removal in the absence of complications.

This study has some noteworthy limitations. First, the small sample size and lack of long-term follow-up warrant future multicenter prospective studies for final evaluation. Second, our analysis was based on clinical cases in the prediction of the stability of the fixation technique, and a biomechanical study is necessary for more convincing conclusions. Third, this study does not report functional outcomes, and a long-term functional score analysis is necessary. Fourth, the MPSRF technique used US Food and Drug Administration-approved implants for cervical spinal fixation for an unapproved method in the pelvis. It is thus an off-label use.

Conclusions

The operative time of the MPSRF technique was relatively longer than that in previous subcutaneous techniques, which might be explained by the deeper approach of dissection, the more complex implants used, and bilateral anterior pelvic ring fractures. The blood loss in our series was not as low as that in other subcutaneous techniques, which might be due to the open direct reduction methods we employed and the longer surgical time of the MPSRF technique.

The MPSRF technique afforded satisfactory clinical and radiological outcomes with fewer complications in the present study. We believe that the modified technique represents a novel minimally invasive procedure for the treatment of anterior pelvic ring instability and offers a reliable and effective alternative to current surgical techniques.

Abbreviations

AIIS: Anterior inferior iliac spine; ASIS: Anterior superior iliac spine; CT: Computed tomography; LFCN: Lateral femoral cutaneous nerve; MPSRF: Minimally invasive modified pedicle screw-rod fixation

Authors' contributions

TTY contributed to the investigation, methodology, data curation, and preparation of the original draft. CCH contributed to the formal analysis, data curation, and preparation of the original draft. JLW contributed to the data curation and preparation of the original draft. YWC prepared the original draft. CCW did the validation of data. HCS contributed to the visualization of data. YTL contributed to the project administration. TTY edited and reviewed the manuscript. All authors read and approved the final manuscript.

Competing interests

The authors declare that they have no competing interests.

Author details

[1]Department of Orthopedic Surgery, Tri-Service General Hospital and National Defense Medical Center, 325 Cheng-Kung Road, Section 2, Taipei 114, Taiwan. [2]Department of Orthopedics, School of Medicine, College of Medicine, Taipei Medical University, Taipei, Taiwan. [3]Department of Orthopedics, Taipei Medical University Hospital, Taipei, Taiwan.

References

1. Giannoudis PV, Pape HC. Damage control orthopaedics in unstable pelvic ring injuries. Injury. 2004;35:671–7.
2. Bi C, Wang Q, Nagelli C, Wu J, Wang Q, Wang J. Treatment of unstable posterior pelvic ring fracture with pedicle screw-rod fixator versus locking compression plate: a comparative study. Med Sci Monit. 2016;22:3764–70.
3. Tile M. Pelvic ring fractures: should they be fixed? J Bone Joint Surg. (Br). 1988;70- B:1–12.
4. Starr AJ, Nakatani T, Reinert CM, Cederberg K. Superior pubic ramus fractures fixed with percutaneous screws: what predicts fixation failure? J Orthop Trauma. 2008;22:81–7.
5. Tucker MC, Nork SE, Simonian PT, Routt ML Jr. Simple anterior pelvic external fixation. J Trauma. 2000;49(6):989–94.
6. Vaidya R, Colen R, Vigdorchik J, Tonnos F, Sethi A. Treatment of unstable pelvic ring injuries with an internal anterior fixator and posterior fixation: initial clinical series. J Orthop Trauma. 2012;26:1–8.
7. Mason WT, Khan SN, James CL, Chesser TJ, Ward AJ. Complications of temporary and definitive external fixation of pelvic ring injuries. Injury. 2005; 36:599–604.
8. Cole PA, Gauger EM, Anavian J, Ly TV, Morgan RA, Heddings AA. Anterior pelvic external fixator versus subcutaneous internal fixator in the treatment of anterior ring pelvic fractures. J Orthop Trauma. 2012;26:269–7.
9. Hiesterman TG, Hill BW, Cole PA. Surgical technique: a percutaneous method of subcutaneous fixation for the anterior pelvic ring: the pelvic bridge. Clin Orthop Relat Res. 2012;470:2116–23.

10. Gardner MJ, Mehta S, Mirza A, Ricci WM. Anterior pelvic reduction and fixation using a subcutaneous internal fixator. J Orthop Trauma. 2012;26: 314–21.

11. Scheyerer MJ, Zimmermann SM, Osterhoff G, Tiziani S, Simmen HP, Wanner GA, et al. Anterior subcutaneous internal fixation for treatment of unstable pelvic fractures. BMC Res Notes. 2014;7:133.

12. Wu X, Liu Z, Fu W, Zhao S, Feng J. Modified pedicle screw-rod fixation as a minimally invasive treatment for anterior pelvic ring injury: an initial case series. J Orthop Surg Res. 2017;12:84.

13. Cole PA, Dyskin EA, Gilbertson JA. Minimally-invasive fixation for anterior pelvic ring disruptions. Injury. 2015;46:S27–34.

14. Fang C, Alabdulrahman H, Pape HC. Complications after percutaneous internal fixator for anterior pelvic ring injuries. Int Orthop. 2017;41:1785–90.

15. Doklamyai P, Agthong S, Chentanez V, Huanmanop T, Amarase C, Surunchupakorn P, et al. Anatomy of the lateral femoral cutaneous nerve related to inguinal ligament, adjacent bony landmarks, and femoral artery. Clin Anat. 2008;21:769–74.

16. Matta JM. Indications for anterior fixation of pelvic fractures. Clin Orthop Relat Res. 1996;329:88–96.

17. Yu X, Tang M, Zhou Z, Peng X, Wu T, Sun Y. Minimally invasive treatment for pubic ramus fractures combined with a sacroiliac joint complex injury. Int Orthop. 2013;37:1547–54.

18. Vaidya R, Kubiak EN, Bergin PF, Dombroski DG, Critchlow RJ, Sethi A, et al. Complications of anterior subcutaneous internal fixation for unstable pelvis fractures: a multicenter study. Clin Orthop Relat Res. 2012b;470:2124–31.

19. Haidukewych GJ, Kumar S, Prpa B. Placement of half-pins for supra-acetabular external fixation: an anatomic study. Clin Orthop Relat Res. 2003; 411:269–73.

20. Moazzam C, Heddings A, Moodie P, Cole PA. Anterior pelvic subcutaneous internal fixator application: an anatomic study. J Orthop Trauma. 2012;26:263–8.

21. Hoskins W, Bucknill A, Wong J, Britton E, Judson R, Gumm K, et al. A prospective case series for a minimally invasive internal fixation device for anterior pelvic ring fractures. J Orthop Surg Res. 2016;11:135.

22. Apivatthakakul T, Rujiwattanapong N. Anterior subcutaneous pelvic internal fixator (INFIX), Is it safe? A cadaveric study. Injury. 2016;47:2077–80.

23. Kuttner M, Klaiber A, Lorenz T, Füchtmeier B, Neugebauer R. The pelvic subcutaneous cross-over internal fixator. Unfallchirurg. 2009;112:661–9.

24. Owen MT, Tinkler B, Stewart R. Failure and salvage of "INFIX" instrumentation for pelvic ring disruption in a morbidly obese patient. J Orthop Trauma. 2013;27:e243–6.

25. Vigdorchik JM, Esquivel AO, Jin X, Yang KH, Onwudiwe NA, Vaidya R. Biomechanical stability of a supra-acetabular pedicle screw internal fixation device (INFIX) vs external fixation and plates for vertically unstable pelvic fractures. J Orthop Surg Res. 2012;7:31.

26. Eagan M, Kim H, Manson TT, Gary JL, Russell JP, Hsieh AH. Internal anterior fixators for pelvic ring injuries: do monaxial pedicle screws provide more stiffness than polyaxial pedicle screws? Injury. 2015;46:996–1000.

27. Shetty AP, Bosco A, Perumal R, Dheenadhayalan J, Rajasekaran S. Midterm radiologic and functional outcomes of minimally-invasive fixation of unstable pelvic fractures using anterior internal fixator (INFIX) and percutaneous iliosacral screws. J Clin Orthop Trauma. 2017;8:241–8.

28

Pigmented villonodular synovitis does not influence the outcome following cementless total hip arthroplasty using ceramic-on-ceramic articulation: a case-control study with middle-term follow-up

Chi Xu[1], Heng Guo[1,2], Kerri L. Bell[3], Feng-Chih Kuo[4*] and Ji-Ying Chen[1*]

Abstract

Background: Pigmented villonodular synovitis (PVNS) is a relatively rare, locally aggressive, and potentially recurrent synovial disease of large joints. The purpose of this study was to investigate (1) the disease recurrence rate and (2) the treatment outcomes including Harris hip scores, complications, and revision following cementless total hip arthroplasty (THA) with ceramic-on-ceramic (CoC) articulation in patients with PVNS.

Methods: Twenty-two patients (14 females and 8 males) with histologically confirmed PVNS underwent cementless THA using CoC bearings between 2000 and 2013. Three patients with less than 5-year follow-up were excluded. The mean age was 35.2 years (range, 22–58 years) with a mean follow-up of 8.6 years (range, 6.9–10.8 years). A control group was matched in a 2:1 ratio with the PVNS group for age, sex, body mass index (BMI), year of surgery, and American Society of Anesthesiologists score (ASA). Postoperative outcome variables included disease recurrence, Harris Hip Scores (HHS) at the latest follow-up, complications (dislocation, squeaking, ceramic fracture), and any-cause revision. A Kaplan-Meier implant survivorship curve with 95% confidence interval (CI) of the two groups was generated.

Results: No recurrence of PVNS was noted in the follow-up period. The HSS in the PVNS group was 92.6 ± 5.5, which was similar to the control group (93.4 ± 4.6, $p = 0.584$) at the last follow-up visit. No patients sustained dislocation, osteolysis, or any ceramic fracture within the study duration. One patient in the PVNS group had a complication of squeaking, but did not require revision. Another patient in the PVNS group underwent revision surgery due to aseptic loosening. There was no significant difference in revision rates between the two groups ($p = 1.000$). The implant survivorship free of any revision was 90.0% (95% CI, 73.2% to 100%) in the PVNS group and 92.5% (95% CI, 82.6% to 100%) in the control group at 10 years ($p = 0.99$).

Conclusions: For young and active patients with end-stage PVNS of the hips, cementless THA using CoC bearing has similar functional outcome scores, a low complication rate, and similar implant survivorship compared to the control group.

Keywords: Synovitis, pigmented villonodular, Total hip arthroplasty, Ceramic-on-ceramic, Cementless

---

* Correspondence: fongchikuo@cgmh.org.tw; jiying_chen301@163.com
[4]Department of Orthopaedic Surgery, Kaohsiung Chang Gung Memorial Hospital, and Chang Gung University, College of Medicine, No. 123, Dapi Rd., Niaosong Dist, Kaohsiung 833, Taiwan
[1]Department of Orthopaedic Surgery, General Hospital of People's Liberation Army, No.28 Fuxing Road, Haidian District, Beijing 100853, China
Full list of author information is available at the end of the article

Background

Pigmented villonodular synovitis (PVNS) of the hip is a benign, but potentially locally aggressive and recurrent monoarticular disorder which typically affects large joints; 80% of the time it involves the knee, while hips are affected only 15% of the time [1]. It is an uncommon disorder, with an estimated incidence of 1.8 per million patients [2–4]. It is characterized by a proliferation of synovial villi and nodules within joint spaces, bursa, or tendon sheaths [5]. As synovial hyperplasia pervades the hip, it causes discomfort by narrowing the joint space, leading to sharp hip pain [3]. A radical synovectomy, whether via arthroscopy or an open surgical approach, has been utilized as a treatment for hips with mild cartilage degeneration. However, in cases demonstrating severe end-stage arthritis due to disease progression, total hip arthroplasty (THA) plus radical synovectomy is the preferred treatment choice [6].

PVNS of the hip commonly affects patients in their third or fourth decade of life [7]. A recent study reported that complications and revision rates following THA are high in patients with PVNS due to the youth of patients and the utilization of conventional polyethylene [8]. Given the likelihood of requiring revision surgery for younger patients undergoing THA, the concern of implant survivorship, wear performance, and functionality should be considered when selecting a fixation technique and a bearing surface. As one of the most popular combinations, cementless implants with ceramic-on-ceramic (CoC) articulation have shown potential benefits in young patients, as they have low wear rates with excellent clinical outcomes [9–13]. Although several studies have suggested acceptable outcomes with a low recurrence rate following THA in PVNS patients during the long-term follow-up [1, 6, 8, 14], there is a paucity of data focusing on cementless implants using CoC articulation in these patients. Moreover, these previous studies were limited by small sample sizes and lacked a control group in their evaluation of outcomes.

Therefore, the purpose of this study was to investigate the disease recurrence rate and the treatment outcomes including Harris Hip Scores, complications, and revision rates following cementless THA with CoC articulation in patients with PVNS.

Materials and methods

Study cohort

After the Institutional Review Board approval, we retrospectively reviewed 22 patients with a diagnosis of PVNS of the hip who underwent cementless THA with CoC articulation between 2000 and 2013. The diagnosis of diffuse PVNS was made for all patients by histological confirmation in accordance with Jaffé's classification [15]. Three patients with follow-up less than 5 years were excluded. In all, 19 patients with a mean follow-up of 8.6 years (range, 6.9 to 10.8 years) were enrolled in this study (Table 1). There were 7 males and 12 females with a mean age of 35.2 (range, 22 to 58) years.

These patients were matched with a control group of patients; the controls were patients diagnosed with either osteoarthritis of the hip or femoral head necrosis who underwent cementless THA using CoC articulation. The patients in the control group were matched with the patients in the study group for age (± 5 years), sex, body mass index (BMI, ± 1 kg/m^2), year of surgery (within 1 year), and American Society of Anesthesiologists Score (ASA) (± 1) in a 2:1 ratio.

Clinical and radiographic features of patients with PVNS before THA

The mean time from onset of symptoms to arthroplasty was 2.9 years (range, 1–6.2 years). All patients presented hip pain as the primary complaint. One patient, a 28-year-old woman (case 13), was diagnosed with Crowe Type III developmental hip dysplasia. Four patients had hip trauma before THA, while another patient had undergone internal fixation with cannulated screws for a fracture of the femoral neck. Five patients had undergone arthroscopic synovectomy before THA; the mean time from the last synovectomy to THA was 2.4 years (range, 0.8–3.6 years). A limitation of hip motion (ranging between 10 and 30°) was identified in eight patients. Average flexion was 91.1° (range, 35–130°). Elevation of both C-reactive protein (CRP) and erythrocyte sedimentation rate (ESR) was identified in two patients. The serum white blood count, CRP, and ESR were normal in the other 17 patients.

Radiographs showed the typical characteristics of end-stage PVNS of the hip including cystic erosions and joint space narrowing (Fig. 1). Eight patients had the nearly complete disappearance of the joint space. Seven patients underwent preoperative magnetic resonance imaging, which showed the characteristic low signal intensity on the T2-weighted sequences and blooming artifact from the high hemosiderin on the gradient-echo sequences.

Surgical treatment

An institutional standard protocol for total hip arthroplasty was performed for all cases by experienced arthroplasty surgeons. A posterolateral approach was utilized for all patients within the study. For patients with PVNS, complete radical excision of the diseased synovium was performed and pathologic synovial tissues were submitted for histologic evaluation. Removal of the femoral head and neck provided enough space between the pelvis and the femur for a synovectomy. The tissue contained within the cystic areas of the acetabulum and

Table 1 The patients with pigmented villonodular synovitis of the hip

Case	Age	Gender	Duration of symptoms (years)	Surgery before THA	Cup	Stem	FU (years)	Complications
1	28	Male	1	N/A	Pinnacle	Corail	8.6	–
2	26	Female	1.3	N/A	Betacup	Corail	9.3	Aseptic loosening
3	39	Female	2.4	N/A	Combicup	Ribbed	7.6	–
4	35	Female	3	Arthroscopic synovectomy	Pinnacle	Corail	8.8	–
5	53	Male	2.7	N/A	Betacup	Ribbed	10.6	–
6	24	Female	2	N/A	Combicup	Ribbed	8.5	–
7	40	Male	2.3	Internal fixation	Betacup	Ribbed	10.3	Squeaking
8	48	Female	2	N/A	Pinnacle	Corail	7.4	–
9	26	Male	4	N/A	Betacup	Ribbed	7.9	–
10	30	Female	6.2	N/A	Betacup	LCU	7.7	–
11	32	Female	3.8	Arthroscopic synovectomy	Pinnacle	Corail	8.3	–
12	58	Female	2.5	N/A	Pinnacle	Corail	7.7	–
13	28	Female	3	N/A	Combicup	LCU	6.9	–
14	47	Male	1.2	N/A	Combicup	Ribbed	10.8	–
15	35	Male	4.2	N/A	Pinnacle	Corail	7.9	–
16	22	Female	1.8	Arthroscopic synovectomy	Pinnacle	Corail	9.1	–
17	29	Female	2.8	Arthroscopic synovectomy	Betacup	LCU	9.7	–
18	37	Female	4.3	N/A	Betacup	LCU	7.8	–
19	31	Male	4	Arthroscopic synovectomy	Combicup	LCU	9.5	–

THA total hip arthroplasty, *LCU* link classic uncemented, *FU* follow-up, *N/A* not applicable

the femur was carefully removed. Cementless implants using ceramic-on-ceramic bearings were inserted in all patients. Pinnacle* (DePuy, Warsaw, IN, USA) or Betacup*/Combicup* (Link, Hamburg, Germany) were used for cup components, while Corail* (DePuy, Warsaw, IN, USA) or Ribbed*/LCU* Link Classic Uncemented (Link, Hamburg, Germany) were used for stem components.

The postoperative protocol included a drainage tube and prophylactic administration of antibiotics for 24 h. The patients were allowed partial weight-bearing with a walking aid after a postoperative radiographic evaluation on the first postoperative day, and then were allowed full weight-bearing at 6–8 weeks. The duration of prophylaxis for deep vein thrombosis was for 30 days.

Clinical and radiologic evaluation

Hip function was evaluated using Harris Hip Scores (HHS) before THA and at the last follow-up of each patient [16]. Questionnaire responses regarding the need for walking aids and the ability to perform moderate and strenuous activities were also recorded. Radiographic loosening was defined in accordance with previously published studies: a loose acetabular component was defined if the cup had ≥ 2 mm migration, ≥ 5° changes in tilting, shedding of metal particles, or a continuous radiolucent line across all zones, as described by Delee

and Charnley [17, 18]; a loose femoral stem was characterized by ≥ 5 mm progressive subsidence, pedestal formation, the shedding of metal particles, or a continuous radiolucent line around the stem, as defined by Gruen et al. [19]. Periprosthetic osteolysis was determined to be present if there were periprosthetic lesions ≥ 2 mm in diameter on follow-up radiographs [20]. Local recurrence of PVNS was determined by a series of radiological changes in adjacent bone (e.g., cystic erosions without calcification or sclerosis, demineralization of surrounding bone) [21]. All radiologic evaluations were performed by two experienced orthopedic surgeons. Complications related to CoC THA included infection, dislocation, squeaking, or ceramic fracture were recorded.

Statistical analysis

Categorical variables were presented as frequencies and percentages, and continuous variables as means and standard deviations. The clinical characteristics between groups were compared with the use of the independent t test or the Mann-Whitney test for continuous variables and the chi-squared test or Fisher's exact test for categorical variables. A Kaplan-Meier implant survival curve was generated with 95% confidence intervals (CI) at 10 years. The end point was set at the any-cause revision of CoC THA (e.g., aseptic loosening, infection, osteolysis, recurrent dislocation, ceramic fracture, or

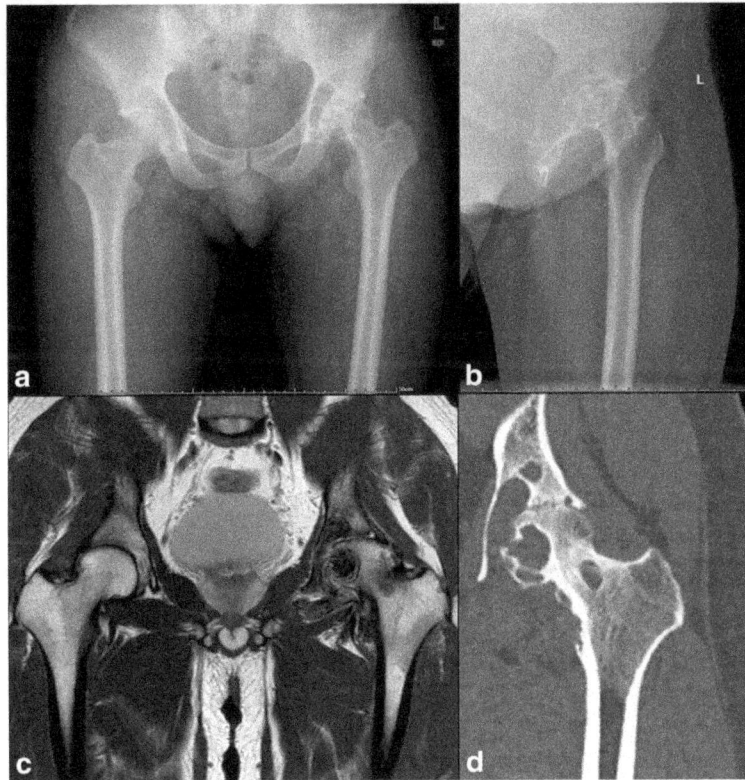

Fig. 1 The typical appearance of PVNS as seen in radiography of the hip, magnetic resonance imaging (MRI), and computed tomography (CT). Anteroposterior radiograph of case 5 (**a**) and lateral radiograph of the case 16 (**b**) show erosions and cysts in both the femoral head and the acetabulum of left hip with nearly complete obliteration of the joint space. CT (**c**) and MRI (**d**) of case 14 show the characteristic cyst-like structure of the femoral head

Table 2 Patient characteristics and follow-up between the PVNS group and the control group

	PVNS (n = 19)	Controls (n = 38)	p value
Age (year), mean ± SD	35.2 ± 10.2	35.2 ± 10.0	1.000
Gender, n (%)			1.000
Female	12 (63.2%)	24 (63.2%)	
Male	7 (36.8%)	14 (36.8%)	
Body mass index (kg/m^2), mean ± SD	24.6 ± 2.2	24.5 ± 1.9	0.975
American Society of Anesthesiologists score			1.000
1	14	28	
2	4	8	
3	1	2	
Diagnosis, n (%)			—
Osteonecrosis	0 (0%)	27 (71%)	
Osteoarthritis	0 (0%)	11 (29%)	
PVNS	19 (100%)	0 (0%)	
Follow-up (years), mean ± SD	8.7 ± 1.3	8.6 ± 1.1	0.902

PVNS pigmented villonodular synovitis, *SD* standard deviation

squeaking). A *p* value of < 0.05 was considered significant. All of the statistical analyses were performed with the statistical software packages R (http://www.R-project.org, The R Foundation) and EmpowerStats (http://www.empowerstats.com, X&Y Solution, Inc., Boston, MA).

Results

Cohort and specimen characteristics

Due to strict matching, the age, sex, BMI, and ASA scores were similar between the two groups (Table 2). Of the 38 controls, 27 were patients with osteonecrosis of the femoral head while 11 were diagnosed with osteoarthritis of the hip. The mean follow-up for the PVNS and the control group was 8.6 ± 1.1 years and 8.7 ± 1.3 years, respectively. The diagnosis of PVNS was made by pathological examination of all 19 patients. Macroscopically, the pathologic synovial tissues were brown or yellowish. Histologically, there were numerous synovial cell and multinucleated giant cells (Fig. 2). Hemosiderin-laden macrophages were found in 13 of 19 patients. We did not identify any malignant changes or atypical cytology.

PVNS and outcomes following THA

The outcomes following cementless CoC THA between groups are presented in Table 3. At the most recent follow-up, there were no clinical or radiological signs of osteolysis or loosing after CoC THA in PVNS patients, which indicated no recurrence of PVNS (Fig. 3). The results of radiologic evaluations by the two different surgeons were consistent. There was no significant difference between the PVNS group and the control group for HHS scores prior to the THA and at the most recent follow-up. In the PVNS group, the mean HHS

Table 3 The outcomes following cementless ceramic-on-ceramic total hip arthroplasty between the PVNS group and the control group

	PVNS ($n = 19$)	Controls ($n = 38$)	p value
Mean HHS, point, SD			
Preoperative	48.7 ± 3.8	48.2 ± 4.1	0.612
Latest follow-up	92.6 ± 5.5	93.4 ± 4.6	0.584
Aseptic loosening, *n* (%)	1 (5.3%)	1 (2.6%)	0.614
Infection, *n* (%)	0 (0%)	1 (2.6%)	0.480
Osteolysis, *n* (%)	0 (0%)	0 (0%)	–
Dislocation, *n* (%)	0 (0%)	0 (0%)	–
Ceramic fracture, *n* (%)	0 (0%)	0 (0%)	–
Squeaking, *n* (%)	1 (5.3%)	0 (0%)	–
Any revision, *n* (%)	1 (5.3%)	2 (5.3%)	1.000

PVNS pigmented villonodular synovitis, *HHS* Harris Hip Score, *SD* standard deviation

improved from 48.7 (range 39–62) points preoperatively to 92.6 (range 81–99) at the last follow-up, and was statistically significant ($P < 0.001$). All patients could perform moderate physical activities without crutches, and five patients could perform strenuous activities regularly, including running, sports, and climbing.

One patient (case 2) underwent revision due to aseptic loosening in the PVNS group, while another patient (case 7) developed a squeaking complication 2 years postoperatively, but did not require revision. In the control group, two patients underwent revision (one aseptic revision and one infection) ($p = 1.000$). For the patient who underwent aseptic revision in the PVNS group, no pathological evidence of recurrence of PVNS was found by histological examination. None of the patients experience osteolysis, dislocation, or ceramic fracture in either group. The implant survivorship free of any revision was

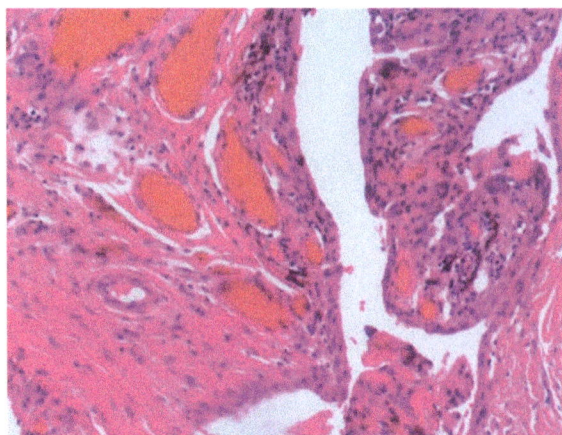

Fig. 2 A photomicrograph of case 14 showing synovial hypertrophy and histiocyte proliferation with multinucleated giant cells. (hematoxylin and eosin, original magnification × 200)

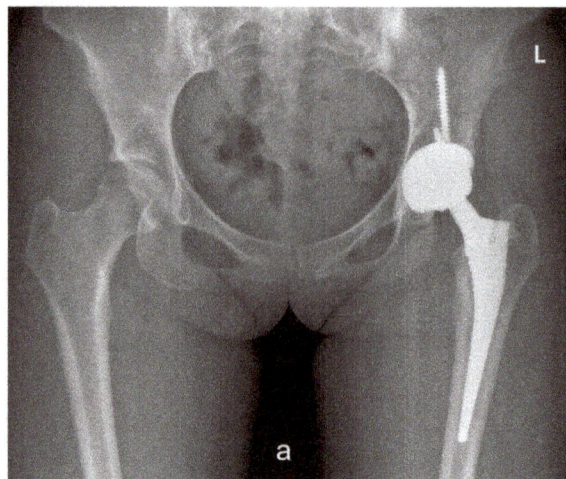

Fig. 3 A radiograph was taken 9.1 years after THA showed well-fixed prosthesis (case 16)

90.0% (95% CI, 73.2% to 100%) in the PVNS group and 92.5% (95% CI, 82.6% to 100%) in the control group at 10 years ($p = 0.99$) (Fig. 4).

Discussion

This study demonstrated that patients with PVNS undergoing cementless CoC THA had similar survivorship and functionality compared to those with the diagnosis of osteonecrosis of femoral heads or osteoarthritis of hips. None of the patients with PVNS experienced infection, osteolysis, dislocation, or ceramic fracture after a mean follow-up of 8.6 years. Moreover, there was no evidence of recurrent PVNS during the middle-term follow-up in the present study.

PVNS is a proliferative disorder characterized by infiltration of hemosiderin-laden macrophages, multinucleated giant cells, and inflammatory cells which carry a high risk of recurrence [22–24]. Due to its low incidence, PVNS is not well understood. While a consensus regarding the pathogenesis of PVNS has not yet been established, some researchers have hypothesized that trauma-induced hemorrhage could be a causative factor [25, 26]; in previously published case series, prior trauma ranged from 3 to 53% [27] In our study, 4 of

19 patients with PVNS (21.1%) had had a history of hip trauma before the diagnosis of PVNS. Although other researchers suggested patients with PVNS commonly have abnormal serum inflammation markers [28], there were only two patients with PVNS (10.5%) with elevated ESR and CRP in our study. However, our results correspond to those reported by Gitelis et al. who initially documented a lack of an inflammatory syndrome associated with PVNS [27].

Despite improved imaging, definitive preoperative diagnosis of PVNS is difficult without histopathology. At the early stage of PVNS, the treatment primarily includes either open or arthroscopic synovectomy. However, PVNS has a high recurrence rate, up to 25%, likely due to incomplete debridement without neck cutting [2]. In the present study, five patients with PVNS had undergone previous arthroscopic synovectomy; the duration between the last synovectomy and the primary THA were 0.8, 2, 2.5, 3.1, and 3.6 years (mean 2.4 years). We hypothesize that the short-term recurrence may be related to incomplete synovectomy by arthroscopy technique.

At end-stage PVNS, THA is the most effective treatment option, with lower PVNS recurrence rates and

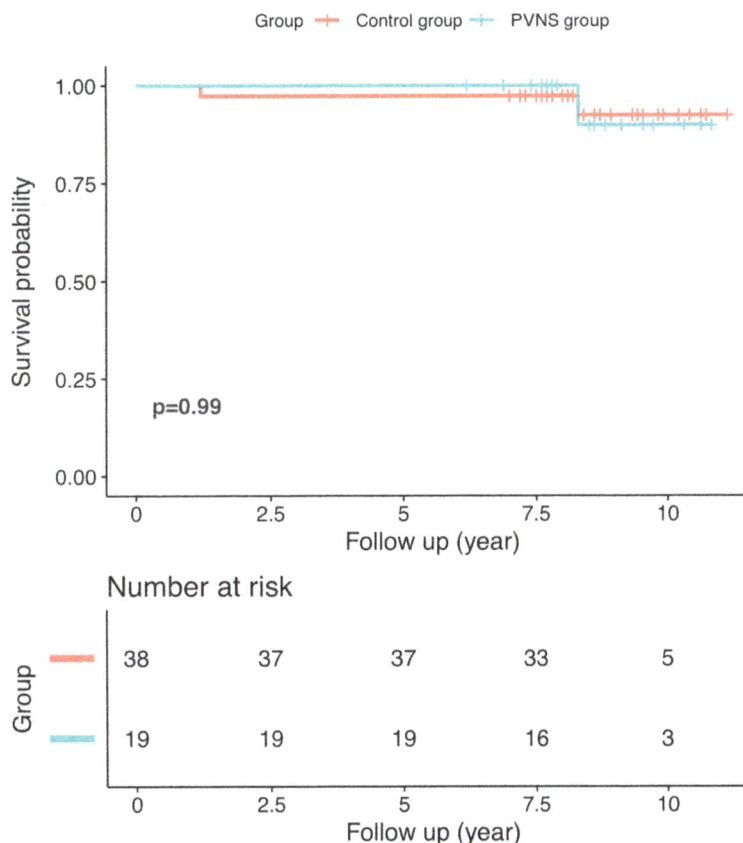

Fig. 4 A Kaplan-Meier implant survivorship curve of patients with and without PVNS

lower revision rates than synovectomy alone [8]. The lifespan of the primary THA is of significant concern, as patients with PVNS are typically younger and will therefore retain the implants for a longer duration of time. The two most important aspects of implant longevity are the method of implant fixation and the type of bearing surface [14]. While case studies of PVNS of the hip are limited, both cemented and cementless THA have been reported to result in good outcomes [14].

No recurrent PVNS was found during the follow-up in the present study, which is similar to prior studies [5, 7, 13, 14]. Yoo et al. [5] reported eight PVNS patients with cementless THA and none of the patients had clinical or radiographic evidence of recurrent PVNS for an average of 8.9 years follow-up. Recently, Tibbo et al. [7] reviewed 25 patients PVNS who underwent THA with conventional polyethylene or highly crosslinked polyethylene bearings during a mean of 10 years follow-up. Of them, only one patient (4%, 1/25) occurred recurrence at 24 years postoperatively.

Of the studies involving cementless THAs, most of the studies, however, only reported on polyethylene or metal bearing surfaces [5, 7, 14, 27]. Hoberg et al. [29] reported two cases of metal-on-metal hip resurfacing in patients with PVNS. Yoo et al. [6] described revisions due to prosthesis loosening and osteolysis in two of eight patients who had undergone THA using metal-non-cross-linked polyethylene bearing and periprosthetic osteolysis; additionally, two other patients had loosening with zirconia-non-cross-linked polyethylene. The need for revisions and the shorter implant survivorship in these cases is thought to be due to conventional polyethylene induced-wear and metal ion-induced osteolysis resulting in aseptic loosening [28, 29]. Recently, Tibbo et al. reported the 10-year survivorship free from any revision was 100% for highly crosslinked polyethylene liners and 66% for conventional polyethylene liners [8]. The Ceramic-on-ceramic bearing surface, characterized by its superior hardness and smoothness, has the lowest wear rates in comparison to all other bearing surfaces in THA [30, 31]. In our study, only one patient underwent a revision arthroplasty due to aseptic loosening. The 10-year implant survivorship free of any revision after CoC THA was 90.0% in the PVNS group, which was similar to that in the control group (92.5%, $p = 0.99$). Moreover, we did not identify any local recurrence in the PVNS cohort.

There are several limitations in our study. A major limitation was the retrospective case-control design of the study, which is subject to inherent biases of the design. Additionally, we did not sort the disease manifestations (diffuse vs. focal) based on pathological classification, although all cases were diagnosed by histological evaluations. Another limitation is that we cannot compare outcomes of different bearing surfaces, such as metal-on-metal, metal-on-polyethylene, or ceramic-on-polyethylene articulation, as PVNS patients in this study were all treated with CoC THA.

Conclusions
In conclusion, end-stage PVNS of hip treated with cementless CoC THA had a low complication rate with similar implant survivorship and restoration of function in comparison to other young patients with osteonecrosis or osteoarthritis. These findings indicate that utilization of cementless THA ceramic-on-ceramic bearings could be a viable option for young patients with PVNS.

Abbreviations
ASA: American Society of Anesthesiologists; CI: Confidence interval; CoC: Ceramic-on-ceramic; CRP: C-reactive protein; ESR: Erythrocyte sedimentation rate; HHS: Harris Hip Scores; PVNS: Pigmented villonodular synovitis; THA: Total hip arthroplasty

Acknowledgments
The authors would like to thank all staff from the participating departments and clinics.

Funding
Not applicable.

Authors' contributions
CX drafted the manuscript. CX, HG, KB, FK, and CY performed data collection and data analysis. CX, GH, FK, and CY conceived of the study, participated in the design of the study, performed data interpretation, and participated in coordination. All authors read and approved the final manuscript.

Competing interests
The authors declare that they have no competing interests.

Author details
[1]Department of Orthopaedic Surgery, General Hospital of People's Liberation Army, No.28 Fuxing Road, Haidian District, Beijing 100853, China. [2]Department of Orthopaedic Surgery, Beijing Mentougou District Hosptial, Beijing, China. [3]The Rothman Institute at Thomas Jefferson University, Philadelphia, PA, USA. [4]Department of Orthopaedic Surgery, Kaohsiung Chang Gung Memorial Hospital, and Chang Gung University, College of Medicine, No. 123, Dapi Rd., Niaosong Dist, Kaohsiung 833, Taiwan.

References

1. Hufeland M, Gesslein M, Perka C, Schröder JH. Long-term outcome of pigmented villonodular synovitis of the hip after joint preserving therapy. Arch Orthop Trauma Surg. 2018;138:471–7.

2. Levy DM, Haughom BD, Nho SJ, Gitelis S. Pigmented Villonodular synovitis of the hip: a systematic review. Am J Orthop. 2016;45:23–8.

3. Startzman A, Collins D, Carreira D. A systematic literature review of synovial chondromatosis and pigmented villonodular synovitis of the hip. Phys Sportsmed. 2016;44:425–31.

4. Lu H, Chen Q, Shen H. Pigmented villonodular synovitis of the elbow with rdial, median and ulnar nerve compression. Int J Clin Exp Pathol. 2015;8:14045–9.

5. Byrd JWT, Jones KS, Maiers GP. Two to 10 years' follow-up of arthroscopic management of pigmented villonodular synovitis in the hip: a case series. Arthroscopy. 2013;29:1783–7.

6. Yoo JJ, Kwon YS, Koo K-H, Yoon KS, Min BW, Kim HJ. Cementless Total hip arthroplasty performed in patients with pigmented villonodular synovitis. J Arthroplast. 2010;25:552–7.

7. Li LM, Jeffery J. Exceptionally aggressive pigmented villonodular synovitis of the hip unresponsive to radiotherapy. J Bone Joint Surg Br. 2011;93:995–7.

8. Tibbo ME, Wyles CC, Rose PS, Sim FH, Houdek MT, Taunton MJ. Long-term outcome of hip arthroplasty in the setting of pigmented villonodular synovitis. J Arthroplast. 2018;33:1467–71.

9. Atrey A, Wolfstadt JI, Hussain N, Khoshbin A, Ward S, Shahid M, et al. The ideal total hip replacement bearing surface in the young patient: a prospective randomized trial comparing alumina ceramic-on-ceramic with ceramic-on-conventional polyethylene: 15-year follow-up. J Arthroplast. 2018;33:1752–6.

10. Swarup I, Lee Y-Y, Chiu Y-F, Sutherland R, Shields M, Figgie MP. Implant survival and patient-reported outcomes after total hip arthroplasty in young patients. J Arthroplast. 2018;33:2893–8.

11. Costi K, Solomon LB, McGee MA, Rickman MS, Howie DW. Advantages in using cemented polished tapered stems when performing total hip arthroplasty in very young patients. J Arthroplast. 2017;32:1227–33.

12. Archibeck MJ, Surdam JW, Schultz SC, Junick DW, White RE. Cementless total hip arthroplasty in patients 50 years or younger. J Arthroplast. 2006;21:476–83.

13. Kuo F-C, Liu H-C, Chen W-S, Wang J-W. Ceramic-on-ceramic total hip arthroplasty: incidence and risk factors of bearing surface-related noises in 125 patients. Orthopedics. 2012;35:e1581–5.

14. Elzohairy MM. Pigmented villonodular synovitis managed by total synovectomy and cementless total hip arthroplasty. Eur J Orthop Surg Traumatol. 2018;28:1375–80. [cited 2018 May 31]; Available from: http://link.springer.com/10.1007/s00590-018-2214-y

15. JAFFE H. Pigmented villonodular synovitis, bursitis, and tenosynovitis. Arch Pathol. 1941;31:731–65.

16. Williams VG, Whiteside LA, White SE, McCarthy DS. Fixation of ultrahigh-molecular-weight polyethylene liners to metal-backed acetabular cups. J Arthroplast. 1997;12:25–31.

17. Charnley J, Halley DK. Rate of wear in total hip replacement. Clin Orthop Relat Res. 1975;112:170–9.

18. DeLee JG, Charnley J. Radiological demarcation of cemented sockets in total hip replacement. Clin Orthop Relat Res. 1976;121:20–32.

19. Gruen TA, McNeice GM, Amstutz HC. "Modes of failure" of cemented stem-type femoral components: a radiographic analysis of loosening. Clin Orthop Relat Res. 1979;141:17–27.

20. Joshi RP, Eftekhar NS, McMahon DJ, Nercessian OA. Osteolysis after Charnley primary low-friction arthroplasty. A comparison of two matched paired groups. J Bone Joint Surg Br. 1998;80:585–90.

21. Smith JH, Pugh DG. Roentgenographic aspects of articular pigmented villonodular synovitis. Am J Roentgenol Radium Therapy, Nucl Med. 1962;87:1146–56.

22. Colman MW, Ye J, Weiss KR, Goodman MA, McGough RL. Does combined open and arthroscopic synovectomy for diffuse PVNS of the knee improve recurrence rates? Clin Orthop Relat Res. 2013;471:883–90.

23. Shoji T, Yasunaga Y, Yamasaki T, Nakamae A, Mori R, Hamanishi M, et al. Transtrochanteric rotational osteotomy combined with intra-articular procedures for pigmented villonodular synovitis of the hip. J Orthop Sci. 2015;20:943–50.

24. Chiari C, Pirich C, Brannath W, Kotz R, Trieb K. What affects the recurrence and clinical outcome of pigmented villonodular synovitis? Clin Orthop Relat Res. 2006;450:172–8.

25. Ma X, Shi G, Xia C, Liu H, He J, Jin W. Pigmented villonodular synovitis: a retrospective study of seventy five cases (eighty one joints). Int Orthop. 2013;37:1165–70.

26. Baba S, Motomura G, Fukushi J, Ikemura S, Sonoda K, Kubo Y, et al. Osteonecrosis of the femoral head associated with pigmented villonodular synovitis. Rheumatol Int. 2017;37:841–5.

27. Steinmetz S, Rougemont A-L, Peter R. Pigmented villonodular synovitis of the hip. EFORT Open Rev. 2016;1:260–6.

28. Xie G, Jiang N, Liang C, Zeng J, Chen Z, Xu Q, et al. Pigmented villonodular synovitis: a retrospective multicenter study of 237 cases. PLoS One. 2015;10:e0121451.

29. Hoberg M, Amstutz HC. Metal-on-metal hip resurfacing in patients with pigmented villonodular synovitis: a report of two cases. Orthopedics. 2010;33:50.

30. Hannouche D, Devriese F, Delambre J, Zadegan F, Tourabaly I, Sedel L, et al. Ceramic-on-ceramic THA implants in patients younger than 20 years. Clin Orthop Relat Res. 2016;474:520–7.

31. Cai Y, Yan S. Development of ceramic-on-ceramic implants for total hip arthroplasty. Orthop Surg. 2010;2:175–81.

29

Correlation of serum cartilage oligomeric matrix protein with knee osteoarthritis diagnosis: a meta-analysis

Xiaoyang Bi ⓘ

Abstract

Background: The measurement of cartilage oligomeric matrix protein (COMP) has become a novel way for the diagnosis of knee osteoarthritis (OA). However, no conclusive correlation has been drawn between COMP and knee OA. The purpose of this study was to examine the utility of serum COMP as biomarker for knee OA and its relation with disease severity.

Methods: A systematic search on PubMed, ScienceDirect, and EMBASE was conducted in January 2018 using certain keywords. Initial search yielded a total of 285 publications, and 35 articles were reviewed in full-text. Eventually, nine studies were included in the analysis. All the retrieved studies used Kellgren-Lawrence (K-L) classification for knee OA and provided available data of serum COMP in OA patients and healthy controls. Sensitivity analysis was performed by removing one study result at a time to detect the impact of each study have on the overall effect and to test the stability of the cumulative result. Subgroup study based on K-L grade system was also conducted to disclose the correlation between serum COMP and knee OA disease severity.

Results: Pooled analysis of nine studies demonstrated a significant elevation of serum COMP in knee OA patients (SMD 0.81, [95% CI, 0.36, 1.25], $P = 0.0004$) compared with controls. In comparisons between K-L 1–4 and controls, significantly higher serum COMP was detected in all three subgroups except K-L grade 1 versus control. Comparisons among K-L grades 1–4 revealed significantly higher serum COMP levels in patients with more serious than less serious disease stage. However, the elevation in patients with K-L grade 3 did not reach statistical significance when compared with K-L grade 1 patients.

Conclusion: The overall analysis showed significantly higher serum COMP in knee OA patients compared to controls which indicate the potential ability of serum COMP in differentiating knee OA patients from healthy subjects. Pooled statistic of our meta-analysis showed that serum COMP levels were effective in distinguishing patients with K-L ≥ 2.

Keywords: Knee osteoarthritis, Cartilage oligomeric matrix protein, Kellgren-Lawrence

Background

Osteoarthritis (OA) is one of the most common joint diseases worldwide, affecting approximately 9.6% of men and 18% of women in the elderly [1]. It is characterized by progressive destruction of the articular cartilage and substantial abnormalities in the subchondral bone, ligaments, synovial membrane, articular capsule, and periarticular muscles. OA can be triggered by various factors like inflammation, physical injury, and other metabolic causes [2]. A number of environmental risk factors such as obesity and trauma can also initiate diverse pathological pathways which may eventually lead to OA [3].

Until now, the most reliable method for OA assessment is joint space width (JSW) measurement using radiography [4, 5]. However, since the disease is initiated long before the plain X-rays can be detected, irreversible joint damages have often already occurred at the time radiological diagnosis is established. Therefore, more sensitive techniques for early diagnosis of OA are needed. Magnetic resonance imaging (MRI) is well-established for this purpose. However, there are still

Correspondence: xiaoyangbi123@163.com
Department of Orthopedic Medicine, Tianjin Hospital, No 406 JieFangNan Road , Hexin District, Tianjin City 300211, China

obstacles in availability and cost of this imaging approach [6]. Biomarkers, molecules that are secreted into biological fluids during matrix metabolism of articular cartilage, subchondral bone, and synovial tissue, have received increased research attention for the diagnosis of OA. A variety of biomarkers, such as proinflammatory and anti-inflammatory cytokines, catabolic enzymes, and markers of cartilage and bone turnover, can be applied to OA diagnosis. According to the "BIPED" classification, each biomarkers can be classified to one or more of the following five categories: burden of disease, investigative, prognostic, efficacy of intervention, and diagnostic [7]. A study reviewing the status of available biochemical markers for OA suggests that cartilage markers are the most extensively investigated and well-performed type in comparison with the bone or synovial tissue biomarkers [8].

Cartilage oligomeric matrix protein (COMP), a 524-kd pentameric glycoprotein related to the thrombospondin family, is one of the cartilage markers [9]. COMP is found predominantly in cartilage, and recent studies have demonstrated that COMP expression can also be identified in other structures such as the ligaments, tendons, menisci, and synovial membrane [10, 11]. Since its appearance, the diagnostic value of serum COMP for OA as well as its correlation with disease progression and severity has been frequently and broadly assessed [9, 12–14]. However, the efficiency of serum COMP as biomarker for OA diagnosis is still in controversy. Several previous studies suggested that serum COMP had the ability to distinguish OA patients from healthy controls, as significant higher serum COMP levels were detected when compared with controls [15, 16]. Some research suggested that more rapid knee, hip, or hand joint destruction would occur in patients with higher levels of COMP in serum in comparison to that in patients with lower levels [17, 18]. Other studies, however, found no correlation between serum COMP and OA presence at all [19, 20]. One possible reason for such discrepancy could be the limited statistical power of studies due to their relatively small sample sizes.

Thus, by collecting and combining all available data, the primary objective of the present meta-analysis is to assess the diagnostic performance of serum COMP as biomarker for knee OA as well as the correlation between serum COMP levels and knee OA disease severity classified by Kellgren-Lawrence (K-L) grade.

Methods
Search strategy
Electronic databases, PubMed, ScienceDirect, and EMBASE, were systematically searched for relevant publications till January 2018. The search terms were as follows: osteoarthritis, cartilage oligomeric matrix protein,

serum, knee OA, diagnosis, and all of the combinations. Reviewer screened all abstracts retrieved from the initial search results. Study was reviewed in full-text if it is relevant to our topic or the abstracts did not provide enough information to include or exclude the study from the review. Further manual search of all reference lists and other relevant meta-analysis were conducted for additional studies which were not included in the original search. There was no restriction on studies in terms of their year, region, or language of publication. However, all the selected non-English articles must contain an English abstract.

Eligibility criteria
All the studies need to fulfill the following criteria to be included in the meta-analysis:

- Studies involved patients with radiographic diagnosis of knee OA.
- Studies with a disease free control group for comparison.
- The severity of knee OA was graded using K-L classification.
- Studies provided extractable serum COMP levels in both knee OA and control group.
- All enrolled participant were adult (age > 18).
- Levels of serum COMP were quantified using enzyme-linked immunosorbent assay (ELISA) regardless of type and manufacture company.

Studies that did not match the above requirements, review papers, case reports, and other non-related studies were excluded. We only included publications that applied K-L severity grade system for knee OA. Studies that used other OA severity classification systems were excluded to guarantee consistent comparisons across studies.

Data extraction
Reviewer inspected and extracted all the relevant data according to predefined form. In case of discrepancies, a second reviewer was reached and solved them. The outcome of interest for this study was differences of serum COMP levels between the knee OA patients and controls. A majority of studies reported serum COMP in unit of measure nanograms per milliliter or milligram per milliliter [9, 18, 19, 21–23], but some studies used the unit units per liter [17, 20, 24]. For this analysis, serum COMP in all units of measure was extracted, and data were combined using a standardized mean differences (SMD) model. Other study characteristics, including sample size, number of woman patients, patients' body mass index, number of patients in different K-L grade group, type and manufacture information of the ELIAS kits, and the region in which the study take place, were also extracted.

Statistical analysis

Inter-group analysis of serum COMP was based on the difference in the levels of COMP between knee OA patients and healthy controls. Statistical analysis was performed using chi-squared test and manifested by forest plot where Q and I^2 were presented. A random effects model was used when considerable heterogeneity ($I^2 >$ 50%) existed among studies. A fixed-effects model was applied when $I^2 < 50\%$. Since the included studies measured the levels of serum COMP with different scales, pooled results of this meta-analysis were calculated using SMD with 95% confidence intervals (CIs). Sensitivity analysis were performed by removing one study result at a time to determine the influence of individual study have on the overall estimate and to test the stability of the cumulative result across the included studies [25]. Subgroup analysis based on different unit of measure was performed to explore the source of heterogeneity across study, and outcomes were presented as mean difference (MD) with 95% CI. To further reveal the mechanism of serum COMP in different OA severity, subgroup analysis was also conducted by comparing serum COMP levels among different K-L grades. All statistical analyses were processed using Review Manager (Version 5.3. Copenhagen: The Nordic Cochrane Centre, The Cochrane Collaboration, 2014). We considered P value < 0.05 as statistically significant.

Results

Study selection

The electronic databases and manual cross-checking of reference lists identified 285 articles for the initial review.

After examining all the tiles and abstracts by one reviewer, 35 studies satisfied the most crucial and basic criterion which was assessing the efficiency of serum COMP as a biomarker for knee OA remained and went through full-text review. Excluding studies that did not use K-L grade for OA classification and studies that did not provide necessary data, nine studies were included in this meta-analysis. Figure 1 presented the flow diagram of study selection.

Study description

Our analysis only included studies that involved patients with radiological defined knee OA classified by K-L severity grade and measured COMP concentrations in serum. The variables in terms of joint and type of OA, source of COMP, and OA classification system were restricted. Other characteristics, such as sample size, patients' age, body mass index (BMI), and ethnic groups, were varied from individual study. Eventually, 9 studies with a total of 1694 participant were included in this study [9, 17–24]. Overall, the sample size of the enrolled studies ranged from 48 to 769 patients. Selected participants were more than 20 years old. Most of the study applied a sandwich ELISA kits while competitive and two-site ELISA were also used by one study respectively [9, 24]. Manufacture of the ELISA assays were also varied from study to study, and several trials applied an ELIAS kit modified by authors [9, 18, 22]. For outcome measurement, three studies expressed serum COMP in the unit units per liter [17, 20, 24]. Other six used the unit of measure nanograms per milliliter or milligram

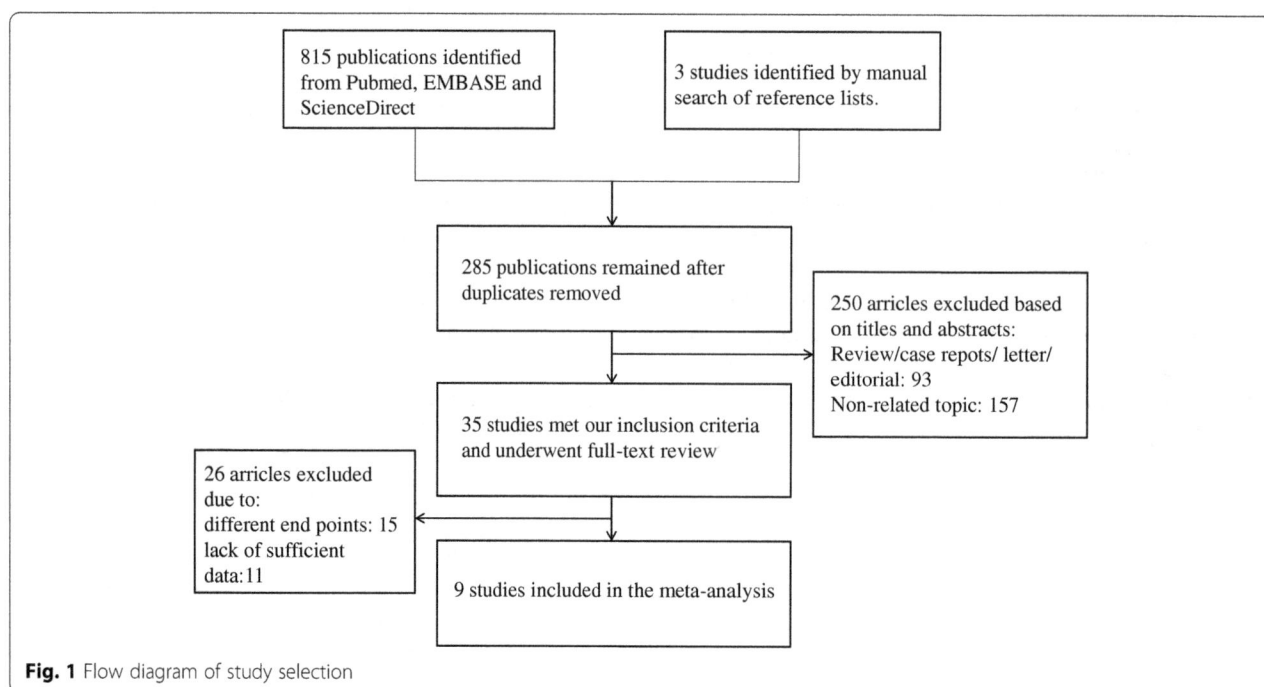

Fig. 1 Flow diagram of study selection

per milliliter. Table 1 summarized all relevant detailed characteristics of the included studies.

Correlation between serum COMP levels and knee OA

Pooled results of nine studies revealed a significant elevation of serum COMP in OA patients compared with healthy controls (SMD 0.81, [95% CI, 0.36, 1.25], $P = 0.0004$, Fig. 2). Considering high heterogeneity existed among studies ($I^2 = 93\%$), sensitivity analysis was also conducted. The pooled SMD ranged from 0.51 to 0.90 when removing each given study, and all the outcomes still remained statistical significant. The forest plot figure and results of the sensitivity analysis indicated that the study of Li might be the source of heterogeneity. When omitting the study result of Li et al., the pooled SMD changed from 0.81 (95% CI, 0.36, 1.25) to 0.51 (95% CI, 0.25, 0.78) with I^2 value dropped from 93% to 79%. Subgroup analysis based on different measure of units was also performed. Results showed increased serum COMP in knee OA patients compared to controls in both units per liter unit (MD 2.13, [95% CI, 0.11, 4.16], $P = 0.04$, Table 2) and microgram per milliliter unit subgroups (MD 0.73, [95% CI, 0.02, 1.44], $P = 0.04$, Table 2).

Correlation between serum COMP levels and OA severity

For studies providing serum COMP data in different K-L grades, comparisons were performed between K-L grades 1–4 and controls. Significant differences in serum COMP were observed comparing patients with K-L grades 2–4 with healthy controls (K-L 2: SMD = 0.86, 95% CI, 0.09, 1.62, $P = 0.03$; K-L 3: SMD = 1.05, 95% CI, 0.01, 2.08, $P = 0.05$; K-L 4: SMD = 0.99, 95% CI, 0.33, 1.65, $P = 0.003$) (Fig. 3) Sensitivity analysis further showed that the study of Li might be the reason of high heterogeneity. When removing the result of Li, the outcomes still showed significant higher serum COMP levels in knee OA patients with K-L grades 2–4 compared with controls, while the I^2 value changed from > 90% to < 50%. Patients with OA of K-L grade 1 tended to have higher serum COMP concentrations than healthy participants, although the differences were not significant (Fig. 3).

Comparisons within different K-L grades were also conducted. In the comparison between K-L grades 2–4 and K-L grade 1, significant differences were found in K-L grade 2 and K-L grade 4 compared with K-L grade 1. Serum COMP levels tended to be higher in patient with K-L grade 3 than with K-L grade 1; however, the result did not reach statistical significance. A significant elevated

Table 1 Characteristics of included studies for COMP

Author	Group	N	Age (years)	Female (n)	BMI (kg/m2)	Region	K-L 0~4 of patients (n)	ELISA manufacture information	Type of ELISA
Clark1999	Control	148	60 ± 20	144		USA	K-L 0 = 148, K-L2 = 109 K-L 3,4 = 34	In-house method	Competitive
	OA	143	60 ± 20						
Das Gupta E2017	Control	30	62.5 ± 12	15	25.01 ± 6.31	Malaysia	K-L 2 = 30 K-L 3 = 23 K-L 4 = 7	R&D Systems	Solid-phase sandwich
	OA	60	57.5 ± 9	46	26.72 ± 5.35				
Fernandes2007	Control	40	53.8 ± 8.5	24		Brazil	K-L 0,1 = 40 K-L 2–4 = 75	AnaMar Medical (Uppsala, Sweden)	Sandwich
	OA	75	56.6 ± 7.6	51					
Jordan JM2003	Control	302	63.3 ± 10.8	258	31.5 ± 7.4	USA	K-L 0 = 302, K-L 2 = 313, K-L 3 = 110, K-L 4 = 44	AnaMar Medical (Lund, Sweden)	Sandwich
	OA	467	60.6 ± 9.6	190	28.9 ± 6.1				
Li2012	Control	35	53 ± 12.53	19	21.8 ± 4.9	China	K-L 1 = 28, K-L 2 = 36, K-L 3 = 27, K-L 4 = 24	AnaMar Medical AB (Lund, Sweden)	Sandwich
	OA	115	55 ± 13.32	60	22.3 ± 5.7				
Mündermann A2009	Control	41	57.5 ± 7	20	25.7 ± 4.2	USA	K-L 1 = 11, K-L 2 = 7, K-L 3 = 12, K-L 4 = 12	AnaMar Medical AB (Lund, Sweden)	Sandwich
	OA	42	60.7 ± 8.6	22	27.0 ± 3.8				
Author	Group	N	Age (years)	Female (n)	BMI (kg/m2)	Region	K-L 0~4 of patients (n)	ELISA manufacture information	Type of ELISA
Senolt L2005	Control	38	58.3 ± 9.1	23		Czech Republic	K-L 1 = 2, K-L 2 = 18 K-L 3 = 14, K-L 4 = 4	In-house method	Sandwich
	OA	38	64.1 ± 10.1	25					
Sowers MF2009	Control	36	47.5 ± 2.6	36	29.7 ± 6.2	France	K-L 0,1 = 36 K-L 2 = 16 K-L 3,4 = 20	AnaMar Medical (COMPTM ELISA kit)	A two-site ELISA
	OA	36	47.5 ± 2.6	36	39.15 ± 8.22				
Wakitani2007	Control	24	20–54	8		Japan	K-L 1 = 7, K-L 2 = 4 K-L 3 = 6, K-L 4 = 7	Kamiya Biomedical Company, Seattle, WA, USA	Sandwich
	OA	24	40–80	20					

COMP cartilage oligomeric matrix protein, *K-L* Kellgren-Lawrence classification, *ELISA* enzyme-linked immunosorbent assay

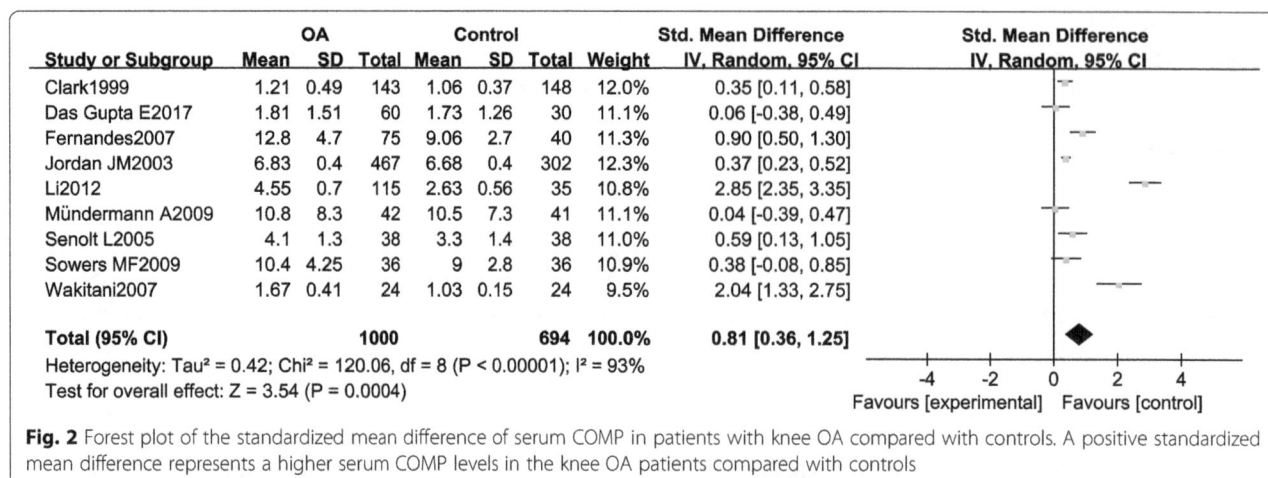

Fig. 2 Forest plot of the standardized mean difference of serum COMP in patients with knee OA compared with controls. A positive standardized mean difference represents a higher serum COMP levels in the knee OA patients compared with controls

serum COMP levels were found in subgroups K-L grades 3–4 versus K-L grade 2 and K-L grade 4 versus K-L grade 3. Pooled statistics revealed that serum COMP levels had a tendency to increase as OA symptom became more serious (Table 2).

Discussion

Biomarkers have risen as a non-invasive and more sensitive measurement in detecting subtle changes in bone, cartilage, and synovial tissues, which is more capable of diagnosing early sight of OA [26–28]. The measurement of serum COMP becomes popular among researchers as a potential indicator for OA [8, 9, 29, 30]. It is believed that changes in serum COMP can reflect changes in cartilage breakdown [10, 31]. Some researchers also put forward that the presence of OA might induce more active cartilage turnover, resulting in a greater percentage increase in serum COMP levels [32]. However, the conclusions from previous investigations were differed from study to study, and a single study could not provide enough evidence to confirm to usefulness of serum

COMP in diagnosing knee OA. Thus, we performed the current meta-analysis to systematically combine all available information and assess the correlation of serum COMP levels with knee OA and disease severity. The combined result from 9 studies involved 1000 knee OA patients and 694 healthy participants demonstrated a significant elevation in serum COMP levels in knee OA patients compared to controls. Although considerable heterogeneity existed, sensitivity analysis still revealed significantly higher levels of serum COMP in knee OA group compared to controls when we removed each study result. Also, we found that the study of Li might be the source of heterogeneity as the I^2 value dropped when we omitted its outcome. Comparisons were made between Li et al. and other included studies. However, the study of Li did not differ much from the others in study design, patients demographic, and biomarker quantify method, except that it was the only included study assessed serum COMP in Chinese patients and the article was published in Chinese. The different body structure of participant or the differential expression of the Chinese language might be the distributions of heterogeneity. Future analysis might need to restrict the population and language of the included study. Nevertheless, our finding supported the perspective that serum COMP levels could serve as effective biomarker for diagnosing knee OA.

As part of the inclusion criteria, the present analysis must include study that used K-L severity grade system for the classification of knee OA patients. This classification system was chosen because it was the most widely and commonly used classification tool in clinical practice and in research, especially in grading OA [33]. To further prove whether serum COMP was correlated with knee OA disease severity, subgroup analyses between K-L grades 1–4 and control group and comparisons among K-L grades 1–4 were carried out. Significant differences were found in all the subgroups except the

Table 2 Subgroup analysis of serum COMP with different unit of measure and disease severity

Subgroups	Number of study	Mean difference	95% CI	P
Unit of measure				
U/L	3	2.13	0.11, 4.16	0.04
µg/ml	6	1.00	0.37, 1.63	0.002
Disease severity				
K-L 1 VS K-L 2	3	0.79	0.34, 1.25	0.0007
K-L 1 VS K-L 3	3	1.08	0.44, 2.60	0.16
K-L 1 VS K-L 4	3	1.61	0.57, 2.65	0.002
K-L 2 VS K-L 3	6	0.44	0.04, 0.85	0.03
K-L 2 VS K-L 4	7	0.61	0.17, 1.05	0.007
K-L 3 VS K-L 4	5	0.41	0.15, 0.68	0.002

K-L Kellgren-Lawrence classification, *CI* confidence intervals

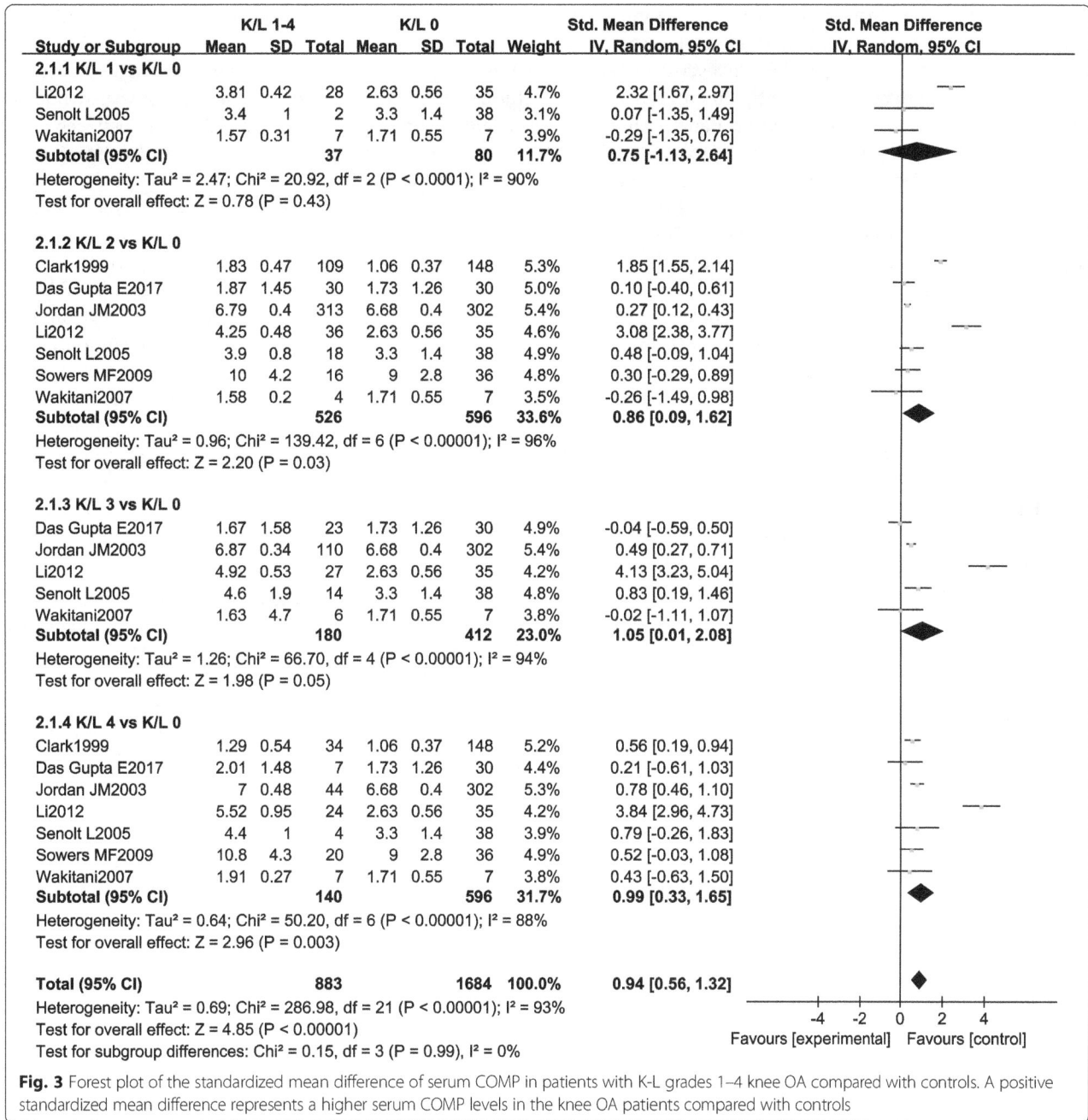

Fig. 3 Forest plot of the standardized mean difference of serum COMP in patients with K-L grades 1–4 knee OA compared with controls. A positive standardized mean difference represents a higher serum COMP levels in the knee OA patients compared with controls

comparison of K-L grade 1 versus control and K-L grade 3 versus grade 1. Although the result of the two subgroups did not reach statistical significance, data still showed that compared with patients with a lower severity, patients with higher disease severity had higher serum COMP. However, only three studies provided COMP levels in K-L grade 1 patients [21–23], the limited data might be insufficient to define the relationship between K-L grade 1 and other groups. These uncertain results might also cause by the different definitions for each of the K-L classifications used to assess OA severity in each study. A recent review of K-L

classifications used in published study reported grade 2 definitions are different throughout the reported literature [34]. Only four studies recruited in this study provided specific K-L classifications. Future investigation should confirm the definition of K-L grade system allowing better comparisons to be made across the studies. According to the outcome of our analysis, we observed a potential correlation between serum COMP and knee OA severity. The levels of serum COMP trend to rise as the disease become more serious. However, whether serum COMP is useful in diagnosing early knee OA need further evidence.

Previous research suggested that ethnic differences could affect the symptom manifestations in knee OA population [35]. A study by GANDHI investigating the influence of ethnic differences on joint pain and function in knee OA patients reported that joint pain and dysfunction were greater in Asian patients than in Caucasians [36]. In assessing the correlation between serum COMP and knee OA, researchers also point out the influence of ethnicity have on the levels of COMP. In the study of Jordan et al., higher levels of serum COMP were found in African American women compared with that in Caucasian women in both controls and knee OA patients [18]. Three of the included studies assessed serum COMP in specific ethnic group, Caucasian, Brazilian, and Malaysian [17–19]. Results showed that serum COMP was significantly elevated in Caucasian and Brazilian patients versus controls [9, 17]. Whereas no difference in serum COMP levels between healthy controls and knee OA patients were found in Malaysian population [19]. Notably, in overall analysis, sensitivity analysis showed that Li et al. and Wakitani et al. affected mostly on the overall effect [21, 23]. When removing the data of Li and Wakitani, the SMD effect size dropped from 0.81 to 0.51, and from 0.81 to 0.67. Interestingly, both studies were performed in Asian population. This observation put us to further consideration that the diagnostic performance of serum COMP might be preferable in certain ethnic group. However, comparisons among different ethnicities could not be conducted in our analysis due to the limited and insufficient information. These factors should be considered in the derivation of standards using this, and possibly other, potential biomarkers of OA.

There are still some limitations. First of all, although sensitivity and subgroup analyses were performed to confirm the statistic power of the study, the effect of heterogeneity still cannot be eliminated completely. We assumed that the inclusion of small sample size studies might be the reason causing inconclusive and imprecise results. However, only nine publications met all our inclusion criteria, it is impossible to omit the outcomes of small sample size studies in this meta-analysis. Furthermore, the use of different ELISA kits might be another reason causing heterogeneity and discrepancy. Some researchers put forward that certain ELISAs were more appropriate for detecting human serum COMP than others. A study comparing three ELISA kits for measuring COMP in serum concluded that an in-house method utilizing MAb's 16F12 and 17C10 and the Biovendor kit (Modrice, Czech Rep.) were more suitable for detecting serum COMP than Anamar kit (Gothenburg, Sweden) [37]. A previous meta-analysis reported that the ELISA kit manufactured by Kamiya Biomedical Company was preferable than other ELISA kits in the measurement of serum COMP [30]. However, due to the diverse ELISA kits involved in our study, subgroup analysis could not be performed to prove which ELISA kit is the best choice. Yet, by examining the results of the nine enrolled studies, we observed that two of them revealed no significant difference in serum COMP levels between knee OA patients and controls [19, 23]. These two studies applied a R&D Systems ELISA and a Kamiya Biomedical ELISA respectively, while other studies utilized in-house method or AnaMar Medical kit manufactured by different company. However, the direct comparison among studies is less rigorous. To ascertain the best ELISA kits for assessing serum COMP, the only way is to compare the serum sample quantified by the each technique from the same subjects. Future experiments should investigate in this field. Our study only estimates the diagnostic value of serum COMP in knee OA. The effectiveness of synovial fluid COMP in predicting knee OA and the usefulness of serum COMP in detecting other joints of OA remain to be established.

Conclusion

The overall analysis revealed a significant elevation of serum COMP in knee OA patients compared to controls. The overall effect showed that serum COMP had the potential to differentiate knee OA patients from healthy subjects. In assessing the correlation between serum COMP and knee OA disease severity, although the result of K-L 1 versus control and K-L grade 3 versus K-L 1 did not reach statistical significance, serum COMP still showed elevation toward patients with more serious OA stage. Pooled statistic of our meta-analysis showed that serum COMP levels were better in distinguishing patients with K-L grades ≥ 2. Future rigorous prospective study is required in order to strengthen our findings.

Abbreviations

CI: Confidence intervals; COMP: Cartilage oligomeric matrix protein; ELISA: Enzyme-linked immunosorbent assay; JSW: Joint space width; K-L: Kellgren-Lawrence; MD: Mean differences; OA: Osteoarthritis; SMD: Standardized mean differences

Acknowledgements

I shall extend my thanks to Haiyuan Li and Qianqian Lu for their kind help in the data extraction and statistical analysis processes.

Funding

This research did not receive any specific grant from funding agencies.

Author's contributions

XYB conceived the study and reviewed all the included publications. XYB extracted participants' data from patients group and control group, and performed statistical analysis. XYB finally wrote and approved the manuscript.

Competing interests

The author declares that he has no competing interests.

References

1. Woolf AD, Pfleger B. Burden of major musculoskeletal conditions. Bull World Health Organ. 2003;81:646–56.
2. Ashkavand Z, Malekinejad H, Vishwanath BS. The pathophysiology of osteoarthritis. J Pharm Res. 2013;7:132–8.
3. Verma P, Dalal K. Serum cartilage oligomeric matrix protein (COMP) in knee osteoarthritis: a novel diagnostic and prognostic biomarker. J Orthop Res. 2013;31:999–1006.
4. Buckland-Wright JC, Macfarlane DG, Lynch JA, Jasani MK, Bradshaw CR. Joint space width measures cartilage thickness in osteoarthritis of the knee: high resolution plain film and double contrast macroradiographic investigation. Ann Rheum Dis. 1995;54:263–8.
5. Jo E. Osteoarthritic disorders. J Bone Joint Surg Br Vol. 1996;78-B:170.
6. Podlipská J, Guermazi A, Liukkonen E, Lammentausta E, Niinimäki J, Nieminen MT, Tervonen O, Koski JM, Saarakkala S. Diagnostic performance of semi-quantitative knee ultrasonography – comparison with magnetic resonance imaging osteoarthritis knee score (MOAKS): data from the Oulu osteoarthritis study. Osteoarthr Cartil. 2015;23:A76–7.
7. Bauer DC, Hunter DJ, Abramson SB, Attur M, Corr M, Felson D, Heinegård D, Jordan JM, Kepler TB, Lane NE. Classification of osteoarthritis biomarkers: a proposed approach 1. Osteoarthr Cartil. 2006;14:723–7.
8. Spil WEV, Degroot J, Lems WF, Lafeber FP. Serum and urinary biochemical markers for knee and hip osteoarthritis: a systematic review applying the consensus biped criteria. Osteoarthr Cartil. 2010;18:605.
9. Clark AG, Jordan JM, Vilim V, Renner JB, Dragomir AD, Luta G, Kraus VB. Serum cartilage oligomeric matrix protein reflects osteoarthritis presence and severity: the Johnston County Osteoarthritis Project. Arthritis Rheum. 1999;42:2356–64.
10. Neidhart M, Hauser N, Paulsson M, Dicesare PE, Michel BA, Häuselmann HJ. Small fragments of cartilage oligomeric matrix protein in synovial fluid and serum as markers for cartilage degradation. Br J Rheumatol. 1997;36:1151.
11. Muller G, Michel A, Altenburg E. COMP (cartilage oligomeric matrix protein) is synthesized in ligament, tendon, meniscus, and articular cartilage. Connect Tissue Res. 1998;39:233–44.
12. Sharif M, Saxne T, Shepstone L, Kirwan JR, Elson CJ, Heinegård D, Dieppe PA. Relationship between serum cartilage oligomeric matrix protein levels and disease progression in osteoarthritis of the knee joint. Br J Rheumatol. 1995;34:306.
13. Vilím V, Olejárová M, Machácek S, Gatterová J, Kraus VB, Pavelka K. Serum levels of cartilage oligomeric matrix protein (COMP) correlate with radiographic progression of knee osteoarthritis. Osteoarthr Cartil. 2002;10:707–13.
14. Song SY, Han YD, Hong SY, Kim K, Yang SS, Min BH, Yoon HC. Chip-based cartilage oligomeric matrix protein detection in serum and synovial fluid for osteoarthritis diagnosis. Anal Biochem. 2012;420:139.
15. Blumenfeld O, Williams FM, Hart DJ, Spector TD, Arden N, Livshits G. Association between cartilage and bone biomarkers and incidence of radiographic knee osteoarthritis (RKOA) in UK females: a prospective study. Osteoarthr Cartil. 2013;21:923–9.
16. El-Arman MM, El-Fayoumi G, El-Shal EW, El-Boghdady I, El-Ghaweet A. Aggrecan and cartilage oligomeric matrix protein in serum and synovial fluid of patients with knee osteoarthritis. HSS J. 2010;6:171–6.
17. Fernandes FA, Pucinelli MLC, Silva NPD, Feldman D. Serum cartilage oligomeric matrix protein (COMP) levels in knee osteoarthritis in a Brazilian population: clinical and radiological correlation. Scand J Rheumatol. 2007;36:211.
18. Jordan JM, Luta G, Stabler T, Renner JB, Dragomir AD, Vilim V, Hochberg MC, Helmick CG, Kraus VB. Ethnic and sex differences in serum levels of

19. cartilage oligomeric matrix protein: the Johnston County osteoarthritis project. Arthritis Rheum. 2003;48:675–81.
19. Das GE, Ng WR, Wong SF, Bhurhanudeen AK, Yeap SS. Correlation of serum cartilage oligometric matrix protein (COMP) and interleukin-16 (IL-16) levels with disease severity in primary knee osteoarthritis: a pilot study in a Malaysian population. PLoS One. 2017;12:e0184802.
20. Mündermann A, King KB, Smith RL, Andriacchi TP. Change in serum COMP concentration due to ambulatory load is not related to knee OA status. J Orthop Res. 2010;27:1408–13.
21. Li H, Wang D, Wu ZQ, Zhong JM, Yuan YJ. Serum levels of cartilage oligomeric matrix protein in the diagnosis of knee osteoarthritis. Zhongguo Gu Shang. 2012;25:380.
22. Šenolt L, Braun M, Olejárová M, Forejtová Š, Gatterová J, Pavelka K. Increased pentosidine, an advanced glycation end product, in serum and synovial fluid from patients with knee osteoarthritis and its relation with cartilage oligomeric matrix protein. Ann Rheum Dis. 2005;64:886–90.
23. Wakitani S, Nawata M, Kawaguchi A, Okabe T, Takaoka K, Tsuchiya T, Nakaoka R, Masuda H, Miyazaki K. Serum keratan sulfate is a promising marker of early articular cartilage breakdown. Rheumatology. 2007;46:1652.
24. Sowers MF, Karvonengutierrez CA, Yosef M, Jannausch M, Jiang Y, Garnero P, Jacobson J. Longitudinal changes of serum COMP and urinary CTX-II predict x-ray defined knee osteoarthritis severity and stiffness in women. Osteoarthr Cartil. 2009;17:1609–14.
25. Borenstein M. Introduction to meta-analysis. Paediatr Perinat Epidemiol. 2009;24:91572T-91572T-91574.
26. Schmidt-Rohlfing B, Gavenis K, Kippels M, Schneider U. New potential markers for cartilage degradation of the knee joint. Acta Rheumatol Scand. 2002;31:151–7.
27. Thonar EJ, Shinmei M, Lohmander LS. Body fluid markers of cartilage changes in osteoarthritis. Rheum Dis Clin N Am. 1993;19:635–57.
28. Jch R, Garnero P. Biological markers in osteoarthritis. Nat Clin Pract Rheumatol. 2007;3:346–56.
29. Kumm J, Tamm A, Veske K, Lintrop M, Tamm A. Associations between cartilage oligomeric matrix protein and several articular tissues in early knee joint osteoarthritis. Rheumatology. 2006;45:1308.
30. Hoch JM, Mattacola CG, Medina McKeon JM, Howard JS, Lattermann C. Serum cartilage oligomeric matrix protein (sCOMP) is elevated in patients with knee osteoarthritis: a systematic review and meta-analysis. Osteoarthr Cartil. 2011;19:1396–404.
31. Lohmander LS, Saxne T, Heinegård DK. Release of cartilage oligomeric matrix protein (COMP) into joint fluid after knee injury and in osteoarthritis. Ann Rheum Dis. 1994;53:8–13.
32. Saxne T, Heinegård D. Cartilage oligomeric matrix protein: a novel marker of cartilage turnover detectable in synovial fluid and blood. Br J Rheumatol. 1992;31:583.
33. Kohn MD, Sassoon AA, Fernando ND. Classifications in Brief: Kellgren-Lawrence classification of osteoarthritis. Clin Orthop Relat Res. 2016;474: 1886–93.
34. Schiphof D, Boers M, Bierma-Zeinstra SM. Differences in descriptions of Kellgren and Lawrence grades of knee osteoarthritis. Ann Rheum Dis. 2008; 67:1034.
35. Joshi R, Ganguli N, Carvalho C, Leon FD, Pope J. Varus and valgus deformities in knee osteoarthritis among different ethnic groups (Indian, Portuguese and Canadians) within an urban Canadian rheumatology practice. Indian J Rheumatol. 2010;5:180–4.
36. Gandhi R, Razak F, Mahomed NN. Ethnic differences in the relationship between obesity and joint pain and function in a joint arthroplasty population. J Rheumatol. 2008;35:1874–7.
37. Stabler T, Fang F, Jordan J, Vilim V, Kraus VB. A comparison of methods for measuring cartilage oligomeric protein (comp) in human subjects with knee OA. Osteoarthr Cartil. 2007;15:C81–2.

30

Tibiofemoral joint contact area and stress after single-bundle anterior cruciate ligament reconstruction with transtibial versus anteromedial portal drilling techniques

Chunhui Liu[1†], Yingpeng Wang[2†], Zhongli Li[1*], Ji Li[1], Hao Zhang[1], Yangmu Fu[1] and Kuan Zhang[2]

Abstract

Background: During single-bundle ACLR, femoral tunnel location plays an important role in restoring the intact knee mechanisms, whereas malplacement of the tunnel was cited as the most common cause of knee instability. The objective of this study is to evaluate, objectively, the tibiofemoral contact area and stress after single-bundle (SB) anterior cruciate ligament reconstruction (ACLR) with femoral tunnel positions drilled by transtibial (TT) or anteromedial (AM) portal techniques.

Methods: Seven fresh human cadaveric knees underwent ACLR by the use of TT or AM portal techniques in a randomized order. These specimens were reused for ACL-R (TT and AM). The tibiofemoral contact area and stresses were gauged by an electronic stress-sensitive film inserted into the joint space. The knee was under the femoral axial compressive load of 1000 N using a biomechanics testing machine at 0°, 10°, 20°, and 30° of flexion. Three conditions were compared: (1) intact ACL, (2) ACLR by the use of the TT method, and (3) ACLR by the use of the AM portal method.

Results: Compared with AM portal ACL-reconstructed knees, a significantly decreased tibiofemoral contact area on the medial compartment was detected in the TT ACL-reconstructed knees at 20°of knee flexion ($P = .047$). Compared with the intact group, the TT ACLR group showed a higher mean stress at 20° and 30° of flexion on the medial compartments ($P = .001$, $P = .003$, respectively), while the AM portal ACLR group showed no significant differences at 30° of flexion ($P = .073$). The TT ACLR group also showed a higher mean maximum stress at 20° of flexion on the medial compartments ($P = .047$), while the AM portal ACLR group showed no significant differences at this angle($P = .319$).

Discussion: The alternation of the tibiofemoral joint contact area and stress in reconstructed knees may be caused by the mismatch of the tibiofemoral joint during knee movement procedures compared with intact knees.

Conclusions: SB ACLR by the use of the AM portal method and TT method both alter the tibiofemoral contact area and stress when compared with the intact knee. When compared with the TT technique, ACLR by the AM portal technique more closely restores the intact tibiofemoral contact area and stress at low flexion angles.

Keywords: Anterior cruciate ligament reconstruction, Transtibial technique, Anteromedial portal technique, Tibiofemoral, Contact area, Contact stress

* Correspondence: lizhongli@263.net
†Chunhui Liu and Yingpeng Wang contributed equally to this work.
[1]Department of Orthopedics, General Hospital of PLA, No. 28 Fuxing Road, Haidian District, Beijing 100853, China
Full list of author information is available at the end of the article

Background

Among the current methods of anterior cruciate ligament reconstruction (ACLR), single-bundle(SB) reconstruction is performed by most surgeons [1, 2]. During single-bundle ACLR, femoral tunnel location plays an important role in restoring the intact knee mechanisms, whereas malplacement of the tunnel was cited as the most common cause of knee instability [3–5]. As a result, the best location of the femoral tunnel during single-bundle ACLR is subject to extensive exploration with the development of anatomic studies [6–9]. There are mainly two methods for femoral tunnel creation: transtibial versus anteromedial portal techniques. The current femoral tunnel preparation focus has shifted from the TT method(with femoral tunnel location at the "over-the-top" position approximately 11 o'clock in the femoral notch of the right knee) toward the independent drilling method(with the femoral tunnel location at the center of the AM bundle of the ACL footprint approximately 9 o'clock in the femoral notch of the right knee) with restoration of the native ACL knee kinematics. The use of the AM portal drilling technique has increased in recent years from 68% of surgeons using this technique in 2013 [1] to 89.6% in 2016 [2]. Although the anatomic single-bundle ACLR procedure is currently in use, it remains controversial whether the AM technique is biomechanically superior compared with the TT method. Investigators focusing on the femoral tunnel position have shown improvements in knee stability by placing the femoral tunnel into the native femoral footprint [5, 10–12]. However, not all of the results supported the advantages of anatomical reconstruction. Other studies have demonstrated that no significant knee kinematic changes were found between the TT versus AM portal drilling techniques [13–15].In addition, two meta-analyses showed that there were no significant clinical differences found between the two techniques [13, 16]. As a result of these conflicting outcomes, the best technique of femoral tunnel creation for restoring intact knee kinematics remains unclear. Therefore, the purposes of this study were (1) to quantify the effect of two femoral tunnel creation methods on the tibiofemoral joint contact area and stress after single-bundle ACL reconstruction, (2) to identify the optimal femoral tunnel creation method, and (3) to give new evidence to the present conflicting results. The hypothesis was that SB ACLR by the use of the AM portal method would better restore the intact tibiofemoral contact area and stress compared with the TT method.

Methods

Preparation of cadaveric knees

Seven intact fresh-frozen human cadaveric knees (mean age, 58 years; range, 46 to 71 years,4 males and 3 females) without macroscopic degenerative changes were used in this study. Lateral and anteroposterior X-ray films were taken for each knee with the aim of assessing signs of osteoarthritis or bony deformities. No cadaveric knees were excluded from the study. The specimens were stored in sealed plastic bags at − 20 °C and thawed 24 h at room temperature when they were prepared to be tested. The gracilis and semitendinosus tendons were harvested from each knee for ACL reconstruction. The proximal tibia and distal femur were then cut approximately 20 cm from the joint line. The skin and all subcutaneous tissues were removed, leaving all but the posterior portion of the joint capsule, with the cruciate and collateral ligaments intact. The soft tissues 13 to 15 cm away from the joint line were subsequently cut off so that the proximal and distal bones were exposed not less than 5 cm [5]. The proximal and distal bone stumps were then embedded in custom-made plastic cylinders using acrylic resin polymer (Anyang Eagle Dental Material Co., Ltd., Products, China, Anyang City). The femoral cylinder was fixed to the top of the testing machine using custom-made fixtures, while the tibial cylinder was connected to a specially designed knee simulator that allows 6 degrees of freedom of movement of the knee (anterior-posterior, medial-lateral, and internal rotation-external rotation) (Fig. 1).

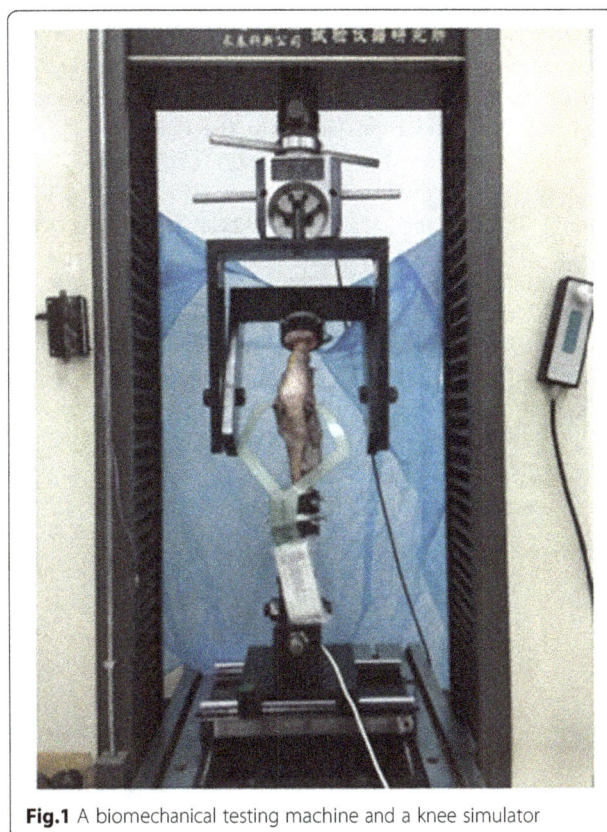

Fig.1 A biomechanical testing machine and a knee simulator

Normal gait simulator

For this study, combined external conditions simulating normal gait were applied to the knee: (1) considering that some of the specimens were skinny, an axial load of 1000 N was applied by a biomechanical testing machine (Electronic Universal Material Testing Machine, WDW4100, China, Changchun City) from the femoral side to the tibia along the direction of the tibial longitudinal axis (2) at 0°, 10°, 20°, and 30°of knee flexion. This protocol was based on the work of Kumar et al. and Kutzner et al. [17, 18] in which the authors analyzed the tibiofemoral reactive stress that the knee experiences during normal gait. The custom-designed knee simulator allows 6 degrees of freedom of movement of the knee that can simulate the normal gait closely. For knee flexion, the flexion angles were achieved by moving the femur on the sagittal plane locked in position by two screw fixtures at each side of the normal gait simulator. The axial testing machine and knee simulator helped to achieve these goals perfectly (Fig. 1).

Tibiofemoral contact area and stress measurement

Stress-sensitive film (K-Scan 4000, Tekscan Inc., Boston, MA) of 0.1 mm was used in this system. Before insertion into the joint spaces, the sensors were calibrated according to the standardized protocols provided by the manufacturer [19]. An incision between the meniscus and femoral condyle was made along the joint line through the anteromedial and anterolateral arthrotomy. The film was then carefully inserted into the joint and then spread on top of the cartilage and the meniscus [20]. The contact area and peak and mean stress in the tibiofemoral joint were measured at the knee flexion angles of 0°, 10°, 20°,and 30° combined with axial load simulating the joint motion during normal walking [21]. The knees were loaded axially for 20 cycles to simulate various phases of

the gait cycle for each testing condition and flexion angle. To assess changes in the tibiofemoral contact area and stress, the same external conditions previously applied to the intact knees were again applied to the ACLR knees, and the results were measured. The experimental testing system is shown in Fig. 2.

Surgical procedures and testing groups

Graft preparation and fixation

The distal 3 cm of the semitendinosus and gracilis tendon grafts were stitched by a polyester thread (No. 5 TiCron suture, Covidien plc, Dublin, Ireland) and placed on a tensioning board under the tension of 10 N for 15 min. Subsequently, a 15- to 30-mm EndoButton CL was used to suspend at the middle of the semitendinosus and gracilis tendons, and then the grafts were folded into four bundles with a diameter of 7–8 mm. The graft in the femoral tunnel was suspended fixed by the use of the EndoButton CL (Smith & Nephew Endoscopy). After 10 flexion-extension cycles under 80 N of graft tension, the graft fixation at the tibial side was accomplished under 30° of knee flexion with the maintained tension [22] by the use of an interference screw (Arthrex, Naples, FL). The interference screw diameter was 1 mm up from the graft. The graft was then released by loosening the tibial screw after biomechanical testing of the first reconstruction, and the first femoral tunnel was backfilled with bone cement (Link, Germany). The alternate femoral tunnel was then drilled, partially overlapping the first tunnel occasionally. The two methods of femoral tunnel creation were performed in an alternating order, with the aim of randomizing the possible influences of previous reconstructions [22]. The graft fixation methods were subsequently repeated to perform the second reconstruction with the same graft with one exception: previous screws were substituted for 1-mm up

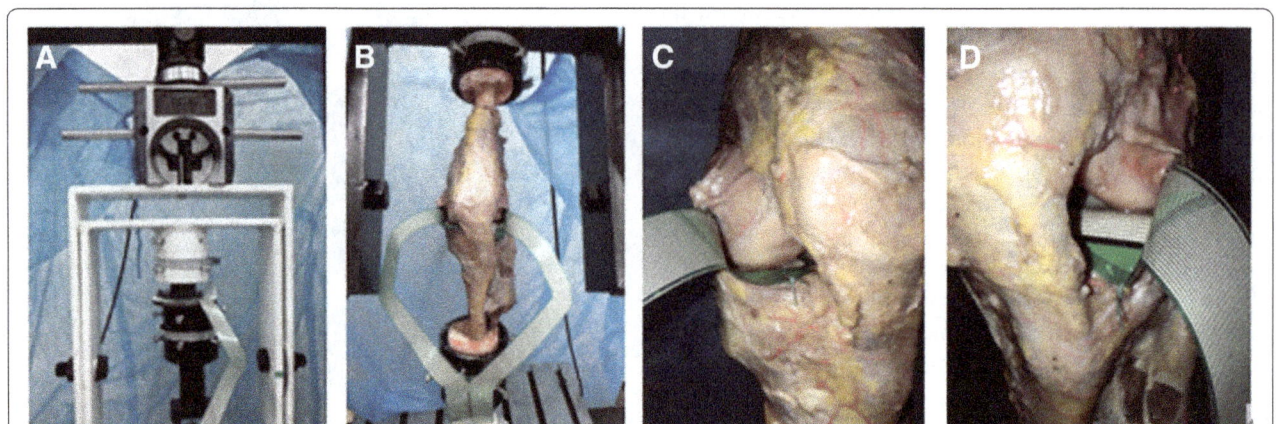

Fig. 2 The experimental testing system (a sensor was calibrated according to the standardized protocols provided by the manufacturer (**a**), a left knee mounted onto the machine (**b**), a film was carefully inserted into the joint and then spread on top of the cartilage and the meniscus (**c**, **d**)) presented in this study with a left knee

screws in the tibia to compensate for any bone tunnel deformity that may have occurred during the initial reconstruction [23]. We used the same graft for the limited source of the tendon. We placed the tendons on a tensioning board under the tension of 10 N for 15 min in order to reduce the difference caused by reuse.

Tibial tunnel preparation for the initial reconstruction

The tibial tunnel was placed using a commercial tibial ACL guide (Smith & Nephew, ACUFEX DIRECTOR™ Drill Guide) set at 55°with the tip aimed at the center of the tibial footprint of the ACL and the sleeve positioned at the midpoint of the anterior margin of the medial collateral ligament and the medial margin of the tibial tubercle [24]. A K-wire was drilled into the tibia along the ACL guide, and a tibial tunnel was then reamed over by the use of a cannulated drill along the K-wire. The tunnel diameter was finally created with regard to the graft diameter prepared previously.

SB-TT technique group

For the TT method of ACL reconstruction, the inside entrance of the femoral tunnel was located using an offset guide (EndoButton Guide; Smith & Nephew), which was passed through the tibial tunnel and hooked at the "over-the-top" position, assuring that the posterior edge of the femoral tunnel was placed 2 mm anterior from the posterior edge of the intercondylar notch. With the aim of positioning the guidewire for the most possible approximation of the anatomic femoral ACL footprint, the offset guide was then laterally rotated [24]. After the desirable position was located, a guidewire was drilled into the femur, and then a 4.5-mm-diameter cannulated drill (EndoButton Drill; Smith & Nephew Endoscopy) was reamed along the guidewire until it pierced through the femoral cortex. The length of the graft inserted into the tunnel was not less than 15 cm and was decided by the total femoral tunnel length measured by a depth probe (Depth Probe; Smith & Nephew Endoscopy). A blunt head reamer was then used to create a graft diameter femoral tunnel with 10 mm more than the inserted graft length. The graft fixation technique described previously was used finally to accomplish the SB-ACLR.

SB-AM portal technique group

The AM portal method was performed by the use of an offset guide inserted through the independent AM portal. The hook of the femoral offset guide was placed behind the posterior notch and adjusted in order to place the pointer at the center of the femoral AM bundle footprint of the ACL at 90°of knee flexion. The knee was then flexed to 110°, and a 2.4-mm guidewire was drilled into the lateral condyle with the offset guide. The femoral tunnel preparation for EndoButton fixation was then accomplished, as described above. The graft fixation was performed as described previously.

The testing groups were as follows: intact knee group, SB-TT technique reconstruction group and SB-AM portal technique reconstruction group. These specimens were reused for ACL-R (TT and AM).

Statistical analyses

Because all variables were measured within each specimen, the tibiofemoral contact area and stress data were analyzed using a two-way analysis of variance (SPSS, version 17.0 Chicago, IL). This analysis has the advantage of minimized specimen variability and being very sensitive to relative changes occurring within an individual knee. Multiple contrasts were detected by the post hoc Tukey multiple comparisons test for all experiments performed on the same knee at each knee flexion angle tested. $P < .05$ was set as the level of significance a priori.

Results

Tibiofemoral contact area

Compared with the intact ACL group, the tibiofemoral contact area was decreased in the AM portal ACLR group at 20° and 30° of flexion on both the medial and lateral compartments, respectively ($P = .004$ for medial at 20°, $P = .014$ for medial at 30°, $P = .001$ for lateral at 20°, and $P = .01$ for lateral at 30°). For the TT ACL-reconstructed knees, a significantly decreased tibiofemoral contact area was also observed at 20° and 30° of flexion on both the medial and lateral compartments, respectively($P < .001$ for medial at 20°, $P = .001$ for medial at 30°, $P < .001$ for lateral at 20°, and $P = .038$ for lateral at 30°). Both the AM portal and TT ACLR groups showed no significant difference from the intact ACL group at 0° and 10°, respectively, of knee flexion. When comparing the contact area between the two ACLR groups, however, a significantly decreased contact area was detected in the TT ACL-reconstructed knees at 20° of knee flexion on the medial compartment ($P = .047$) (Fig. 3). There were no significant differences between the TT and AM portal ACL-reconstructed knees on the medial contact area at other angles of flexion and the lateral contact area at all angles of flexion. The values for the contact area are shown in Table 1.

Mean tibiofemoral stress

For the AM portal ACL-reconstructed knees, there were no significant differences in mean tibiofemoral stress from the intact knees on both the lateral and medial knee joint compartments, except at 20° of flexion ($P = .045$ for medial and $P = .006$ for lateral). The TT ACLR group showed a higher mean stress at 20° and 30° of flexion on the medial compartment and at 20° of flexion on the lateral compartment compared with the intact ACL group ($P = .001$ for medial at 20°, $P = .003$ for

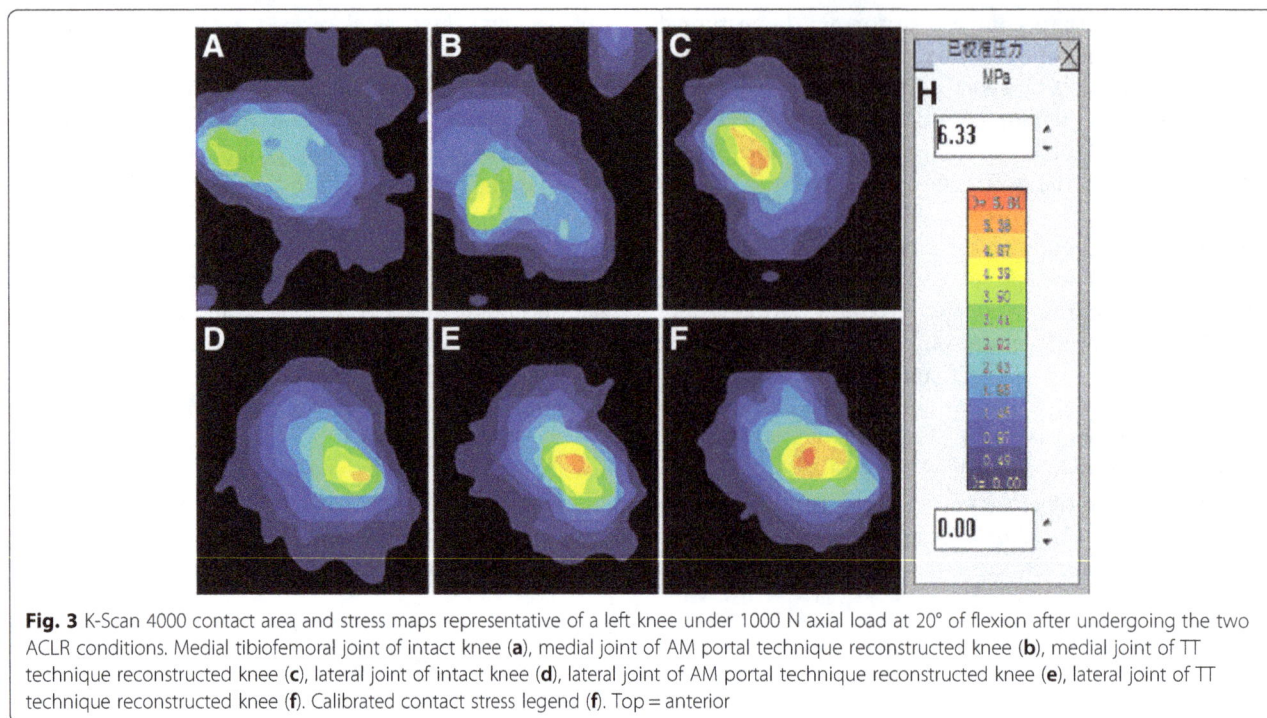

Fig. 3 K-Scan 4000 contact area and stress maps representative of a left knee under 1000 N axial load at 20° of flexion after undergoing the two ACLR conditions. Medial tibiofemoral joint of intact knee (**a**), medial joint of AM portal technique reconstructed knee (**b**), medial joint of TT technique reconstructed knee (**c**), lateral joint of intact knee (**d**), lateral joint of AM portal technique reconstructed knee (**e**), lateral joint of TT technique reconstructed knee (**f**). Calibrated contact stress legend (**f**). Top = anterior

medial at 30°, and $P < .001$ for lateral at 20°), but no significant differences at 0° and 10°of flexion on the medial compartment and at 0°, 10°, and 30° of flexion on the lateral compartment were found. When comparing the mean tibiofemoral stress between the two ACLR groups, however, no significant differences were observed at all angles of knee flexion on both the medial and lateral compartments (Fig. 3). The values for mean stress are shown in Fig. 4.

Maximum tibiofemoral stress
When compared with the intact ACL, the AM portal ACLR altered the maximum stress only on the lateral joint compartment at 20°of flexion($P = .022$) (Fig. 3). No significant differences were observed at other angles of flexion on the lateral compartment and at all angles of flexion on the medial compartment. For the TT ACL-reconstructed knees, a higher maximum stress was

detected at 20° of flexion on both the lateral and medial compartments ($P = .047$ for medial and $P = .005$ for lateral) (Fig. 5). There were no significant differences at all in other flexion angles when compared with the intact ACL knees. Although no significant differences were observed at all angles of knee flexion on both the medial and lateral compartments when comparing the maximum tibiofemoral stress between the two ACLR groups, the results of AM portal ACLR knees were more similar to the intact knees. The values for maximum stress are shown in Fig. 5.

Discussion
In this study, the tibiofemoral joint contact area and stress of the knees after ACL reconstruction by the AM portal and TT techniques were measured and compared. Specifically, the experimental data collected from the same cadaveric knee specimen under different experimental

Table 1 Contact area results in intact and two different reconstruction groups

	Contact area (mm^2) (mean ± SD)					
	Medial tibiofemoral joint			Lateral tibiofemoral joint		
	Intact ACL	AM portal technique	TT technique	Intact ACL	AM portal technique	TT technique
0°	515.29 ± 123.43	467.86 ± 119	461.43 ± 117.62	390.29 ± 99.75	358.71 ± 72.86	363.71 ± 79.64
10°	501.71 ± 105.26	456.29 ± 97.68	432.86 ± 101.89	378.14 ± 102.55	335.29 ± 77.98	326.71 ± 76.22
20°	454.57 ± 104.83	381 ± 79.89*	332.86 ± 76.76*■	358.14 ± 70.11	305.43 ± 72.48*	285 ± 57.51*
30°	445.71 ± 103.02	400.43 ± 92.16*	383.29 ± 100.17*	393.86 ± 79.26	353.86 ± 78.81*	362.14 ± 73.23*

Tibiofemoral contact area results in intact and two different reconstruction groups (intact, TT technique, and AM portal technique). Single asterisk (*) denotes the difference between the intact state with other states and square symbol (■) denotes the difference between TT technique and AM portal technique

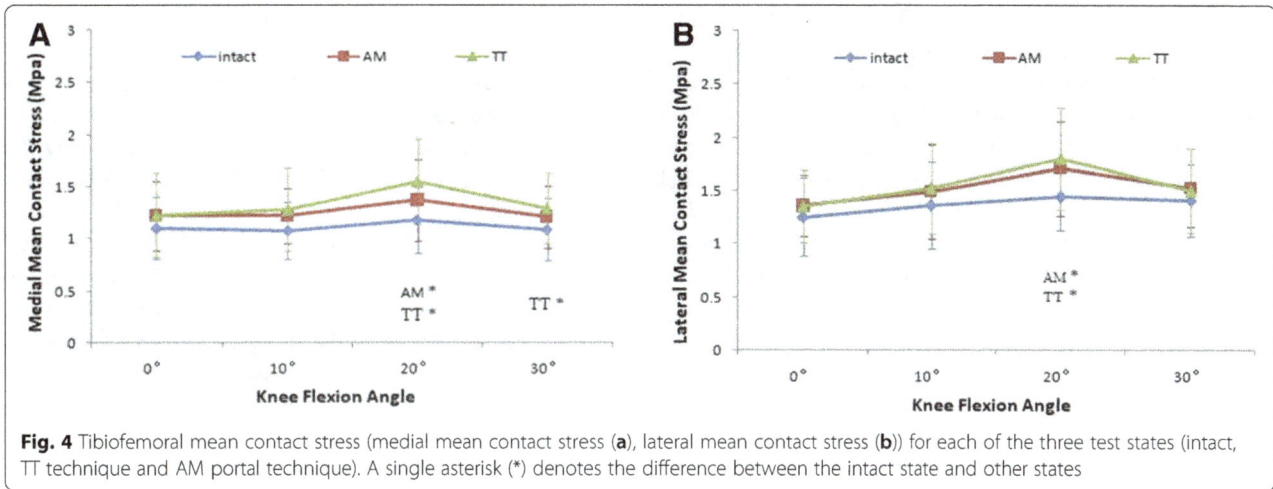

Fig. 4 Tibiofemoral mean contact stress (medial mean contact stress (**a**), lateral mean contact stress (**b**)) for each of the three test states (intact, TT technique and AM portal technique). A single asterisk (*) denotes the difference between the intact state and other states

conditions (ACL-intact and ACL-reconstructed with TT and AMP methods) reduced the effect of interspecimen variation [5]. The results supported that SB ACL reconstruction via the AM portal technique restored the tibiofemoral joint contact area and stress more closely to the intact knee than SB ACL reconstruction via the TT technique. Until now, there have been few studies comparing the changes in tibiofemoral contact mechanics between TT and AM portal ACLR groups to the authors' knowledge. In one prior study, Lee et al. [25] investigated the contact area and stress in knees with serial posterior medial meniscectomies. In Lee et al., the outcomes of contact area, mean contact stress, and peak contact stress, which were measured in intact knees, were similar to our studies. Another prior study has evaluated the effects of SB ACLR and double-bundle ACLR. In that study, Morimoto et al. [26] tested knees after undergoing SB ACLR and double-bundle ACLR and pointed out that SB ACL reconstruction resulted in a significantly smaller tibiofemoral

contact area and higher stress. The peak stress and contact areas measured in their study were also comparable to our data in intact ACL knees, while the mean contact stress reported is higher than our outcomes. This difference may be explained by the type of stress-sensor used in the joint space. And the various experimental conditions and methods for measuring knee contact stress made the comparisons between studies complicated. In their study, the TT or AM portal method was used for femoral tunnel placing. However, in our experience, the femoral tunnel position cannot be placed at the center of the AM bundle position via the TT method. Nevertheless, our study confirms the observation that the SB ACLR condition resulted in decreasing contact area and increasing mean tibiofemoral contact stress and peak contact stress compared with the intact knee.

The alternation of the tibiofemoral joint contact area and stress in reconstructed knees may be caused by the mismatch of the tibiofemoral joint during knee movement

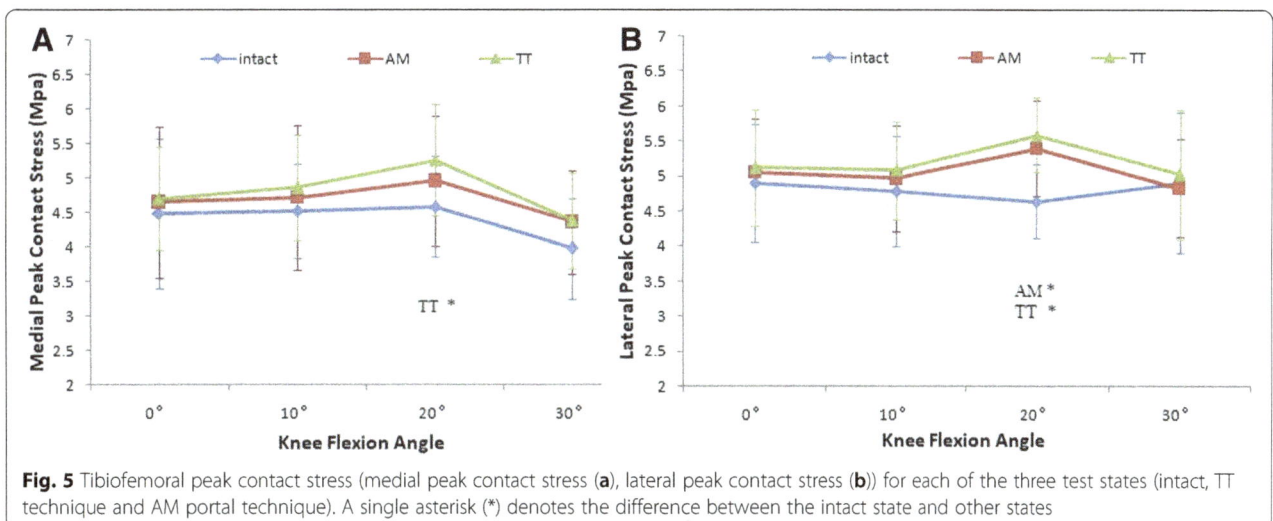

Fig. 5 Tibiofemoral peak contact stress (medial peak contact stress (**a**), lateral peak contact stress (**b**)) for each of the three test states (intact, TT technique and AM portal technique). A single asterisk (*) denotes the difference between the intact state and other states

procedures compared with intact knees. And the reconstructed ACL, which cannot provide original biomechanics compared with the original ACL, may have resulted in the mismatch of the tibiofemoral joint. Anatomic studies of the ACL indicated that the ligament consists of two grossly distinguishable components: the anteromedial (AM) bundle and posterolateral (PL) bundle [27, 28]. Comparing the in situ forces between the two bundles, the PL bundle has higher in situ forces from full extension to 30° of flexion, whereas the AM bundle has higher in situ forces from 30° of flexion to further flexion under anterior tibial loads [29]. The PL bundle also shows an important role, especially at lower flexion angles under rotatory loads [30]. Such anatomic complexity of the ACL cannot be restored by non-anatomic SB ACLR, which may alter the tibiofemoral joint matching relationship during knee movement procedures and results in a significant alternation of the tibiofemoral joint contact area and stress.

The alternation of the tibiofemoral joint contact area and stress between SB ACL- reconstructed knees via TT versus AM portal drilling techniques may be caused by different femoral tunnel positions. Previous studies indicated that the tunnel location plays an important role in ACL reconstruction, and small variations in the femoral tunnel placement significantly influence the resulting knee kinematics and clinical outcomes [10, 22, 31–33]. Biomechanical studies using cadavers indicated that the AM portal technique placed the femoral tunnel more closely to the anatomic femoral footprint [24, 34, 35], and this may be the reason why SB ACLR by the use of the AM portal method more closely restores the intact tibiofemoral contact area and stress compared with the TT method. There are numerous studies that indicated that the AM portal technique reconstruction provided better rotatory stability at low flexion angles [36–38] without sacrificing anteroposterior stability compared with TT ACL reconstruction [10, 39–42]. Guler et al. [34] and Lee et al. [43] evaluated the femoral tunnel positions created by the AM portal or TT technique in their study and indicated that the AM portal technique is superior to the TT technique in terms of anatomical graft positioning. In a meta-analysis, Riboh et al. [16] reported that there are biomechanical data suggesting improved knee stability and more anatomic graft placement with independent drilling. This literature may also help to explain the superiority of the AM portal technique reconstruction, which better restored the normal knee kinematics, resulting in closer normal contact area and stress, when compared with TT technique reconstruction.

Other studies also have shown that the ACL reconstruction by the use of the TT technique could not effectively prevent the prevalence of secondary knee OA [44–48]. Leiter et al. [49] shown in their meta-analysis that

ACL-reconstructed knees using the TT technique had a higher incidence of normal and serious OA than control knees, especially in patients combined with medial meniscus repair or excision. Hart et al. [48] reported in their article that the patellar tender ACL reconstruction using the TT method did not lead to prevention of the occurrence of radiological OA after 10 years by the use of the Kellgren and Fairbank classifications. Janssen et al. [50] found that the radiological signs of OA were detected in 53.5% of the patients with transtibial ACL reconstruction using four-strand hamstring autograft at the 10-year follow-up. However, all of the studies mentioned above were based on the TT technique of ACL reconstruction. With regard to ACL reconstruction using the AM portal method, there are some studies that indicated that anatomic ACL reconstruction showed favorable results regarding OA [51, 52]. Alentorn-Geli et al. [13] indicated in their study that patients in the TT ACLR group had greater long-term knee osteoarthritic changes (greater space narrowing) compared with the AM portal ACLR group when the radiographic parameters were statistically analyzed with a KT-1000 arthrometer. According to Wolff's law, osteoclasia and bone resorption may be triggered by a low bone stress and an overloading bone stress [53]. Therefore, the ACL reconstructed knee with altered contact area and stress may result in undesirable bone remodeling and predisposition of the knee joint, which finally lead to the occurrence of OA. In this study, ACL reconstruction using the AM portal technique better restored the normal tibial-femoral contact area and stress when compared with the TT technique and may help to explain the favorable results regarding the OA after AM portal technique ACL reconstruction. However, there are too few studies to confirm whether the ACL reconstruction using the AM portal technique will better prevent the occurrence of knee arthritis, and long-term clinical follow-up studies are necessary to verify our hypothesis.

Limitations

As for the limitations of this study, the number of cadaveric knees used in the experiment was relatively limited, and the donor age and specimen tissue quality were variable. Another limitation of this study is the reuse of the specimens, both the grafts and cemented femoral condyles. Reusing the graft after it has already been tested and fixated on the tibia via screws may have led to some compromising of the tissue itself. The additional cycling will also introduce some additional creep between the tests. Besides, due to the lack of freedom of the varus/valgus moment, a slight deviation of varus/valgus positioning may have resulted in an unequal load between the medial and lateral compartments when putting and positioning the knee into the knee simulator. Moreover, this controlled laboratory experiment cannot simulate muscle load, and we conducted an extensive soft tissue dissection to the posteromedial capsule in order to insert the Tekscan stress sensors, which may be different from the in vivo research. Although all of the conditions mentioned above may affect the knee joint contact area and stress, the conclusions of this study remain valid; the main purpose was to observe the biomechanical variations of the two ACLR conditions within each specimen.

Conclusions

SB ACLR by the use of the AM portal method and TT method both alter the tibiofemoral contact area and stress when compared with the intact knee. When compared with the TT technique, ACLR by the AM portal technique more closely restores the intact tibiofemoral contact area and stress at low flexion angles.

Abbreviations

ACL: Anterior cruciate ligament; ACLR: Anterior cruciate ligament reconstruction; AM: Anteromedial; SB: Single-bundle; TT: Transtibial

Acknowledgements

The authors acknowledge Jinfeng Li, Yu Wei, Yichen Zhu, and Ketao Wang who contributed toward the analysis and interpretation of data involved in drafting the manuscript.

Authors' contributions

CH carried out the data analysis and drafted the manuscript. ZL conceived of the study, participated in its design and coordination, and helped to draft the manuscript. YP and JL participated in the design of the study and performed the statistical analysis. HZ, KZ, and YM helped to collect data and performed the statistical analysis. All authors have been actively involved in the drafting and critical revision of the manuscript, and each provided final approval of the version to be published.

Competing interests

The authors declare that they have no competing interests.

Author details

[1]Department of Orthopedics, General Hospital of PLA, No. 28 Fuxing Road, Haidian District, Beijing 100853, China. [2]School of Biomedical Engineering, Capital Medical University, Beijing 100069, China.

References

1. Chechik O, Ama E, Khashan M, Lador R, Eyal G, Gold A. An international survey on anterior cruciate ligament reconstruction practices. Int Orthop. 2013;37:201–6.
2. Vaishya R, Agarwal AK, Ingole S, Vijay V. Current practice variations in the management of anterior cruciate ligament injuries in Delhi. J Clin Orthop Trauma. 2016;7:193–9.
3. Marchant BG, Noyes FR, Barber-Westin SD, Fleckenstein C. Prevalence of nonanatomical graft placement in a series of failed anterior cruciate ligament reconstructions. Am J Sports Med. 2010;38:1987–96.
4. Diamantopoulos AP, Lorbach O, Paessler HH. Anterior cruciate ligament revision reconstruction: results in 107 patients. Am J Sports Med. 2008;36:851–60.
5. Loh JC, Fukuda Y, Tsuda E, Steadman RJ, Fu FH, Woo SL. Knee stability and graft function following anterior cruciate ligament reconstruction: comparison between 11 o'clock and 10 o'clock femoral tunnel placement. Arthroscopy. 2003;19:297–304.
6. Mochizuki T, Muneta T, Nagase T, Shirasawa S, Akita KI, Sekiya I. Cadaveric knee observation study for describing anatomic femoral tunnel placement for two-bundle anterior cruciate ligament reconstruction. Arthroscopy. 2006;22:356–61.
7. Dhaher YY, Salehghaffari S, Adouni M. Anterior laxity, graft-tunnel interaction and surgical design variations during anterior cruciate ligament reconstruction: a probabilistic simulation of the surgery. J Biomech. 2016;49:3009–16.
8. Au AG, Raso VJ, Liggins AB, Otto DD, Amirfazli A. A three-dimensional finite element stress analysis for tunnel placement and buttons in anterior cruciate ligament reconstructions. J Biomech. 2005;38:827–32.
9. Salehghaffari S, Dhaher YY. A phenomenological contact model: understanding the graft-tunnel interaction in anterior cruciate ligament reconstructive surgery. J Biomech. 2015;48:1844–51.
10. Musahl V, Plakseychuk A, VanScyoc A, et al. Varying femoral tunnels between the anatomical footprint and isometric positions: effect on kinematics of the anterior cruciate ligament-reconstructed knee. Am J Sports Med. 2005;33:712–8.
11. Scopp JM, Jasper LE, Belkoff SM, Moorman CT. The effect of oblique femoral tunnel placement on rotational constraint of the knee reconstructed using patellar tendon autografts. Arthroscopy. 2004;20:294–9.
12. Yamamoto Y, Hsu WH, Woo SL, Van Scyoc AH, Takakura Y, Debski RE. Knee stability and graft function after anterior cruciate ligament reconstruction: a comparison of a lateral and an anatomical femoral tunnel placement. Am J Sports Med. 2004;32:1825–32.
13. Alentorn-Geli E, Lajara F, Samitier G, Cugat R. The transtibial versus the anteromedial portal technique in the arthroscopic bone-patellar tendon-bone anterior cruciate ligament reconstruction. Knee Surg Sports Traumatol Arthrosc. 2010;18:1013–37.
14. Asai S, Maeyama A, Hoshino Y, et al. A comparison of dynamic rotational knee instability between anatomic single-bundle and over-the-top anterior cruciate ligament reconstruction using triaxial accelerometry. Knee Surg Sports Traumatol Arthrosc. 2014;22:972–8.
15. Markolf KL, Jackson SR, Mcallister DR. A comparison of 11 o'clock versus oblique femoral tunnels in the anterior cruciate ligament-reconstructed knee: knee kinematics during a simulated pivot test. Am J Sports Med. 2010;38:912–7.
16. Riboh JC, Hasselblad V, Godin JA, Mather RC. Transtibial versus independent drilling techniques for anterior cruciate ligament reconstruction: a systematic review, meta-analysis, and meta-regression. Am J Sports Med. 2013;41:2693–702.
17. Kutzner I, Heinlein B, Graichen F, et al. Loading of the knee joint during activities of daily living measured in vivo in five subjects. J Biomech. 2010;43:2164–73.
18. Kumar D, Manal KT, Rudolph KS. Knee joint loading during gait in healthy controls and individuals with knee osteoarthritis. Osteoarthr Cartil. 2013;21:298–305.
19. Beamer BS, Walley KC, Okajima S, et al. Changes in contact area in meniscus horizontal cleavage tears subjected to repair and resection. Arthroscopy. 2017;33:617–24.

20. Agneskirchner JD, Hurschler C, Stukenborg-Colsman C, Imhoff AB, Lobenhoffer P. Effect of high tibial flexion osteotomy on cartilage stress and joint kinematics: a biomechanical study in human cadaveric knees. Arch Orthop Trauma Surg. 2004;124:575–84.

21. Bedi A, Kelly NM, Fox AJ, et al. Dynamic contact mechanics of the medial meniscus as a function of radial tear, repair, and partial meniscectomy. J Bone Joint Surg Am. 2010;92:1398–408.

22. Herbort M, Domnick C, Raschke MJ, et al. Comparison of knee kinematics after single-bundle anterior cruciate ligament reconstruction via the medial portal technique with a central femoral tunnel and an eccentric femoral tunnel and after anatomic double-bundle reconstruction a human cadaveric study. Am J Sports Med. 2016;44:126–32.

23. Driscoll MD, Isabell GP Jr, Conditt MA et al. Comparison of 2 femoral tunnel locations in anatomic single-bundle anterior cruciate ligament reconstruction: a biomechanical study[J]. Arthroscopy 2012, 28(10): 1481–1489.

24. Gadikota HR, Sim JA, Hosseini A, Gill TJ, Li G. The relationship between femoral tunnels created by the transtibial, anteromedial portal, and outside-in techniques and the anterior cruciate ligament footprint. Am J Sports Med. 2012;40:882–8.

25. Lee SJ, Aadalen KJ, Malaviya P, et al. Tibiofemoral contact mechanics after serial medial meniscectomies in the human cadaveric knee. Am J Sports Med. 2006;34:1334–44.

26. Morimoto Y, Ferretti M, Ekdahl M, Smolinski P, Fu FH. Tibiofemoral joint contact area and stress after single- and double-bundle anterior cruciate ligament reconstruction. Arthroscopy. 2009;25:62–9.

27. Clark JM, Sidles JA. The interrelation of fiber bundles in the anterior cruciate ligament. J Orthop Res. 1990;8:180–8.

28. Colombet P, Robinson J, Christel P, et al. Morphology of anterior cruciate ligament attachments for anatomic reconstruction: a cadaveric dissection and radiographic study. Arthroscopy. 2006;22:984–92.

29. Sakane M, Fox RJ, Woo SL, Livesay GA, Li G, Fu FH. In situ forces in the anterior cruciate ligament and its bundles in response to anterior tibial loads. J Orthop Res. 1997;15:285–93.

30. Gabriel MT, Wong EK, Woo SL, Yagi M, Debski RE. Distribution of in situ forces in the anterior cruciate ligament in response to rotatory loads. J Orthop Res. 2004;22:85–9.

31. Bedi A, Musahl V, O'Loughlin P, et al. A comparison of the effect of central anatomical single-bundle anterior cruciate ligament reconstruction and double-bundle anterior cruciate ligament reconstruction on pivot-shift kinematics. Am J Sports Med. 2010;38:1788–94.

32. Zaffagnini S, Bruni D, Martelli S, Imakiire N, Marcacci M, Russo A. Double-bundle ACL reconstruction: influence of femoral tunnel orientation in knee laxity analysed with a navigation system – an in-vitro biomechanical study. BMC Musculoskelet Disord. 2008;9:25.

33. Bedi A, Musahl V, Steuber V, et al. Transtibial versus anteromedial portal reaming in anterior cruciate ligament reconstruction: an anatomic and biomechanical evaluation of surgical technique. Arthroscopy. 2011;27: 380–90.

34. Guler O, Mahırogulları M, Mutlu S, Cerci MH, Seker A, Cakmak S. Graft position in arthroscopic anterior cruciate ligament reconstruction: anteromedial versus transtibial technique. Arch Orthop Trauma Surg. 2016;136:1–10.

35. Robin BN, Lubowitz JH. Disadvantages and advantages of transtibial technique for creating the anterior cruciate ligament femoral socket. J Knee Surg. 2014;27:327–30.

36. Franceschi F, Papalia R, Rizzello G, Del Buono A, Maffulli N, Denaro V. Anteromedial portal versus transtibial drilling techniques in anterior cruciate ligament reconstruction: any clinical relevance? A retrospective comparative study. Arthroscopy. 2013;29:1330–7.

37. Seo SS, Kim CW, Kim JG, Jin SY. Clinical results comparing transtibial technique and outside in technique in single bundle anterior cruciate ligament reconstruction. Knee Surg Relat Res. 2013;25:133–40.

38. Wang H, Fleischli JE, Zheng NN. Transtibial versus anteromedial portal technique in single-bundle anterior cruciate ligament reconstruction: outcomes of knee joint kinematics during walking. Am J Sports Med. 2013; 41:1847–56.

39. Tudisco C, Bisicchia S. Drilling the femoral tunnel during ACL reconstruction: transtibial versus anteromedial portal techniques. Orthopedics. 2012;35:1166–72.

40. Kato Y, Maeyama A, Lertwanich P, et al. Biomechanical comparison of different graft positions for single-bundle anterior cruciate ligament reconstruction. Knee Surg Sports Traumatol Arthrosc. 2013;21:816–23.

41. Sim JA, Gadikota HR, Li JS, Li G, Gill TJ. Biomechanical evaluation of knee joint laxities and graft forces after anterior cruciate ligament reconstruction by anteromedial portal, outside-in, and transtibial techniques. Am J Sports Med. 2011;39:2604–10.

42. Steiner ME, Battaglia TC, Heming JF, Rand JD, Festa A, Baria M. Independent drilling outperforms conventional transtibial drilling in anterior cruciate ligament reconstruction. Am J Sports Med. 2009;37:1912–9.

43. Lee DH, Kim HJ, Ahn HS, Bin SI. Comparison of femur tunnel aperture location in patients undergoing transtibial and anatomical single-bundle anterior cruciate ligament reconstruction. Knee Surg Sports Traumatol Arthrosc. 2016;24:3713–21.

44. Holm I, Oiestad BE, Risberg MA, Aune AK. No difference in knee function or prevalence of osteoarthritis after reconstruction of the anterior cruciate ligament with 4-strand hamstring autograft versus patellar tendon-bone autograft: a randomized study with 10-year follow-up. Am J Sports Med. 2010;38:448–54.

45. Kessler MA, Behrend H, Henz S, Stutz G, Rukavina A, Kuster MS. Function, osteoarthritis and activity after ACL-rupture: 11 years follow-up results of conservative versus reconstructive treatment. Knee Surg Sports Traumatol Arthrosc. 2008;16:442–8.

46. Qiestad BE, Holm I, Engebretsen L, Risberg MA. The association between radiographic knee osteoarthritis and knee symptoms, function and quality of life 10-15 years after anterior cruciate ligament reconstruction. Br J Sports Med. 2011;45:583–8.

47. Lohmander LS, Östenberg A, Englund M, Roos H. High prevalence of knee osteoarthritis, pain, and functional limitations in female soccer players twelve years after anterior cruciate ligament injury. Arthritis Rheum. 2004;50: 3145–52.

48. van der Hart CP, van den Bekerom MPJ, Patt TW. The occurrence of osteoarthritis at a minimum of ten years after reconstruction of the anterior cruciate ligament. J Orthop Surg. 2008;3:24.

49. Leiter JRS, Gourlay R, McRae S, de Korompay N, MacDonald PB. Long-term follow-up of ACL reconstruction with hamstring autograft. Knee Surg Sports Traumatol Arthrosc. 2014;22:1061–9.

50. Janssen RPA, du Mée AWF, van Valkenburg J, Sala HA, Tseng CM. Anterior cruciate ligament reconstruction with 4-strand hamstring autograft and accelerated rehabilitation: a 10-year prospective study on clinical results, knee osteoarthritis and its predictors. Knee Surg Sports Traumatol Arthrosc. 2013;21:1977–88.

51. Gerhard P, Bolt R, Duck K, Mayer R, Friederich NF, Hirschmann MT. Long-term results of arthroscopically assisted anatomical single bundle anterior cruciate ligament reconstruction using patellar tendon autograft: are there any predictors for the development of osteoarthritis? Knee Surg Sports Traumatol Arthrosc. 2013;21:957–64.

52. Wipfler B, Donner S, Zechmann CM, Springer J, Siebold R, Paessler HH. Anterior cruciate ligament reconstruction using patellar tendon versus hamstring tendon: a prospective comparative study with 9-year follow-up. Arthroscopy. 2011;27:653–65.

53. Frost HM. A 2003 update of bone physiology and Wolff's law for clinicians. Angle Orthod. 2004;74:3–15.

Permissions

All chapters in this book were first published in JOSR, by BioMed Central; hereby published with permission under the Creative Commons Attribution License or equivalent. Every chapter published in this book has been scrutinized by our experts. Their significance has been extensively debated. The topics covered herein carry significant findings which will fuel the growth of the discipline. They may even be implemented as practical applications or may be referred to as a beginning point for another development.

The contributors of this book come from diverse backgrounds, making this book a truly international effort. This book will bring forth new frontiers with its revolutionizing research information and detailed analysis of the nascent developments around the world.

We would like to thank all the contributing authors for lending their expertise to make the book truly unique. They have played a crucial role in the development of this book. Without their invaluable contributions this book wouldn't have been possible. They have made vital efforts to compile up to date information on the varied aspects of this subject to make this book a valuable addition to the collection of many professionals and students.

This book was conceptualized with the vision of imparting up-to-date information and advanced data in this field. To ensure the same, a matchless editorial board was set up. Every individual on the board went through rigorous rounds of assessment to prove their worth. After which they invested a large part of their time researching and compiling the most relevant data for our readers.

The editorial board has been involved in producing this book since its inception. They have spent rigorous hours researching and exploring the diverse topics which have resulted in the successful publishing of this book. They have passed on their knowledge of decades through this book. To expedite this challenging task, the publisher supported the team at every step. A small team of assistant editors was also appointed to further simplify the editing procedure and attain best results for the readers.

Apart from the editorial board, the designing team has also invested a significant amount of their time in understanding the subject and creating the most relevant covers. They scrutinized every image to scout for the most suitable representation of the subject and create an appropriate cover for the book.

The publishing team has been an ardent support to the editorial, designing and production team. Their endless efforts to recruit the best for this project, has resulted in the accomplishment of this book. They are a veteran in the field of academics and their pool of knowledge is as vast as their experience in printing. Their expertise and guidance has proved useful at every step. Their uncompromising quality standards have made this book an exceptional effort. Their encouragement from time to time has been an inspiration for everyone.

The publisher and the editorial board hope that this book will prove to be a valuable piece of knowledge for researchers, students, practitioners and scholars across the globe.

List of Contributors

Kuan-Ting Wu and Wen-Yi Chou
Department of Orthopaedic Surgery, Kaohsiung Chang Gung Memorial Hospital, No.123, Dapi Rd., Niaosong Dist., Kaohsiung city 833, Taiwan, Republic of China

Pei-Shan Lee and Shu-Hua Chen
Department of Orthopedics Operation Room, Kaohsiung Chang Gung Memorial Hospital, No.123, Dapi Rd., Niaosong Dist., Kaohsiung city 833, Taiwan, Republic of China

Yee-Tzu Huang
Department of Hospital and Health Care Administration, Chia Nan University of Pharmacy and Science, No.60, Sec. 1, Erren Rd., Rende Dist, Tainan city 717, Taiwan, Republic of China

Zhiqiang Zhang, Hao Li, Hai Li, Qing Fan, Xuan Yang, Pinquan Shen, Ting Chen, Qixun Cai, Jing Zhang and Ziming Zhang
Department of Pediatric Orthopedics, Xinhua Hospital, School of Medicine, Shanghai Jiao Tong University, 1665 Kongjiang Road, Yangpu District, Shanghai 20092, China

Michael Beverly and David Murray
Botnar Research Centre, Nuffield Department of Orthopaedics, Rheumatology and Musculoskeletal Sciences, University of Oxford, Nuffield Orthopaedic Centre, Headington, Oxford OX3 7LD, UK

Jae-Hwa Kim, Soohyun Lee, Kyunghun Jung and Wonchul Choi
Department of Orthopaedic Surgery, CHA Bundang Medical Center, CHA University, 351 Yatap-dong, Bundang-gu, Seongnam-si, Gyeonggi-do, Republic of Korea

Doo Hoe Ha and Sang Min Lee
Department of Radiology, CHA Bundang Medical Center, CHA University, 351 Yatap-dong, Bundang-gu, Seongnam-si, Gyeonggi-do, Republic of Korea

Yangquan Hao, Hao Guo, Zhaochen Xu and Chao Lu
Department of Osteonecrosis and Joint Reconstruction, Honghui Hospital Xi'an Jiao Tong University Health Science Center, No. 555 Youyi East Road, Xi'an, Shaanxi 710054, People's Republic of China

Handeng Qi, Yugui Wang, Jie Liu and Puwei Yuan
Shaanxi University of Chinese Medicine, Shiji Ave, New Economic Zone, Xi'an-Xianyang, Shaanxi 712046, People's Republic of China

Stavros Oikonomidis and Rolf Sobottke
Department of Orthopaedics and Trauma Surgery, Rhein-Maas Klinikum GmbH, Mauerfeldchen 25, 52146 Wuerselen, Germany
Department of Orthopaedics and Trauma Surgery, University Hospital Cologne, Joseph-Stelzmann-Str. 24, 50931 Cologne, Germany

Ghazi Ashqar and Thomas Kaulhausen
Department of Orthopaedics and Trauma Surgery, Rhein-Maas Klinikum GmbH, Mauerfeldchen 25, 52146 Wuerselen, Germany

Christian Herren
Department of Trauma and Reconstructive Surgery, University Hospital RWTH Aachen, Pauwelsstraße 30, 52074 Aachen, Germany

Jan Siewe
Department of Orthopaedics and Trauma Surgery, University Hospital Cologne, Joseph-Stelzmann-Str. 24, 50931 Cologne, Germany

Hai-Dong Li, Qiang-Hua Zhang, Shi-Tong Xing and Ji-Kang Min
Department of Spine Surgery, First People's Hospital affiliated to the Huzhou University Medical College, 158 GuangChang Hou Road, Huzhou, Zhejiang Province, China

Jian-Gang Shi and Xiong-Sheng Chen
Department of Spine Surgery, Changzheng Hospital, 415 Fengyang Road, Huangpu District, Shanghai, China

Qiang Liang, Guangwei Sun, Wenxin Ma, Jiandang Shi and Weidong Jin
Department of Spinal Surgery, General Hospital of Ningxia Medical University, 804 Shengli Street, Yinchuan 750004, China

Shiyuan Shi
Department of Orthopedics, Hospital of Integrated Traditional Chinese and Western Medicine in Zhejiang Province, Hangzhou 310003, Zhejiang, China

Zili Wang
Department of Spinal Surgery, General Hospital of Ningxia Medical University, 804 Shengli Street, Yinchuan 750004, China
Hillsborough Community College, Tampa, USA

Qian Wang
Hillsborough Community College, Tampa, USA

Cong Wang, Chenhe Zhou, Hao Qu, Shigui Yan and Zhijun Pan
Department of Orthopaedic Surgery, The Second Affiliated Hospital, Zhejiang University School of Medicine, No. 88 Jiefang Road, Hangzhou 310009, China

Xiu-hua Mao
Department of Pain Treatment, Ningbo No.2 Hospital, Ningbo 315000, Zhejiang, China

Ye-jun Zhan
Physical Health and Sports, College of Education, Lishui University, 1. No, Xueyuan Road, Liandu District, Lishui City 323000, Zhejiang, China

Yi-Ming Ren, Yuan-Hui Duan, Yun-Bo Sun, Tao Yang, Wen-Jun Zhao, Dong-Liang Zhang, Zheng-Wei Tian and Meng-Qiang Tian
Department of Joint and Sport Medicine, Tianjin Union Medical Center, Jieyuan Road 190, Hongqiao District, Tianjin 300121, People's Republic of China

Zhao Wang, Jing-zhao Hou, Can-hua Wu, Yue-jiang Zhou, Xiao-ming Gu, Hai-hong Wang, Wu Feng, Yan-xiao Cheng, Xia Sheng and Hong-wei Bao
Department of orthopaedics, Jingjiang People's Hospital, 28 No, Zhongzhou Road, Jingjiang, Taizhou City 214500, Jiangsu Province, China

Junyan Cao, Bowen Zheng, Yan Lv, Kun Wang, Dongmei Huang and Jie Ren
Department of Medical Ultrasonics, The Third Affiliated Hospital of Sun Yat-sen University, 600 Tianhe Road, Guangzhou 510630, People's Republic of China

Xiaochun Meng
Department of Radiology, The Third Affiliated Hospital of Sun Yat-sen University, 600 Tianhe Road, Guangzhou 510630, People's Republic of China

Huading Lu
Department of Orthopedics, The Third Affiliated Hospital of Sun Yat-sen University, 600 Tianhe Road, Guangzhou 510630, People's Republic of China

Bin Zhang, Shen Liu, Bingbing Yu, Wei Guo, Yongjin Li, Yang Liu, Wendong Ruan, Guangzhi Ning and Shiqing Feng
Department of Orthopedics, Tianjin Medical University General Hospital, No. 154 Anshan Road, Heping District, Tianjin 300052, People's Republic of China

Jun Liu
Department of Orthopedics, First Affiliated Hospital of Gannan Medical University General Hospital, No. 23 Qingnian Road, Zhanggong District, Ganzhou 341000, People's Republic of China

Qiuke Wang, Junjie Guan, Yunfeng Chen and Lei Wang
Department of Orthopedic Surgery, Shanghai Jiao Tong University Affiliated Sixth People's Hospital, 600 Yishan Road, Shanghai 200233, People's Republic of China

Jian Hu
Department of Pathology, Shanghai Eighth People's Hospital, 8 Caobao Road, Shanghai 200233, People's Republic of China

Mathias Donnez
Aix Marseille Univ, CNRS, ISM, Marseille, France
Aix Marseille Univ, APHM, CNRS, ISM, Sainte-Marguerite Hospital, Institute for Locomotion, Department of Orthopaedics and Traumatology, Marseille, France
Newclip Technics, Haute-Goulaine, France

Matthieu Ollivier, Patrick Chabrand and Sébastien Parratte
Aix Marseille Univ, CNRS, ISM, Marseille, France
Aix Marseille Univ, APHM, CNRS, ISM, Sainte-Marguerite Hospital, Institute for Locomotion, Department of Orthopaedics and Traumatology, Marseille, France

Maxime Munier
Aix Marseille Univ, APHM, CNRS, ISM, Sainte-Marguerite Hospital, Institute for Locomotion, Department of Orthopaedics and Traumatology, Marseille, France

Philippe Berton and Jean-Pierre Podgorski
Newclip Technics, Haute-Goulaine, France

Sorawut Thamyongkit
Department of Orthopaedic Surgery, The Johns Hopkins University, 4940 Eastern Avenue, Baltimore, MD 21224, USA
Chakri Naruebodindra Medical Institute, Faculty of Medicine Ramathibodi Hospital, Mahidol University, 270 Rama VI Road, Ratchatewi, Bangkok 10400, Thailand

Laura M. Fayad
Russell H. Morgan Department of Radiology and Radiological Science, The Johns Hopkins University, 601 North Caroline Street, Baltimore, MD 21224, USA

Lynne C. Jones, Erik A. Hasenboehler and Norachart Sirisreetreerux
Department of Orthopaedic Surgery, The Johns Hopkins University, 4940 Eastern Avenue, Baltimore, MD 21224, USA

Babar Shafiq
Department of Orthopaedic Surgery, The Johns Hopkins University, 4940 Eastern Avenue, Baltimore, MD 21224, USA
Department of Orthopaedic Surgery, The Johns Hopkins University, 601 N. Caroline St., Fl. 5, Baltimore, MD 21205, USA

Marco Viganò, Irene Tessaro, Alessandra Colombini and Laura de Girolamo
IRCCS Istituto Ortopedico Galeazzi, via Riccardo Galeazzi 4, 20161 Milan, Italy

Letizia Trovato
Human Brain Wave, corso Galileo Ferraris 63, 10128 Turin, Italy

Marco Scala
Primus Gel srl, Via Casaregis, 30, 16129 Genoa, Italy

Alberto Magi and Andrea Toto
Clinica Veterinaria San Rossore, via delle cascine 149, 56100 Pisa, Italy

Giuseppe Peretti
IRCCS Istituto Ortopedico Galeazzi, via Riccardo Galeazzi 4, 20161 Milan, Italy
Department of Biomedical Sciences for Health, Università degli Studi di Milano, via Mangiagalli 31, 20133 Milan, Italy

Edgar A Wakelin, Linda Tran, Willy Theodore and Brad P Miles
360 Knee Systems, Suite 3, Building 1, Sydney, NSW 2073, Australia

Joshua G Twiggs
360 Knee Systems, Suite 3, Building 1, Sydney, NSW 2073, Australia
Department of Biomedical Engineering, University of Sydney, Sydney, NSW 2006, Australia

Justin P Roe
North Sydney Orthopaedic and Sports Medicine Centre, The Mater Hospital, North Sydney, NSW 2065, Australia

Michael I Solomon
Prince of Wales Private Hospital, Barker Street, Kensington, NSW 2030, Australia

Brett A Fritsch
Sydney Orthopaedic Research Institute, 445 Victoria Ave, Sydney, NSW 2067, Australia.

Yen-Jung Chou
Department of Traditional Chinese Medicine, MacKay Memorial Hospital, Taipei City, Taiwan
Department of Life Science, Fu Jen Catholic University, New Taipei City, Taiwan. 3Graduate Institute of Applied Science and Engineering, Fu Jen Catholic University, No. 510, Zhongzheng Rd., Xinzhuang Dist., New Taipei City 24205, Taiwan

Jiunn-Jye Chuu and Yu-Hsuan Cheng
Department of Biotechnology, College of Engineering, Southern Taiwan University, Tainan City, Taiwan

Yi-Jen Peng
Department of Pathology, Tri-Service General Hospital, National Defense Medical Center, Taipei City, Taiwan

Chin-Hsien Chang
Department of Cosmetic Science, Chang Gung University of Science and Technology, Tao-Yuan City, Taiwan
Department of Traditional Chinese Medicine, En Chu Kong Hospital, New Taipei City 237, Taiwan

Chieh-Min Chang
Department of Traditional Chinese Medicine, En Chu Kong Hospital, New Taipei City 237, Taiwan

Hsia-Wei Liu
Department of Life Science, Fu Jen Catholic University, New Taipei City, Taiwan. 3Graduate Institute of Applied Science and Engineering, Fu Jen Catholic University, No. 510, Zhongzheng Rd., Xinzhuang Dist., New Taipei City 24205, Taiwan

Mingqing Li, Can Xu, Jie Xie, Yihe Hu and Hua Liu
Department of Orthopedics, Xiangya Hospital, Central South University, Changsha, Hunan 410008, People's Republic of China

Song-bo Shi, Xing-bo Wang, Jian-min Song, Shi-fang Guo, Zhi-xin Chen and Yin Wang
Orthopaedics Department, Gansu Provincial Hospital, Lanzhou 730000, Gansu, China

Qi-fang He, Hui Sun, Yu Zhan, Yi Zhu, Bin-bin Zhang and Cong-feng Luo
Department of Orthopaedic Surgery, Shanghai Jiao Tong University Affiliated Sixth People's Hospital, 600 YiShan Road, Shanghai 200233, China

Lin-yuan Shu
Department of Emergency, Shanghai Jiao Tong University Affiliated Sixth People's Hospital, 600 YiShan Road, Shanghai 200233, China

Chun-yan He
Chongqing Health Center for Women and Children, 64 Jintang Street, Yuzhong District, Chongqing 400013, China

Wenbin Hua, Xinghuo Wu, Yukun Zhang, Yong Gao, Shuai Li, Kun Wang, Xianzhe Liu, Shuhua Yang and Cao Yang
Department of Orthopaedics, Union Hospital, Tongji Medical College, Huazhong University of Science and Technology, Wuhan 430022, China

Yun-Peng Huang, Jian-Hua Lin, Gui Wu and Xuan-Wei Chen
Department of Spine Surgery, The First Affiliated Hospital of Fujian Medical University, 20 Chazhong Road, Fuzhou City 350005, Fujian Province, China

Xiao-Ping Chen
School of Mathematics and Informatics, Fujian Normal University, Fuzhou City 350117, Fujian Province, China

Werner Schmoelz, Alexander Keiler and Richard A Lindtner
Department of Trauma Surgery, Medical University of Innsbruck, Anichstraße 35, 6020 Innsbruck, Austria

Alessandro Gasbarrini
Instituto Orthopedic Rizzoli, Bologna, Italy

Marko Konschake
Department of Anatomy, Histology and Embryology, Medical University of Innsbruck, Innsbruck, Austria

Chun-Chi Hung, Yuan-Ta Li, Yung-Wen Cheng, Chia-Chun Wu, Hsain-Chung Shen and Tsu-Te Yeh
Department of Orthopedic Surgery, Tri-Service General Hospital and National Defense Medical Center, 325 Cheng-Kung Road, Section 2, Taipei 114, Taiwan

Jia-Lin Wu
Department of Orthopedics, School of Medicine, College of Medicine, Taipei Medical University, Taipei, Taiwan
Department of Orthopedics, Taipei Medical University Hospital, Taipei, Taiwan

Chi Xu and Ji-Ying Chen
Department of Orthopaedic Surgery, General Hospital of People's Liberation Army, No.28 Fuxing Road, Haidian District, Beijing 100853, China

Heng Guo
Department of Orthopaedic Surgery, General Hospital of People's Liberation Army, No.28 Fuxing Road, Haidian District, Beijing 100853, China
Department of Orthopaedic Surgery, Beijing Mentougou District Hosptial, Beijing, China

Kerri L. Bell
The Rothman Institute at Thomas Jefferson University, Philadelphia, PA, USA

Feng-Chih Kuo
Department of Orthopaedic Surgery, Kaohsiung Chang Gung Memorial Hospital, and Chang Gung University, College of Medicine, No. 123, Dapi Rd., Niaosong Dist, Kaohsiung 833, Taiwan

Xiaoyang Bi
Department of Orthopedic Medicine, Tianjin Hospital, No 406 JieFangNan Road, Hexin District, Tianjin City 300211, China

Chunhui Liu, Zhongli Li, Ji Li, Hao Zhang and Yangmu Fu
Department of Orthopedics, General Hospital of PLA, No. 28 Fuxing Road, Haidian District, Beijing 100853, China

Yingpeng Wang and Kuan Zhang
School of Biomedical Engineering, Capital Medical University, Beijing 100069, China

Index

www.ingramcontent.com/pod-product-compliance
Lightning Source LLC
Chambersburg PA
CBHW080458200326
41458CB00012B/4018